Environmental Exposures and Human Health Challenges

Paraskevi Papadopoulou
Deree - The American College of Greece, Greece

Christina Marouli
Deree - The American College of Greece, Greece

Anastasia Misseyanni
Deree - The American College of Greece, Greece

A volume in the Advances in Human Services and Public Health (AHSPH) Book Series

Published in the United States of America by
IGI Global
Medical Information Science Reference (an imprint of IGI Global)
701 E. Chocolate Avenue
Hershey PA, USA 17033
Tel: 717-533-8845
Fax: 717-533-8661
E-mail: cust@igi-global.com
Web site: http://www.igi-global.com

Library of Congress Cataloging-in-Publication Data

Names: Papadopoulou, Paraskevi, 1961- editor. | Marouli, Christina, 1961- editor. | Misseyanni, Anastasia, 1962- editor.
Title: Environmental exposures and human health challenges / Paraskevi Papadopoulou, Christina Marouli, and Anastasia Misseyanni, editors.
Description: Hershey PA : Medical Information Science Reference, [2019] | Includes bibliographical references.
Identifiers: LCCN 2018031961| ISBN 9781522576358 (h/c) | ISBN 9781522576365 (eISBN)
Subjects: | MESH: Environmental Exposure--adverse effects | Environmental Pollutants--toxicity | Hazardous Substances--toxicity
Classification: LCC RA566 | NLM WA 670 | DDC 363.73--dc23 LC record available at https://lccn.loc.gov/2018031961

This book is published in the IGI Global book series Advances in Human Services and Public Health (AHSPH) (ISSN: 2475-6571; eISSN: 2475-658X)

British Cataloguing in Publication Data
A Cataloguing in Publication record for this book is available from the British Library.

For electronic access to this publication, please contact: eresources@igi-global.com.

Advances in Human Services and Public Health (AHSPH) Book Series

Jennifer Martin
RMIT University, Australia

ISSN:2475-6571
EISSN:2475-658X

Mission

The well-being of the general public should be a primary concern for any modern civilization. Ongoing research in the field of human services and public healthcare is necessary to evaluate, manage, and respond to the health and social needs of the global population.

The **Advances in Human Services and Public Health (AHSPH)** book series aims to publish high-quality reference publications focused on the latest methodologies, tools, issues, and strategies for managing the health and social welfare of the public. The AHSPH book series will be especially relevant for healthcare professionals, policy makers, government officials, and students seeking the latest research in this field.

Coverage

- Health policy
- Assistance Programs
- Medicare and Medicaid
- Poverty
- Social Welfare Policy
- Public Funding
- Healthcare Reform
- Public Welfare
- Youth Development
- Social Work

IGI Global is currently accepting manuscripts for publication within this series. To submit a proposal for a volume in this series, please contact our Acquisition Editors at Acquisitions@igi-global.com or visit: http://www.igi-global.com/publish/.

The Advances in Human Services and Public Health (AHSPH) Book Series (ISSN 2475-6571) is published by IGI Global, 701 E. Chocolate Avenue, Hershey, PA 17033-1240, USA, www.igi-global.com. This series is composed of titles available for purchase individually; each title is edited to be contextually exclusive from any other title within the series. For pricing and ordering information please visit http://www.igi-global.com/book-series/advances-human-services-public-health/102256. Postmaster: Send all address changes to above address.

Titles in this Series

For a list of additional titles in this series, please visit: www.igi-global.com/book-series

Forecasting and Managing Risk in the Health and Safety Sectors
Luisa Dall'Acqua (Scientific Lyceum TCO, Italy & University of Bologna, Italy)
Medical Information Science Reference • copyright 2019 • 304pp • H/C (ISBN: 9781522579038) • US $245.00 (our price)

Psycho-Socio-Physical Dimensions of Adolescent Health Management Emerging Research and Opportunities
Sapna Nanda (Panjab University, India)
Medical Information Science Reference • copyright 2019 • 202pp • H/C (ISBN: 9781522573845) • US $195.00 (our price)

Mental Health Policy, Practice, and Service Accessibility in Contemporary Society
Jennifer M. Martin (Swinburne University, Australia)
Medical Information Science Reference • copyright 2019 • 323pp • H/C (ISBN: 9781522574026) • US $245.00 (our price)

Socio-Cultural Influences on Teenage Pregnancy and Contemporary Prevention Measures
Devi Akella (Albany State University, USA)
Information Science Reference • copyright 2019 • 349pp • H/C (ISBN: 9781522561088) • US $195.00 (our price)

Nutraceutical and Functional Foods in Disease Prevention
Raj K. Keservani (Chhatrapati Shahu Ji Maharaj Group of Institutions, India) Anil K. Sharma (Delhi Institute of Pharmaceutical Sciences and Research, India) and Rajesh K. Kesharwani (Nims University Rajasthan, India)
Medical Information Science Reference • copyright 2019 • 569pp • H/C (ISBN: 9781522532675) • US $215.00 (our price)

Ethical Issues in Social Work Practice
Antonio Sandu (Ştefan cel Mare University of Suceava, Romania) and Ana Frunza (LUMEN Research Center in Social and Humanistic Sciences, Romania)
Information Science Reference • copyright 2018 • 328pp • H/C (ISBN: 9781522530909) • US $195.00 (our price)

Global Perspectives on Human Migration, Asylum, and Security
Christina M. Akrivopoulou (Hellenic Open University, Greece)
Information Science Reference • copyright 2018 • 268pp • H/C (ISBN: 9781522528173) • US $185.00 (our price)

IGI Global
DISSEMINATOR OF KNOWLEDGE

701 East Chocolate Avenue, Hershey, PA 17033, USA
Tel: 717-533-8845 x100 • Fax: 717-533-8661
E-Mail: cust@igi-global.com • www.igi-global.com

Editorial Advisory Board

List of Reviewers

Table of Contents

Detailed Table of Contents

Connectivity introduces a new exposome based paradigm in environmental health. This denotes an approach that builds on the exploration of the interconnections between the co-existence of multiple exogenous and endogenous stressors and the different scales of biological organization. Coupling the two results in the final adverse health effect. This differs from the conventional paradigm, which seeks to shed light on the identification of singular cause-effect relationships between stressors and health outcomes. It creates a new way of combining health-relevant information coming from different disciplines, treating all factors affecting internal and external exposome are as covariates. Their functional integration into results in understanding the complex interaction between genome and exposome. The applicability of the exposome (and more specifically the connectivity) approach towards a better understanding of the exposure, sociodemographic and biological factors interplay in the association between environment and disease, is demonstrated in two different case studies.

Autism spectrum disorder (ASD) is a developmental condition characterized by impaired social interactions and communication, as well as by stereotypic movements, that affects 1 in 59 children. ASD is expected to reach 1 in about 40 children by 2020, yet it remains without distinct pathogenesis and effective treatment. Children with ASD respond with high anxiety to almost any unknown stimulus and appear to misread danger/threat signals, and may not experience anxiety in situations where normotypic children do. The authors propose that environmental stimuli stimulate the unique immune cells, known as mast cells (MC), which then trigger microglia, leading to dysfunctional neuronal connectivity in the

In the entire world, about 200 million people are exposed to arsenic poisoning in groundwater. In Bihar, India, about 50 million people are drinking arsenic contaminated water. Humans are exposed to elevated levels of inorganic arsenic mainly through the consumption of arsenic contaminated groundwater as drinking water and food crops are irrigated with high-arsenic water resources. This has caused various health-related problems in the population like skin diseases, anemia, bronchitis, gastrointestinal problems, hormonal imbalance and cancer. According to recent study, cancer risk is associated with daily consumption of 2 litres of water with inorganic arsenic 50 µg/L has been estimated to be 1/100 denotes that elevated blood arsenic levels in population can lead to cause various diseases including cancer. Skin and several types of internal cancers, including, bladder, kidney, liver, gall bladder, lung, uterus, and prostate, have been found associated with arsenic ingestion. This hospital-based study also correlates the cause of cancer due to arsenic contamination.

Chemsensors have been playing a crucial role in various aspects of biomedical science, analytical and environmental chemistry. The toxic metal ions like Zn, Cd, Cu, Pb and Hg have increased gradually but now have reached an alarming situation, crossing the threshold value. Due to high toxicity of these heavy metals there is an obvious need for a sensor system to detect their presence. Chemsensors including surface acoustic wave sensors, enzymes, carbon nanotubes, nanoparticles, and chromophore-based sensors have attracted increasing attention over the last few years. Chemsensors prove very promising as the system is rapid, selective, sensible, low-cost, easy-to-use, and has the ability to provide real-time signals. However, recently, considerable effort has been devoted to the synthesis of sterically encumbered selenium containing species reported to display strong affinities with Hg2+ or Ag2+. This chapter reviews the basic principles involved in the design of chemsensors, their variety and applications in various established and emerging fields.

Occupational epidemiology studies the distribution of health events and health related determinants and its relation to the working environment. Environmental epidemiology focuses on the involuntary exposure to physical and chemical factors in the indoor or outdoor environment that may affect health patterns. Occupational and environmental epidemiology use similar methodology although the conditions differ. The environmental epidemiology studies beyond the health effect of exposure to specific environmental factors and must consider the long-term impact of the ecosystems to nearby populations. Molecular technologies allow the detection of effects at the molecular level originated by very low levels of exposure. The concept of an exposome is a kind of database with information concerning environmental exposure measurements in a life time and corresponding biomarkers concentrations in different biospeciments, considering internal individual genetic characteristics.

As climate change threatens human life and health by causing severe storms, floods, temperature fluctuations and droughts, it is predicted that in the coming decades, most of the global population will be impacted and the lives of millions will be at risk. In this context, the article investigates the existence of a symmetric and asymmetric causality between climate change and health between 1990 and 2015 for European countries, including EU, EFTA member and EU candidate states. In the first stage of the analysis, health scores are estimated by cluster and discriminant analyses; in the second stage, the relationships among these scores and climate variables are examined. The country-specific findings are obtained for the health effects of climate change variables according to factors such as geographical structure and seasonal characteristics. According to the results, while the health effects of changes in temperature and greenhouse emissions differ from country to country, the reduction in precipitation for nearly half of the countries is found to have a negative effect on health.

Section 2
Social and Political Aspects of Environmental Health

Supporters of agricultural biotechnology have maintained a high enthusiasm for its role in improving agricultural yields and enhancing sustainability, for instance, in Africa. However, critics are deeply skeptical. This chapter sketches some of the main arguments on both sides to provide a summary analysis. The discussion includes multiple climatic, socioeconomic, and public policy drivers that have collided with the ability of the average person to achieve food security. If food security is to be understood as a matter of human health, then its definitions and designs must recognize food's many roles in creating positive public health outcomes. Hence, the discussion expands to include an integrative model of food security linking sociocultural, public policy, and ecological aspects to public health. The chapter concludes that extensive work must be done to steer policy initiatives toward common sense sustainability paths to achieve food security and/or sovereignty.

Pharmaceuticals and personal care products (PPCPs) constitute an integral part of modern healthcare systems which enter the environment through various routes. Because of their inherent biological activity, their presence in soil and the aquatic environment poses several eco-toxicological problems. Antibiotic contamination of soil and water bodies is leading to the development of microbial resistance to antibiotics and this has been recognized by several global bodies like WHO and EPA. Effective steps need to be taken in this regard including increased awareness, reduced pharmaceutical discharges in environment, green and sustainable pharmaceutical practice by pharmaceutical industry and healthcare professionals and improved remediation/bioremediation methods. This chapter outlines the various anticipated routes of exposure of pharmaceuticals to the environment along with their detrimental effects, fate and degradation in aquatic and terrestrial environments. The chapter also dwells upon the role of various regulatory bodies and plausible measures that may be adopted to alleviate the problem.

Preface

Despite noteworthy developments and technological advances in the health and biomedical sciences in the last decades, with obvious improvements in the prevalence of some communicable diseases and in disease treatment in general, contemporary societies continue facing very significant health challenges. The average human life span has increased but individual wellbeing is challenged by an array of "contemporary" diseases. Differences in the health challenges industrialized nations and less developed countries face persist. Life expectancy at birth continues being higher in North America, Oceania and Europe, while mortality continues to be significantly higher in poor countries (European Environment Agency, 2013; United Nations, 2017), while the health issues that constitute priorities in these two broad categories of countries are also different (Prüss-Üstün, Wolf, Corvalán, Bos & Neira, 2016; European Environment Agency, 2013). Communicable diseases are a major concern in developing countries, while non-communicable diseases like cancers, diabetes, asthma, Autism Spectrum Disorders (ASDs) or heart attacks are on the rise in the industrialized world.

Albeit these disparities, there is a common trend relating to health issues worldwide. Environmental exposures or pressures constitute a major cause of contemporary diseases (Prüss-Üstün et al., 2016; European Environment Agency, 2013). WHO highlights the significance of environmental factors – which it defines as "factors external to a person, and all related behaviours, but excluding those natural environments that cannot be reasonably modified" (Prüss-Üstün et al., 2016) – for the state of human health.

In this context, environmental health arose as a science that studies the relation of different environmental factors with health impacts or correlates diseases with environmental exposures. It is a field of rising interest and particular relevance in our times, with important insights for environmental and health policy making. Given our increasing understanding of the intricate network of interrelated factors that contribute to environmental concerns as well as of the multiple impacts on human health, environmental health is a body of knowledge that draws from a variety of disciplines: medicine and public health, environmental sciences, sociology and communications, technology, policy-making, and legislation. As a consequence, it is a multidisciplinary field with noteworthy challenges and significant, much-promising developments.

Exposures to a great variety of environmental toxins and stressors pose serious risks to individual and public health. Environmental hazards include biological, chemical, physical and cultural ones, as well as some lifestyle choices (Prüss-Üstün et al., 2016). Biological hazards refer to disease-causing organisms such as bacteria, fungi and parasites including diseases caused by viruses. Chemical hazards include all harmful chemicals to which people get exposed in their environment via air, water, soil, food or human made products. Physical hazards can be natural phenomena such as fires, floods, earthquakes, hurricanes and volcanic eruptions, but also physical agents such as electromagnetic radiation (ultraviolet, radio waves), noise, nanoparticles and climate change effects. Cultural hazards are associated with the social environment of an individual; e.g. conditions such as an unhealthy workplace, poverty and criminality. Lifestyle choices refer to those hazards that are a matter of individual choice, or at least are influenced by choice, like smoking, over-eating, alcohol or drug abuse. In contemporary societies, malaria and respiratory infections such as tuberculosis, diarrhea and various parasitic intestinal diseases constitute significant biological hazards. Humans get exposed to a wide and increasing range of chemical hazards; carcinogenic and mutagenic chemicals, heavy metals, persistent organic pollutants and endocrine disruptors are among the groups of chemicals that are of particular concern. Climate change, nanoparticles, noise and exposure to electromagnetic radiation (from radiofrequencies and infrared to UV and X-rays), constitute significant and disconcerting new physical hazards. Workplace exposures and stresses continue being an issue of concern, although technological approaches have contributed to the control of such hazards; however, new challenges arising from socio-political changes such as migration and ageing societies need to be addressed.

Due to the massive amount of health-related issues, scientific literature related to environmental health issues has increased significantly. Recent developments in the human genome, in epigenetics (Bollati & Baccarelli, 2010; Herceg, 2016; Lin, Liu, Hu, Cottrell, & Kass, 2018) and different omics (e.g. transcriptomics, metabolomics) and in environmental sciences, along with increased and more systematic environmental and biological monitoring have made invaluable contributions to our understanding of environmental challenges and human diseases. However, additional research investigating the interrelations of environment and health is required to improve the wellbeing of citizens worldwide. A primary challenge in the environmental health field is the effective combination of environmental monitoring data and bio-monitoring information (Dennis et al., 2017) taking into account many and diverse parameters such as genetic predisposition, environmental exposures, the processes that constitute these exposures and various threats throughout one's life time starting from conception. Thus, recent developments such as the exposome (Wild, 2005; Rappaport, 2011; Lioy & Rappaport, 2011; Wild, Scalbert & Herceg, 2013; Vrijheid, 2014; Buck Louis, Smarr & Patel, 2017; Johnson et al., 2017; Stingone, Buck Louis, Nakayama, Vermeulen, Kwok et. al., 2017; Sarigiannis, 2017; Sarigiannis, Karakitsios et al., 2018; Sarigiannis, Gotti, Handakas & Karakitsios, 2018) and the use of data analytics are promising future directions in the field (Lytras, & Papadopoulou, 2018). Now, massive amounts of medical and public health data related to numerous human health issues are available and there is an urgent need to apply big data analytics in healthcare (Papadopoulou, Lytras & Marouli 2018). Hot issues in the relevant sciences include single gene polymorphisms, genome sequences, gene expression data, exposure to carcinogens, endocrine disruptors, heavy metals (Ellis, et al., 2012) and other toxins, their metabolism and health impacts, exposome analysis (Larkin & Hystad 2017), risk analysis, (Turner et al., 2017) bioinformatics and data storage and handling (Papadopoulou, Lytras, & Marouli, 2018).

However, understanding only the science of the intricate relation between the environment and human health, a daunting task by itself, is limited. The uneven distribution of environmental health hazards and the marriage of informatics with health science and management make a discussion of social inequalities and injustices particularly relevant. Environmental health is a political and cultural issue, and these dimensions need to be understood and effectively addressed if we are to transition to sustainable and healthy societies (Papadopoulou, Lytras, & Marouli, 2018; Spruit & Lammertink, 2018). Environmental justice literature relating to a great variety of environmental issues, from waste management, air pollution, water pollution, to food, Genetically Modified Organisms (GMOs) or climate change, emphasize the different level of environmental risks various social groups are exposed to, the differential impact of environmental exposures to human health in relation to social inequalities, as well as the differential access of marginalized peoples to the benefits healthy environments offer (Masuda, Poland & Baxter, 2010; indicatively, see also: Walker, 2012; Carmin & Agyeman, 2011; Gaffron, 2012; Wolch, Byrne & Newell, 2014; Cutts, Darby, Boone & Brewis, 2009; Bardsley & Wiseman, 2012). Social and power inequalities are important parameters that influence health. These beg for close consideration in the exploration of environmental health issues, and especially for the drafting of policies that promote healthy communities for all. Discourses from the environmental health sciences and the environmental justice field underline the need for contemporary societies to focus on interrelations, adopting a systemic view that incorporates knowledge from the environmental, bio-medical and socio-political sciences, and to develop integrative policies and other mechanisms – like education and public accountability. Given the increasing use of data analytics, policy, ethical and justice issues related with bio-data management and use are also important parameters that should be considered (Papadopoulou, Lytras, & Marouli, 2018).

This publication contributes to this challenging scene and presents some major contemporary environmental health hazards and their impacts. It approaches the contemporary exciting developments in the environmental health fields in an interdisciplinary manner covering from cutting-edge scientific developments to environmental justice and policy issues.

THE CHALLENGES

Human health hazards are intricate, their causes multi-faceted and health impacts are influenced by both individual characteristics and practices – like genetics or lifestyle choices – and social structures and inequalities. The challenges environmental health science faces are:

- **Research:** Establishing research efforts that are multi-disciplinary in terms of design, goals and methods is a persisting challenge, as well as the effective dissemination of the results to all stakeholders via good academic and management practices in a geographically dispersed environment.
- **Policies:** Establishing policies, legislation and procedures that aim for both a clean environment and health and wellness for all, while adequately reflecting the local and global organizational context and processes, is a prerequisite for the transition towards healthy societies.
- **Privacy and Security of Personal Health Data:** Establishing appropriate information technology precaution measures and socially appropriate policies for the handling and storage of health-related big data is a major challenge of our times. Securing personal privacy in the age of connected health data is a big challenge.
- **Social Inequalities:** Addressing social inequalities in exposure to environmental hazards and in access to proper health care with appropriate socio-political processes, policies, strategies, structures and institutions, as well as education for a wellness- and social solidarity-oriented culture and ethos.
- **Points of Intervention:** Identifying the most effective points of intervention in the spectrum society-politics-environment-health for sustainable and healthy communities, which requires further multidisciplinary and integrative research and inclusive governance processes. Establishing appropriate information technology precaution plans and disaster recovery plans is also a big challenge.

Numerous studies have been carried out toward meeting those challenges and continue onto providing good and sustainable solutions. Back in 2009 the International Life Sciences Institute (ILSI) Health and Environmental Sciences Institute (HESI) scientific portfolio, groups of experts of key government, academic, and industry scientists from around the world were assembled with the main goal to map the human and environmental health challenges for the decade (2010–2020) and offer suggestions and develop tools on the current and future landscape of scientific and regulatory challenges. This scientific mapping could serve as a valuable tool indeed which "HESI, individual companies, research institutions, government agencies, and regulatory authorities could use to anticipate key challenges, place them into context, and thus strategically refine and expand scientific project portfolios into the future" (Bonnefoi et al., 2010). As we are heading to the end of the decade it would be interesting to examine if such goals were met. The challenges of high or medium priority as defined at the January 2009 HESI Scientific Mapping Meeting in Japan are outlined and their present status is considered in comparison to what has been planned and what seems to have been achieved. Overall, it appears that whereas the goals and objectives were set in a clear way by the International Life Sciences Institute (ILSI) Health and Environmental Sciences Institute (HESI) scientific portfolio, groups of experts, the implementation for most of the plans is far from being materialized in most parts of the world despite some additional serious efforts to achieve such goals. Furthermore, many policies have been adopted for the protection of the environment, sustainable development and better health, but their implementation has still not brought about the desired results.

SEARCHING FOR SOLUTIONS: RECOMMENDATIONS

The book "Environmental Exposures and Human Health Challenges" aims to provide interdisciplinary insights into concepts and theories related to environmental health, and environmental exposures via chemical, biological or physical factors in the air, water, soil or food (Prüss-Üstün et al., 2016). It covers a diversity of environmental health topics of concern today. The exposome approach is one of the latest and very promising developments in the field, as it aims to connect both environmental and biological monitoring for a more holistic understanding of the way different exposures affect health. Autism spectrum disorders (ASDs) (Theoharides, Tsilioni, Patel & Doyle, 2016) and various autoimmune and inflammatory disorders have increased in the recent years, and it has been shown that environmental exposures, such as neurotoxins in commonly used synthetic fragrances, endocrine disruptors, (Braun et al., 2014) various molds and viruses among a number of other harmful exposures at critical stages of a human's life are main parameters contributing to their prevalence. Heavy metals constitute an important category of environmental health hazards in contemporary societies. Arsenic is one of these health risks and due to its serious health impacts, it has been investigated in several situations. Genetically modified food is another major challenge of our times, with health consequences that require further research and exploration. This need is further enhanced by recent research on the effects of Glyphosate on human health, a major constituent of the widely used pesticide Roundup, including research on toxicity of formulants and heavy metals in glyphosate-based herbicides and other pesticides. (Mesnage, Defarge, Spiroux de Vendomois & Seralini, 2015; Myers et al., 2016; Townsend, Peck, Meng, Heaton, Robison & O'Neill, 2017; Séralini et al., 2014; Defarge, Spirouxde Vendômois & Séralini, 2018). Food is generally a main issue of concern for human health, both in terms of food security – availability of adequate and good quality food - and of food quality. Cotton is a frequently used material in the world and its production with conventional agricultural practices, including the use of pesticides, constitute a significant threat to human health. Appropriate methods for investigating environmental health issues are also discussed. The book also addresses environmental health policies as well as inequalities and injustices in relation to environmental exposures and health impacts.

This book examines in a cross-cutting way, how various environmental exposures affect individuals, workers, professions and populations from different regions of the world. It offers suggestions and recommendations so as to help increase awareness on issues of sustainability and to help improve human health and healthcare. Grounded on scientific evidence and up-to-date socio-political discourses on environmental health issues, this book aspires to contribute to the improvement of health, wellbeing and healthcare of citizens worldwide. This publication is designed for public health professionals, preventive medicine specialists, clinicians, data scientists, environmentalists, academicians, practitioners, researchers, and students. The book can also stimulate sharing opinions and ideas, so as to facilitate a better fusion of health-related issues and challenges including health informatics and other big data emerging technologies, including exposome analytics, to the academic and industry research, which combined, can lead to improvements in the quality of people's daily life.

ORGANIZATION OF THE BOOK

The book is organized into two sections. The first section focuses on the science of environmental exposures and their health impacts, while the second one delves into a discussion of policy and environmental justice aspects of selected environmental health issues.

The book includes 15 chapters. A brief description of each of the chapters follows:

Chapter 1 identifies how connectivity introduces a new exposome based paradigm in environmental health. This denotes an approach that builds on the exploration of the interconnections between the coexistence of multiple exogenous and endogenous stressors and the different scales of biological organization. Coupling the two results in the final adverse health effect. This differs from the conventional paradigm, which seeks to shed light on the identification of singular cause-effect relationships between stressors and health outcomes. It creates a new way of combining health-relevant information coming from different disciplines, treating all factors affecting internal and external exposome as covariates. Their functional integration results in understanding the complex interaction between genome and exposome. The connectivity approach is applied on toxicity assessment of nanomaterials; here multiple assays, human multi-omics and *in vitro* data are used to elucidate toxicity mechanisms.

Chapter 2 presents Autism Spectrum Disorder (ASD) as a developmental condition characterized by impaired social interactions and communication, as well as by stereotypic movements, that affects 1 in 59 children. The authors state that ASD is expected to reach 1 in about 40 children by 2020, yet it remains without distinct pathogenesis and effective treatment. Children with ASD respond with high anxiety to almost any unknown stimulus and appear to misread danger/threat signals, and may not experience anxiety in situations where normotypic children do. The authors propose that environmental stimuli stimulate the unique immune cells, known as mast cells (MC), which then trigger microglia, leading to dysfunctional neuronal connectivity in the amygdala. This process lowers or disrupts the "fear response" and leads to an exaggerated "fight-or-flight" reaction. Corticotropin-releasing hormone (CRH) could have a synergistic effect with environmental stimuli, especially mycotoxins. The authors propose that recognizing this association and preventing stimulation of mast cells/microglia could lead to effective treatment of ASD.

Chapter 3 explores how the human brain develops and what the critical stages are in which a fetal brain may acquire genetic and developmental abnormalities through environmental agents. The authors summarize the prevailing theories regarding the etiologies of autism and present scientific data supporting the thesis that some of the most commonly used environmental agents that we have so easily accepted into our social fabric of life may be major contributors in the development of autism spectrum disorders (ASD). They provide a large body of scientific data carried out in their laboratory, utilizing developing human neurons exposed to femtomolar concentrations of chemicals found in fragrances. Their studies, the authors argue, demonstrate that synthetic fragrances can impart profound neuromodifications at the morphologic, immunologic and molecular levels. They hypothesize that high exposure to teratogenic neurotoxins in our environment during critical periods of development best explains the rapid rise of autism spectrum disorder diagnosis over the past three decades.

Chapter 4 focuses on the possible sources of arsenic (As), leading to environmental contamination, followed by its hazardous effects which pave the way to various human health manifestations. The authors explore how arsenic can cause various health disorders through acute and chronic exposures such as gastrointestinal, hepatic, respiratory, cardiovascular, integumentary, renal, neurological and reproductive disorders including stillbirth and infant mortality.

Chapter 5 is a specific case study of Arsenic exposure via contaminated water in Bihar, India of about 50 million people. In addition to health-related problems in the population like skin diseases, anemia, bronchitis, gastrointestinal problems, hormonal imbalance, according to the author's recent study, cancer risk is associated with daily consumption of 2 litres of water with inorganic arsenic 50 μg/L which has been estimated to be 1/100 denoting that elevated blood arsenic levels in a population can lead to various diseases including cancer. Skin and several types of internal cancers, including bladder, kidney, liver, gall bladder, lung, uterus and prostate cancers have been found associated with arsenic ingestion. Their hospital- based study also correlates the cause of cancer with arsenic contamination.

Chapter 6 reviews chemsensors and their role in various aspects of biomedical science, analytical and environmental chemistry. The toxic metal ions like Zn, Cd, Cu, Pb and Hg have increased gradually but now have reached an alarming situation, crossing the threshold value. Due to high toxicity of these heavy metals, there is an obvious need for a sensor system to detect their presence. The authors argue that chemsensors including surface acoustic wave sensors, enzymes, carbon nanotubes, nanoparticles and chromophore-based sensors have attracted increasing attention during the last few years. Chemsensors prove very promising as the system is rapid, selective, sensible, low cost, easy to use and has the ability to furnish real time signals. However, during recent times, considerable efforts have been devoted to the synthesis of sterically encumbered selenium containing species reported to display strong affinities with Hg^{2+} or Ag^{+}. This chapter overall, reviews the basic principles involved in the design of chemsensors, their variety and applications in various established and emerging fields.

Chapter 7 examines occupational epidemiology studies in terms of the distribution of health events and health-related determinants and its relation to the working environment. Environmental epidemiology focuses on the involuntary exposure to physical and chemical factors in the indoor or outdoor environment that may affect health patterns. Occupational and environmental epidemiology use similar methodology although the conditions differ. The environmental epidemiology studies, beyond the health effect of exposure to specific environmental factors, must consider the long-term impact of the environment on the populations. Molecular technologies allow to detect effects at the molecular level originated by very low levels of exposure. The concept of the exposome is also briefly discussed as a kind of database with information concerning environmental exposure measurements in a life time and corresponding biomarkers concentrations in different biospecimen, considering internal individual genetic characteristics.

Chapter 8 seeks to highlight general concerns and potential lifelong effects of consuming GM plant-based food. The author argues that consumption of GM plant-based food is as risky as consuming conventional plant-based food. However, the alien genes in these products may be unstable leading to antinutritional and unintended short-term consequences. The author believes that due to the paucity of research, no long-term effects have been attributed to the lifelong consumption of these products. Nonetheless, possible lifelong health and socioeconomic effects may result from outcrossing of genes, increasing antibiotic resistance, development of new diseases, as well as potential effects on the environment and biodiversity. The author advises biotechnology companies to invest more in interdisciplinary research addressing the potential lifelong effects of these products. Although GM foods are safe for consumption, the author believes that clarification of current risks and lifelong effects is required.

Chapter 9 addresses the issue of the world dairy consumption. The author examines the impact the use of dairy products has on sustainability and health. This chapter provides an overview of milk consumption around the world, sustainability, health concerns, and dairy milk alternatives. In addition, advantages and disadvantages are discussed, as individuals are often faced with choosing the option that best meets their individual needs.

Chapter 10 informs the reader about cotton uses for the production of cotton textiles and apparel and the three different possibilities for cotton growth in the world: production of conventional, organic or genetically modified cotton. Their influence on human health, due to the application of pesticides, is discussed by the author. The influence of the pesticides on the environment, which, in turn, affects the human health through the water, soil, and food chain, is also discussed. The preferable cotton sector is presented, giving a chance to the customers of cotton textiles and apparel, to assess the positive influence of the existing initiatives in the cotton field on the human health and the environment.

Chapter 11 explores climate change and how it threatens human life and health by causing severe storms, floods, temperature fluctuations and droughts. The authors hold the belief, as predicted for the coming decades, that most of the global population will be impacted and the lives of millions will be at risk. In this context, the chapter investigates the existence of a symmetric and asymmetric causality between climate change and health between 1990 and 2015 for European countries, including EU, EFTA member and EU candidate states. In the first stage of the analysis, health scores are estimated by cluster and discriminant analyses; in the second stage, the relationships among these scores and climate variables are examined. The country-specific findings are obtained for the health effects of climate change variables according to factors such as geographical structure and seasonal characteristics. According to the results, while the health effects of changes in temperature and greenhouse gas emissions differ from country to country, the reduction in precipitation for nearly half of the countries is found to have a negative effect on health.

Chapter 12 examines how supporters of agricultural biotechnology have maintained a high enthusiasm for its role in improved agricultural yields and enhanced sustainability, for instance, in Africa. However, according to the author, critics are deeply skeptical. This chapter sketches some of the main arguments on both sides to provide a summary analysis. The discussion includes multiple climatic, socioeconomic, and public policy drivers that have collided with the ability of the average person to achieve food security. If food security is to be understood as a matter of human health, then the author argues, definitions and designs must recognize food's many roles in creating positive public health outcomes. Hence, the discussion expands to include an integrative model of food security linking sociocultural, public policy, and ecological aspects to public health. The chapter concludes that extensive work must be done to steer policy initiatives toward common sense sustainability paths to achieve food security and/or sovereignty.

Chapter 13 explores how pharmaceuticals and personal care products (PPCPs) constitute an integral part of modern healthcare system which enter environment through various routes. Because of their inherent biological activity, their presence in soil and aquatic environment poses several eco-toxicological problems. Antibiotic contamination of soil and water bodies is leading to development of microbial resistance to antibiotics and this has been recognized by several global bodies like WHO and EPA. Effective steps need to be taken in this regard including increased awareness, reduced pharmaceutical discharges in environment, green and sustainable pharmaceutical practice by pharmaceutical industry and healthcare professionals and improved remediation/bioremediation methods. This chapter outlines the various anticipated routes of exposure of pharmaceuticals to the environment along with their detrimental effects, fate and degradation in aquatic and terrestrial environments. The chapter also dwells upon the role of various regulatory bodies and plausible measures that may be adopted to alleviate the problem.

Chapter 14 addresses the main issues that pertain to the health burden from waste management and energy resource use by highlighting the aspects that determine actual exposures and the socio-economic conditions that underlie them. Case studies covering biomass burning, acute and chronic exposure to urban and industrial waste are described by the authors. They refer to different areas in Europe and socio-economic strata focusing on susceptible population groups, which may be affected by enhanced exposure to environmental toxicants stemming from municipal and industrial waste management and domestic heating or cooking using biomass. These features, the authors argue, make socio-economic status and the consequent social (in)justice a key determinant of overall exposure early in life. The latter results in a high probability of onset or exacerbation of adverse health outcomes both in the medium term and later in life. Additional factors that affect the health impacts of environmental exposures comprise choice of diet, education level of parents, access to green or blue space and housing condition.

Chapter 15 explores the glaring scientific differences in the human health assessment of the popular herbicide glyphosate between European and American institutions. The International Agency for Research on Cancer (IARC) classified glyphosate as a probable human carcinogen, while the U.S. Environmental Protection Agency (EPA) concluded that glyphosate is not likely to be carcinogenic to humans. Both IARC's and the EPA's carcinogenic risk assessment processes are discussed by the author. With this work the author argues that uncertainties are reviled in the sciences of toxicology and epidemiology, as well as assumptions made in their applications for evaluating glyphosate. These uncertainties, along with the political context of chemical risk assessment, the author believes, are at the root of the divergent findings on the carcinogenic risks of glyphosate.

Paraskevi Papadopoulou
Deree – The American College of Greece, Greece

Christina Marouli
Deree – The American College of Greece, Greece

Anastasia Misseyanni
Deree – The American College of Greece, Greece

REFERENCES

Bardsley, D. K., & Wiseman, N. D. (2012). Climate change vulnerability and social development for remote indigenous communities of South Australia. *Global Environmental Change*, *22*(3), 713–723. doi:10.1016/j.gloenvcha.2012.04.003

Bollati, V., & Baccarelli, A. (2010). Environmental epigenetics. *Heredity*, *105*(1), 105–112. doi:10.1038/hdy.2010.2 PMID:20179736

Bonnefoi, M. S., Belanger, S. E., Devlin, D. J., Doerrer, N. G., Embry, M. R., Fukushima, S., ... van der Laan, J. W. (2010). Human and environmental health challenges for the next decade (2010–2020). *Critical Reviews in Toxicology*, *40*(10), 893–911. doi:10.3109/10408444.2010.506640 PMID:20854192

Braun, J. M., Kalkbrenner, A. E., Just, A. C., Yolton, K., Calafat, A. M., Sjödin, A., ... Lanphear, B. P. (2014). Gestational exposure to endocrine-disrupting chemicals and reciprocal social, repetitive, and stereotypic behaviors in 4- and 5-year-old children: The HOME study. *Environmental Health Perspectives*, *122*(5), 513–520. doi:10.1289/ehp.1307261 PMID:24622245

Buck Louis, G. M., Smarr, M. M., & Patel, C. J. (2017). The Exposome Research Paradigm: An Opportunity to Understand the Environmental Basis for Human Health and Disease. *Current Environmental Health Reports*, *4*(1), 89–98. doi:10.100740572-017-0126-3 PMID:28194614

Carmin, J., & Agyeman, J. (Eds.). (2011). *Environmental Inequalities Beyond Borders: Local Perspectives on Global Injustices*. Boston, MA: MIT Press. doi:10.7551/mitpress/8759.001.0001

Cutts, B. B., Darby, K. J., Boone, C. G., & Brewis, A. (2009). City structure, obesity, and environmental justice: An integrated analysis of physical and social barriers to walkable streets and park access. *Social Science & Medicine*, *69*(9), 1314–1322. doi:10.1016/j.socscimed.2009.08.020 PMID:19751959

Defarge, N., Spirouxde Vendômois, J., & Séralini, G. E. (2018). Toxicity of formulants and heavy metals in glyphosate-based herbicides and other pesticides. *Toxicology Reports*, *5*, 156–163. doi:10.1016/j.toxrep.2017.12.025 PMID:29321978

Dennis, K. K., Marder, E., Balshaw, D. M., Cui, Y., Lynes, M. A., Patti, G. J., ... Barr, D. B. (2017). Biomonitoring in the Era of the Exposome. *Environmental Health Perspectives*, *125*(4), 502–510. Epub-2016Jul6. doi:10.1289/EHP474 PMID:27385067

Ellis, J., Athersuch, T., Thomas, L., Teichert, F., Perez-Trujillo, M., Svendsen, C., ... Keun, H. C. (2012). Metabolic profiling detects early effects of environmental and lifestyle exposure to cadmium in a human population. *BMC Medicine*, *10*(1), 61. doi:10.1186/1741-7015-10-61 PMID:22713677

European Environment Agency. (2013). *Environment and human health*. EEA Report No 5/2013. doi:10.2800/9092

Gaffron, P. (2012). Urban transport, environmental justice and human daily activity patterns. *Transport Policy*, *20*, 114–127. doi:10.1016/j.tranpol.2012.01.011

Herceg, Z. (2016). Epigenetic Mechanisms as an Interface Between the Environment and Genome. *Advances in Experimental Medicine and Biology*, *903*, 3–15. doi:10.1007/978-1-4899-7678-9_1 PMID:27343085

Johnson, C. H., Athersuch, T. J., Collman, G. W., Dhungana, S., Grant, D. F., Jones, D. P., ... Vasiliou, V. (2017). Yale school of public health symposium on lifetime exposures and human health: The exposome; summary and future reflections. *Human Genomics*, *11*(1), 32. doi:10.118640246-017-0128-0 PMID:29221465

Larkin, A., & Hystad, P. (2017). Towards Personal Exposures: How Technology Is Changing Air Pollution and Health Research. *Current Environmental Health Reports*, *4*(4), 463–471. doi:10.100740572-017-0163-y PMID:28983874

Lin, D., Liu, J., Hu, Z., Cottrell, J. E., & Kass, I. S. (2018). Neonatal anesthesia exposure impacts brain microRNAs and their associated neurodevelopmental processes. *Scientific Reports*, *8*(1), 10656. doi:10.103841598-018-28874-0 PMID:30006558

Lioy, P. J., & Rappaport, S. M. (2011). Exposure science and the exposome: An opportunity for coherence in the environmental health sciences [Editorial]. *Environmental Health Perspectives*, *119*(11), A466–A467. doi:10.1289/ehp.1104387 PMID:22171373

Lytras, M. D., & Papadopoulou, P. (2018). *Applying Big Data Analytics in Bioinformatics and Medicine*. Hershey, PA: IGI Global. doi:10.4018/978-1-5225-2607-0

Masuda, J. R., Poland, B., & Baxter, J. (2010). Reaching for environmental health justice: Canadian experiences for a comprehensive research, policy and advocacy agenda in health promotion. *Health Promotion International*, *25*(4), 453–463. doi:10.1093/heapro/daq041 PMID:20615911

Mesnage, R., Defarge, N., Spiroux de Vendomois, J., & Seralini, G.-E. (2015). Potential toxic effects of glyphosate and its commercial formulations below regulatory limits. *Food and Chemical Toxicology*, *84*, 133–153. doi:10.1016/j.fct.2015.08.012 PMID:26282372

Myers, P. J., Antoniou, M. N., Blumberg, B., Carroll, L., Colborn, T., Everett, L. G., … Benbrook, C. M. (2016). Concerns over use of glyphosate-based herbicides and risks associated with exposures: a consensus statement, *Environmental Health, 15*. doi:10.118612940-016-0117-0

Papadopoulou, P., Lytras, M., & Marouli, C. (2018). Bioinformatics as Applied to Medicine: Challenges Faced Moving from Big Data to Smart Data to Wise Data. In M. Lytras & P. Papadopoulou (Eds.), *Applying Big Data Analytics in Bioinformatics and Medicine* (pp. 1–25). Hershey, PA: IGI Global. doi:10.4018/978-1-5225-2607-0.ch001

Prüss-Üstün, A., Wolf, J., Corvalán, C. F., Bos, R., & Neira, M. P. (2016). *Preventing disease through healthy environments: a global assessment of the burden of disease from environmental risks*. World Health Organization. Retrieved from http://www.who.int/iris/handle/10665/204585

Rappaport, S. M. (2011). Implications of the exposome for exposure science. *Journal of Exposure Science & Environmental Epidemiology*, *21*(1), 5–9. doi:10.1038/jes.2010.50 PMID:21081972

Sarigiannis, D. A. (2017). Assessing the impact of hazardous waste on children's health: The exposome paradigm. *Environmental Research*, *158*, 531–541. doi:10.1016/j.envres.2017.06.031 PMID:28711809

Sarigiannis, D. A., Gotti, A., Handakas, E., & Karakitsios, S. P. (2018). Informatics and Data Analytics to Support Exposome-Based Discovery: Part 2 - Computational Exposure Biology. In M. Lytras & P. Papadopoulou (Eds.), *Applying Big Data Analytics in Bioinformatics and Medicine* (pp. 145–187). Hershey, PA: IGI Global. doi:10.4018/978-1-5225-2607-0.ch007

Sarigiannis, D. A., Karakitsios, S. P., Handakas, E., Papadaki, K., Chapizanis, D., & Gotti, A. (2018). Informatics and Data Analytics to Support Exposome-Based Discovery: Part 1 - Assessment of External and Internal Exposure. In M. Lytras & P. Papadopoulou (Eds.), *Applying Big Data Analytics in Bioinformatics and Medicine* (pp. 115–144). Hershey, PA: IGI Global. doi:10.4018/978-1-5225-2607-0.ch006

Séralini, G.-E., Clair, E., Mesnage, R., Gress, S., Defarge, N., Malatesta, M., ... Spiroux de Vendômois, J. (2014). Republished study: Long-term toxicity of a Roundup herbicide and a Roundup-tolerant genetically modified maize. *Environmental Sciences Europe*, *26*(1), 14. doi:10.118612302-014-0014-5 PMID:27752412

Spruit, M., & Lammertink, M. (2018). Effective and Efficient Business Intelligence Dashboard Design: Gestalt Theory in Dutch Long-Term and Chronic Healthcare. In M. Lytras & P. Papadopoulou (Eds.), *Applying Big Data Analytics in Bioinformatics and Medicine* (pp. 243–271). Hershey, PA: IGI Global. doi:10.4018/978-1-5225-2607-0.ch010

Stingone, J. A., Buck Louis, G. M., Nakayama, S. F., Vermeulen, R. C., Kwok, R. K., Cui, Y., ... Teitelbaum, S. L. (2017). Toward Greater Implementation of the Exposome Research Paradigm within Environmental Epidemiology. *Annual Review of Public Health*, *20*(38), 315–327. Epub2017Jan6. doi:10.1146/annurev-publhealth-082516-012750 PMID:28125387

Theoharides, T. C., Tsilioni, I., Patel, A. B., & Doyle, R. (2016). Atopic diseases and inflammation of the brain in the pathogenesis of autism spectrum disorders. *Translational Psychiatry*, *6*(6), e844. doi:10.1038/tp.2016.77 PMID:27351598

Townsend, M., Peck, C., Meng, W., Heaton, M., Robison, R., & O'Neill, K. (2017). Evaluation of various glyphosate concentrations on DNA damage in human Raji cells and its impact on cytotoxicity. *Regulatory Toxicology and Pharmacology*, *85*, 79–85. doi:10.1016/j.yrtph.2017.02.002 PMID:28185844

Turner, M. C., Nieuwenhuijsen, M., Anderson, K., Balshaw, D., Cui, Y., Dunton, G., ... Turner, M. C. (2017). Assessing the Exposome with External Measures: Commentary on the State of the Science and Research Recommendations. *Annual Review of Public Health*, *20*(38), 215–239. doi:10.1146/annurev-publhealth-082516-012802 PMID:28384083

United Nations. (2017). *World Mortality 2017: Data Booklet*. Retrieved from http://www.un.org/en/development/desa/population/publications/pdf/mortality/World-Mortality-2017-Data-Booklet.pdf

Vrijheid, M. (2014). The exposome: A new paradigm to study the impact of environment on health. *Thorax*, *69*(9), 876–878. doi:10.1136/thoraxjnl-2013-204949 PMID:24906490

Walker, G. (2012). *Environmental Justice: Concepts, Evidence and Politics*. Routledge. doi:10.4324/9780203610671

Wild, C. P. (2005). Complementing the genome with an "exposome": The outstanding challenge of environmental exposure measurement in molecular epidemiology. *Cancer Epidemiology, Biomarkers & Prevention*, *14*(8), 1847–1850. doi:10.1158/1055-9965.EPI-05-0456 PMID:16103423

Wild, C. P., Scalbert, A., & Herceg, Z. (2013). Measuring the exposome: A powerful basis for evaluating environmental exposures and cancer risk. *Environmental and Molecular Mutagenesis*, *54*(7), 480–499. doi:10.1002/em.21777 PMID:23681765

Wolch, J., Byrne, J., & Newell, J. P. (2014). Urban green space, public health, and environmental justice: The challenge of making cities 'just green enough.' *Landscape and Urban Planning*, *125*, 234–244. doi:10.1016/j.landurbplan.2014.01.017

Acknowledgment

The editors would like to acknowledge the help of all the people involved in this project and, more specifically, the authors, the Editorial Advisory Board (EAB) and the reviewers that took part in the review process. Without their support, this book would not have become a reality.

First, the editors would like to thank each one of the authors for their contributions. Our sincere gratitude goes to the chapters' authors who contributed their time and expertise to this book.

Second, the editors wish to acknowledge the valuable contributions of the EAB and the reviewers regarding the improvement of quality, coherence, and content presentation of chapters. Most of the authors also served as referees; we highly appreciate their double task.

Paraskevi Papadopoulou
Deree – The American College of Greece, Greece

Christina Marouli
Deree – The American College of Greece, Greece

Anastasia Misseyanni
Deree – The American College of Greece, Greece

Section 1

Contemporary Environmental Health Challenges

Chapter 1
The Exposome Paradigm in Environmental Health

Denis Andreas Sarigiannis
Aristotle University of Thessaloniki, Greece

ABSTRACT

Connectivity introduces a new exposome based paradigm in environmental health. This denotes an approach that builds on the exploration of the interconnections between the co-existence of multiple exogenous and endogenous stressors and the different scales of biological organization. Coupling the two results in the final adverse health effect. This differs from the conventional paradigm, which seeks to shed light on the identification of singular cause-effect relationships between stressors and health outcomes. It creates a new way of combining health-relevant information coming from different disciplines, treating all factors affecting internal and external exposome are as covariates. Their functional integration into results in understanding the complex interaction between genome and exposome. The applicability of the exposome (and more specifically the connectivity) approach towards a better understanding of the exposure, sociodemographic and biological factors interplay in the association between environment and disease, is demonstrated in two different case studies.

INTRODUCTION

The exposome (Wild, 2005) refers to all the exposures – exogenous and endogenous - throughout a person's life starting from conception, and it simultaneously identifies, characterizes and quantifies them along with modifiable risk factors in order to understand the person's predisposition to diseases.

The human genome preceded the exposome. Decoding the human genome (Schmutz et al., 2004) significantly contributed to a deeper understanding of the underlying causes of disease. However, its explanatory power regarding the health burden of the population is limited, as environmental factors are equally or eventually more important than genetic characteristics.

What is actually critical is the interaction of environmental factors with biological systems. Towards a better understanding of the causal links among the genome, the environment and human disease,

DOI: 10.4018/978-1-5225-7635-8.ch001

unraveling the exposome implies that both environmental exposures and genetic variation are reliably measured simultaneously (Sarigiannis et al., 2019a).

Given the enormous amount of information that needs to be integrated, unraveling the exposome is daunting. Various efforts have taken place (e.g. COPHES (harmonization of HBM), EHES (harmonization of Health Surveys), EU-menu (harmonization of data collection on food consumption), CHICOS (harmonization of child cohort studies) or U-BIOPRED (unbiased biomarkers in prediction of respiratory disease outcomes)) aiming to harmonise existing, often disparate information. At the moment, the largest exposome ongoing project is HEALS; HEALS employees a large array of technologies for both external (Asimina et al., 2018; Loh et al., 2017b) and internal (Sarigiannis et al., 2016) exposome, that involve multiple sensors for monitoring exposure, biomonitoring analysis, physiology based biokinetic modelling, multi-omics and advanced bioinformatics and advanced statistics for environment health associations, that support the efficient design and execution of large-scale exposome studies. The other two key projects that comprised the EU exposome initiative, include Exposomics (led by Imperial College, in London, UK) and HELIX (led by CREAL in Barcelona, Spain). In Exposomics, a personal exposure monitoring system that involved sensors, smartphones, geo-referencing and remote sensing has been developed for constructing external exposome, followed by biological samples analysis. The aim was to identify associations between external exposure and molecular fingerprints (through omics analysis) of cancer (Chadeau-Hyam et al., 2013; Vineis et al., 2013; Vineis and Wild, 2014). On the other hand, the Human Early-Life Exposome (HELIX) project (Vrijheid et al., 2014) aims at the association of early-life cumulative exposure with omics and child health outcomes. Finally, CROME (Cross-Mediterranean Environment and Health Network) is a fourth exposome EU project, with a particular focus on environmental health issues of Mediterranean countries. CROME paid particular attention on integrating human biomonitoring for developing individual exposome, highlighting associations among environmental, dietary and genetic factors with adverse health outcomes such as child neurodevelopment (Snoj Tratnik et al., 2017) and cancer (Sarigiannis et al., 2015b), paying a particular attention to toxicokinetics (Andra et al., 2015; Sarigiannis et al., 2016; Sarigiannis et al., 2019b).

The two key exposome-related initiatives in USA were funded by NIEHS, including the HERCULES center at Emory University in Georgia and the Exposome Research Center at the University of California at Berkeley. The approach of HERCULES is based on a multi-faceted approach to the exposome (Miller, 2014), aiming at the estimation of allostatic load related to environmental factors over individual lifetime (Miller and Jones, 2014; Niedzwiecki and Miller, 2017). The UC Berkeley Center has a different approach, paying more attention on exploiting untargeted metabolomics (Rappaport et al., 2014) for developing individual exposome profiles for identifying the associations among environmental factors and adverse health effects (Rappaport, 2018), employing a top-down approach (Rappaport and Smith, 2010).

The progressive digestion of the exposome concept by the scientific community, impacted significantly the domain of environmental health. Firstly, it was very important that additional information than typical exposure biomarkers can be retrieved from biomonitoring, serving the needs for an exposome approach (Dennis et al., 2017). A key component of exposome studies is that they include the full picture of stressors that are relevant for health, coming from both endogenous and/or exogenous sources. The full array of human biosample analysis that involves exposure biomarker analysis and multi-omics (transcriptomics, proteomics, metabolomics, adductomics and epigenomics), results in the generation of big data that has to be put into a plausible biological context through appropriate computational tools (Manrai et al., 2017); these include both the ones aiming at elucidating the link of both external-internal exposure association (Sarigiannis et al., 2015a; Sarigiannis et al., 2016), but also the ones that highlight the underlying biology that explain toxic versus adaptive effects, culminating in health adversities (Sarigiannis, 2015a; Sarigiannis, 2015b; Sarigiannis and Salifoglou, 2016). With regard to external exposome, a key advance offered by exposome studies is related to the use of personal sensors (Loh et al., 2017a), especially the ones that provide information about space-time lines at a personal level. Considering the inherent deficiencies of the current sensor technologies in terms of accuracy, machine learning techniques (Sarigiannis et al., 2009; Stamatelopoulou et al., 2018), provide an interesting option for maximizing their exploitation. One thing that needs to be further discussed is the need for the functional integration of the various technological options that could serve the exposome approach and in particular the large-scale population studies (Cui et al., 2016). Towards this aim, it is essential to focus on untargeted data-driven approaches that involve dimension reduction techniques. Approaching the environmental-health interaction in such an agnostic way, we are able to overcome some of the major limitations related to classic epidemiology, that pertain to exposure misclassification, cumulative exposure and multiple stressors and factors such as diet or sociodemographic characteristics (Sarigiannis and Karakitsios, 2018b), and more importantly, to identify causality (Kim and Hong, 2017). It worth also to be highlighted that exposome by definition addresses one of the key issues of the modern environmental-health nexus, which is cumulative exposure; overall, risk assessment process is moving away from a one-chemical one-health outcome model, toward a new paradigm of monitoring the totality of exposures that individuals may experience over their lifetime (Johnson et al., 2017). The mechanistic understanding on how cumulative exposure results in health effects, is greatly facilitated by the adverse outcome pathways (AOPs) concept; this allows the identification of common key events among intersecting pathways of toxicity (Escher et al., 2017), thus, enhancing our mechanistic understanding.

The exposome has contributed to invaluable methodological advances in risk and health impact assessment. The exposome concept was initially proposed in 2005; however, scientific interest in the exposome increased rapidly only after 2011 (Kiossoglou et al., 2017). The broad inclusion of various exposure components in its definition, resulted in equally broad interpretations by the experts in the field; unfortunately, these interpretations are usually limited by the capacities (know-how, infrastructure) of the various research groups. For a methodology to be consistent with the original exposome definition while addressing the individual exposome, it should be broadly inclusive. This should account for the contribution of integrated and cumulative exposure during the lifecourse and how this relates to the various disease states, as well as for the understanding of the molecular mechanisms that describe the continuous interaction of environmental and genetic factors towards the deployment of adverse outcome pathways. Such an approach that involves a large array of methodological approaches and tools covering the different levels of complexity in environmental and biological organization and governed by the interconnections between these complexity levels is the so-called connectivity approach. Connectivity has been shown to be one of the most comprehensive concepts for developing the individual exposome (Sarigiannis et al., 2019a). The following figure schematically demonstrates the connectivity approach as well as the wide variety of information that is used for the assessment of both external and internal exposome.

The connectivity approach combines a variety of state-of-the-art technologies from all relevant disciplines of environmental sciences, biochemistry, molecular biology, toxicology, bioinformatics and epidemiology.

The exposome stands as toolbox with interconnecting elements, aiming at the integration of different elements that formulate the lifelong individual exposure profiles towards a better understanding of the

Figure 1. Conceptual representation of the connectivity approach
Source: (Sarigiannis et al., 2019a)

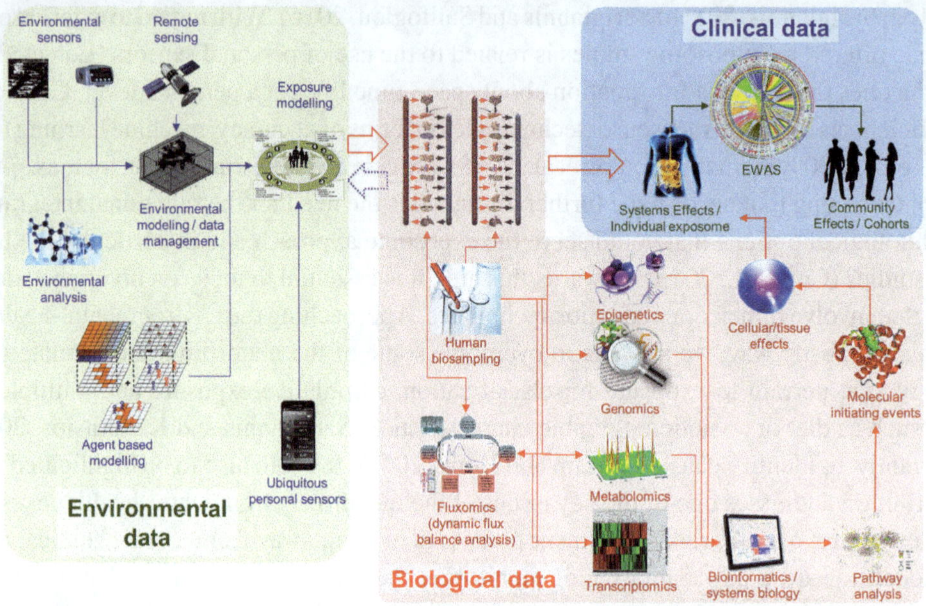

environmental origins of disease. Towards this direction, it is important to describe the sequencing of key intermediate events; environmental exposure is able to initiate perturbations on biological system function on the genetic and gene expression level; however it is important to identify whether this is going to result in adaptive or toxic responses in order to mechanistically connect environmental exposure to adverse health outcomes. To better understand the interaction of the continuously changing exposure dynamics with the biological systems, genetics have to be accounted as well. Their result will define the level of biological perturbations at different levels of biological organization, which can be described by effect biomarkers and especially effect biomarkers derived using -omics (i.e. high throughput) techniques. When cumulative exposure levels are able to sustain the activation of toxicity pathways and to overcome the homeostatic capacity, adverse health outcomes are to be observed. In this sense, various pieces of information involving different technological platforms (personalized sensors, environmental analysis, exposure modelling, omics analysis, toxicokinetics and bioinformatics) are equally important in order to properly identify the link between environmental exposure and disease. Environmental and micro-environmental monitoring, sensors, Agent-Based Models (ABM), human bio-monitoring, multiple –omics, internal dose modeling, bioinformatics and environment wide association studies (EWAS) are all important contributors to an exposome analysis[1].

To better understand how the exposome (and more specifically the connectivity approach towards unraveling it) result in a better understanding of the exposure, sociodemographic and biological factors interplay in the association between environment and disease two different case studies are described below.

APPLICATIONS OF THE CONNECTIVITY APPROACH

Application on the REPRO_PL Cohort

Problem Identification

The Polish Mother and Child Cohort (REPRO_PL, www.repropl.com), is a multicenter prospective cohort study of environmental factors contributing to pregnancy outcomes, children's health and neurodevelopment, established in 2007 (Polańska et al., 2009; Polańska et al., 2011). Briefly, women were recruited during the first trimester of pregnancy at maternity units or clinics in selected regions of Poland if they fulfilled the following inclusion criteria:

- Single pregnancy up to 12 weeks of gestation
- No assisted conception
- No pregnancy complications
- No chronic diseases as specified in the study protocol

The women were interviewed 3 times during the pregnancy (once in each trimester) in order to collect and update demographic and socio-economic data, medical and reproductive history, and information about occupational exposure and lifestyle factors. After delivery, detailed information regarding pregnancy outcomes and children's health was obtained. Two years after birth, assessment of exposure, health status as well as neurodevelopment of each child was performed by a pediatrician as well as a psychologist/child development specialist (Polanska et al., 2013). At that time also information concerning socio-demographic, environmental and lifestyle factors have been updated by conducting interviews with mothers. Current analysis was restricted to 149 mother-child pairs from Lodz (central Poland) district.

Exposure Factors

For the association, several exposure factors have been investigated, including:

- Prenatal phthalate exposure (Polanska et al., 2014; Polanska et al., 2016), by measuring phthalate metabolites in the urine collected from the mothers during the third trimester of pregnancy (range 30–34 weeks)
- Postnatal exposure was determined by measuring phthalate metabolites in the urine from children at around the 24th month of age (range 23– 28 months). In both cases the following 11 phthalate metabolites were measured: a) five Low-MWP: monoethyl phthalate (MEP) (metabolite of diethyl phthalate; DEP), mono-iso-butyl phthalate (MiBP) (metabolite of di-iso-butyl phthalate; DiBP), mono-n-butyl phthalate (MnBP) (metabolite of di-n-butyl phthalate; DnBP), 3OH-mono-n-butyl phthalate (3OH-MnBP) (secondary metabolite of DnBP), and monobenzyl phthalate (MBzP) (metabolite of butyl-benzyl phthalate; BBzP), and b) six High-MWP: mono(2- ethylhexyl) phthalate (MEHP) (metabolite of di(2-ethylhexyl) phthalate; DEHP), 5OH-mono(2-ethylhexyl) phthalate (5OH-MEHP) and 5oxo-mono(2-ethylhexyl) phthalate (5oxo-MEHP) (secondary metabolites of DEHP), 7OH-mono-methyloctyl phthalate (OH-MiNP) and 7oxo-mono-methyloctyl phthalate

(oxo-MiNP) (secondary metabolites of di-iso-nonyl phthalate; DiNP), and mono-n-octyl phthalate (MnOP) (metabolite of di-n-octyl phthalate; DnOP).

- Prenatal exposure to tobacco constituents was assessed based on the cotinine level in saliva collected from the women during the third trimester of pregnancy
- Child exposure to environmental tobacco smoke (ETS) was assessed based on the cotinine level in the urine collected during the visit scheduled for assessment of child health and neurodevelopment
- Pb in the mother plasma during during pregnancy, delivery and in cord blood (Polańska et al., 2014)
- Hg in maternal hair during the 30-34th week of pregnancy
- Se, Cu and Zn in the mother plasma during the 8-12th, 20-24th, 30-34th week and day of newborn birth (Polanska et al., 2017)
- 1-HP in mother urine during the 20-24th week of pregnancy

Exposure and Effect Modifiers

Additional factors considered as exposure and effects modifiers were included as well. These included:

- Sociodemographic parameters such as
    - Socioeconomic status
    - Mother education
    - Marital status
    - Day-care attendance at one and two years of age
- Mother and child anthropometric parameters
    - Mother bodyweight
    - Mother height
    - Mother age at birth
    - Child birth weight
    - Child gender
- Other gestational and post-delivery factors
    - Child birth weight
    - Mode of delivery
    - Breastfeeding
- Presence of micronutrients, minerals and vitamins
    - Zn in the mother plasma during pregnancy, delivery and in cord blood
    - Se in the mother plasma during pregnancy, delivery and in cord blood
    - Cu in the mother plasma during pregnancy, delivery and in cord blood
    - Vitamin D2
    - Vitamin D3
- Enzymatic activity
    - Thiobarbituric acid reactive substances in the mother plasma during pregnancy
    - GPX3 glutathione peroxidase 3 in the mother plasma during pregnancy
    - GPX1 glutathione peroxidase 1 in the mother plasma during pregnancy
    - Superoxide dismutase in the mother plasma during pregnancy
    - Ceruloplasmin in the mother plasma during pregnancy

Health Outcomes

The health outcomes investigated in this study included children neurodevelopment, assessed at around the 24th (±1.2) month of age (range, 23 to 28 months) using the Bayley Scales of Infant and Toddler Development, third edition (Bayley-III). Examination was performed at pediatric medical centers at two University Hospitals in Lodz. The testing was done in the presence of the mother or a relative by a psychologist or a child development specialist. Before commencement of the examination the training of examiners in the field of the Bayley-III was performed by a professional. Bayley-III is an individually applied examination that assesses the developmental functioning of children up to 42 months of age. The test presents child with situations and tasks designed to produce an observable set of behavioral responses. In the current analysis, focus was on child cognitive, motor and language development. The child psychomotor development measured by row score/chronologic age was yielded with each subtest, and composite scores for language, motor scales, and composite score equivalent for cognitive scale were generated based on such data.

EWAS Analysis of Exposure, Socioeconomic, Biochemical, and Health Outcomes

Metabolic Pathway Analysis

The metabolites are reactants, products and intermediates of enzymatic reactions which are modified by a sequence of chemical reactions catalyzed by enzymes (Acid, 2004). In the field of biochemistry a metabolic pathway is a linked series of chemical reactions occurring within a cell (Alonso et al., 2015). The metabolic pathways can be divined according to their ability to synthesize, to break down molecules or both of them to anabolic, catabolic and amphibolic pathways (Reece et al., 2011). A wide range of metabolic pathway libraries are available aiming at connected metabolites with metabolic pathways. Such libraries are the Kyoto Encyclopedia of Genes and Genomes (KEGG) (Kanehisa et al., 2012), the Small Molecule Pathway Database (SMPDB) (Jewison et al., 2014), the Edinburgh human metabolic network (EHMN) (Ma et al., 2007), WikiPathways (Kelder et al., 2012) and MetaCyc (Caspi et al., 2014).

In this study the used pathways arose using the Agilent Tecnhologies software Mass Profiler Professional (https://www.agilent.com). This software first tries to find direct matches between the pathway entities (pathways from databases) and the entities in the selected entity list (input data). A direct match can only occur when entities from both pathways and entity lists have identifiers from the same annotation. The advanced algorithms used by Mass Profiler provide the ability to specify several filter criteria for input data and relations. As input data will be used the identified biomarkers (Table 1) and metabolic pathways will be created with Natural Language Processing (NLP) Network discovery:

- **Workflow:** NLP Network Discover
    - Direct Interpretations
    - Matching statistics (Matched and redundant)
- **Analysis Filters:** Relation score ≥ 9
- **Relation Types:** Member, transport, expression, regulation, binding, promoter binding, metabolism, protein modification.
- **Pathways From:** WikiPathways, KEGG, BioCyc.

Table 1. Identified biomarkers

Isocitrate dehydrogenase (NADP(+))	IDP	Riboflavin
IDH1	Istidina	Rize
IDH2	LNAC	Saccharin
1-Methylhistidine	Mefloquine	Salicylurate
2'-deoxyinosine	Methoxyhydroxyphenylglycol	Sirup
3'-SL	Mimosine	Sorbo
3-Chlorotyrosine	N-benzoylglycine	Sulfalene
3008-B	NARIGENIN	Thiothixene
4'-Hydroxyflurbiprofen	Nevirapine	Tinidazole
4-Pyridoxic acid	Glumin	Tobrex
5-HTP	Guaifenesin	Tryptophan
5-acetamido-6-formamido-3-methyluracil	H-Asp-OH	Uridine
5-oxoproline	HPPA	Usaf hc-1
6-Mercaptopurine	Hgln	Vasc
6-Sulfatoxymelatonin	GENOP	WSQR DQ CVQ
7,9-dihydro-1H-purine-2,6,8(3H)-trione	Glumin	Xanthurenate
734571A	Beflavin	Xylose
AAMU	CATECHOL	Zeranol
APAP	CF3COO(-)	acetaminophen O-glucuronide
Ac-Try	CF3COOH	androsterone 3-glucosiduronic acid
Acetaminophen	CRESOL	cis-Aconitate
Acetylcysteine	Catechin	estrone 3-glucosiduronic acid
Adrin	Cerulenin	ketoglutarate
Afalanine	Clavulanic Acid	meletin
Alna	Clonidine	testosterone 3-glucosiduronic acid
Amifostine	D-glucono-1,5-lactone	Niflumic Acid
Andros-S	DHLA	Noname
Asp-Phe	DOPAC	Nystatin
Azadc	Depas	O-Due
Dexfenfluramine	Dicid	Edetic Acid
Dihydroxymandelic acid	Ecgonine methyl ester	Enalaprilat
Epinephrine	Ethacrynic acid	Flunarizine

The Pathway entities of Experiment Type columns contain the number of entities in the pathway that are of the experiment type: the number of genes and proteins in the pathway if the experiment type is Genomics/Proteomics/Transcriptomics and the number of metabolites if the experiment type is Metabolomics, regardless of whether the entities are present in the technology or not.

Data Clustering

The two different clustering techniques described above were used to cluster the data. The cluster analysis has been carried out using R language and Hmisc package (Harrell Jr and Dupont, 2006). The results are graphically illustrated in Figure 2 and Figure 3 respectively.

A remarkable result of Pearson's hierarchical clustering is that in the same branch of the tree co-exist breastfeeding and neurodevelopment test (Figure 3). In addition, Figure 3 illustrates that according to the results, motor development test and day care at the 1st age were strongly associated as their distance in the hierarchical tree was short but the r^2 is not high. However, it is noted that Rogan and Gladen (1993) examined the effect of breastfeeding to the child neurodevelopment and concluded that breast-fed children scored slightly better than those bottle fed. Moreover, Andres (Andres et al., 2012) identified that breast-fed children had higher Psychomotor Development Index scores than protein–based formula–fed infants at age of 6 months and slightly higher Preschool Language Scale-3 scores than milk-based formula–fed infants at ages of 3 and 6 months. Also, it is worth mentioning that Anderson et al., 1999 (Anderson et al., 1999) concluded that breast-feeding was associated with significantly higher scores for cognitive development than formula feeding.

The correlations of the various parameters are also illustrated with a heatmap in Figure 4. However, because of the size of the dataset the explanation of the figure could become tedious. Hence, the heatmap results were presented using a globe diagram (Figure 5).

Results and Interpretation of EWAS Analysis

EWAS analysis allowed to investigate the negative or beneficial contribution between various neurodevelopment and environmental indices. The neurodevelopment indices are based on Bayley test (Bayley, 2006). The overall analysis came up a wide range of associations that are illustrated in Figure 5.

With regard to cognitive development at one year of life, it was found that child exposure to metals result in lower cognitive scores, while the same occurs for the levels of inosine 5 phosphate and asparagine in the mother plasma during pregnancy. In addition, the results reveal that gestational age of the mother has negative effect (Figure 5 and Figure 6).

Moreover, EWAS correlations between Bayley test and metabolic pathways divulge that the Nitric oxide (NO^-) can have effects on the children neurodevelopment (Figure 6). According to literature, NO produces reactive oxygen species (ROS) and is also involved in the production of a neurotransmitter in the central (CNS) and peripheral (PNS) nervous system (Atmaca et al., 2007). It is produced by the family of nitric oxide synthase (NOS) and is known to affect neurodevelopmental process in the CNS (Black et al., 1999). Moreover, NO^- is described as an atypical neurotransmitter in the nervous system (Schulman, 1997). It is also remarked that NO is synthesized from arginine by nitric oxide synthase (NOS) (Hecker et al., 1990). However, a by- product of this synthesis is L-citrulline (Figure 6), as part of the L-citrulline-nitric oxide cycle and regulates the argininosuccinate synthase. According the study of Haas et al. (2002) mRNA levels of inducible nitric oxide synthase (iNOS) and arginine regenerating enzyme argininosuccinate synthetase (ASS) is related to pathogenesis of local inflammation and neuronal cell death. This is observed in patients experiencing neurological disorders (Braissant et al., 1999; Haas et al., 2002; Heneka et al., 2001); the latter association has also been confirmed by the Pearson's hierarchical cluster tree (Figure 3). Indeed, according to the results, L-citrulline, asparagine and inosine

Figure 2. Hierarchical clustering using the Hoeffding D method

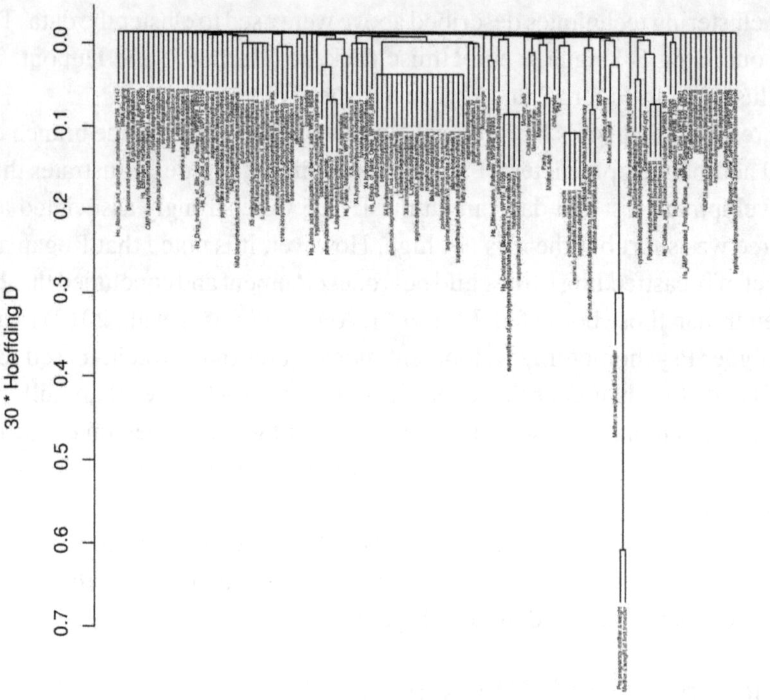

Figure 3. Hierarchical clustering using Pearson correlation

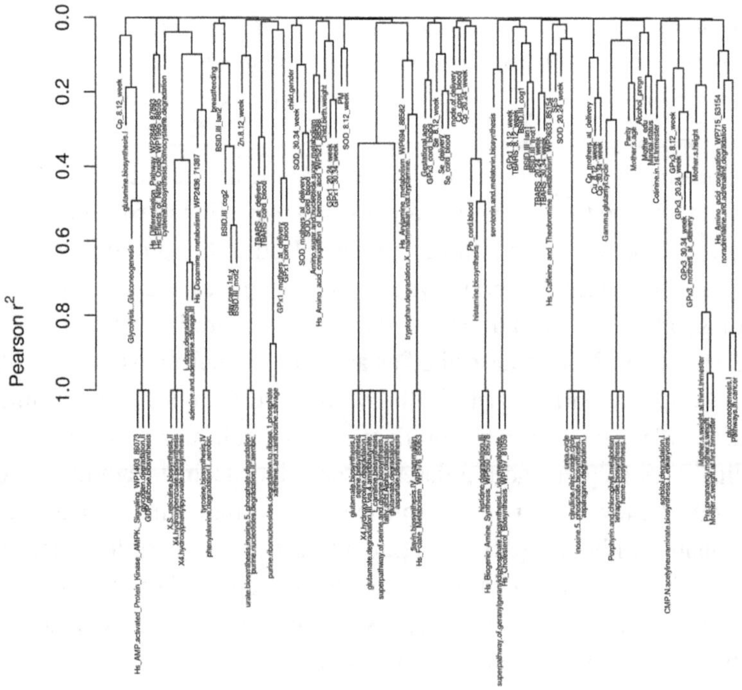

Figure 4. Heatmap of the exposure, environmental parameters and metabolic pathways of the REPRO_PL study

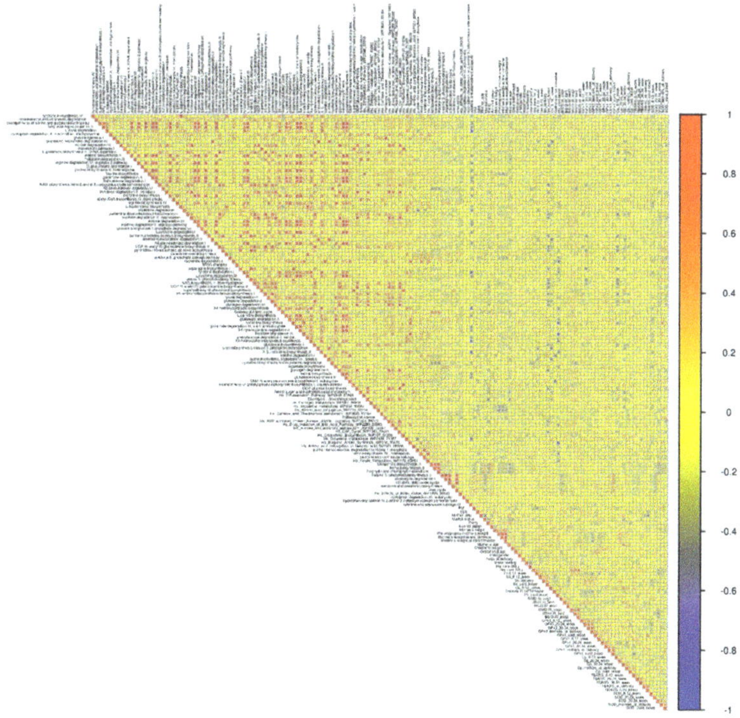

5 appeare in the same branch of the cluster (Figure 3) and EWAS analysis through the Volcano plot (Figure 6) associates them with cognitive development.

It is also very important to highlight that according to the EWAS analysis, cognitive development strongly depends on the attendance of day care center by the child; children hosted in day care centers present higher cognitive skills (Figure 7).

According to the followed methodology, at two years of age, SOD is unfavorably associated with cognitive development (Figure 5, Figure 7). This could be associated to lipid peroxidation that is increased due to exposure in Lead (Monteiro et al., 1991). It is remarkable that glutathione peroxidases (GPx) (EC 1.11.1.9), that belong to a family of enzymes of main biological role, are responsible for the maintenance of homeostasis from oxidative damage. Moreover, exposure to lead can decrease the activity of tissue SOD and brain GPx (glutathione peroxidase) (Tripathi et al., 2001).

Language development at the 1st year (Figure 8) as well as cognitive development (Figure 7) and motor development (Figure 12) at the 2nd year of age are correlated with SOD and GPx levels, as well as with Se. Hence, a significant result of EWAS is the association between Se and motor development (Figure 11). It is a fact that selenium has an important roles in regulating antioxidant status because it acts through the selenoprotein glutathione peroxidases (Nehru and Dua, 1996).

It is evident that selenium has complex peculiarities physiopathology and metabolism in the brain that have been related to neurological diseases (Bou-Resli et al., 2002; Buckman et al., 1993; Vinceti et al., 2001). Also, a wide range of stuies depicted the crucial role of Se in biological activity and protective

Figure 5. Correlation globe plot of the REPRO_PL study. With blue and red lines are illustrated the correlations that appear negative and positive correlation between them respectively. The green and the dark yellow connection lines are subsets of the blue and red lines respectively. These subsets have been calculated taking into account the q value of the EWAS analysis, applying as validation method the false discovery rate (Benjamini and Hochberg, 1995) on 4 random subsets of the investigated dataset.

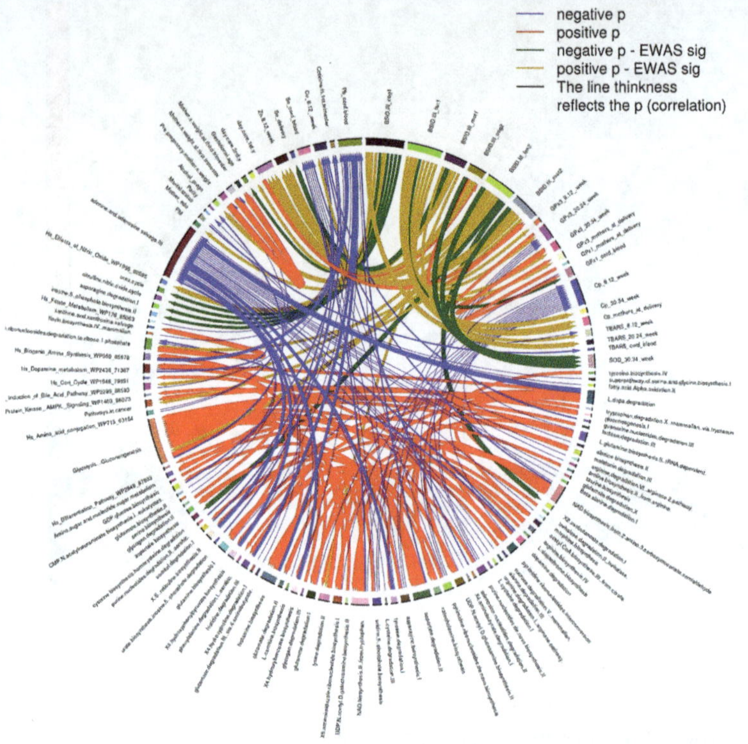

role against the toxicity implied by the concurrent exposure to toxic chemicals (Michalke and Berthele, 2011; Zwolak and Zaporowska, 2012). Moreover, Se has a beneficial effect on the activity of antioxidant enzymes insulted by chromium, vanadium and arsenic in animal cells (Zwolak and Zaporowska, 2012). The molecular antagonism between inorganic arsenic and selenium compounds, as well as mercury and selenium has also been studied (Gailer, 2007; Gailer, 2009), allowing the comprehension of the potential effects of this interaction on human health. According to the EWAS analysis, it is worth mentioning that the presence of selenium during the third semester of pregnancy seems to be a significant beneficial parameter, followed by glutathione peroxidase 1 in the mother plasma during pregnancy.

With regard to language development, the presence of Zn in maternal plasma (Figure 6) (during all the trimesters of pregnancy) and Cu (Figure 8) act beneficially. It is also known that, a wide range of metals are involved in cellular metabolism (Classen et al., 2011; Powell, 2000). Zn especially, is stored in specific synaptic vesicles by glutamatergic neurons, modulating the brain excitability (Bitanihirwe and Cunningham, 2009). The absence of Zn could lead to emotional disturbances because of atrophy to the brain cortex. In addition, Cu can neutralize free radicals that result in adverse effects to human health (Bonham et al., 2002). However, it is remarkable that an abnormal ratio between Zn and Cu could also result in neurolodevelpmental disorders (Osredkar and Sustar, 2011; Plum et al., 2010).

Figure 6. Association of the cognitive development at one year of age with exposure and modifiers

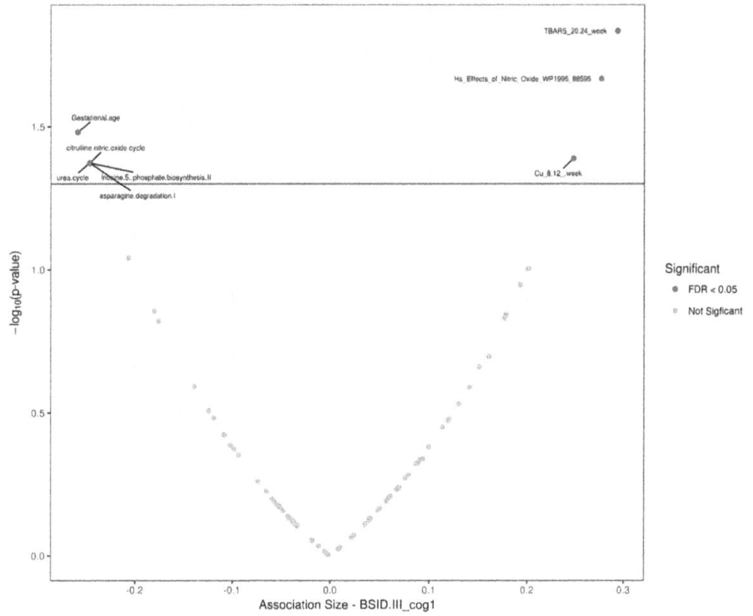

Figure 7. Association of the cognitive development at two years of age with exposure and modifiers

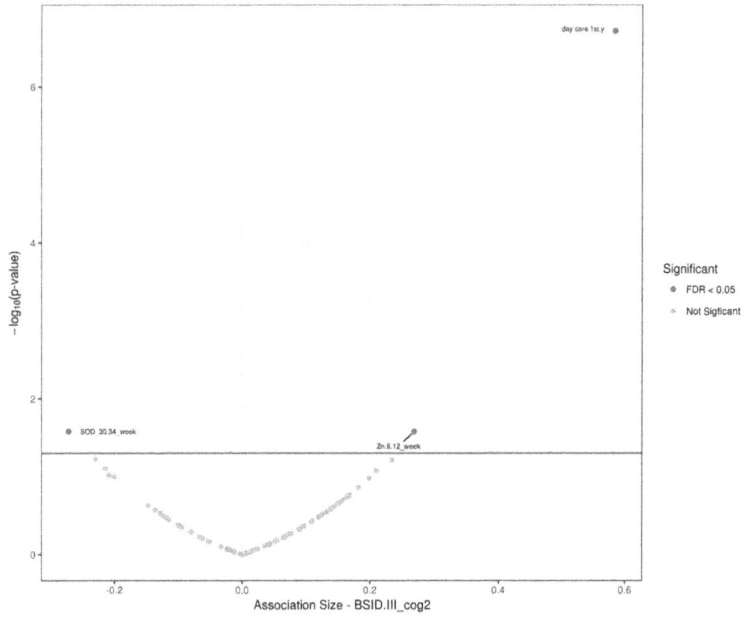

Figure 8. Association of the language development at one year of age with exposure and modifiers

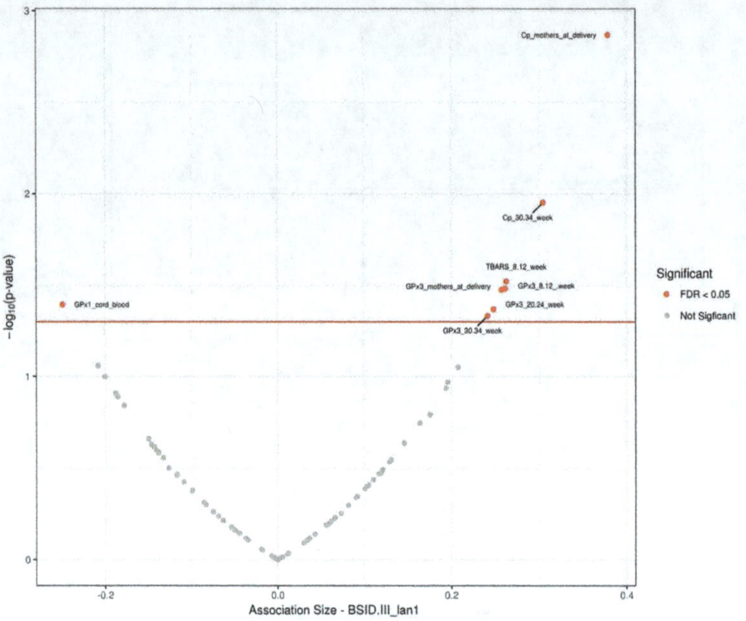

According to the EWAS results, neurodevelopmental effects are also related to TBARS (Thiobarbituric acid reactive substances) (Figure 6 and Figure 8). In particular, linguistic and cognitive development at the first year of life appear to correlate with TBARs and this could be attributed to lipid peroxidation. TBARs are generated during oxidative stress (Saugstad, 2005) as well as during the lipid peroxidation (Polydoro et al., 2004), that is the oxidative degradation of lipids, and actually. Since ROS are involved in a wide range of mechanisms such as the metabolism of glutathione, the role of antioxidants (Ji et al., 1992) and nitric oxide (Lee et al., 2012), they can potentially result in neurodevelopmental disorders. Especially, glutathione prevents the damage of important cellular components (Ji et al., 1992) caused by reactive oxygen species such as lipid peroxides and heavy metals (Pompella et al., 2003). At the same time, several mechanisms have been proposed as being implicated in the neurotoxic effects of metals exposure such induction of oxidative stress or brain inflammation (Aschner et al., 2000) and how these are conjugated with biological systems (Faro et al., 2005) and associated to protein inactivation and consequently to cell death in the central nervous system (Crespo-López et al., 2007).

A strong correlation according to EWAS analysis appears between language development at second year and glycogenesis and glycogenolysis (Figure 10). These processes control the synthesis of the macromolecule glycogen (for glucose storage) and degrade glycogen into glucose-1-phosphate (and glucose) (Tirone and Brunicardi, 2001). In this process of metabolism glycine is produced. glycine is a cytoprotective agent that it scavenges ROS and inhibits inflammatory responses (Bonvallot et al., 2013). On the other hand, glycine is that acts as inhibitory neurotransmitter in the central nervous system (Petrat et al., 2012).

Furthermore, EWAS reveals an association between 2-oxobutyrate degradation and language development. 2-oxobutyrate is produced during glycine, serine and threonine metabolism (KEGG). It is worth mentioning that threonine holds an important role in Tricarboxylic Acid (TCA) cycle because its

Figure 9. Serine, Theorine and Glycine metabolism (KEGG)

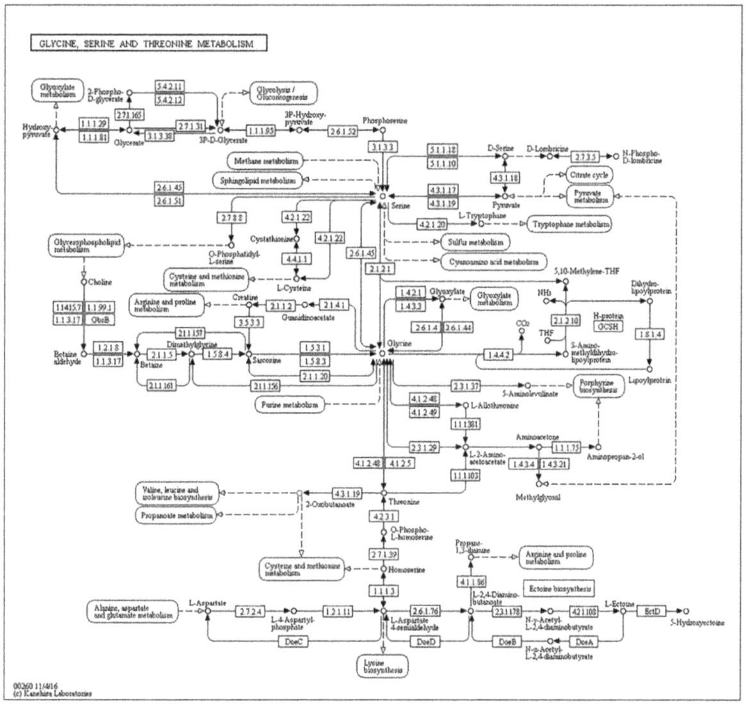

Figure 10. Association of the language development at two years of age with exposure and modifiers

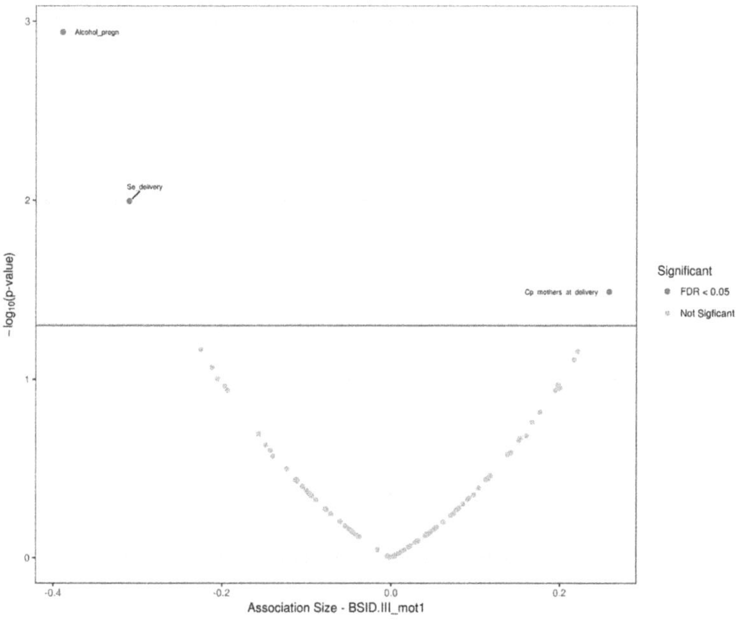

catabolism in mammals produces 2-oxobutyrate, glycine and acetylCoA (Boehm et al., 1998). Threonine is an α-amino acid that its incensement could be linked with a disruption in the TCA cycle (Regnault et al., 2005). According to Boehm et al. (1998), there is a significant positive correlation between threonine and glycine ratio (Figure 9). Consequently, threonine concentrations in plasma exert some effects on the glycinergic neurotransmitter system of the brain.

There is also evidence that threonine and glycine levels are not similar in the various tissues such as liver, muscles or plasma, inferring that threonine metabolism and/or glycine utilization are different in the brain in comparison with the other peripheral tissues (Boehm et al., 1998). In addition, several studies reveal that imbalance in the uptake of amino acids by the fetus results in various neurodevelopment (Ronzoni et al., 1999; Ronzoni et al., 2002).

It has to be noted that the presence of metals does not act (in terms of physiology) positively in motor development; it is rather an indicator of high consumption of food items (e.g. fish), rich in Hg, but also in other nutrients (e.g. omega 3 fatty acids) that are beneficial for child neurodevelopment (Andreji et al., 2005).

With regard to motor development, none of the environmental exposure factors seem to hold a key role. At year one (Figure 11), maternal alcohol consumption during pregnancy results in lower scores of motor development, while the presence of selenium (during the 1st and the 3rd trimester), contributes beneficially. In addition, child attendance in a day care center contributes beneficially as well.

Figure 12 illustrates the significant correlation of the purine ribonucleotides degradation to ribose 1 phosphate and motor development. Indeed, purines play an essential role in many cellular processes such cellular signaling and energy metabolism (biocyc.org) and they can potentially lead to neurodevelopmental abnormality (Simmonds et al., 1985). In addition, it is worth mentioning that xanthine and xanthosine are generated to the purine metabolism (Figure 13) and a disturbance on their synthesis can cause adverse effects in multiple cellular processes.

Figure 11. Association of the motor development at one year of age with exposure and modifiers

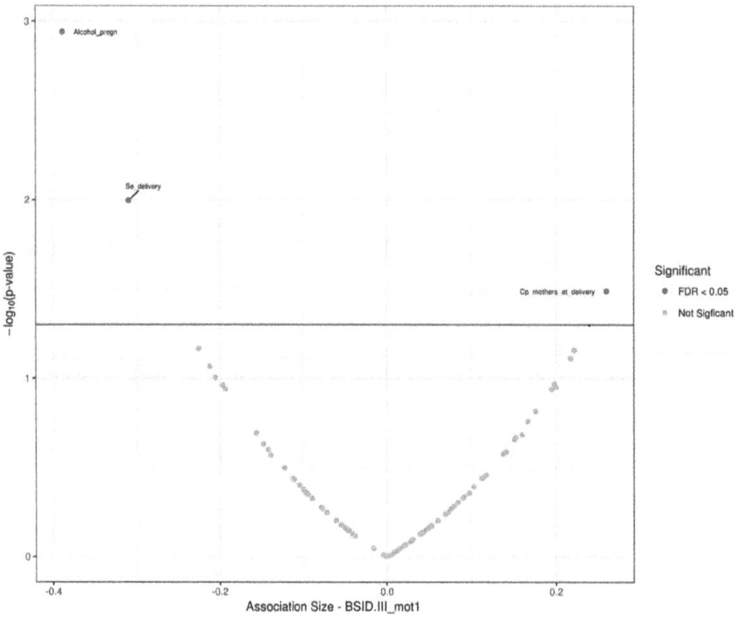

Figure 12. Association of the motor development at two years of age with exposure and modifiers

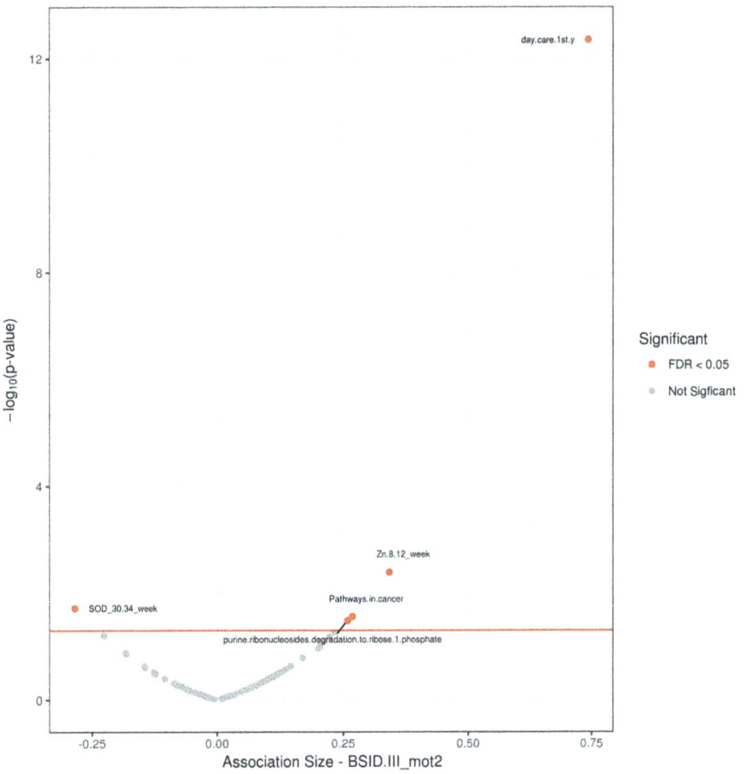

Figure 13. Purine metabolism (KEGG)

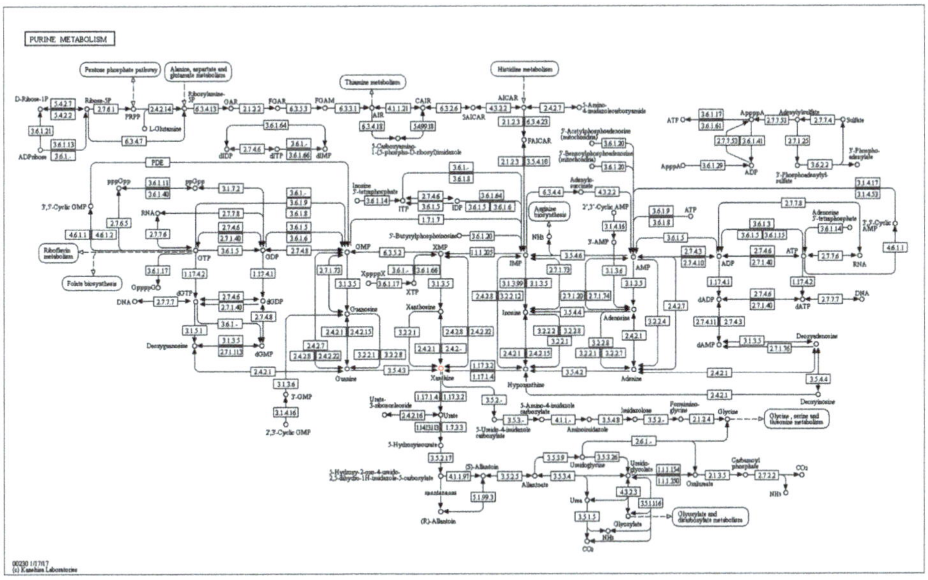

Last but not least, using graph theory (Bondy and Murty, 1976), a network community analysis was applied to EWAS results, in order to detected as well as to evaluate the identified associations. For this reason, an algorithm based on label propagation (Raghavan et al., 2007) was applied, allowing the detection of localized communities without imposing restrictions to the size of the community networks. The analysis was carried out in R using the *i-graph* package (Csardi and Nepusz, 2006). The results (Figure 14) disclose the existence of network community between neurodevelopment and metabolic pathways and they are in compliance with the overall approach.

The Heracles Waste Case Study

The exposome methodology proposed above has been applied for assessing the health impacts related to waste management in the area of Athens, the capital of Greece, which is populated with around 5 million inhabitants. The HERACLES (Waste Management) Greek cohort is a study aiming at assessing the contribution of environmental contamination due to waste management practices in the urban and periurban environment associated to children neurodevelopment. The study was initiated in 2012. In the study, 350 children between 3 to 8 years old living in the proximity of the Fili landfill (between 0.5 to 12 km) were participating (Sarigiannis, 2017; Sarigiannis and Karakitsios, 2018a). In order to identify the links among child neurodevelopment and exposure to waste contaminants, a number of exposure factors were included, such as:

- Toxic heavy metals, such as Cd, Hg and As in urine, Pb in blood, Mn and Hg in hair

Figure 14. Undirected community network. Cluster on the correlation results of EWAS analysis

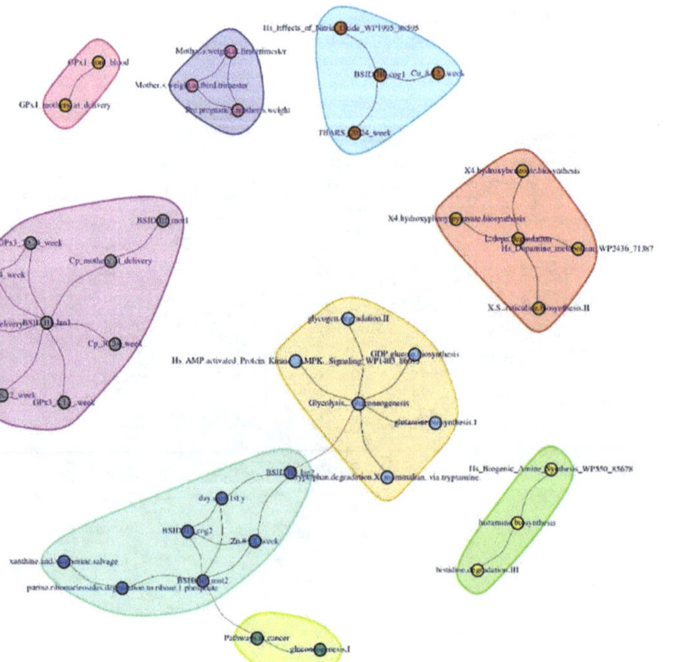

- More generic exposure metrics, like the distance of the residential address from the contaminated sites, in addition to levels of toxic heavy metals in the soil of the residence.
- Some other factors that eventually modify exposure and effect:
    - Parameters related to socioeconomic status, education level of parents as well as stress events.
    - Parameters related to anthropometric characteristics, such as child gender and body mass index, breastfeeding, presence of micronutrients, minerals and vitamins, and selenium levels during in utero life.
    - All type of diet components
- Omics analysis included metabolomics that was further used for metabolic pathway analysis, aiming at identifying the perturbations associated with deficient neurodevelopment.
- Child neurodevelopment using the Wechsler Intelligence Scale.

From the analysis it was found that a detrimental factor inversely associated with child neurodevelopment is the distance of the living address to the waste management site. Also, it was found that diet might contribute in both s positive or a negative way in child neurodevelopment. Consumption of tomatoes is positively associated with QI, Verbal Comprehension index and Working Memory index, while cereal consumption is strongly associated with the Perceptual Reasoning index. These properties are attributed to lycopene; additional evidence from epidemiology suggests that consumption of lycopene, a natural antioxidant present in tomatoes, is able to reduce the risk of chronic diseases such as cancer, cardiovascular diseases as well as psychiatric syndromes. An interesting conclusion has been drawn regarding fish consumption, depending on the type of fish and the neurodevelopmental indicator considered. Thus, higher consumption of white fish appears to have positive effects on the IQ and Verbal Comprehension index (p-value <0.001) while on the other hand affects negatively (p-value <0.01) the Perceptual Reasoning and Working Memory indexes. As expected, sociodemographic parameters are also important for child neurodevelopment; parental educational level was found to be positively associated with IQ, comprising the second (mother educational level) and third (father educational level) most significant parameters. Metabolomics and related bioinformatics analysis helped us identify the involvement of various metabolic pathways associated with child neurodevelopment. In a nutshell, it was found that autophagy may degrade the glycogen in neurons, in a way similar to many other tissues. Defects in lysosomal enzyme acid alpha-glucosidase are linked to accumulation of glycogen in several tissues, including neurons; it is well established that glycogen in neurons provokes neurodegenaration. Trehalose promotes the stabilization of proteins, resulting in higher levels of protein structural integrity, reducing aggregation of pathologically misfolded proteins. Trehalose is an mTOR-independent inducer of autophagy and, together with TSC, form a complex which is the key regulator of protein synthesis, controlling the growth of cell. TSC1/2 complex influences neural polarity as shown by recent evidence. Finally, the mevalonate cascade regulates several cellular functions and is associated in the progress of various brain related adverse outcomes including both neurodevelopmental and neurodegenerative disorders.

CONCLUSION

Despite the worldwide awareness about introducing the exposome perspective in environmental health studies, there is still lack of understanding the opportunities for interdisciplinary research, aiming at understanding the complex gene and environment interaction. Although significant advances are proposed by molecular epidemiology and statistical approached based on gene-environment wide associations, a more in depth and synthetic approach is required to understand the causality of environmental burden of disease. It has to be noted, that the case studies described above, are based on cohorts that are re-evaluated through the exposome point of view (including re-analysis of existing samples towards an alignment with the exposome concept) and they were not initially designed having in mind the full connectivity approach. However, the reanalysis of existing data using the association tools provided by exposome (such as EWAS) and more importantly the reanalysis of existing biobanked samples (that allowed metabolomics and pathway analysis) provided a more in depth understanding of the associations among the various patterns and child neurodevelopment than the initial analysis. In practice, the only currently ongoing cohort build upon the exposome approach is the EXHES study within the frame of HEALS project, which is currently ongoing. However, based on what has been done and what is currently missing, useful conclusions on the importance of the various aspects that comprise the exposome concept can be drawn.

Firstly, it is important to capture individual lifetime exposure and to quantify differences in exposure among individuals liming in phenomenally similar environments. This will be greatly facilitated by using personal sensors and developing the algorithms for translating the acquired information into personalized activity patterns. This will allow us to draw a more accurate timeline of environments and microenvironments encountered, as well as to the physiological conditions (inhalation and cardiac rate) occurring to the contact medium. Considering that it is impossible to have the detailed full picture of large population groups, extrapolation from the detailed individual profiles to population groups have to be wisely executed, accounting for the different parameters resulting in different behavioral patterns such as age, gender and socioeconomic status; agent-based modelling seems a promising tool towards this direction.

Translating external exposure into internal exposure and biological responses is the next step. Firstly, we need to take into account that internal dose resulting from the same external exposure might vary significantly among individuals; this is the result of differences in the physiology (developmental stage, bodyweight, inhalation rate, obesity status), co-exposure to other compounds (environmental or pharmaceutical) and also to polymorphisms related to exposure to xenobiotics. Before moving forward to genome and environment wide associations, all these parameters have to be taken into account for, utilizing PBBK modelling and the SNPs profiling related to genes regulating xenobiotics metabolism. Thus, association between exposure and response have to be initiated after "adjusting" external exposure into individual internal dose profiles.

The connectivity approach functionally integrates the broadest array of technologies involved in exposome studies. Although collection of HBM data is the starting point of the assessment, bi-directional mechanistic links (external exposure to HBM and from HBM to disease) should be in equally investigated in depth; misclassification of exposure or its translation into actual biologically effective dose results in loss of valuable information. From the other side, analysis of internal exposome should be more comprehensive, explaining how the exogenous molecules identified result in changes in endogenous molecules, both found in HBM samples (Rappaport et al., 2014). Moving from associations to disease causality results the mechanistic understanding of all intermediate events related to human homeostasis unbalancing. Identifying these perturbations requires data acquisition (multi-omics, with a special focus on transcriptomics and metabolomics) and data interpretation and this can be effectively described by regulatory and pathway analysis (Roede et al., 2014). It is also very important to highlight the importance of cumulative exposure to the environmental disease burden. The results of the agnostic transcriptome and metabolome search on biological samples with regard to the identification of potential genomic signatures that can serve as exposure biomarkers. Even when exposure to single compounds only shows intermediate results, it has been found that co-exposure to a real-life mixture may have more than additive effects on gene expression modulation. After the agnostic tier it is possible to identify not only single genes that have shown significant modulation in expression levels, but also determine the biological pathways that are regulated by gene networks that were significantly modulated with regard to their induction levels from exposure to xenobiotics. Combined with the changes in metabolomics profile, pathway analysis can reveal the key pathways involved in each perturbation, (e.g. regulation of p53 or induction of oxidative stress) and how these are differentially modulated from specific chemical families, while specific genes or gene sequences as well as combination of other small molecules could be characterized as molecular markers of exposure. By further proceeding with the targeted analysis described in the exposure biology workflow described above, causalities among genome, environment and specific endotypes or disease phenotypes can be deciphered.

Overall, connectivity introduces a new exposome based paradigm for interdisciplinary scientific work in the area of environment and health. This denotes an approach that builds on the exploration of the interconnections between the co-existence of multiple stressors and the different scales of biological organization that together produce the final adverse health effect. This marks a clear departure from the conventional paradigm, which seeks to shed light on the identification of singular cause-effect relationships between stressors and health outcomes. It entails creating a new way of combining health-relevant information coming from different disciplines, including (but not limited to) environmental science, epidemiology, toxicology, physiology, molecular biology, biochemistry, mathematics and computer science. According to the connectivity approach, all factors affecting internal and external exposome are treated as co-variates, rather than just as confounders. The functional integration of these different information classes into a unique framework will result in understanding the complex interaction between the genome and exposure to environmental factors.

REFERENCES

Acid, S. A. (2004). Lehninger principles of biochemistry.

Alonso, A., Marsal, S., & Julia, A. (2015). Analytical methods in untargeted metabolomics: State of the art in 2015. *Frontiers in Bioengineering and Biotechnology*, *3*, 23. doi:10.3389/fbioe.2015.00023 PMID:25798438

Anderson, J. W., Johnstone, B. M., & Remley, D. T. (1999). Breast-feeding and cognitive development: A meta-analysis. *The American Journal of Clinical Nutrition*, *70*(4), 525–535. doi:10.1093/ajcn/70.4.525 PMID:10500022

Andra, S. S., Charisiadis, P., Karakitsios, S., Sarigiannis, D. A., & Makris, K. C. (2015). Passive exposures of children to volatile trihalomethanes during domestic cleaning activities of their parents. *Environmental Research, 136*, 187–195. doi:10.1016/j.envres.2014.10.018 PMID:25460636

Andreji, J., Stránai, I., Massanyi, P. & Valent, M. (2005). Concentration of selected metals in muscle of various fish species. *Journal of environmental science and health, 40*, 899-912.

Andres, A., Cleves, M. A., Bellando, J. B., Pivik, R., Casey, P. H., & Badger, T. M. (2012). Developmental status of 1-year-old infants fed breast milk, cow's milk formula, or soy formula. *Pediatrics, 129*(6), 1134–1140. doi:10.1542/peds.2011-3121 PMID:22641754

Aschner, M., Yao, C. P., Allen, J. W., & Tan, K. H. (2000). Methylmercury alters glutamate transport in astrocytes. *Neurochemistry International, 37*(2-3), 199–206. doi:10.1016/S0197-0186(00)00023-1 PMID:10812205

Asimina, S., Chapizanis, D., Karakitsios, S., Kontoroupis, P., Asimakopoulos, D. N., Maggos, T., & Sarigiannis, D. (2018). Assessing and enhancing the utility of low-cost activity and location sensors for exposure studies. *Environmental Monitoring and Assessment, 190*(3), 155. doi:10.100710661-018-6537-2 PMID:29464404

Atmaca, M., Tezcan, E., & Ustundag, B. (2007). Plasma nitric oxide and leptin values in patients with olanzapine-induced weight gain. *Journal of Psychiatric Research, 41*(1-2), 74–79. doi:10.1016/j.jpsychires.2005.12.003 PMID:16426639

Bayley, N. (2006). *Bayley scales of infant and toddler development: administration manual*. Harcourt Assessment.

Benjamini, Y., & Hochberg, Y. (1995). Controlling the false discovery rate: A practical and powerful approach to multiple testing. *Journal of the Royal Statistical Society. Series B. Methodological*, 289–300.

Biocyc.org. (2017). Pathway: inosine-5'-phosphate biosynthesis.

Bitanihirwe, B. K., & Cunningham, M. G. (2009). Zinc: The brain's dark horse. *Synapse (New York, N.Y.), 63*(11), 1029–1049. doi:10.1002yn.20683 PMID:19623531

Black, M. D., Selk, D. E., Hitchcock, J., Wettstein, J. G., & Sorensen, S. M. (1999). On the effect of neonatal nitric oxide synthase inhibition in rats: A potential neurodevelopmental model of schizophrenia. *Neuropharmacology, 38*(9), 1299–1306. doi:10.1016/S0028-3908(99)00041-6 PMID:10471083

Boehm, G., Cervantes, H., Georgi, G., Jelinek, J., Sawatzki, G., Wermuth, B., & Colombo, J.-P. (1998). Effect of increasing dietary threonine intakes on amino acid metabolism of the central nervous system and peripheral tissues in growing rats. *Pediatric Research, 44*(6), 900–906. doi:10.1203/00006450-199812000-00013 PMID:9853925

Bondy, J. A., & Murty, U. S. R. (1976). *Graph theory with applications*. Citeseer. doi:10.1007/978-1-349-03521-2

Bonham, M., O'Connor, J. M., Hannigan, B. M., & Strain, J. (2002). The immune system as a physiological indicator of marginal copper status? *British Journal of Nutrition, 87*(05), 393–403. doi:10.1079/BJN2002558 PMID:12010579

Bonvallot, N., Tremblay-Franco, M., Chevrier, C., Canlet, C., Warembourg, C., Cravedi, J.-P., & Cordier, S. (2013). Metabolomics tools for describing complex pesticide exposure in pregnant women in Brittany (France). *PLoS One*, *8*(5), e64433. doi:10.1371/journal.pone.0064433 PMID:23704985

Bou-Resli, M., Mathew, T., Dashti, H., & Al-Zaid, N. (2002). Brain selenium accumulation in rat pups of selenium supplemented mothers. *Anatomia, Histologia, Embryologia*, *31*(4), 228–231. doi:10.1046/j.1439-0264.2002.00400.x PMID:12196265

Braissant, O., Honegger, P., Loup, M., Iwase, K., Takiguchi, M., & Bachmann, C. (1999). Hyperammonemia: Regulation of argininosuccinate synthetase and argininosuccinate lyase genes in aggregating cell cultures of fetal rat brain. *Neuroscience Letters*, *266*(2), 89–92. doi:10.1016/S0304-3940(99)00274-8 PMID:10353334

Buckman, T. D., Sutphin, M. S., & Eckhert, C. D. (1993). A comparison of the effects of dietary selenium on selenoprotein expression in rat brain and liver. Biochimica et Biophysica Acta (BBA)-. *Protein Structure and Molecular Enzymology.*, *1163*(2), 176–184. doi:10.1016/0167-4838(93)90179-U PMID:8490049

Caspi, R., Altman, T., Billington, R., Dreher, K., Foerster, H., Fulcher, C. A., ... Karp, P. D. (2014). The MetaCyc database of metabolic pathways and enzymes and the BioCyc collection of Pathway/Genome Databases. *Nucleic Acids Research*, *42*(D1), D459–D471. doi:10.1093/nar/gkt1103 PMID:24225315

Chadeau-Hyam, M., Campanella, G., Jombart, T., Bottolo, L., Portengen, L., Vineis, P., ... Vermeulen, R. C. H. (2013). Deciphering the complex: Methodological overview of statistical models to derive OMICS-based biomarkers. *Environmental and Molecular Mutagenesis*, *54*(7), 542–557. doi:10.1002/em.21797 PMID:23918146

Classen, H., Gröber, U., Löw, D., Schmidt, J., & Stracke, H. (2011). Zinc deficiency. Symptoms, causes, diagnosis and therapy. *Medizinische Monatsschrift fur Pharmazeuten*, *34*, 87–95. PMID:21736013

Crespo-López, M. E., De Sa, A. L., Herculano, A. M., Burbano, R. R., & do Nascimento, J. L. M. (2007). Methylmercury genotoxicity: A novel effect in human cell lines of the central nervous system. *Environment International*, *33*(2), 141–146. doi:10.1016/j.envint.2006.08.005 PMID:17007929

Csardi, G., & Nepusz, T. (2006). The igraph software package for complex network research. InterJournal. *Complex Systems*, *1695*, 1–9.

Cui, Y., Balshaw, D. M., Kwok, R. K., Thompson, C. L., Collman, G. W., & Birnbaum, L. S. (2016). The Exposome: Embracing the Complexity for Discovery in Environmental Health. *Environmental Health Perspectives*, *124*(8), A137–A140. doi:10.1289/EHP412 PMID:27479988

Dennis, K. K., Marder, E., Balshaw, D. M., Cui, Y., Lynes, M. A., Patti, G. J., ... Barr, D. B. (2017). Biomonitoring in the Era of the Exposome. *Environmental Health Perspectives*, *125*(4), 502–510. doi:10.1289/EHP474 PMID:27385067

Escher, B. I., Hackermüller, J., Polte, T., Scholz, S., Aigner, A., Altenburger, R., ... Wambaugh, J. F. (2017). From the exposome to mechanistic understanding of chemical-induced adverse effects. *Environment International*, *99*, 97–106. doi:10.1016/j.envint.2016.11.029 PMID:27939949

Faro, L., do Nascimento, J., Campos, F., Vidal, L., Alfonso, M., & Durán, R. (2005). Protective effects of glutathione and cysteine on the methylmercury-induced striatal dopamine release in vivo. *Life Sciences, 77*(4), 444–451. doi:10.1016/j.lfs.2004.11.033 PMID:15894013

Gailer, J. (2007). Arsenic–selenium and mercury–selenium bonds in biology. *Coordination Chemistry Reviews, 251*(1-2), 234–254. doi:10.1016/j.ccr.2006.07.018

Gailer, J. (2009). Chronic toxicity of As III in mammals: The role of (GS) 2 AsSe−. *Biochimie, 91*(10), 1268–1272. doi:10.1016/j.biochi.2009.06.004 PMID:19539009

Haas, J., Storch-Hagenlocher, B., Biessmann, A., & Wildemann, B. (2002). Inducible nitric oxide synthase and argininosuccinate synthetase: Co-induction in brain tissue of patients with Alzheimer's dementia and following stimulation with β-amyloid 1–42 in vitro. *Neuroscience Letters, 322*(2), 121–125. doi:10.1016/S0304-3940(02)00095-2 PMID:11958858

Harrell, F.E. Jr. & Dupont, M. C. (2006). The Hmisc Package. R package version. 3, 0-12.

Hecker, M., Sessa, W. C., Harris, H. J., Anggård, E., & Vane, J. R. (1990). The metabolism of L-arginine and its significance for the biosynthesis of endothelium-derived relaxing factor: Cultured endothelial cells recycle L-citrulline to L-arginine. *Proceedings of the National Academy of Sciences of the United States of America, 87*(21), 8612–8616. doi:10.1073/pnas.87.21.8612 PMID:2236071

Heneka, M. T., Wiesinger, H., Dumitrescu-Ozimek, L., Riederer, P., Feinstein, D. L., & Klockgether, T. (2001). Neuronal and glial coexpression of argininosuccinate synthetase and inducible nitric oxide synthase in Alzheimer disease. *Journal of Neuropathology and Experimental Neurology, 60*(9), 906–916. doi:10.1093/jnen/60.9.906 PMID:11556547

Jewison, T., Su, Y., Disfany, F. M., Liang, Y., Knox, C., Maciejewski, A., ... Wishart, D. S. (2014). SMPDB 2.0: Big improvements to the Small Molecule Pathway Database. *Nucleic Acids Research, 42*(D1), D478–D484. doi:10.1093/nar/gkt1067 PMID:24203708

Ji, L., Fu, R., & Mitchell, E. W. (1992). Glutathione and antioxidant enzymes in skeletal muscle: Effects of fiber type and exercise intensity. *Journal of Applied Physiology, 73*(5), 1854–1859. doi:10.1152/jappl.1992.73.5.1854 PMID:1474061

Johnson, C. H., Athersuch, T. J., Collman, G. W., Dhungana, S., Grant, D. F., Jones, D. P., ... Vasiliou, V. (2017). Yale school of public health symposium on lifetime exposures and human health: The exposome; summary and future reflections. *Human Genomics, 11*(1), 32. doi:10.118640246-017-0128-0 PMID:29221465

Kanehisa, M., Goto, S., Sato, Y., Furumichi, M., & Tanabe, M. (2012). KEGG for integration and interpretation of large-scale molecular data sets. *Nucleic Acids Research, 40*(D1), D109–D114. doi:10.1093/nar/gkr988 PMID:22080510

KEGG. (2017). *2-Oxobutanoate. Vol.* KEGG, Purine Metabolism.

KEGG. (n.d.). Citrate cycle (TCA cycle).

Kelder, T., van Iersel, M. P., Hanspers, K., Kutmon, M., Conklin, B. R., Evelo, C. T., & Pico, A. R. (2012). WikiPathways: Building research communities on biological pathways. *Nucleic Acids Research*, *40*(D1), D1301–D1307. doi:10.1093/nar/gkr1074 PMID:22096230

Kim, K. N. & Hong, Y. C. (2017). The exposome and the future of epidemiology: a vision and prospect.

Kiossoglou, P., Borda, A., Gray, K., Martin-Sanchez, F., Verspoor, K., & Lopez-Campos, G. (2017). Characterising the Scope of Exposome Research: A Generalisable Approach. *Studies in Health Technology and Informatics*, *245*, 457–461. PMID:29295136

Lee, R., Margaritis, M. M., Channon, K., & Antoniades, C. (2012). Evaluating oxidative stress in human cardiovascular disease: Methodological aspects and considerations. *Current Medicinal Chemistry*, *19*, 2504–2520. doi:10.2174/092986712800493057 PMID:22489713

Loh, M., Sarigiannis, D., Gotti, A., Karakitsios, S., Pronk, A., Kuijpers, E., ... Cherrie, J. (2017a). How Sensors Might Help Define the External Exposome. *International Journal of Environmental Research and Public Health*, *14*(4), 434. doi:10.3390/ijerph14040434 PMID:28420222

Loh, M., Sarigiannis, D., Gotti, A., Karakitsios, S., Pronk, A., Kuijpers, E., ... Cherrie, J. W. (2017b). How Sensors Might Help Define the External Exposome. *International Journal of Environmental Research and Public Health*, *14*(4), 434. doi:10.3390/ijerph14040434 PMID:28420222

Ma, H., Sorokin, A., Mazein, A., Selkov, A., Selkov, E., Demin, O., & Goryanin, I. (2007). The Edinburgh human metabolic network reconstruction and its functional analysis. *Molecular Systems Biology*, *3*, 135–135. doi:10.1038/msb4100177 PMID:17882155

Manrai, A. K., Cui, Y., Bushel, P. R., Hall, M., Karakitsios, S., Mattingly, C. J., ... Patel, C. J. (2017). Informatics and Data Analytics to Support Exposome-Based Discovery for Public Health. *Annual Review of Public Health*, *38*(1), 279–294. doi:10.1146/annurev-publhealth-082516-012737 PMID:28068484

Michalke, B., & Berthele, A. (2011). Contribution to selenium speciation in cerebrospinal fluid samples. *Journal of Analytical Atomic Spectrometry*, *26*(1), 165–170. doi:10.1039/C0JA00106F

Miller, G. W. (2014). The Exposome: Purpose, Definition, and Scope. In G. W. Miller (Ed.), *The Exposome* (pp. 1–12). San Diego, CA: Academic Press. doi:10.1016/B978-0-12-417217-3.00001-X

Miller, G. W., & Jones, D. P. (2014). The nature of nurture: Refining the definition of the exposome. *Toxicological Sciences*, *137*(1), 1–2. doi:10.1093/toxsci/kft251 PMID:24213143

Monteiro, H. P., Bechara, E. J., & Abdalla, D. S. (1991). Free radicals involvement in neurological porphyrias and lead poisoning. *Molecular and Cellular Biochemistry*, *103*(1), 73–83. doi:10.1007/BF00229595 PMID:1857346

Nehru, B., & Dua, R. (1997). The effect of dietary selenium on lead neurotoxicity. *Journal of Environmental Pathology, Toxicology and Oncology*, *16*(1), 47–50.

Niedzwiecki, M. M., & Miller, G. W. (2017). The Exposome Paradigm in Human Health: Lessons from the Emory Exposome Summer Course. *Environmental Health Perspectives*, *125*(6), 064502. doi:10.1289/EHP1712 PMID:28669935

Osredkar, J., & Sustar, N. (2011). Copper and zinc, biological role and significance of copper/zinc imbalance. *J. Clinic. Toxicological Sciences*, *3*, 2161–0495.

Petrat, F., Boengler, K., Schulz, R., & de Groot, H. (2012). Glycine, a simple physiological compound protecting by yet puzzling mechanism (s) against ischaemia–reperfusion injury: Current knowledge. *British Journal of Pharmacology*, *165*(7), 2059–2072. doi:10.1111/j.1476-5381.2011.01711.x PMID:22044190

Plum, L. M., Rink, L., & Haase, H. (2010). The essential toxin: Impact of zinc on human health. *International Journal of Environmental Research and Public Health*, *7*(4), 1342–1365. doi:10.3390/ijerph7041342 PMID:20617034

Polańska, K., Hanke, W., Gromadzińska, J., Ligocka, D., Gulczyńska, E., Sobala, W., & Wąsowicz, W. (2009). Polish mother and child cohort study - Defining the problem, the aim of the study and methodological assumptions. *International Journal of Occupational Medicine and Environmental Health*, *22*(4), 383–391. doi:10.2478/v10001-009-0037-0 PMID:20053622

Polańska, K., Hanke, W., Jurewicz, J., Sobala, W., Madsen, C., Nafstad, P., & Magnus, P. (2011). Polish mother and child cohort study (REPRO-PL) -Methodology of follow-up of the children. *International Journal of Occupational Medicine and Environmental Health*, *24*(4), 391–398. doi:10.247813382-011-0026-y PMID:22086452

Polanska, K., Hanke, W., Krol, A., Gromadzinska, J., Kuras, R., Janasik, B., ... Calamandrei, G. (2017). Micronutrients during pregnancy and child psychomotor development: Opposite effects of Zinc and Selenium. *Environmental Research*, *158*, 583–589. doi:10.1016/j.envres.2017.06.037 PMID:28715787

Polanska, K., Hanke, W., Sobala, W., Trzcinka-Ochocka, M., Ligocka, D., Brzeznicki, S., ... Magnus, P. (2013). Developmental effects of exposures to environmental factors: The polish mother and child cohort study. *BioMed Research International*. PMID:24191247

Polańska, K., Hanke, W., Sobala, W., Trzcinka-Ochocka, M., Ligocka, D., Strugała-Stawik, H., & Magnus, P. (2014). Predictors of environmental lead exposure among pregnant women - A prospective cohort study in Poland. *Annals of Agricultural and Environmental Medicine*, *21*, 49–54. PMID:24738496

Polanska, K., Ligocka, D., Sobala, W., & Hanke, W. (2014). Phthalate exposure and child development: The Polish Mother and Child Cohort Study. *Early Human Development*, *90*(9), 477–485. doi:10.1016/j.earlhumdev.2014.06.006 PMID:25038557

Polanska, K., Ligocka, D., Sobala, W., & Hanke, W. (2016). Effect of environmental phthalate exposure on pregnancy duration and birth outcomes. *International Journal of Occupational Medicine and Environmental Health*, *29*(4), 683–697. doi:10.13075/ijomeh.1896.00691 PMID:27443763

Polydoro, M., Schröder, N., Lima, M. N. M., Caldana, F., Laranja, D. C., Bromberg, E., ... Dal-Pizzol, F. (2004). Haloperidol-and clozapine-induced oxidative stress in the rat brain. *Pharmacology, Biochemistry, and Behavior*, *78*(4), 751–756. doi:10.1016/j.pbb.2004.05.018 PMID:15301931

Pompella, A., Visvikis, A., Paolicchi, A., De Tata, V., & Casini, A. F. (2003). The changing faces of glutathione, a cellular protagonist. *Biochemical Pharmacology*, *66*(8), 1499–1503. doi:10.1016/S0006-2952(03)00504-5 PMID:14555227

Powell, S. R. (2000). The antioxidant properties of zinc. *The Journal of Nutrition, 130*(5), 1447S–1454S. doi:10.1093/jn/130.5.1447S PMID:10801958

Raghavan, U. N., Albert, R., & Kumara, S. (2007). Near linear time algorithm to detect community structures in large-scale networks. *Physical Review. E, 76*(3), 036106. doi:10.1103/PhysRevE.76.036106 PMID:17930305

Rappaport, S. M. (2018). Redefining environmental exposure for disease etiology. *NPJ Syst Biol Appl., 4*(1), 30. doi:10.103841540-018-0065-0 PMID:30181901

Rappaport, S. M., Barupal, D. K., Wishart, D., Vineis, P., & Scalbert, A. (2014). The Blood Exposome and Its Role in Discovering Causes of Disease. *Environmental Health Perspectives, 122*(8), 769–774. doi:10.1289/ehp.1308015 PMID:24659601

Rappaport, S. M., & Smith, M. T. (2010). Environment and disease risks. *Science, 330*(6003), 460–461. doi:10.1126cience.1192603 PMID:20966241

Reece, J. B., Urry, L. A., Cain, M. L., Wasserman, S. A., Minorsky, P. V., & Jackson, R. B. (2011). *Campbell biology*. Pearson Boston.

Regnault, T., Friedman, J., Wilkening, R., Anthony, R., & Hay, W. Jr. (2005). Fetoplacental transport and utilization of amino acids in IUGR—A review. *Placenta, 26*, S52–S62. doi:10.1016/j.placenta.2005.01.003 PMID:15837069

Roede, J. R., Uppal, K., Park, Y., Tran, V., & Jones, D. P. (2014). Transcriptome–metabolome wide association study (TMWAS) of maneb and paraquat neurotoxicity reveals network level interactions in toxicologic mechanism. *Toxicology Reports, 1*, 435–444. doi:10.1016/j.toxrep.2014.07.006 PMID:27722094

Rogan, W. J., & Gladen, B. C. (1993). Breast-feeding and cognitive development. *Early Human Development, 31*(3), 181–193. doi:10.1016/0378-3782(93)90194-Y PMID:8444137

Ronzoni, S., Marconi, A. M., Cetin, I., Paolini, C. L., Teng, C., Pardi, G., & Battaglia, F. C. (1999). Umbilical amino acid uptake at increasing maternal amino acid concentrations: Effect of a maternal amino acid infusate. *American Journal of Obstetrics and Gynecology, 181*(2), 477–483. doi:10.1016/S0002-9378(99)70581-8 PMID:10454703

Ronzoni, S., Marconi, A. M., Paolini, C. L., Teng, C., Pardi, G., & Battaglia, F. C. (2002). The effect of a maternal infusion of amino acids on umbilical uptake in pregnancies complicated by intrauterine growth restriction. *American Journal of Obstetrics and Gynecology, 187*(3), 741–746. doi:10.1067/mob.2002.124291 PMID:12237657

Sarigiannis, D. (2015a). Exposome science for public health protection and innovation. *Toxicology Letters, 238*(2), S12–S13. doi:10.1016/j.toxlet.2015.08.154

Sarigiannis, D. (2015b). Unravelling the Exposome through integrated exposure biology. *Toxicology Letters, 238*(2), S229–S230. doi:10.1016/j.toxlet.2015.08.680

Sarigiannis, D., Karakitsios, S., Gotti, A., Handakas, E., & Papadaki, K. (2015a). INTEGRA: Advancing risk assessment using internal dosimetry metrics. *Toxicology Letters, 238*(2), S110–S111. doi:10.1016/j.toxlet.2015.08.359

Sarigiannis, D. A. (2017). Assessing the impact of hazardous waste on children's health: The exposome paradigm. *Environmental Research, 158*, 531–541. doi:10.1016/j.envres.2017.06.031 PMID:28711809

Sarigiannis, D. A., Gotti, A., & Karakitsios, S. P. (2019a). Indoor Air and Public Health. In B. Roig & ... (Eds.), *Management of Emerging Public Health Issues and Risks* (pp. 3–29). Academic Press. doi:10.1016/B978-0-12-813290-6.00001-9

Sarigiannis, D. A., & Karakitsios, S. P. (2018a). Addressing complexity of health impact assessment in industrially contaminated sites via the exposome paradigm. *Epidemiologia e Prevenzione, 42*, 37–48. PMID:30322234

Sarigiannis, D. A., & Karakitsios, S. P. (2018b). Modeling Complex Exposures. In C. V. Rider & J. E. Simmons (Eds.), *Chemical Mixtures and Combined Chemical and Nonchemical Stressors: Exposure, Toxicity, Analysis, and Risk* (pp. 81–125). Cham: Springer International Publishing. doi:10.1007/978-3-319-56234-6_4

Sarigiannis, D. A., Karakitsios, S. P., Gotti, A., Papaloukas, C. L., Kassomenos, P. A., & Pilidis, G. A. (2009). Bayesian algorithm implementation in a real time exposure assessment model on benzene with calculation of associated cancer risks. *Sensors (Basel), 9*(2), 731–755. doi:10.339090200731 PMID:22399936

Sarigiannis, D. A., Karakitsios, S. P., Handakas, E., Simou, K., Solomou, E., & Gotti, A. (2016). Integrated exposure and risk characterization of bisphenol-A in Europe. *Food and Chemical Toxicology, 98*, 134–147. doi:10.1016/j.fct.2016.10.017 PMID:27769850

Sarigiannis, D. A., & Salifoglou, A. (2016). Research directives toward deciphering adverse outcome pathways induced by environmental metallotoxins. *Current Opinion in Chemical Engineering, 13*, 161–169. doi:10.1016/j.coche.2016.09.010

Sarigiannis, D. A., Tratnik, J. S., Mazej, D., Kosjek, T., Heath, E., Horvat, M., ... Karakitsios, S. P. (2019b). Risk characterization of bisphenol-A in the Slovenian population starting from human biomonitoring data. *Environmental Research, 170*, 293–300. doi:10.1016/j.envres.2018.12.056 PMID:30605834

Sarigiannis, D. A., Karakitsios, S. P., Zikopoulos, D., Nikolaki, S., & Kermenidou, M. (2015b). Lung cancer risk from PAHs emitted from biomass combustion. *Environmental Research, 137*, 147–156. doi:10.1016/j.envres.2014.12.009 PMID:25543545

Saugstad, O. D. (2005). Oxidative stress in the newborn–a 30-year perspective. *Neonatology, 88*(3), 228–236. doi:10.1159/000087586 PMID:16210845

Schmutz, J., Wheeler, J., Grimwood, J., Dickson, M., Yang, J., Caoile, C., ... Myers, R. M. (2004). Quality assessment of the human genome sequence. *Nature, 429*(6990), 365–368. doi:10.1038/nature02390 PMID:15164052

Schulman, H. (1997). Nitric oxide: A spatial second messenger. *Molecular Psychiatry, 2*(4), 296–299. doi:10.1038j.mp.4000197 PMID:9246669

Simmonds, H., Webster, D., Lingam, S., & Wilson, J. (1985). An inborn error of purine metabolism, deafness and neurodevelopmental abnormality. *Neuropediatrics*, *16*(02), 106–108. doi:10.1055-2008-1052552 PMID:2989725

Snoj Tratnik, J., Falnoga, I., Trdin, A., Mazej, D., Fajon, V., Miklavčič, A., ... Horvat, M. (2017). Prenatal mercury exposure, neurodevelopment and apolipoprotein E genetic polymorphism. *Environmental Research*, *152*, 375–385. doi:10.1016/j.envres.2016.08.035 PMID:27616663

Stamatelopoulou, A., Chapizanis, D., Karakitsios, S., Kontoroupis, P., Asimakopoulos, D., Maggos, T., & Sarigiannis, D. (2018). Assessing and enhancing the utility of low-cost activity and location sensors for exposure studies. *Environmental Monitoring and Assessment*. PMID:29464404

Tirone, T. A., & Brunicardi, F. C. (2001). Overview of glucose regulation. *World Journal of Surgery*, *25*(4), 461–467. doi:10.1007002680020338 PMID:11344399

Tripathi, R., Raghunath, R., Mahapatra, S., & Sadasivan, S. (2001). Blood lead and its effect on Cd, Cu, Zn, Fe and hemoglobin levels of children. *The Science of the Total Environment*, *277*(1-3), 161–168. doi:10.1016/S0048-9697(00)00871-8 PMID:11589396

Vinceti, M., Wei, E. T., Malagoli, C., Bergomi, M., & Vivoli, G. (2001). Adverse health effects of selenium in humans. *Reviews on Environmental Health*, *16*(4), 233–252. doi:10.1515/REVEH.2001.16.4.233 PMID:12041880

Vineis, P., van Veldhoven, K., Chadeau-Hyam, M., & Athersuch, T. J. (2013). Advancing the application of omics-based biomarkers in environmental epidemiology. *Environmental and Molecular Mutagenesis*, *54*(7), 461–467. doi:10.1002/em.21764 PMID:23519765

Vineis, P., & Wild, C. P. (2014). Global cancer patterns: Causes and prevention. *Lancet*, *383*(9916), 549–557. doi:10.1016/S0140-6736(13)62224-2 PMID:24351322

Vrijheid, M., Slama, R., Robinson, O., Chatzi, L., Coen, M., van den Hazel, P., ... Nieuwenhuijsen, M. J. (2014). The Human Early-Life Exposome (HELIX): Project Rationale and Design. *Environmental Health Perspectives*, *122*(6), 535–544. doi:10.1289/ehp.1307204 PMID:24610234

Wild, C. P. (2005). Complementing the genome with an "exposome": The outstanding challenge of environmental exposure measurement in molecular epidemiology. *Cancer Epidemiology, Biomarkers & Prevention*, *14*(8), 1847–1850. doi:10.1158/1055-9965.EPI-05-0456 PMID:16103423

Zwolak, I., & Zaporowska, H. (2012). Selenium interactions and toxicity: A review. *Cell Biology and Toxicology*, *28*(1), 31–46. doi:10.100710565-011-9203-9 PMID:21913064

ENDNOTE

1 For further analysis of the different technological arrays used in the connectivity approach and their functional integration, please check Sarigiannis et al. (2019).

Chapter 2
Autism Spectrum Disorder, Fear Response, and Environmental Exposures

Theoharis C. Theoharides
Tufts University, USA

Jaanvi Sant
Tufts University, USA

Maria-Eleni Giota
National and Kapodistrian University of Athens, Greece

ABSTRACT

Autism spectrum disorder (ASD) is a developmental condition characterized by impaired social interactions and communication, as well as by stereotypic movements, that affects 1 in 59 children. ASD is expected to reach 1 in about 40 children by 2020, yet it remains without distinct pathogenesis and effective treatment. Children with ASD respond with high anxiety to almost any unknown stimulus and appear to misread danger/threat signals, and may not experience anxiety in situations where normotypic children do. The authors propose that environmental stimuli stimulate the unique immune cells, known as mast cells (MC), which then trigger microglia, leading to dysfunctional neuronal connectivity in the amygdala. This process lowers or disrupts the "fear response" and leads to an exaggerated "fight-or-flight" reaction. corticotropin-releasing hormone (CRH) could have a synergistic effect with environmental stimuli, especially mycotoxins. Recognizing this association and preventing stimulation of mast cells/microglia could lead to effective treatment of ASD.

INTRODUCTION

Autism Spectrum Disorder (ASD) is a developmental condition characterized by impaired social interactions and communication, as well as by stereotypic movements. It affects 1 in 59 children (Centers for Disease Control and Prevention, 2018; Fombonne, 2009; Lai et al., 2014; McPartland & Volkmar,

DOI: 10.4018/978-1-5225-7635-8.ch002

2012), but is projected to reach 1 in 40 children by 2020. In spite of the discovery of numerous gene mutations in patients with ASD, no direct link has so far been uncovered (Abrahams & Geschwind, 2008; Geschwind & State, 2015; Willsey & State, 2015). The lack of reliable biomarkers (Ruggeri et al., 2014) and a specific pathogenesis (Theoharides et al., 2008), as well as the existence of subgroups and comorbidities (Bauman, 2010), complicates the diagnosis and treatment of ASD. Increasing evidence indicates that microglia, responsible for innate immunity of the brain (Aguzzi et al., 2013; Ransohoff & Brown, 2012), are activated in ASD (Gupta et al., 2014; Koyama & Ikegaya, 2015; Rodriguez & Kern, 2011; Takano, 2015), but the triggers are not known.

Neuroinflammation (Theoharides et al., 2016) may result from stimulation of unique tissue immune cells called mast cells (MC) (Theoharides et al., 2015c), which are located around blood vessels and nerves in the brain (Edvinsson et al., 1977; Goldschmidt et al., 1984; Marathias et al., 1991; Matsumoto et al., 2001; Taiwo et al., 2005), especially at the amygdala, the thalamus and the hypothalamus (Pang et al., 1996). Mediators derived from MC (Mukai et al., 2018; Theoharides et al., 2012, 2015c) could then activate microglia (Patel et al., 2016; Zhang et al., 2016), causing localized inflammation (Girolamo et al., 2017; Skaper et al., 2014; Theoharides et al., 2015a, 2015b) and leading to symptoms of ASD (Theoharides et al., 2016). Mast cells act as sensors of environmental and psychological stress (Theoharides, 2017), secreting danger signals (Theoharides, 2016) such as mitochondrial DNA (mtDNA) (Zhang et al., 2012), which acts as an "innate pathogen" (Theoharides et al., 2013) that causes auto-inflammatory responses (Collins et al., 2004; Marques et al., 2012; Sun et al., 2013). In fact, we reported that mtDNA is increased in the serum of children with ASD (Zhang et al., 2010).

Indirect evidence of the role of MC in ASD stems from the recognition that ASD has been significantly associated with atopic diseases (Theoharides et al., 2016) such as allergies (Liao et al., 2016; Lyall et al., 2015), asthma (Kotey et al., 2014) and eczema (Billeci et al., 2015), all of which involve MC. In addition, we reported that the incidence of ASD is 10 times higher in children with mastocytosis than in the general population (Theoharides, 2009). Moreover, most patients with mastocytosis complain of a variety of neuropsychological symptoms, including fatigue (Georgin-Lavialle et al., 2016a), cognitive impairment (Moura et al., 2012) and depression (Georgin-Lavialle et al., 2016b).

Immune-neural connections regulate responses to environmental and infectious agents, leading to altered behavior (McCusker & Kelley, 2013). We propose that stimulation of brain MC by environmental, neural, immune, pathogenic or stress triggers disrupt the normal "fear threshold" in the amygdala and the hypothalamic-pituitary-adrenal axis (HPA) (Chrousos, 1995). Mast cells act as sensors of environmental and psychological health (Theoharides et al., 2004) via corticotrophin-releasing hormone (CRH) together with the peptide neurotensin (NT) (Donelan et al., 2006). Triggers of MC can reach the hypothalamus from the nasal cavity through the cribriform plexus (Kalogeromitros et al., 2007), or may reach the brain through the lymphatics (Louveau et al., 2015). In addition, mast cell-derived mediators, especially cytokines (Abbott, 2000; Pan et al., 2011), increase the permeability of the gut-blood and blood-brain barriers (BBB) (Esposito et al., 2002; Fiorentino et al., 2016; Theoharides & Doyle, 2008). As a result, circulating and environmental toxins are allowed to pass into the brain, trigger microglia (Patel et al., 2016; Zhang et al., 2016), and disrupt neuronal connectivity, especially in the amygdala (Cowan et al., 2018; Rozniecki et al., 2009; Theoharides et al., 2016).

BACKGROUND

Fear Response

Infants are well-known to instinctively recognize threatening images, an innate fear response programmed in the amygdala (Choi & Kim, 2010; Moscarello & LeDoux, 2013). Considerable evidence indicates that patients with ASD have inappropriate responses to threatening images (Philip et al., 2010). This heightened reaction to stress may be rooted in a maladaptive lowering of the "fear response," which could become even more dysregulated when unfavorable environmental factors are present (Hollocks et al., 2014). Synergism between stress and environmental factors has been implicated at both the prenatal and the perinatal time periods (Tottenham & Sheridan, 2009). One such example is the effect of maternal immune activation (MIA) together with prenatal exposure to vehicle exhaust particles in mice, which leads to autism-like behavior (Bilbo et al., 2018). Postnatal stress-environment interactions may also affect the amygdala, especially its basolateral (BLA) and medial nuclei, both of which are involved in predator odor-induced fear in cats (Takahashi et al., 2007). For example, fear-induced activation of the BLA was reported to change how the brain processes environmental stimuli in rats (Holmes et al., 2013). The glucocorticoid receptor has been suggested as a potential target for toxins (Marketon & Sternberg, 2010).

It is important that ASD has been associated with dysfunctional connectivity in the amygdala, as well between the amygdala, the prefrontal cortex, and the hypothalamus (Layton et al., 1981; Merzhanova et al., 2000). Excitation of the nucleus amygdalae centralis in rats activated other nuclei in the amygdala via CRH and SP, leading to heightened responses and to prolonged emotional stress (Wu et al., 1999). The neuropeptides SP and NT also interact with other pathways in the limbic system, leading to altered homeostatic responses that may impact nervous system arousal (Lenard et al., 2018). Atypical patterns of amygdala development are also implicated in ASD. For example, the amygdala undergoes rapid early growth compared to normotypic children, as evidenced by higher spine density than age-matched controls (Parratt & Sturgess, 1977). Moreover, children with ASD show an initial excess of neurons in the basal amygdala with a reduction in adulthood, while normal controls have fewer neurons in childhood, but a greater number in adulthood (Avino et al., 2018). These differences in brain volume and circuitry central to emotional processing may be at the root of the dysregulated "fear response" that many ASD patients exhibit (Bauman & Kemper, 2003; Ressler, 2010).

There is extensive literature from animals and humans connecting the amygdala to social behavior (Bauman & Kemper, 2003; Bliss-Moreau et al., 2017) and to pathophysiologic responses to stress (Bondarenko et al., 2014). Bauman and Kemper (2003) first identified neuropathologic changes in the amygdala of postmortem brains (Bauman & Kemper, 2003), and even though the amygdala may not be essential for processing necessary for social behavior, amygdala are critical for responses to normally fear-inducing stimuli (Amaral et al., 2003; Bauman et al., 2004). Studies in non-human primates also showed that neonatal amygdala lesions compromise emotional processing (Bliss-Moreau et al., 2011a, 2011b). Furthermore, recent studies reported that amygdala lesions in rhesus monkeys generate more frequent stress-related behaviors (Bliss-Moreau et al., 2017). Such findings could further enhance our understanding of the pathogenesis of ASD (Bauman et al., 2004). It was found that disruption of the inhibitory tone of the BLA by administering the CRH analogue urocortin-1 to rats led to persistent social inhibition (Truitt et al., 2007).

The importance of stress and the HPA axis cannot be overemphasized, as suggested by numerous human studies. Prenatal stress was recently reported to be an independent risk factor for offspring having hyperactivity and conduct disorders (MacKinnon et al., 2018). Another study examined the effect of a sudden onset flood that occurred in Queensland, Australia in 2011. The findings showed that maternal stress during pregnancy predicted, at 30 months of age of the offspring, worse theory of mind, an important aspect of child development and successful social functioning (Simcock et al., 2017). Prenatal stress was linked to increased risk of ASD (Beversdorf et al., 2005; Ronald et al., 2010). There is also evidence that stress related to migration of pregnant mothers resulted in higher risk of giving birth to children with ASD (Crafa & Warfa, 2015). A study of genome-wide DNA methylation in paternal semen samples from the Early Autism Risk Longitudinal Investigation cohort concluded that epigenetic differences in paternal sperm may contribute to increased risk of the offspring developing ASD (Feinberg et al., 2015). In addition, prenatal and perinatal stress could lead to epigenetic changes in regulatory genes responsible for coping with stressful experiences and hostile environmental factors (Babenko et al., 2015). Such epigenetic changes are possibly due to interactions between genes and environmental triggers (Tordjman et al., 2014). One recent study of Danish men and women, for example, showed that prenatal and early postnatal stress were associated with increased serum levels of IL-6 (Pedersen et al., 2018).

Animal models of stress and epigenetics may also enhance our understanding of ASD. For example, prenatal stress was reported to decrease neuron excitability in the amygdala and social behavior in rats (Ehrlich & Rainnie, 2015), reinforcing the link between parent-offspring health. Another study showed that maternal deprivation stress induces long-term colonic nerve-MC interactions in rats (Barreau et al., 2008). Prereproductive stress in female rats altered CRHR-1 expression in ova and its expression in the brain of the offspring (Zaidan et al., 2013). The combined exposure of pregnant rats to a stressful insult and the drug terbutaline (used to arrest preterm labor) resulted in synergistic development of severe autism-like behavior (Bercum et al., 2015). This effect could be mediated via changes in the placenta that may contribute to the development of ASD (Wong et al., 2015). While many studies focus on maternal health history, paternal stress can also affect offspring. One study showed that paternal stress altered sperm micro RNA and reprogrammed the offspring stress response in mice (Rodgers et al., 2013).

Postnatal anxiety may have lasting consequences, too. A few studies, for example, focused on the importance of cortisol as an index of HPA axis activation. Children with ASD have higher peak cortisol levels and longer recovery time, suggesting increased HPA activation (Spratt et al., 2012). ASD patients are prone to stress, and their experience of anxiety was strongly correlated with repetitive behaviors (Rodgers et al., 2012). In fact, a meta-analysis showed a significant association between the presence of anxiety disorders and ASD (van Steensel et al., 2011). Anxiety in children with ASD was consistent with sympathetic over–arousal, which may be implicated in an exaggerated fear response (Kushki et al., 2013). Studies with non-humans have also shed light on the neurobiology of anxiety. For instance, increased anxiety in rats led to increased expression of glutamic acid decarboxylase and increased γ-aminobutyric acid transporter 1 (Olexova et al., 2016).

Post-stress cortisol levels were also associated with gut symptoms in children with ASD (Ferguson et al., 2016). Many children with ASD have abnormal gut function (Buie et al., 2010). The gut microbiome is well-known to exert a major effect on brain development and behavior (Sampson & Mazmanian, 2015), and is considered to contribute to the pathogenesis of neurodevelopmental disorders (Petra et al., 2015; Hsiao et al., 2013). One study from children with ASD in Slovakia reported a strong, positive correlation between autism severity and GI dysfunction, suggesting a role of gut microbiota and brain connection (Tomova et al., 2015). Another recent study investigated MRI images and fecal 16S ribosomal RNA indicative of bacterial presence from normal children, and reported a significant association between higher microbiota and lower cognition, but no association with brain volume at one and two years of age (Carlson et al., 2018).

MOLD EXPOSURE

The possible contribution of environmental triggers to ASD has been reviewed (Deth et al., 2008) (Herbert, 2010; Modabbernia et al., 2017; Rossignol & Frye, 2012; Sealey et al., 2016), but no specific pathogenetic mechanism has been proposed. Many studies have reported that exposure to air pollutants, both prenatally and during childhood, can lead to cognitive development deficits in children (McCall, 1977; Moffitt et al., 1981). Another key environmental trigger could be mold.

Mold is not uncommon, and its effects may be far-reaching. One study of Caucasian children (n = 13,369, 8 to 12 years old) in 24 communities across North America reported that the prevalence of indoor mold growth was between 22% to 57%, affecting more than 50% of households in five communities (Spengler et al., 1994). Many studies reported that mold-exposed groups had altered neurological functions compared to controls (Baldo et al., 2002; Brown et al., 2005; Campbell et al., 2004; Crago et al., 2003). Some indoor molds, including *Trichoderma*, *Fusarium*, and *Stachybotrys*, produce mycotoxins (Andersson et al., 1997; Bennett & Klich, 2003; da Rocha et al., 2014; Etzel, 2002; Fog, 2003; Gorny et al., 2002; Ismaiel & and Papenbrock, 2015; Peltola et al., 2001). Mold is usually associated with release of spores that can survive drought and other harsh environmental conditions. In contrast, mycotoxins can be released when moisture is present, and appear at approximately 300 times the concentration of spores (Brasel et al., 2005a). Absorption of mycotoxins occurs through dermal contact, inhalation, and ingestion (Fromme et al., 2016), and exposed persons have significantly more mycotoxins in their sera as compared to controls (Brasel et al., 2004, 2005b; Hendry & Cole, 1993; Ziats et al., 2015). These molecules can induce multisystemic effects, including gastrointestinal, cardiovascular, and neuropsychiatric complications (Campbell et al., 2003; Doi & Uetsuka, 2011; Hope, 2013).

Many studies have documented the risks of mycotoxin exposure. Ochratoxin A is the most common mycotoxin found in foods and water-damaged buildings, and has been associated with serious health problems (Hope & Hope, 2012), including severe neurological issues in humans (Sava et al., 2006a, 2006b). Furthermore, individuals exposed to mold reported multiple symptoms, including cognitive impairment, which appeared to be related to the length of exposure (Baldo et al., 2002; Brown et al., 2005; Campbell et al., 2004; Crago et al., 2003). Other studies have also stressed the pathogenic potential of mycotoxins (Brasel et al., 2005a, 2005b; Charpin-Kadouch et al., 2006; Hope, 2013), especially with respect to neuropsychiatric symptoms (Ratnaseelan et al., 2018; Theoharides, 2018) and neurological dysfunction (Kilburn, 2003; Rea et al., 2003). While a single mycotoxin may not produce any effect, a combination of mycotoxins could induce toxicity at very low levels (Alassane-Kpembi et al., 2013). For instance, exposure to Satratoxin H increased susceptibility to other neurotoxic mycotoxins (Karunasena et al., 2010; Thrasher & Crawley, 2009). Thus, the synergistic actions of these molecules may render exposed individuals more vulnerable.

Evidence suggests that mold-exposed children are at a greater risk of suffering cognitive deficits than are controls (Anyanwu et al., 2003; Casas et al., 2013; Gordon et al., 2004). One study of six-year-old children found that exposure to mold-contaminated homes for over two years in the early postnatal period was associated with deficits in intelligence quotient (Jedrychowski et al., 2011). Other studies showed an association between mold with depression and emotional distress (Hopton & Hunt, 1996; Hyndman, 1990; Martin et al., 1987; Packer et al., 1994). Mycotoxins have also been specifically associated with ASD (Deth et al., 2008; Herbert, 2010; Rzhetsky et al., 2014; Wong et al., 2015). For example, one study reported that boys with ASD exposed to mold had significantly more neurobehavioral abnormalities than either non-exposed children with ASD or unrelated normotypic controls (Kilburn et al., 2009). In another study, researchers found a strong association between levels of Ochratoxin A in urine and serum of children with ASD (De et al., 2017). Similarly, a subsequent study reported that levels of Ochratoxin A, Aflatoxin M1, and Fumonisin B1 were significantly higher in serum and urine of children with ASD as compared to healthy controls (von Tobel et al., 2014).

SOLUTIONS AND RECOMMENDATIONS

The mechanism via which mycotoxins can affect the "fear response" or the HPA axis is not presently known. However, mycotoxins were shown to bind to proteins involved in neuronal plasticity (Scafuri et al., 2017), which could be a promising avenue of research. If amygdala and hypothalamic connections are disrupted, especially during a critical period of development, an individual may become predisposed to maladaptive fear processing (Amaral et al., 2003; Bauman & Kemper, 2003; Ressler, 2010). In addition, the effect of mycotoxins and other peptide triggers could be at least partially explained via stimulation of MC (Doebler et al., 1992; Saluja et al., 2012; Yarom et al., 1987) and/or microglia (von Tobel et al., 2014). For instance, CRH augmented the effect of mtDNA on allergic stimulation of human cultured MC (Asadi & Theoharides, 2012). The combination of CRH and NT synergistically stimulated vascular endothelial growth factor (VEGF) secretion from human MC (Donelan et al., 2006), and induced the expression of each other's receptors on human MC (Alysandratos et al., 2012). We also showed that NT (Alysandratos et al., 2012) and SP (Asadi et al., 2012) increased expression of CRHR-1 on human MC. Evidence from rodents supports the possibility that environment-stress interactions trigger inflammation, and, in turn, affect brain regions that govern the "fear response" (Frank et al., 2016; Kim et al., 2018; Li et al., 2018; Michopoulos et al., 2017).

Studies are needed investigating the comorbid presence of emotional stressors and environmental triggers in children with ASD.

CONCLUSION

Stimulation of brain MC and/or microglia by a combination of environmental and stress triggers may disrupt neuronal connectivity and the HPA axis, thereby lowering of the normal "fear threshold." This process could explain at least part of the pathogenesis of ASD. Identifying ways to inhibit inflammation in the amygdala/hypothalamus may constitute a novel approach to the treatment of ASD.

ACKNOWLEDGMENT

This research was partly supported by an Anonymous grant to TCT.

REFERENCES

Abbott, N. J. (2000). Inflammatory mediators and modulation of blood-brain barrier permeability. *Cellular and Molecular Neurobiology*, *20*(2), 131–147. doi:10.1023/A:1007074420772 PMID:10696506

Abrahams, B. S., & Geschwind, D. H. (2008). Advances in autism genetics: On the threshold of a new neurobiology. *Nature Reviews. Genetics*, *9*(5), 341–355. doi:10.1038/nrg2346 PMID:18414403

Aguzzi, A., Barres, B. A., & Bennett, M. L. (2013). Microglia: Scapegoat, saboteur, or something else? *Science*, *339*(6116), 156–161. doi:10.1126cience.1227901 PMID:23307732

Alassane-Kpembi, I., Kolf-Clauw, M., Gauthier, T., Abrami, R., Abiola, F. A., Oswald, I. P., & Puel, O. (2013). New insights into mycotoxin mixtures: The toxicity of low doses of Type B trichothecenes on intestinal epithelial cells is synergistic. *Toxicology and Applied Pharmacology*, *272*(1), 191–198. doi:10.1016/j.taap.2013.05.023 PMID:23735874

Alysandratos, K. D., Asadi, S., Angelidou, A., Zhang, B., Sismanopoulos, N., Yang, H., ... Theoharides, T. C. (2012). Neurotensin and CRH interactions augment human mast cell activation. *PLoS One*, *7*(11), e48934. doi:10.1371/journal.pone.0048934 PMID:23155429

Amaral, D. G., Bauman, M. D., & Schumann, C. M. (2003). The amygdala and autism: Implications from non-human primate studies. *Genes Brain & Behavior*, *2*(5), 295–302. doi:10.1034/j.1601-183X.2003.00043.x PMID:14606694

American Academy of Pediatrics. Committee on Environmental Health. (1998). Toxic effects of indoor molds. *Pediatrics, 101,* 712-714.

Andersson, M. A., Nikulin, M., Koljalg, U., Andersson, M. C., Rainey, F., Reijula, K., & ... . (1997). Bacteria, molds, and toxins in water-damaged building materials. *Applied and Environmental Microbiology*, *63*, 387–393. PMID:9023919

Anyanwu, E. C., Campbell, A. W., & Vojdani, A. (2003). Neurophysiological effects of chronic indoor environmental toxic mold exposure on children. *The Scientific World Journal*, *3*, 281–290. doi:10.1100/tsw.2003.22 PMID:12806113

Asadi, S., Alysandratos, K. D., Angelidou, A., Miniati, A., Sismanopoulos, N., Vasiadi, M., ... Theoharides, T. C. (2012). Substance P (SP) induces expression of functional corticotropin-releasing hormone receptor-1 (CRHR-1) in human mast cells. *The Journal of Investigative Dermatology*, *132*(2), 324–329. doi:10.1038/jid.2011.334 PMID:22089831

Asadi, S., & Theoharides, T. C. (2012). Corticotropin-releasing hormone and extracellular mitochondria augment IgE-stimulated human mast-cell vascular endothelial growth factor release, which is inhibited by luteolin. *J Neuroinflam*, *9*(1), 85. doi:10.1186/1742-2094-9-85 PMID:22559745

Avino, T. A., Barger, N., Vargas, M. V., Carlson, E. L., Amaral, D. G., Bauman, M. D., & Schumann, C. M. (2018). Neuron numbers increase in the human amygdala from birth to adulthood, but not in autism. *Proceedings of the National Academy of Sciences of the United States of America*, *115*(14), 3710–3715. doi:10.1073/pnas.1801912115 PMID:29559529

Babenko, O., Kovalchuk, I., & Metz, G. A. (2015). Stress-induced perinatal and transgenerational epigenetic programming of brain development and mental health. *Neuroscience and Biobehavioral Reviews*, *48*, 70–91. doi:10.1016/j.neubiorev.2014.11.013 PMID:25464029

Baldo, J. V., Ahmad, L., & Ruff, R. (2002). Neuropsychological performance of patients following mold exposure. *Applied Neuropsychology*, *9*(4), 193–202. doi:10.1207/S15324826AN0904_1 PMID:12584073

Barreau, F., Salvador-Cartier, C., Houdeau, E., Bueno, L., & Fioramonti, J. (2008). Long-term alterations of colonic nerve-mast cell interactions induced by neonatal maternal deprivation in rats. *Gut*, *57*(5), 582–590. doi:10.1136/gut.2007.126680 PMID:18194988

Bauman, M. D., Lavenex, P., Mason, W. A., Capitanio, J. P., & Amaral, D. G. (2004). The development of mother-infant interactions after neonatal amygdala lesions in rhesus monkeys. *The Journal of Neuroscience*, *24*(3), 711–721. doi:10.1523/JNEUROSCI.3263-03.2004 PMID:14736857

Bauman, M. L. (2010). Medical comorbidities in autism: Challenges to diagnosis and treatment. *Neurotherapeutics; the Journal of the American Society for Experimental NeuroTherapeutics*, *7*(3), 320–327. doi:10.1016/j.nurt.2010.06.001 PMID:20643385

Bauman, M. L., & Kemper, T. L. (2003). The neuropathology of the autism spectrum disorders: What have we learned? *Novartis Foundation Symposium*, *251*, 112–122. PMID:14521190

Bennett, J. W., & Klich, M. (2003). Mycotoxins. *Clinical Microbiology Reviews*, *16*(3), 497–516. doi:10.1128/CMR.16.3.497-516.2003 PMID:12857779

Bercum, F. M., Rodgers, K. M., Benison, A. M., Smith, Z. Z., Taylor, J., Kornreich, E., ... Barth, D. S. (2015). Maternal Stress Combined with Terbutaline Leads to Comorbid Autistic-Like Behavior and Epilepsy in a Rat Model. *The Journal of Neuroscience*, *35*(48), 15894–15902. doi:10.1523/JNEUROSCI.2803-15.2015 PMID:26631470

Beversdorf, D. Q., Manning, S. E., Hillier, A., Anderson, S. L., Nordgren, R. E., Walters, S. E., ... Bauman, M. L. (2005). Timing of prenatal stressors and autism. *Journal of Autism and Developmental Disorders*, *35*(4), 471–478. doi:10.100710803-005-5037-8 PMID:16134032

Bilbo, S. D., Block, C. L., Bolton, J. L., Hanamsagar, R., & Tran, P. K. (2018). Beyond infection - Maternal immune activation by environmental factors, microglial development, and relevance for autism spectrum disorders. *Experimental Neurology*, *299*, 241–251. doi:10.1016/j.expneurol.2017.07.002 PMID:28698032

Billeci, L., Tonacci, A., Tartarisco, G., Ruta, L., Pioggia, G., & Gangemi, S. (2015). Association Between Atopic Dermatitis and Autism Spectrum Disorders: A Systematic Review. *American Journal of Clinical Dermatology*, *16*(5), 371–388. doi:10.100740257-015-0145-5 PMID:26254000

Bliss-Moreau, E., Bauman, M. D., & Amaral, D. G. (2011a). Neonatal amygdala lesions result in globally blunted affect in adult rhesus macaques. *Behavioral Neuroscience*, *125*(6), 848–858. doi:10.1037/a0025757 PMID:21988521

Bliss-Moreau, E., Moadab, G., Santistevan, A., & Amaral, D. G. (2017). The effects of neonatal amygdala or hippocampus lesions on adult social behavior. *Behavioural Brain Research*, *322*, 123–137. doi:10.1016/j.bbr.2016.11.052 PMID:28017854

Bliss-Moreau, E., Toscano, J. E., Bauman, M. D., Mason, W. A., & Amaral, D. G. (2011b). Neonatal amygdala lesions alter responsiveness to objects in juvenile macaques. *Neuroscience*, *178*, 123–132. doi:10.1016/j.neuroscience.2010.12.038 PMID:21215794

Bondarenko, E., Hodgson, D. M., & Nalivaiko, E. (2014). Amygdala mediates respiratory responses to sudden arousing stimuli and to restraint stress in rats. *American Journal of Physiology. Regulatory, Integrative and Comparative Physiology*, *306*(12), R951–R959. doi:10.1152/ajpregu.00528.2013 PMID:24740655

Brasel, T. L., Campbell, A. W., Demers, R. E., Ferguson, B. S., Fink, J., Vojdani, A., & ... . (2004). Detection of trichothecene mycotoxins in sera from individuals exposed to Stachybotrys chartarum in indoor environments. *Archives of Environmental Health*, *59*, 317–323. PMID:16238166

Brasel, T. L., Douglas, D. R., Wilson, S. C., & Straus, D. C. (2005a). Detection of airborne Stachybotrys chartarum macrocyclic trichothecene mycotoxins on particulates smaller than conidia. *Applied and Environmental Microbiology*, *71*(1), 114–122. doi:10.1128/AEM.71.1.114-122.2005 PMID:15640178

Brasel, T. L., Martin, J. M., Carriker, C. G., Wilson, S. C., & Straus, D. C. (2005b). Detection of airborne Stachybotrys chartarum macrocyclic trichothecene mycotoxins in the indoor environment. *Applied and Environmental Microbiology*, *71*(11), 7376–7388. doi:10.1128/AEM.71.11.7376-7388.2005 PMID:16269780

Brown, R. C., Lockwood, A. H., & Sonawane, B. R. (2005). Neurodegenerative diseases: An overview of environmental risk factors. *Environmental Health Perspectives*, *113*(9), 1250–1256. doi:10.1289/ehp.7567 PMID:16140637

Buie, T., Fuchs, G. J. III, Furuta, G. T., Kooros, K., Levy, J., Lewis, J. D., ... Winter, H. (2010). Recommendations for evaluation and treatment of common gastrointestinal problems in children with ASDs. *Pediatrics*, *125*(Suppl 1), S19–S29. doi:10.1542/peds.2009-1878D PMID:20048084

Campbell, A. W., Thrasher, J. D., Gray, M. R., & Vojdani, A. (2004). Mold and mycotoxins: Effects on the neurological and immune systems in humans. *Advances in Applied Microbiology*, *55*, 375–406. doi:10.1016/S0065-2164(04)55015-3 PMID:15350803

Campbell, A. W., Thrasher, J. D., Madison, R. A., Vojdani, A., Gray, M. R., & Johnson, A. (2003). Neural autoantibodies and neurophysiologic abnormalities in patients exposed to molds in water-damaged buildings. *Archives of Environmental Health*, *58*(8), 464–474. doi:10.3200/AEOH.58.8.464-474 PMID:15259425

Carlson, A. L., Xia, K., Azcarate-Peril, M. A., Goldman, B. D., Ahn, M., Styner, M. A., ... Knickmeyer, R. C. (2018). Infant Gut Microbiome Associated With Cognitive Development. *Biological Psychiatry*, *83*(2), 148–159. doi:10.1016/j.biopsych.2017.06.021 PMID:28793975

Casas, L., Torrent, M., Zock, J. P., Doekes, G., Forns, J., Guxens, M., ... Sunyer, J. (2013). Early life exposures to home dampness, pet ownership and farm animal contact and neuropsychological development in 4 year old children: A prospective birth cohort study. *International Journal of Hygiene and Environmental Health*, *216*(6), 690–697. doi:10.1016/j.ijheh.2012.12.013 PMID:23357052

Centers for Disease Control and Prevention. (2018). CDC estimates 1 in 59 children has been identified with autism spectrum disorder. Retrieved from https://www.cdc.gov/features/new-autism-data/index.html

Charpin-Kadouch, C., Maurel, G., Felipo, R., Queralt, J., Ramadour, M., Dumon, H., ... Charpin, D. (2006). Mycotoxin identification in moldy dwellings. *Journal of Applied Toxicology*, *26*(6), 475–479. doi:10.1002/jat.1164 PMID:17080403

Choi, J. S., & Kim, J. J. (2010). Amygdala regulates risk of predation in rats foraging in a dynamic fear environment. *Proceedings of the National Academy of Sciences of the United States of America*, *107*(50), 21773–21777. doi:10.1073/pnas.1010079108 PMID:21115817

Chrousos, G. P. (1995). The hypothalamic-pituitary-adrenal axis and immune-mediated inflammation. *The New England Journal of Medicine*, *332*(20), 1351–1362. doi:10.1056/NEJM199505183322008 PMID:7715646

Collins, L. V., Hajizadeh, S., Holme, E., Jonsson, I. M., & Tarkowski, A. (2004). Endogenously oxidized mitochondrial DNA induces in vivo and in vitro inflammatory responses. *Journal of Leukocyte Biology*, *75*(6), 995–1000. doi:10.1189/jlb.0703328 PMID:14982943

Cowan, C. S. M., Hoban, A. E., Ventura-Silva, A. P., Dinan, T. G., Clarke, G., & Cryan, J. F. (2018). Gutsy Moves: The Amygdala as a Critical Node in Microbiota to Brain Signaling. *BioEssays*, 40. PMID:29148060

Crafa, D., & Warfa, N. (2015). Maternal migration and autism risk: Systematic analysis. *International Review of Psychiatry (Abingdon, England)*, *27*(1), 64–71. doi:10.3109/09540261.2014.995601 PMID:25738316

Crago, B. R., Gray, M. R., Nelson, L. A., Davis, M., Arnold, L., & Thrasher, J. D. (2003). Psychological, neuropsychological, and electrocortical effects of mixed mold exposure. *Archives of Environmental Health*, *58*(8), 452–463. doi:10.3200/AEOH.58.8.452-463 PMID:15259424

da Rocha, M. E. B., da Chagas, O. F., Maia, F. E. F., Guedes, M. I. F., & Rondina, D. (2014). Mycotoxins and their effects on human and animal health. *Food Control*, *36*(1), 159-165.

De Santis, B., Brera, C., Mezzelani, A., Soricelli, S., Ciceri, F., Moretti, G., ... & Raggi, M. E. (2019). Role of mycotoxins in the pathobiology of autism: A first evidence. Nutritional neuroscience, 22(2), 132-144. PMID:28795659

Deth, R., Muratore, C., Benzecry, J., Power-Charnitsky, V. A., & Waly, M. (2008). How environmental and genetic factors combine to cause autism: A redox/methylation hypothesis. *Neurotoxicology*, *29*(1), 190–201. doi:10.1016/j.neuro.2007.09.010 PMID:18031821

Doebler, J. A., Martin, L. J., Morse, J. D., Ballough, G. P., Strauss, J. A., & Anthony, A. (1992). Mesenteric mast cell degranulation in acute T-2 toxin poisoning. *Toxicology Letters*, *62*(1), 33–38. doi:10.1016/0378-4274(92)90075-U PMID:1509504

Doi, K., & Uetsuka, K. (2011). Mechanisms of mycotoxin-induced neurotoxicity through oxidative stress-associated pathways. *International Journal of Molecular Sciences*, *12*(8), 5213–5237. doi:10.3390/ijms12085213 PMID:21954354

Donelan, J., Boucher, W., Papadopoulou, N., Lytinas, M., Papaliodis, D., & Theoharides, T. C. (2006). Corticotropin-releasing hormone induces skin vascular permeability through a neurotensin-dependent process. *Proceedings of the National Academy of Sciences of the United States of America*, *103*(20), 7759–7764. doi:10.1073/pnas.0602210103 PMID:16682628

Edvinsson, L., Cervos-Navarro, J., Larsson, L. I., Owman, C., & Ronnberg, A. L. (1977). Regional distribution of mast cells containing histamine, dopamine or 5-hydroxytryptamine in the mammalian brain. *Neurology*, *27*(9), 878–884. doi:10.1212/WNL.27.9.878 PMID:408735

Ehrlich, D. E., & Rainnie, D. G. (2015). Prenatal Stress Alters the Development of Socioemotional Behavior and Amygdala Neuron Excitability in Rats. *Neuropsychopharmacology*, *40*(9), 2135–2145. doi:10.1038/npp.2015.55 PMID:25716930

Esposito, P., Chandler, N., Kandere, K., Basu, S., Jacobson, S., Connolly, R., ... & Theoharides, T. C. (2002). Corticotropin-releasing hormone and brain mast cells regulate blood-brain-barrier permeability induced by acute stress. Journal of Pharmacology and Experimental Therapeutics, 303(3), 1061-1066. doi:10.1124/jpet.102.038497 PMID:12438528

Etzel, R. A. (2002). Mycotoxins. *Journal of the American Medical Association*, *287*(4), 425–427. doi:10.1001/jama.287.4.425 PMID:11798344

Feinberg, J. I., Bakulski, K. M., Jaffe, A. E., Tryggvadottir, R., Brown, S. C., Goldman, L. R., ... Feinberg, A. P. (2015). Paternal sperm DNA methylation associated with early signs of autism risk in an autism-enriched cohort. *International Journal of Epidemiology*, *44*(4), 1199–1210. doi:10.1093/ije/dyv028 PMID:25878217

Ferguson, B. J., Marler, S., Altstein, L. L., Lee, E. B., Mazurek, M. O., McLaughlin, A., ... Beversdorf, D. Q. (2016). Associations between cytokines, endocrine stress response, and gastrointestinal symptoms in autism spectrum disorder. *Brain, Behavior, and Immunity*, *58*, 57–62. doi:10.1016/j.bbi.2016.05.009 PMID:27181180

Fiorentino, M., Sapone, A., Senger, S., Camhi, S. S., Kadzielski, S. M., Buie, T. M., ... Fasano, A. (2016). Blood-brain barrier and intestinal epithelial barrier alterations in autism spectrum disorders. *Molecular Autism*, *7*(1), 49. doi:10.118613229-016-0110-z PMID:27957319

Fog, N. K. (2003). Mycotoxin production by indoor molds. *Fungal Genetics and Biology*, *39*(2), 103–117. doi:10.1016/S1087-1845(03)00026-4 PMID:12781669

Fombonne, E. (2009). Epidemiology of pervasive developmental disorders. *Pediatric Research*, *65*(6), 591–598. doi:10.1203/PDR.0b013e31819e7203 PMID:19218885

Frank, M. G., Weber, M. D., Watkins, L. R., & Maier, S. F. (2016). Stress-induced neuroinflammatory priming: A liability factor in the etiology of psychiatric disorders. *Neurobiology of Stress*, *4*, 62–70. doi:10.1016/j.ynstr.2015.12.004 PMID:27981190

Fromme, H., Gareis, M., Volkel, W., & Gottschalk, C. (2016). Overall internal exposure to mycotoxins and their occurrence in occupational and residential settings--An overview. *International Journal of Hygiene and Environmental Health*, *219*(2), 143–165. doi:10.1016/j.ijheh.2015.11.004 PMID:26725999

Georgin-Lavialle, S., Gaillard, R., Moura, D., & Hermine, O. (2016). Mastocytosis in adulthood and neuropsychiatric disorders. *Translational Research; the Journal of Laboratory and Clinical Medicine*, *174*, 77–85.

Georgin-Lavialle, S., Moura, D. S., Salvador, A., Chauvet-Gelinier, J. C., Launay, J. M., Damaj, G., ... Gaillard, R. (2016b). Mast cells' involvement in inflammation pathways linked to depression: Evidence in mastocytosis. *Molecular Psychiatry*, *21*(11), 1511–1516. doi:10.1038/mp.2015.216 PMID:26809839

Geschwind, D. H., & State, M. W. (2015). Gene hunting in autism spectrum disorder: On the path to precision medicine. *Lancet Neurology*, *11*(11), 1109–1120. doi:10.1016/S1474-4422(15)00044-7 PMID:25891009

Girolamo, F., Coppola, C., & Ribatti, D. (2017). Immunoregulatory effect of mast cells influenced by microbes in neurodegenerative diseases. *Brain, Behavior, and Immunity*, *65*, 68–89. doi:10.1016/j.bbi.2017.06.017 PMID:28676349

Goldschmidt, R. C., Hough, L. B., Glick, S. D., & Padawer, J. (1984). Mast cells in rat thalamus: Nuclear localization, sex difference and left-right asymmetry. *Brain Research*, *323*(2), 209–217. doi:10.1016/0006-8993(84)90291-9 PMID:6084538

Gordon, W. A., Cantor, J. B., Johanning, E., Charatz, H. J., Ashman, T. A., Breeze, J. L., ... Abramowitz, S. (2004). Cognitive impairment associated with toxigenic fungal exposure: A replication and extension of previous findings. *Applied Neuropsychology*, *11*(2), 65–74. doi:10.120715324826an1102_1 PMID:15477176

Gorny, R. L., Reponen, T., Willeke, K., Schmechel, D., Robine, E., Boissier, M., & Grinshpun, S. A. (2002). Fungal fragments as indoor air biocontaminants. *Applied and Environmental Microbiology*, *68*(7), 3522–3531. doi:10.1128/AEM.68.7.3522-3531.2002 PMID:12089037

Gupta, S., Ellis, S. E., Ashar, F. N., Moes, A., Bader, J. S., Zhan, J., ... Arking, D. E. (2014). Transcriptome analysis reveals dysregulation of innate immune response genes and neuronal activity-dependent genes in autism. *Nature Communications*, *5*(1), 5748. doi:10.1038/ncomms6748 PMID:25494366

Hendry, K. M., & Cole, E. C. (1993). A review of mycotoxins in indoor air. *Journal of Toxicology and Environmental Health*, *38*(2), 183–198. doi:10.1080/15287399309531711 PMID:8433402

Herbert, M. R. (2010). Contributions of the environment and environmentally vulnerable physiology to autism spectrum disorders. *Current Opinion in Neurology*, *23*(2), 103–110. doi:10.1097/WCO.0b013e328336a01f PMID:20087183

Hollocks, M. J., Howlin, P., Papadopoulos, A. S., Khondoker, M., & Simonoff, E. (2014). Differences in HPA-axis and heart rate responsiveness to psychosocial stress in children with autism spectrum disorders with and without co-morbid anxiety. *Psychoneuroendocrinology*, *46*, 32–45. doi:10.1016/j.psyneuen.2014.04.004 PMID:24882156

Holmes, N. M., Parkes, S. L., Killcross, A. S., & Westbrook, R. F. (2013). The basolateral amygdala is critical for learning about neutral stimuli in the presence of danger, and the perirhinal cortex is critical in the absence of danger. *The Journal of Neuroscience*, *33*(32), 13112–13125. doi:10.1523/JNEUROSCI.1998-13.2013 PMID:23926265

Hope, J. (2013). A review of the mechanism of injury and treatment approaches for illness resulting from exposure to water-damaged buildings, mold, and mycotoxins. *The Scientific World Journal, 2013*, 767482. doi:10.1155/2013/767482 PMID:23710148

Hope, J. H., & Hope, B. E. (2012). A review of the diagnosis and treatment of Ochratoxin A inhalational exposure associated with human illness and kidney disease including focal segmental glomerulosclerosis. *Journal of Environmental and Public Health*. doi:10.1155/2012/835059 PMID:22253638

Hopton, J. L., & Hunt, S. M. (1996). Housing conditions and mental health in a disadvantaged area in Scotland. *Journal of Epidemiology and Community Health*, *50*(1), 56–61. doi:10.1136/jech.50.1.56 PMID:8762355

Hsiao, E. Y., McBride, S. W., Hsien, S., Sharon, G., Hyde, E. R., McCue, T., ... Mazmanian, S. K. (2013). Microbiota modulate behavioral and physiological abnormalities associated with neurodevelopmental disorders. *Cell*, *155*(7), 1451–1463. doi:10.1016/j.cell.2013.11.024 PMID:24315484

Hyndman, S. J. (1990). Housing dampness and health amongst British Bengalis in east London. *Social Science & Medicine*, *30*(1), 131–141. doi:10.1016/0277-9536(90)90336-Q PMID:2305276

Kushki, A., Drumm, E., Mobarak, M. P., Tanel, N., Dupuis, A., Chau, T., & Anagnostou, E. (2013). Investigating the autonomic nervous system response to anxiety in children with autism spectrum disorders. *PLoS One*, *8*(4), e59730. doi:10.1371/journal.pone.0059730 PMID:23577072

Ismaiel, A. A., & Papenbrock, J. (2015). Mycotoxins [Agriculture.]. *Producing Fungi and Mechanisms of Phytotoxicity.*, *5*, 492–537.

Jedrychowski, W., Maugeri, U., Perera, F., Stigter, L., Jankowski, J., Butscher, M., ... Sowa, A.Ref Type. (2011). Cognitive function of 6-year old children exposed to mold-contaminated homes in early postnatal period. Prospective birth cohort study in Poland. *Physiology & Behavior*, *104*(5), 989–995. doi:10.1016/j.physbeh.2011.06.019 PMID:21763705

Kalogeromitros, D., Syrigou, E. I., Makris, M., Kempuraj, D., Stavrianeas, N. G., Vasiadi, M., & Theoharides, T. C. (2007). Nasal provocation of patients with allergic rhinitis and the hypothalamic-pituitary-adrenal axis. *Annals of Allergy, Asthma & Immunology*, *98*(3), 269–273. doi:10.1016/S1081-1206(10)60717-X PMID:17378259

Karunasena, E., Larranaga, M. D., Simoni, J. S., Douglas, D. R., & Straus, D. C. (2010). Building-associated neurological damage modeled in human cells: A mechanism of neurotoxic effects by exposure to mycotoxins in the indoor environment. *Mycopathologia*, *170*(6), 377–390. doi:10.100711046-010-9330-5 PMID:20549560

Kilburn, K. H. (2003). Indoor mold exposure associated with neurobehavioral and pulmonary impairment: A preliminary report. *Archives of Environmental Health*, *58*(7), 390–398. doi:10.1080/00039896.2003.11879139 PMID:15143851

Kilburn, K. H., Thrasher, J. D., & Immers, N. B. (2009). Do terbutaline- and mold-associated impairments of the brain and lung relate to autism? *Toxicology and Industrial Health*, *25*(9-10), 703–710. doi:10.1177/0748233709348391 PMID:19793774

Kim, Y. K., Amidfar, M., & Won, E. (2018). A review on inflammatory cytokine-induced alterations of the brain as potential neural biomarkers in post-traumatic stress disorder. *Progress in Neuro-Psychopharmacology & Biological Psychiatry*. doi:10.1016/j.pnpbp.2018.06.008 PMID:29932946

Kotey, S., Ertel, K., & Whitcomb, B. (2014). Co-occurrence of autism and asthma in a nationally-representative sample of children in the United States. *Journal of Autism and Developmental Disorders*, *44*(12), 3083–3088. doi:10.100710803-014-2174-y PMID:24997632

Koyama, R., & Ikegaya, Y. (2015). Microglia in the pathogenesis of autism spectrum disorders. *Neuroscience Research*, *100*, 1–5. doi:10.1016/j.neures.2015.06.005 PMID:26116891

Lai, M. C., Lombardo, M. V., & Baron-Cohen, S. (2014). Autism. *Lancet*, *383*(9920), 896–910. doi:10.1016/S0140-6736(13)61539-1 PMID:24074734

Layton, B. S., Lafontaine, S., & Renaud, L. P. (1981). Connections of medial preoptic neurons with the median eminence and amygdala. An electrophysiological study in the rat. *Neuroendocrinology*, *33*(4), 235–240. doi:10.1159/000123237 PMID:7290340

Lenard, L., Laszlo, K., Kertes, E., Ollmann, T., Peczely, L., Kovacs, A., ... Karádi, Z. (2018). Substance P and neurotensin in the limbic system: Their roles in reinforcement and memory consolidation. *Neuroscience and Biobehavioral Reviews*, *85*, 1–20. doi:10.1016/j.neubiorev.2017.09.003 PMID:28887225

Li, Y., Missig, G., Finger, B. C., Landino, S. M., Alexander, A. J., Mokler, E. L., ... Bolshakov, V. Y. (2018). Maternal and Early Postnatal Immune Activation Produce Dissociable Effects on Neurotransmission in mPFC-Amygdala Circuits. *The Journal of Neuroscience*, *38*(13), 3358–3372. doi:10.1523/JNEUROSCI.3642-17.2018 PMID:29491010

Liao, T. C., Lien, Y. T., Wang, S., Huang, S. L., & Chen, C. Y. (2016). Comorbidity of Atopic Disorders with Autism Spectrum Disorder and Attention Deficit/Hyperactivity Disorder. *The Journal of Pediatrics*, *171*, 248–255. doi:10.1016/j.jpeds.2015.12.063 PMID:26846570

Louveau, A., Smirnov, I., Keyes, T. J., Eccles, J. D., Rouhani, S. J., Peske, J. D., ... Kipnis, J. (2015). Structural and functional features of central nervous system lymphatic vessels. *Nature*, *523*(7560), 337–341. doi:10.1038/nature14432 PMID:26030524

Lyall, K., Van de Water, J., Ashwood, P., & Hertz-Picciotto, I. (2015). Asthma and Allergies in Children With Autism Spectrum Disorders: Results From the CHARGE Study. *Autism Research*, *8*(5), 567–574. doi:10.1002/aur.1471 PMID:25722050

MacKinnon, N., Kingsbury, M., Mahedy, L., Evans, J., & Colman, I. (2018). The Association Between Prenatal Stress and Externalizing Symptoms in Childhood: Evidence From the Avon Longitudinal Study of Parents and Children. *Biological Psychiatry*, *83*(2), 100–108. doi:10.1016/j.biopsych.2017.07.010 PMID:28893381

Marathias, K., Lambracht-Hall, M., Savala, J., & Theoharides, T. C. (1991). Endogenous regulation of rat brain mast cell serotonin release. *International Archives of Allergy and Applied Immunology*, *95*(4), 332–340. doi:10.1159/000235470 PMID:1720423

Marketon, J. I., & Sternberg, E. M. (2010). The glucocorticoid receptor: A revisited target for toxins. *Toxins*, *2*(6), 1357–1380. doi:10.3390/toxins2061357 PMID:22069642

Marques, P. E., Amaral, S. S., Pires, D. A., Nogueira, L. L., Soriani, F. M., Lima, B. H., ... Menezes, G. B. (2012). Chemokines and mitochondrial products activate neutrophils to amplify organ injury during mouse acute liver failure. *Hepatology (Baltimore, Md.)*, *56*(5), 1971–1982. doi:10.1002/hep.25801 PMID:22532075

Martin, C. J., Platt, S. D., & Hunt, S. M. (1987). Housing conditions and ill health. *British Medical Journal (Clinical Research Ed.)*, *294*(6580), 1125–1127. doi:10.1136/bmj.294.6580.1125 PMID:3107723

Matsumoto, I., Inoue, Y., Shimada, T., & Aikawa, T. (2001). Brain mast cells act as an immune gate to the hypothalamic-pituitary-adrenal axis in dogs. *The Journal of Experimental Medicine*, *194*(1), 71–78. doi:10.1084/jem.194.1.71 PMID:11435473

McCall, R. B. (1977). Childhood IQ's as Predictors of Adult Educational and Occupational Status. *Science*, *197*(4302), 482–483. doi:10.1126cience.197.4302.482 PMID:17783247

McCusker, R. H., & Kelley, K. W. (2013). Immune-neural connections: How the immune system's response to infectious agents influences behavior. *The Journal of Experimental Biology*, *216*(1), 84–98. doi:10.1242/jeb.073411 PMID:23225871

McPartland, J., & Volkmar, F. R. (2012). Autism and related disorders. *Handbook of Clinical Neurology*, *106*, 407–418. doi:10.1016/B978-0-444-52002-9.00023-1 PMID:22608634

Merzhanova, G. K., Dolbakyan, E. E., & Khokhlova, V. N. (2000). Interactions between neurons in the amygdala and hypothalamus during conditioned reflex behavior involving choice of reinforcement quality in cats. *Neuroscience and Behavioral Physiology*, *30*(6), 695–702. doi:10.1023/A:1026654917886 PMID:11127797

Michopoulos, V., Powers, A., Gillespie, C. F., Ressler, K. J., & Jovanovic, T. (2017). Inflammation in Fear- and Anxiety-Based Disorders: PTSD, GAD, and Beyond. *Neuropsychopharmacology*, *42*(1), 254–270. doi:10.1038/npp.2016.146 PMID:27510423

Modabbernia, A., Velthorst, E., & Reichenberg, A. (2017). Environmental risk factors for autism: An evidence-based review of systematic reviews and meta-analyses. *Molecular Autism*, *8*(1), 13. doi:10.118613229-017-0121-4 PMID:28331572

Moffitt, T. E., Gabrielli, W. F., Mednick, S. A., & Schulsinger, F. (1981). Socioeconomic status, IQ, and delinquency. *Journal of Abnormal Psychology*, *90*(2), 152–156. doi:10.1037/0021-843X.90.2.152 PMID:7288005

Moscarello, J. M., & LeDoux, J. E. (2013). Active avoidance learning requires prefrontal suppression of amygdala-mediated defensive reactions. *The Journal of Neuroscience*, *33*(9), 3815–3823. doi:10.1523/JNEUROSCI.2596-12.2013 PMID:23447593

Moura, D. S., Sultan, S., Georgin-Lavialle, S., Barete, S., Lortholary, O., Gaillard, R., & Hermine, O. (2012). Evidence for cognitive impairment in mastocytosis: Prevalence, features and correlations to depression. *PLoS One*, *7*(6), e39468. doi:10.1371/journal.pone.0039468 PMID:22745762

Mukai, K., Tsai, M., Saito, H., & Galli, S. J. (2018). Mast cells as sources of cytokines, chemokines, and growth factors. *Immunological Reviews*, *282*(1), 121–150. doi:10.1111/imr.12634 PMID:29431212

Olexova, L., Stefanik, P., & Krskova, L. (2016). Increased anxiety-like behaviour and altered GABAergic system in the amygdala and cerebellum of VPA rats - An animal model of autism. *Neuroscience Letters*, *629*, 9–14. doi:10.1016/j.neulet.2016.06.035 PMID:27353514

Packer, C. N., Stewart-Brown, S., & Fowle, S. E. (1994). Damp housing and adult health: Results from a lifestyle study in Worcester, England. *Journal of Epidemiology and Community Health*, *48*(6), 555–559. doi:10.1136/jech.48.6.555 PMID:7830009

Pan, W., Stone, K. P., Hsuchou, H., Manda, V. K., Zhang, Y., & Kastin, A. J. (2011). Cytokine signaling modulates blood-brain barrier function. *Current Pharmaceutical Design*, *17*, 3729–3740. doi:10.2174/138161211798220918 PMID:21834767

Pang, X., Letourneau, R., Rozniecki, J. J., Wang, L., & Theoharides, T. C. (1996). Definitive characterization of rat hypothalamic mast cells. *Neuroscience*, *73*(3), 889–902. doi:10.1016/0306-4522(95)00606-0 PMID:8809807

Parratt, J. R., & Sturgess, R. M. (1977). The possible roles of histamine, 5-hydroxytryptamine and prostaglandin F_{2alpha} as mediators of the acute pulmonary effects of endotoxin. *British Journal of Pharmacology*, *60*, 209–219. doi:10.1111/j.1476-5381.1977.tb07743.x PMID:328105

Patel, A. B., Tsilioni, I., Leeman, S. E., & Theoharides, T. C. (2016). Neurotensin stimulates sortilin and mTOR in human microglia inhibitable by methoxyluteolin, a potential therapeutic target for autism. *Proceedings of the National Academy of Sciences of the United States of America*, *113*(45), E7049–E7058. doi:10.1073/pnas.1604992113 PMID:27663735

Pedersen, J. M., Mortensen, E. L., Christensen, D. S., Rozing, M., Brunsgaard, H., Meincke, R. H., ... Lund, R. (2018). Prenatal and early postnatal stress and later life inflammation. *Psychoneuroendocrinology*, *88*, 158–166. doi:10.1016/j.psyneuen.2017.12.014 PMID:29291495

Peltola, J., Andersson, M. A., Haahtela, T., Mussalo-Rauhamaa, H., Rainey, F. A., Kroppenstedt, R. M., ... Salkinoja-Salonen, M. S. (2001). Toxic-metabolite-producing bacteria and fungus in an indoor environment. *Applied and Environmental Microbiology*, *67*(7), 3269–3274. doi:10.1128/AEM.67.7.3269-3274.2001 PMID:11425751

Petra, A. I., Panagiotidou, S., Hatziagelaki, E., Stewart, J. M., Conti, P., & Theoharides, T. C. (2015). Gut-Microbiota-Brain Axis and Its Effect on Neuropsychiatric Disorders With Suspected Immune Dysregulation. *Clinical Therapeutics*, *37*(5), 984–995. doi:10.1016/j.clinthera.2015.04.002 PMID:26046241

Philip, R. C., Whalley, H. C., Stanfield, A. C., Sprengelmeyer, R., Santos, I. M., Young, A. W., ... Hall, J. (2010). Deficits in facial, body movement and vocal emotional processing in autism spectrum disorders. *Psychological Medicine*, *40*(11), 1919–1929. doi:10.1017/S0033291709992364 PMID:20102666

Ransohoff, R. M., & Brown, M. A. (2012). Innate immunity in the central nervous system. *The Journal of Clinical Investigation*, *122*(4), 1164–1171. doi:10.1172/JCI58644 PMID:22466658

Ratnaseelan, A. M., Tsilioni, I., & Theoharides, T. C. (2018). Effects of Mycotoxins on Neuropsychiatric Symptoms and Immune Processes. *Clinical Therapeutics*, *40*(6), 903–917. doi:10.1016/j.clinthera.2018.05.004 PMID:29880330

Rea, W. J., Didriksen, N., Simon, T. R., Pan, Y., Fenyves, E. J., & Griffiths, B. (2003). Effects of toxic exposure to molds and mycotoxins in building-related illnesses. *Archives of Environmental Health*, *58*(7), 399–405. doi:10.1080/00039896.2003.11879140 PMID:15143852

Ressler, K. J. (2010). Amygdala activity, fear, and anxiety: Modulation by stress. *Biological Psychiatry*, *67*(12), 1117–1119. doi:10.1016/j.biopsych.2010.04.027 PMID:20525501

Rodgers, A. B., Morgan, C. P., Bronson, S. L., Revello, S., & Bale, T. L. (2013). Paternal stress exposure alters sperm microRNA content and reprograms offspring HPA stress axis regulation. *The Journal of Neuroscience*, *33*(21), 9003–9012. doi:10.1523/JNEUROSCI.0914-13.2013 PMID:23699511

Rodgers, J., Glod, M., Connolly, B., & McConachie, H. (2012). The relationship between anxiety and repetitive behaviours in autism spectrum disorder. *Journal of Autism and Developmental Disorders*, *42*(11), 2404–2409. doi:10.100710803-012-1531-y PMID:22527704

Rodriguez, J. I., & Kern, J. K. (2011). Evidence of microglial activation in autism and its possible role in brain underconnectivity. *Neuron Glia Biology*, *7*(2-4), 205–213. doi:10.1017/S1740925X12000142 PMID:22874006

Ronald, A., Pennell, C. E., & Whitehouse, A. J. (2010). Prenatal maternal stress associated with ADHD and autistic traits in early childhood. *Frontiers in Psychology*, *1*, 223. PMID:21833278

Rossignol, D. A., & Frye, R. E. (2012). A review of research trends in physiological abnormalities in autism spectrum disorders: Immune dysregulation, inflammation, oxidative stress, mitochondrial dysfunction and environmental toxicant exposures. *Molecular Psychiatry*, *17*(4), 389–401. doi:10.1038/mp.2011.165 PMID:22143005

Rozniecki, J. J., Sahagian, G., Jacobson, S., Kempuraj, D., & Theoharides, T. C. (in press). Acute restraint stress induces brain metastases of luciferase-tagged breast cancer cells in mice. *Brain, Behavior, and Immunity*.

Ruggeri, B., Sarkans, U., Schumann, G., & Persico, A. M. (2014). Biomarkers in autism spectrum disorder: The old and the new 1. *Psychopharmacology*, *231*(6), 1201–1216. doi:10.100700213-013-3290-7 PMID:24096533

Rzhetsky, A., Bagley, S. C., Wang, K., Lyttle, C. S., Cook, E. H. Jr, Altman, R. B., & Gibbons, R. D. (2014). Environmental and state-level regulatory factors affect the incidence of autism and intellectual disability. *PLoS Computational Biology*, *10*(3), e1003518. doi:10.1371/journal.pcbi.1003518 PMID:24625521

Saluja, R., Metz, M., & Maurer, M. (2012). Role and relevance of mast cells in fungal infections. *Frontiers in Immunology*, *3*, 146. doi:10.3389/fimmu.2012.00146 PMID:22707950

Sampson, T. R., & Mazmanian, S. K. (2015). Control of brain development, function, and behavior by the microbiome. *Cell Host & Microbe*, *17*(5), 565–576. doi:10.1016/j.chom.2015.04.011 PMID:25974299

Sava, V., Reunova, O., Velasquez, A., Harbison, R., & Sanchez-Ramos, J. (2006a). Acute neurotoxic effects of the fungal metabolite ochratoxin-A. *Neurotoxicology*, *27*(1), 82–92. doi:10.1016/j.neuro.2005.07.004 PMID:16140385

Sava, V., Reunova, O., Velasquez, A., & Sanchez-Ramos, J. (2006b). Can low level exposure to ochratoxin-A cause parkinsonism? *Journal of the Neurological Sciences*, *249*(1), 68–75. doi:10.1016/j.jns.2006.06.006 PMID:16844142

Scafuri, B., Varriale, A., Facchiano, A., D'Auria, S., Raggi, M. E., & Marabotti, A. (2017). Binding of mycotoxins to proteins involved in neuronal plasticity: A combined in silico/wet investigation. *Scientific Reports*, *7*(1), 15156. doi:10.103841598-017-15148-4 PMID:29123130

Sealey, L. A., Hughes, B. W., Sriskanda, A. N., Guest, J. R., Gibson, A. D., Johnson-Williams, L., ... Bagasra, O. (2016). Environmental factors in the development of autism spectrum disorders. *Environment International*, *88*, 288–298. doi:10.1016/j.envint.2015.12.021 PMID:26826339

Simcock, G., Kildea, S., Elgbeili, G., Laplante, D. P., Cobham, V., & King, S. (2017). Prenatal maternal stress shapes children's theory of mind: The QF2011 Queensland Flood Study. *Journal of Developmental Origins of Health and Disease*, *8*(04), 483–492. doi:10.1017/S2040174417000186 PMID:28337952

Skaper, S. D., Facci, L., & Giusti, P. (2014). Neuroinflammation, microglia and mast cells in the pathophysiology of neurocognitive disorders: A review. *CNS & Neurological Disorders - Drug Targets*, *13*(10), 1654–1666. doi:10.2174/1871527313666141130224206 PMID:25470401

Spengler, J., Neas, L., Nakai, S., Dockery, D., Speizer, F., Ware, J., & Raizenne, M. (1994). Respiratory symptoms and housing characteristics. *Indoor Air*, *4*(2), 72–82.

Spratt, E. G., Nicholas, J. S., Brady, K. T., Carpenter, L. A., Hatcher, C. R., Meekins, K. A., ... Charles, J. M. (2012). Enhanced cortisol response to stress in children in autism. *Journal of Autism and Developmental Disorders*, *42*(1), 75–81. doi:10.100710803-011-1214-0 PMID:21424864

Sun, S., Sursal, T., Adibnia, Y., Zhao, C., Zheng, Y., Li, H., ... Itagaki, K. (2013). Mitochondrial DAMPs increase endothelial permeability through neutrophil dependent and independent pathways. *PLoS One*, *8*(3), e59989. doi:10.1371/journal.pone.0059989 PMID:23527291

Taiwo, O. B., Kovacs, K. J., Sun, Y., & Larson, A. A. (2005). Unilateral spinal nerve ligation leads to an asymmetrical distribution of mast cells in the thalamus of female but not male mice. *Pain*, *114*(1), 131–140. doi:10.1016/j.pain.2004.12.002 PMID:15733638

Takano, T. (2015). Role of Microglia in Autism: Recent Advances. *Developmental Neuroscience*, *37*(3), 195–202. doi:10.1159/000398791 PMID:25998072

Theoharides, T. C. (2009). Autism spectrum disorders and mastocytosis 1. *International Journal of Immunopathology and Pharmacology*, *22*(4), 859–865. doi:10.1177/039463200902200401 PMID:20074449

Theoharides, T. C. (2016). Danger Signals and Inflammation. *Clinical Therapeutics*, *38*(5), 996–999. doi:10.1016/j.clinthera.2016.03.036 PMID:27101818

Theoharides, T. C. (2017). Neuroendocrinology of mast cells: Challenges and controversies. *Experimental Dermatology*, *26*(9), 751–759. doi:10.1111/exd.13288 PMID:28094875

Theoharides, T. C. (2018). Mold and Immunity. *Clinical Therapeutics*, *40*(6), 882–884. doi:10.1016/j.clinthera.2018.05.005 PMID:29859636

Theoharides, T. C., Alysandratos, K. D., Angelidou, A., Delivanis, D. A., Sismanopoulos, N., Zhang, B., ... Kalogeromitros, D. (2012). Mast cells and inflammation. *Biochimica et Biophysica Acta*, *1822*(1), 21–33. doi:10.1016/j.bbadis.2010.12.014 PMID:21185371

Theoharides, T. C., Asadi, S., Panagiotidou, S., & Weng, Z. (2013). The "missing link" in autoimmunity and autism: Extracellular mitochondrial components secreted from activated live mast cells. *Autoimmunity Reviews*, *12*(12), 1136–1142. doi:10.1016/j.autrev.2013.06.018 PMID:23831684

Theoharides, T. C., Donelan, J., Kempuraj, D., & Matsui, M. (in press). Skin mast cells as key sensors of environmental and psychological stress. *Current Opinion in Immunology*.

Theoharides, T. C., & Doyle, R. (2008). Autism, gut-blood-brain barrier and mast cells. *Journal of Clinical Psychopharmacology*, *28*(5), 479–483. doi:10.1097/JCP.0b013e3181845f48 PMID:18794641

Theoharides, T. C., Doyle, R., Francis, K., Conti, P., & Kalogeromitros, D. (2008). Novel therapeutic targets for autism. *Trends in Pharmacological Sciences*, *29*(8), 375–382. doi:10.1016/j.tips.2008.06.002 PMID:18606459

Theoharides, T. C., Stewart, J. M., Hatziagelaki, E., & Kolaitis, G. (2015a). Brain "fog," inflammation and obesity: Key aspects of 2 neuropsychiatric disorders improved by luteolin. *Frontiers in Neuroscience*, *9*, 225. doi:10.3389/fnins.2015.00225 PMID:26190965

Theoharides, T. C., Stewart, J. M., Panagiotidou, S., & Melamed, I. (2015b). Mast cells, brain inflammation and autism. *European Journal of Pharmacology*, *778*, 96–102. doi:10.1016/j.ejphar.2015.03.086 PMID:25941080

Theoharides, T. C., Tsilioni, I., Patel, A. B., & Doyle, R. (2016). Atopic diseases and inflammation of the brain in the pathogenesis of autism spectrum disorders. *Translational Psychiatry*, *6*(6), e844. doi:10.1038/tp.2016.77 PMID:27351598

Theoharides, T. C., Tsilioni, I., Patel, A. B., & Doyle, R. (2016). Atopic diseases and inflammation of the brain in the pathogenesis of autism spectrum disorders. *Translational Psychiatry*, *6*(6), e844. doi:10.1038/tp.2016.77 PMID:27351598

Theoharides, T. C., Valent, P., & Akin, C. (2015c). Mast Cells, Mastocytosis, and Related Disorders. *The New England Journal of Medicine*, *373*(2), 163–172. doi:10.1056/NEJMra1409760 PMID:26154789

Thrasher, J. D., & Crawley, S. (2009). The biocontaminants and complexity of damp indoor spaces: More than what meets the eyes. *Toxicology and Industrial Health*, *25*(9-10), 583–615. doi:10.1177/0748233709348386 PMID:19793773

Tomova, A., Husarova, V., Lakatosova, S., Bakos, J., Vlkova, B., Babinska, K., & Ostatnikova, D. (2015). Gastrointestinal microbiota in children with autism in Slovakia. *Physiology & Behavior*, *138*, 179–187. doi:10.1016/j.physbeh.2014.10.033 PMID:25446201

Tordjman, S., Somogyi, E., Coulon, N., Kermarrec, S., Cohen, D., Bronsard, G., ... Xavier, J. (2014). Gene x Environment interactions in autism spectrum disorders: Role of epigenetic mechanisms. *Frontiers in Psychiatry*, *5*, 53. doi:10.3389/fpsyt.2014.00053 PMID:25136320

Tottenham, N., & Sheridan, M. A. (2009). A review of adversity, the amygdala and the hippocampus: A consideration of developmental timing. *Frontiers in Human Neuroscience*, *3*, 68. PMID:20161700

Truitt, W. A., Sajdyk, T. J., Dietrich, A. D., Oberlin, B., McDougle, C. J., & Shekhar, A. (2007). From anxiety to autism: Spectrum of abnormal social behaviors modeled by progressive disruption of inhibitory neuronal function in the basolateral amygdala in Wistar rats. *Psychopharmacology*, *191*(1), 107–118. doi:10.100700213-006-0674-y PMID:17277936

van Steensel, F. J., Bogels, S. M., & Perrin, S. (2011). Anxiety disorders in children and adolescents with autistic spectrum disorders: A meta-analysis. *Clinical Child and Family Psychology Review*, *14*(3), 302–317. doi:10.100710567-011-0097-0 PMID:21735077

von Tobel, J. S., Antinori, P., Zurich, M. G., Rosset, R., Aschner, M., Gluck, F., ... Monnet-Tschudi, F. (2014). Repeated exposure to Ochratoxin A generates a neuroinflammatory response, characterized by neurodegenerative M1 microglial phenotype. *Neurotoxicology*, *44*, 61–70. doi:10.1016/j.neuro.2014.04.005 PMID:24792326

Willsey, A. J., & State, M. W. (2015). Autism spectrum disorders: From genes to neurobiology. *Current Opinion in Neurobiology*, *30*, 92–99. doi:10.1016/j.conb.2014.10.015 PMID:25464374

Wong, C. T., Wais, J., & Crawford, D. A. (2015). Prenatal exposure to common environmental factors affects brain lipids and increases risk of developing autism spectrum disorders. *The European Journal of Neuroscience*, *42*(10), 2742–2760. doi:10.1111/ejn.13028 PMID:26215319

Wu, J. S., Ku, Y. H., Li, L. S., Lu, Y. C., Ding, X., & Wang, Y. G. (1999). Corticotropin releasing factor and substance P mediate the nucleus amygdaloideus centralis-nucleus ventromedialis-nucleus dorsomedialis pressor system. *Brain Research*, *842*(2), 392–398. doi:10.1016/S0006-8993(99)01862-4 PMID:10526135

Yarom, R., Bergmann, F., & Yagen, B. (1987). Cutaneous injury by topical T-2 toxin: Involvement of microvessels and mast cells. *Toxicon*, *25*(2), 167–174. doi:10.1016/0041-0101(87)90238-8 PMID:3576633

Zaidan, H., Leshem, M., & Gaisler-Salomon, I. (2013). Prereproductive stress to female rats alters corticotropin releasing factor type 1 expression in ova and behavior and brain corticotropin releasing factor type 1 expression in offspring. *Biological Psychiatry*, *74*(9), 680–687. doi:10.1016/j.biopsych.2013.04.014 PMID:23726318

Zhang, B., Angelidou, A., Alysandratos, K. D., Vasiadi, M., Francis, K., Asadi, S., ... Theoharides, T. C. (2010). Mitochondrial DNA and anti-mitochondrial antibodies in serum of autistic children. *Journal of Neuroinflammation*, *7*(1), 80. doi:10.1186/1742-2094-7-80 PMID:21083929

Zhang, B., Asadi, S., Weng, Z., Sismanopoulos, N., & Theoharides, T. C. (2012). Stimulated human mast cells secrete mitochondrial components that have autocrine and paracrine inflammatory actions. *PLoS One*, *7*(12), e49767. doi:10.1371/journal.pone.0049767 PMID:23284625

Zhang, X., Wang, Y., Dong, H., Xu, Y., & Zhang, S. (2016). Induction of Microglial Activation by Mediators Released from Mast Cells. *Cellular Physiology and Biochemistry*, *38*(4), 1520–1531. doi:10.1159/000443093 PMID:27050634

Ziats, M. N., Grosvenor, L. P., & Rennert, O. M. (2015). Functional genomics of human brain development and implications for autism spectrum disorders 1. *Translational Psychiatry*, *5*(10), e665. doi:10.1038/tp.2015.153 PMID:26506051

APPENDIX

Abbreviations

BBB = blood-brain barrier
BLA = basolateral nucleus of amygdala
CRH = corticotrophin-releasing hormone
HPA = hypothalamic-pituitary-adrenal
MC = mast cells
mtDNA = mitochondrial DNA
NT = neurotensin
SP = substance P

Chapter 3
Exposure to Toxic Environmental Agents in the Form of Fragrances and Development of Autism Spectrum Disorders (ASD)

Omar Bagasra
Claflin University, USA

Anisah Bagasra
https://orcid.org/0000-0002-7057-5278
Kennesaw State University, USA

ABSTRACT

In this chapter, the authors explore how the human brain develops and what the critical stages are in which a fetal brain may acquire genetic and developmental abnormalities through environmental agents. They summarize the prevailing theories regarding the etiologies of autism and present scientific data supporting the thesis that some of the most commonly used environmental agents that we have so easily accepted into our social fabric of life may be major contributors in the development of autism spectrum disorders (ASD). They provide a large body of scientific data carried out in their laboratory, utilizing developing human neurons exposed to femtomolar concentrations of chemicals found in fragrances. The studies demonstrate that synthetic fragrances can impart profound neuromodifications at the morphologic, immunologic, and molecular levels. It is hypothesized that high exposure to teratogenic neurotoxins in our environment during critical periods of development best explains the rapid rise of autism spectrum disorder diagnosis over the past three decades.

DOI: 10.4018/978-1-5225-7635-8.ch003

INTRODUCTION

In the process of scientific investigations, new ideas and information emerge that cannot be easily reconciled with the present paradigm. Still, scientists and the medical community are naturally reluctant to adopt new paradigms when established concepts still appear feasible, although they may be in need of major revision. Typically, the effects of such scientific reluctance manifest themselves in enlivened discussions at professional conferences and journals, or in books written by journalists (Silberman, 2016), scientists (Wolff, 2004; Bagasra & Heggen, 2018) and medical professionals (Schopler, Medibov & Kunce, 1998). In the area of autism pathogenesis, however, the consequences of over half-a century of inadequate progress in coming to grips with the basic underlying biology of autism spectrum disorder (ASD) may be calculated not in journal publications or media coverage, but in the quality of human lives for literally millions of autistic children and desperate parents, who find themselves bewildered at the effects of the disorder on both their children and themselves (Bagasra & Heggen, 2018; Chaste et al., 2017). Autism Spectrum Disorder research is at an important crossroads right now, with many pertinent issues being explored including the validity of the current ASD diagnosis criteria, a genetic basis for ASD, and the exploration of epigenetic factors in ASD.

This chapter will review the current research paradigms regarding ASD and focus on new trends in research regarding environmental factors impacting the development and manifestation of ASD. This research is significant in exploring the various prevailing models regarding the development of ASD, and providing pertinent research to argue that environmental factors play a larger contributing role in ASD that previously discussed. This research is important in providing evidence to suggest there are significant concrete ways to reduce rates of ASD by limiting exposure of developing fetuses to toxins in the environment.

BACKGROUND

Autism Spectrum Disorder Definition and History

Autism Spectrum Disorder (ASD) is a psychological disorder defined in the Diagnostic and Statistical Manual (DSM) that has been modified and updated over time. The DSM is a handbook originally published in 1952 to address the needs of clinicians in an attempt to classify mental disorders. The most recent changes occurred from the DSM-IV-TR which was published in 2000, to the newest version the DSM-5 published in 2013 (American Psychiatric Association, 2013). The DSM-IV-TR outlined three unique autism spectrum disorders under the category of pervasive developmental disorders. These were Autistic disorder (AD), Asperger's disorder, and pervasive developmental disorder-not otherwise specified. The criteria for diagnosis of any of the three autism spectrum disorders was wide and varied, and resulted in an inconsistent application of criteria by clinicians and health service providers (McPartland et al., 2012; Robertson et al., 2013). The DSM-V resulted in the combination of those three separate diagnoses into one broad category known as Autism Spectrum Disorder. Kulage, Smaldone & Cohn (2014) analyzed to impact of the changes in diagnostic criteria from the DSM-IV-TR to the DSM-5 and concluded from their review that the changes would likely decrease the number of individuals diagnosed with ASD as a result of a smaller number of possible combinations of criteria for diagnosis, and the elimination of the pervasive developmental disorder-not otherwise specified (PDD-NOS) diagnosis. Currently, a diagnosis of Autism Spectrum Disorder requires an individual to meet three criteria under the area of social communication and interaction, and two under restrictive, repetitive behavior (American Psychiatric Association, 2013).

Autism was established as a separate disorder by Leo Kanner in 1943, who distinguished its symptoms from that of childhood schizophrenia. Hans Asperger introduced a similar disorder in 1944 which was called Autistic Psychopathy and later became known as Asperger's Disorder and categorized as one of the three distinct pervasive developmental disorders included in the DSM up until the revision and publication of the DSM-5. Much controversy has emerged related to who discovered Autism first, Kanner or Asperger, whether Kanner plagiarized Asperger's ideas, or they were documenting distinct disorders (Chown & Hughes, 2016; Wolff, 2004). Regardless of the outcome of this debate, the disorder did not emerge in literature until the 1930s and was not included in the DSM until DSM-III which was published in 1980. The elimination of Asperger's Disorder comes as a result of little evidence to support it as distinct from Autism (Sanders, 2009). In addition, the DSM-5 created a separate Social Communication Disorder for children who display social-communication problems but not repetitive or stereotyped behaviors that must be present in ASD (Ozonoff, 2012). Initial views of Autism included the ideas that Autism was a form of childhood schizophrenia, and earlier accounts linked autistic symptoms to muteness, mental retardation, and dementia. Early literature associated causation of Autism with poor parenting, then later genetic factors, and more recently vaccines (Wolff, 2004). Discussion of causation, treatment, and interventions continue with no clear prognosis and outcome for those impacted by ASD.

Validity of the ASD Diagnosis

Given the continued change to the diagnostic criteria since 1943, it is not surprising that the validity of the ASD diagnosis comes under regular scrutiny (Hassall, 2017). Waterhouse, London and Gillberg's (2016) article brings attention to the reliability and validity in identifying ASD. These authors explain how indecisive professionals and researchers really are when it comes to theoretical stances. In summarizing 14 different theories, the authors were able to conclude that the only consistent finding amongst all of these theories is that none reflect the true nature of the ASD phenomena. Most notably, there are no unifying features that would predict or explain ASD.

Currently, ASD is diagnosed from the perception of our understanding of what is considered deficits in skills which elicit certain behaviors and matching it to an individual's understanding of what those behaviors and functions are under the same findings of the DSM-5 criteria (American Psychiatric Association, 2013). Does a child not look others in the eye because he is uncomfortable with eye contact, or does this child not understand how to use eye contact as a way to communicate with another individual? How we interpret behaviors is what leads to an individual diagnosed with this disorder. Reliability comes from the parents and guardians as well since the most imperative piece of information comes from the historian of the child (McPartland, 2017). How valid is parent reporting if the parents do not understand what a repetitive behavior is? Or if the parents are convinced their child is on the spectrum because they are misunderstanding certain behaviors, or professionals may only consider ASD because nothing else makes sense?

In the past 30 years findings have revealed that the DSM-5 diagnosis is not biologically valid (Waterhouse, London & Gillberg, 2016). While one child may lack eye contact but uses gestures to communicate, another child may have excellent eye contact but does not use descriptive gestures to help others understand what he means. While one child may not use expressive language, he may however use facial expressions and direct them towards others. With another child you may not know when they are happy or sad because their facial expressions never change. Two individuals who may meet criteria will display their behaviors very differently which is why the way we currently diagnosis and understand ASD has to be more concrete than the current process of parent or guardian interviews, observations, assessments and interpretation. For example, the ASD diagnosis would be biologically valid if all individuals diagnosed with ASD shared one or a few related brain impairments. Researchers have tried different means to find a unitary ASD brain impairment but have not been successful. The fact that there are no consistent early behavioral or genetic predictors for an ASD diagnosis is enough to continue more in-depth research.

Molecular Pathogenesis of ASD: A Complex Paradigm

The traditional paradigm regarding the underlying causes of autism declares that it is primarily an autosomal recessive genetic disease that comes about when a child inherits one bad gene from each of the parents. The importance of heritable genetic variability in ASD molecular pathogenesis has been highlighted in twin and family studies. The increased prevalence of the disease in siblings of ASD patients and greater ASD concordance rates in monozygotic twins compared with dizygotic twins has prompted significant efforts toward understanding the genetic architecture of ASD pathophysiology at the molecular level. Although mutations linked to monogenic syndromic forms of ASD (the disorders that result from a single gene defect on the autosomes and are inherited according to Mendel's Laws) have been identified, the mutation can be spontaneous and where there is no previous family history or recessive gene. These rare monogenic syndromes collectively account for only about 5% of ASD cases while 95% of cases of non-syndromic ASD remain mostly unexplainable. There had been numerous attempts to explain the highly heterogeneous disease presentation of non-syndromic ASD including the presence of hundreds of single-nucleotide variants and copy number variants (Geschwind & State, 2015). The use of whole exome sequencing (WES) and whole genome sequencing (WGS) in family cohorts with sporadic ASD (simplex) and with more than one affected individual (multiplex) led to the discovery of both rare inherited and *de novo* ASD risk variants. However, it should be noted that the potential role of inherited variants in ASD generally is not supported when WES in larger cohorts of unrelated families are carried out (Novarino et al., 2012). WES in large cohorts of simplex families (one affected child sequenced together with unaffected parents) provided substantial evidence of *de novo* (or spontaneous) mutation in ASD, strongly suggesting that there may be some mutagenic chemicals that can impart genetic mutations during fetal development. Numerous studies have reported increased rates of rare *de novo* CNVs and SNVs in individuals with ASD and have identified high-confidence ASD genes, including *CHD8*, *SYNGAP1*, *DYRK1A*, and *SCN2A* (Iossifov et al., 2014; Bernier et al., 2014). Moreover, targeted sequencing approaches confirmed the recurrence of some of these *de novo* mutations in independent cohorts, substantiating the role of environmental factors in pathogenesis of ASD (O'Roak et al., 2012). Finally, one very interesting group of genetic variants that has recently been implicated in ASD is somatic mutations (Krupp et al., 2017). Somatic mutations can occur during development in the brain and yield mosaic brain, where individuals have distinct cellular genomes in subsets of their somatic cells (O'Roak et al., 2012). Whereas routine genetic sampling from blood misses the disease-associated somatic variants in the brain, targeted sequencing on ASD post-mortem tissue has detected increased rates of deleterious somatic mutations in cases compared with controls (Poduri et al., 2013).

It should be noted that despite the great progress in genetics analyses, only ~5% of patients carry a genetic alteration unequivocally linked to ASD and very few of them can explain the male excess or the regression to autism that sometimes happens in healthy children between 12 and 36 months (Sealey et al., 2015, 2016). The majority of the ASD cases included in ~ 5% are well-established genetic mutations known before the recent DSM-5 diagnostic criteria therefore, intellectual disability (ID) found in Down's Syndrome, Fragile-X syndrome (FXS) and several others mentioned above are primarily not ASD but fit into the DMS-5 diagnostic criteria of ASD due to ID (American Psychiatric Association, 2013). Of note, many different genetic disorders with many different gene variants produce the same phenotype, or the same phenotypic trait or symptom. In the case of mutations in *SHANK2 and SHANK3* genes, (Waterhouse et al., 2016) results in a variety of phenotypes. A mutation in *SHANK3* has the pleiotropic effect of generating four separate diagnostic phenotypes: ASD, schizophrenia (SCZ), severe ID, and epilepsy (Waterhouse et al., 2016). Hommer and Swedo (2015) noted that *SHANK3* mutations, and the 22q11.2 deletion syndrome and duplications at the Williams syndrome locus (7q11.23) all pleiotropically generated both the ASD and SCZ phenotypes. However, the ASD and SCZ phenotypes disrupted deep layer cortical projection neurons in different brain locations; in ASD, the disruption occurred in the prefrontal and primary motor-somatosensory regions, but in SCZ, the disruption occurred in the dorsolateral and ventrolateral prefrontal cortical regions (Hommer & Swedo, 2015). ASD has frequently been reported with the Phelan- McDermid syndrome caused by the CNV chromosome 22q13 deletion that disrupts the gene *SHANK3*. The SHANK protein regulates synaptic cell adhesion molecules and cell scaffolding in brain development via dendrites and glutamatergic synapses. *SHANK2* and *SHANK3* gene mutations reduce the total number of dendritic spines and synapses on neurons, and the lack of mature glutamatergic synapses appears to cause the impaired brain function that results in ID and ASD symptoms (Waterhouse. London & Gillberg, 2016).

In a meta-analysis of 168 different published studies, Richards et al. (2015) found different rates of ASD across 11 genetic syndromes. For example, individuals diagnosed with Rett's syndrome (RTT), 61% were given an ASD diagnosis, and of those with Cohen's syndrome, 54% were given an ASD diagnosis, and for Cornelia de Lange syndrome, 43% had ASD. Also, individuals with tuberous sclerosis complex (TSC), 36% received an ASD diagnosis. Similarly, individuals with Angelman's syndrome, CHARGE syndrome, FXS with NF1, Down's syndrome, Williams' syndrome, a significant number of individuals received an ASD diagnosis, varying from 16 to 34 percent.

In summary, individuals with numerous genetic diseases are diagnosed with ASD. Therefore, it becomes obvious that we do not know if thousands of SNVs and SNPs have any direct link to etiologies of ASD. Only in 5% of the cases there appears to be genetic links but those genes manifest with varied results (i.e. Ras/MAPK syndromes and SHANK2 and SHANK3) and different neurodevelopment conditions are linked to them (citation). Some researchers have theorized that a network or networks of multiple ASD risk genes disrupt just a few impaired brain circuits or pathways in ASD (Reviewed in Waterhouse L, et al., 2016). As elegantly reviewed by Waterhouse, London and Gillbery (2016), the "Multiple gene-few brain circuits models" are premature and ASD risk gene functions in networks are complex and not yet fully understood. There are thousands of ASD risk genes, and there is evidence for gene-gene and gene-environment interaction in ASD etiology.

The Familial Risk of Autism

One of the most intriguing unsolved issues in ASD is that the disorder aggregates in families, but the individual risk and to what extent this is caused by genetic factors or shared or nonshared environmental factors remains unresolved. The common understand is the high concordance among monozygotic twins

(MZT) strongly suggest a clear-cut genetic link since MZT are genetically identical. In reality this does not prove genetic factors as MZT are exposed to exactly same amount of EFs and are equally at risk for ASD (or other neurodevelopmental risks). A study by Sandin et al. (2014) examined 2,049,973 Swedish children born 1982-2006 and identified 37,570 twin pairs, 2,642,064 full sibling pairs, 432,281 maternal and 445,531 paternal half sibling pairs, and 5,799,875 cousin pairs. They measured relative recurrence risk (RRR) in familial aggregation of disease and calculated RRR for both ASD and autistic disorder adjusting for age, birth year, sex, parental psychiatric history, and parental age and concluded that among children born in Sweden, the individual risk of ASD and autistic disorder increased with increasing genetic relatedness. Heritability of ASD and autistic disorder were estimated to be approximately 50%.

In maternal twins, almost all receive different amounts of blood from their mother during development. How that is possible? There are five different kinds of maternal twins. One of the most unfortunate twin-pair is Twin-to-Twin transfusion syndrome (TTTS), also known as Feto-Fetal Transfusion Syndrome (FFTS). This is a complication of highly disproportionate blood supply, resulting in high morbidity and mortality. It can affect monochorionic twins or triplets where two or more fetuses share a chorion and hence a single placenta. Chorion is the extraembryonic membrane that develops villi and becomes fetal part of the placenta. TTTS is a very serious complication affecting approximately 15% of MZT pregnancies. It affects only MZTs sharing a single placenta and a single chorion. As the placenta develops, the blood vessels form in such a way that vessels from one umbilical cord connect up with vessels from the other. This causes a "short circuit" between the babies resulting in highly disproportionate blood supplies, each twin faces a set of challenges that require expert and experienced urgent care. Most TTTS twins, whether they receive treatment or not, will be born prematurely. TTTS is an extreme form of unequal blood flow in maternal twins. But there are four other conditions that are generally ignored and in reality present subtle situations of unequal blood flows (Figure 1).

The other four types are shown in Figure 1 above that in all cases –maternal or fraternal- the blood supply is slightly uneven, making the exposure to nutritional and environmental factors unequal with differential outcomes.

Role of the Environment in Maternal Twins Revealed by Numerous Methods in Many Conditions

Monozygotic twin pairs provide a valuable opportunity to control for genetic and shared environmental influences while studying the effects of non-shared or partially shared environmental influences, such as unequal blood supply to each of the maternal twin. This unequal sharing or exposure to an environmental chemical can result in unequal manifestation of numerous types in genetically identical twins. There are literally hundreds of reports in peer-reviewed scientific journals that show discordant monozygotic twins with different phenotypes. For example, 'right and left' handedness plays a great role in language and learning. Häberling and her colleagues (2013) have examined the hemispherical asymmetry and callosal morphology in monozygotic twins. Some 20-25% of monozygotic twins are of opposite handedness (Annett, 2002; McManus, 1980) with some even showing reversed cerebral asymmetries (Badzakova-Trajkov, Haberling, & Corballis, 2010). Breckpot et al. (2012) explored the occurrence of copy number differences in monozygotic twins discordant for the presence of a congenital heart defect (CHD).

Most importantly, recent studies have clearly unveiled that monozygotic twins (who are genetically identical) manifest discordant results-where one of the twins has autism and the other one is normal

Figure 1. A) Monochromic Monoamniotic (MCMA) twins have no separating membrane. They share a placenta and share an amniotic sac; B) Monochorionic Diamniotic (MCDA) twins share the same placenta but have a separating membrane of amnion; C) Diaamniotic monochoriatic share share one placenta but have different chorions; D) Dichorionic Diamniotic (DCDA) twins have a separating membrane consisting of both chorion & amnion. They may or may not have separate (or fused) placentae. In each case, the blood flow would be unequal that may result in discordant MZ twins (see text below). As illustrated in the figure above, in each case two monozygotic twins are receiving slightly different amount of blood supply, making ones on the left slightly more vulnerable to environmental factors than the ones on the right
(Bagasra & Heggan 2018)

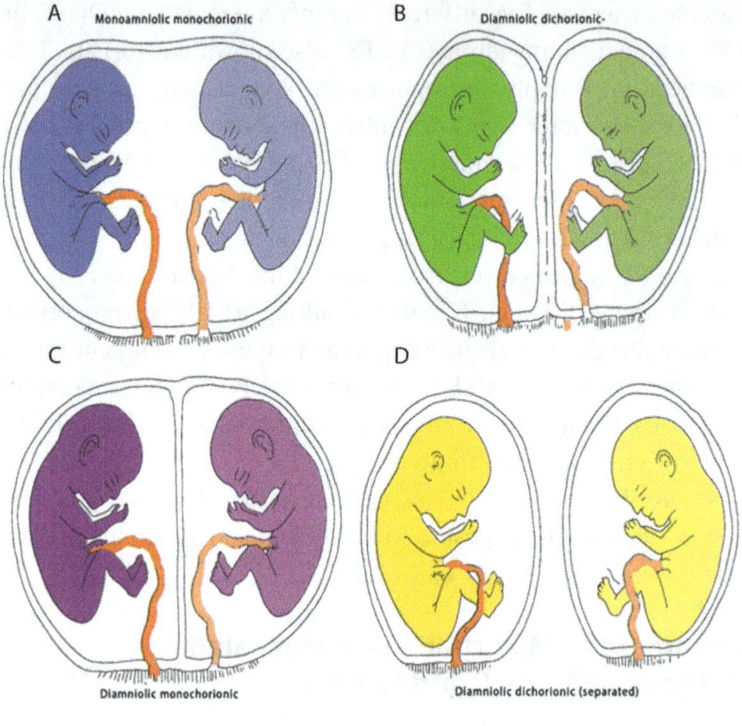

(Hallmayer et al., 2011). Moreover, heritability studies have variably calculated the role of EFs in ASD. Therefore, Colvert et al (2015) put the risk of EFs between 7 to 35%, Tick et al. (2016) between 5 to 44%, Sandin et al. (2014) at 50% and Hallmayer et al. (2011) at 55%. Huguet et al. (2016) reviewed ASD findings and suggested that in ASD risk factors: 49.8% common inherited variants, 2.6% rare inherited CNVs and SNVs, 6.6% de novo SNVs, 2.9% de novo CNVs, and 38.1% environmental risk factors. Huguet et al. (2016) considered the de novo SNVs and CNVs to be environmental and thus 52.4% of ASD had genetic causes, and 47.6% had environmental causes. Most importantly, gene-environment interactions have been identified for ASD (LaSalle 2013; Jeste and Geschwind 2014; Volk et al. 2014).

The spectrum in ASD that shows a broad manifestation of communication disorders can be observed in numerous environmental teratogenic agents that include: heavy metal (i.e. mercury, lead) chemicals (i.e. alcohol), numerous medications prescribed by physicians (i.e. methotrexate, Busuffran, Aminopectin,) even Vitamin A in large doses, antibiotics (i.e. Tetracycline and Trimethadone), infectious agents (i.e.

Herpes simplex virus, Rubella virus, Varicella, Toxoplasma and Treponema pallidum, and Zika virus, among some viruses), and physical agents (i.e. radiation). Some of the most dangerous chemicals that a pregnant woman is exposed to are endocrine disturbing chemicals (EDCs) (Bjørklund et al., 2018). Perfumes contain thousands of synthetic chemicals, many of which are EDCs (Bagasra & Pace, 2013). It should be emphasized that almost all of the EFs mentioned above result in a "spectrum" (Sealey et al., 2015, 2016). Therefore, it depends when during the development a fetus was exposed to an EA and what was the dose of the EA (Bagasra & Heggen, 2018). We will discuss the six principles of Teratogens shortly and show a parallel between various EAs that cause various diseases and ASD. Genetic mutations cannot not clearly explain the spectrum observed in ASD (Bagasra & Pace 2013).

Environmental Syndromic ASD Has Been Found With Varied Brain Impairments

There are fewer well-defined environmental factors (EFs) linked to ASD than genes, CNVs and SNPs associated with ASD (Sealey et al., 2016; Waterhouse et al., 2016). However, there are numerous EFs associated and linked to ASD (Sealey et al., 2016; Waterhouse et al., 2016). These EFs include: significant prenatal, perinatal, and postnatal risk factors. These include maternal inflammation and immune activation, rubella, cytomegalovirus (CMV), influenza, fever, diabetes, folic acid deficiency, toxoplasmosis; exposure to valproic acid, misoprostol, thalidomide, antidepressant serotonin reuptake inhibitors (SSRIs); exposure to pesticides, insecticides, and air pollution, father's age, mother's age, maternal ethanol consumption, cocaine use, maternal hypertension during pregnancy, gestational diabetes, vaginal bleeding, cesarean section, prematurity, induced labor, prolonged labor, lack of infant oxygen during delivery, low birth weight, newborn jaundice, and new- born infection. Kalkbrenner et al. (2014) have linked five chemicals contributed to ASD by disrupting endocrine system development: polychlorinated biphenyls (PCBs), flame retardants, non- stick chemicals, bisphenol A (BPA), and phthalates.

Though not every ASD environmental risk factor is identified as a syndrome, many environmental syndromes have been identified. Our laboratory has concentrated on exposure to fragrances, glyphosate, aluminum, and endocrine disrupting chemicals (EDC) during early stages of pregnancy as important EFs.

Rise of ASD and Rise of Synthetic Chemicals

Autism was relatively rare about four decades ago. In 1960, only one child in 10,000 was diagnosed with autism. By 2011 one in 100 children (1%) was diagnosed with autism spectrum disorders (ASD); in 2013, the ratio worsened to one in 88 and in 2014 according to the Centers for Disease Control (2014), one in 68 children suffered from ASD; and now, in 2018, one in 55 children are autistic (Centers for Disease Control and Prevention, 2018). This sudden rise in ASD, should it continue its upward gallop, could potentially lead to even more devastating results. Where will it end: one child in five; one in two? That is what the Centers for Disease Control and Prevention is predicting (Centers for Disease Control and Prevention, 2018). The genes in humans, or any other large living thing, do not change at the rate that would result in such a rapid rate of new diagnoses of ASD (Zablotsky et al., 2015).

It is illogical to believe that so many, literally thousands of genes, suddenly arose in the human race to cause autism. In the cases of sickle cell anemia, lactose tolerance, and human skin pigmentation— these are each determined by a different single gene. But dozens or even hundreds of genes determine most of the traits that make us who we are as *Homo sapiens*. Human behavior and communication abilities - the majority of the traits that we perceive as causing differences among individuals and among populations - are complex traits. It is against the laws of nature that those genes involved in what "makes us a human" are developing mutations at the speed of light, in evolutionary terms, so we must look for another cause or causes of this disorder (Marco & Skuse, 2006).

The most obvious culprit is changes in the environment. As shown in Figure 2, there are three basic elements that have changed in industrialized nations in the last 50 years. The first and foremost are the introduction of plastics and herbicides (Bagasra & Heggen, 2018). The effects of the active ingredients in plastic polymers on human fetal brains are still not fully researched, however, the active ingredient in herbicide is glyphosate (Morley & Seneff, 2014). When the human gut bacterial (microbiomes) are exposed to glyphosate they cause a major disturbance in gut normal flora and exposure to glyphosate induce the gut normal flora bacterial to secrete neurotoxic chemicals effecting developing fetal brain neurons (unpublished data). Investigators have shown evidence regarding the impact of gut bacteria on neurological outcomes, altering behavior and potentially affecting the onset and/or severity of psychiatric disorders. Pesticides and agrotoxics are also included among this long list of ASD-related environmental stressors. Of note, ingestion of glyphosate (GLY), a broad-spectrum systemic herbicide, can reduce beneficial bacteria in the gastrointestinal tract microbiota without exerting any effects on the Clostridium population, which is highly resistant to this herbicide. The second environmental assault on an unborn child's brain is synthetic fragrances (Bagasra et al., 2013, Sealey et al., 2015, 2016). Most of the synthetic chemicals are made from coal-tar, petroleum by-products and deadly phenolic ring compounds. These innocent, seemingly essential elements that we feel so necessary to use every day, are neurotoxic and can cause genetic mutations in a developing fetal brain at extremely miniscule concentrations, as tested by us by the Ames Test (Ames et al., 1973, Ames et al., 1998, Bagasra et al., 2013). The Ames test, originally described by Bruce Ames et al. (1973), is a well-established biological assay to assess the mutagenic potential of chemical compounds. A positive test indicates that the chemical is mutagenic; therefore, it may act as a carcinogen. The test serves as a convenient screening assay to estimate the carcinogenic potential of a compound. The test utilizes specific strains of *Salmonella typhimurium* that carry mutations in genes involved in histidine synthesis; an auxotrophic mutant, for example, requires histidine for growth. The method tests the capability of mutagenic agents to create mutations that can result in a reversion back to a non-auxotrophic state, which permits cells to grow in a histidine-free medium. In order to carry out the mutagenic potential of perfumes, we mixed one mL of the bacteria in an agar tube containing 1.50 mL of agar at 46°C with 1 mL of histidine (final dilution 1:15,000) in duplicates. This mixture was pipetted on a plate and allowed to culture at 37°C for 48 h. The small amount of histidine in the growth medium allows the bacteria to grow for an initial short period, and have the opportunity to mutate. With histidine depletion, only those bacteria that have a perfume-induced gain-of-function mutation would grow. The mutagenicity of a substance is proportionate to the number of colonies recorded. Each experiment was repeated at least three times. The number of colonies on the negative control (water) was subtracted from the perfume treated and a highly mutagenic chemical 4-nitro-1,2-diaminobenzene (4-NOPD) was used as a positive control.

Our research indicates that every one of the 98 perfumes we tested using Ames test, at dilutions of 1:50,000 (10) showed mutagenic ability. This suggests that synthetic chemical exposure that may appear innocuous are not harmless to highly vulnerable fetal brain cells, and that significant fetal mutations may be linked to such exposure. However, we do not believe that these mutagenic agents are actually responsible for ASD directly. We believe that these are ASD unrelated mutations, thousands of those

SNPs and CNVs, are erroneously claimed to be linked to ASD children. In reality, they are just associated mutations and may not be the cause of ASD. We emphasize the point that over 4,000 synthetic chemicals are used, collectively, in the typical perfumes used in the western world, and that these chemicals are commonly produced by synthetic chemistry, and many are benzene ring products, which is alarming given benzene's well-established reputation as a mutagenic and carcinogenic agent (Bagasra & Pace 2013, Bagasra et al., 2013).

They are selectively neurotoxic to certain special types of neurons that are involved in communication and preferentially eliminate the specific types of brain cells in males more than a female fetal brain. We have shown that human developing brain neurons exposed to femtomolar concentrations of fragrances can preferentially deplete oxytocin receptors (OXYR) and Arginine-Vasopressin receptors (AVPR) expressing neurons in male cell lines as compared to female (Sealey et al., 2015, 2016). Could it be that the highly pleasant-smelling environment in which our society lives is one of the major culprits in this unpleasant outcome? Could it be that the outcome for mothers and their babies would be more pleasant if mothers-to-be breathed air that was free from such pleasant smells? Should prenatal precaution involve not only abstinence from alcohol and other drugs that can be mutagenic to the fetus but also the substances of fragrant smell? Is more actually less in the aromatic arena of life? Of note, many mothers naturally abhor fragrances during early stages of their pregnancy. Is that an evolutionarily defense mechanism to save a fetus from harm? Every single fragrance we have tested on developing fetal neurons can induce a large number of genetic mutations in human fetal brain neurons (Bagasra el al., 2013). To find a major root cause of autism, we may need to look no further than our own noses. It should be noted that as a result of a giant loophole in the Federal Fair Packaging and Labeling Act of 1973, fragrance and cosmetics producers are explicitly exempted from having to enumerate specific ingredients on product labels. Fragrance concealment is not illegal and is often used by the industry to hide from the public the full list of ingredients, even substances that can cause grave health problems. It is a common practice for businesses to list the chemicals as simply "fragrance," which may mean that about half of the ingredients are never revealed to buyers. Even worse, people who use cologne, synthetic fragrances, body spray, baby lotions and other scented cosmetics are blindly exposed to dangerous chemicals since the Food and Drug Administration lacks authority to control mandates to manufacturers that require testing of all synthetic chemicals in fragrances for safety before being released to the public.

The next infringement in our naturally adapted lives was the introduction of endocrine disturbing chemicals (EDCs). EDCs mimic our own natural hormones or bind the receptors found on our cells imitating the natural biochemical and physiological signaling processes. The last one is introduction of vaccines that contain organic mercury (Thimerosal), a known neurotoxin, a real fetal brain damaging agent. Its use is rapidly decreasing in US and EU but it is still widely used in developing nations. We are well aware that the use of these major elements has crept into our way of life, although this creeping has been so silent, so gradual, that we hardly noticed their invasion, and largely overlook the enormous damage they are inflicting on our offspring (Gore et al., 2015). Few pay even the smallest attention to these major shifts that have quietly invaded our lives at global level. The commercially available perfumes for women can contain over 4,000 synthetic chemicals, including many EDCs (Sarantis et al., 2010).

Figure 2. The alarming rise in Autism and life style changes
(https://naturaltothecore.wordpress.com/2013/03/10/autism-head-lag-and-the-core-of-wellbeing/

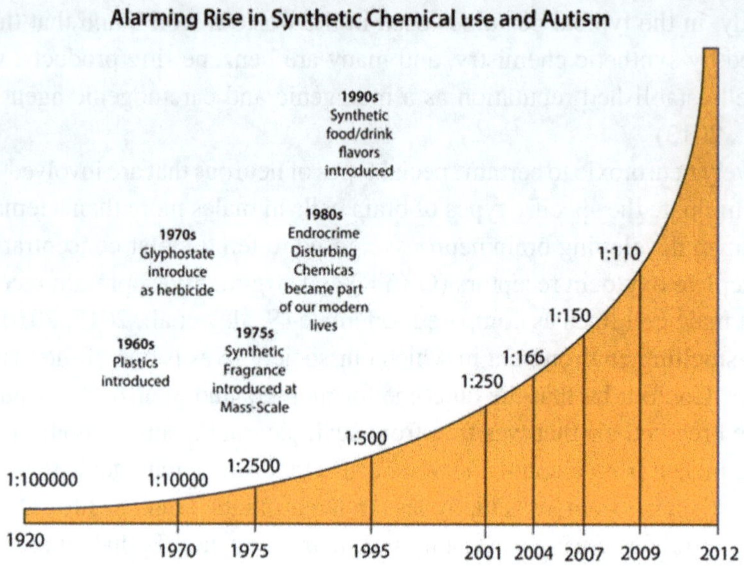

PRESENT RESEARCH

Evidence That Environmental Agents Induce Developmental Neuropathology

It is well documented that in most cases, an autistic child's brain has acquired the genetic and organismal abnormalities during the first trimester of their gestational period (Baron-Cohen et al., 2015; Street et al., 2018). Yet, scientists still don't know what is causing these abnormalities. Here we will summarize the scientific evidence that shows how various well-known EAs can induce major neuropathology. The developing fetal brain is more vulnerable to environmental assaults than an adult brain, especially during week 3 and week 16, a critical period of human fetal brain development (Bagasra & Heggen, 2018). However, the brain's differentiation continues after birth until puberty. Here we will summarize what we know when a developing fetus is exposed to two heavy metals: methylmercury, lead, and one of the most common EAs-alcohol.

In pathology the term neurotoxicity is generally defined as a structural change or a functional alteration of the nervous system, resulting from exposure to a chemical, biological, or physical agent. Neurotoxic effects are the outcome of a series of events during human fetal development which includes entry of the agent into maternal blood and then into fetal blood stream and then transplacental passage to amnion, and subsequent penetration of the agent into the fetal brain. Depending on the stage of gestation, an EA has to gain access to various compartments of the brain and binds to the neurons that express specific receptors on their surface. Interaction with specific cellular targets (i.e. specific types of neurons which subsequently differentiate into various compartments of a newborns brain), and initiation of biological changes (i.e. neuromodifications or eliminations of certain types of neurons via apoptosis) resulting in structural and functional alterations in the nervous system. Although neurotoxicity is known to occur in adult humans, it often involves peripheral nervous system effects because the central nervous system

(CNS) is well protected by the blood- brain barrier (BBB), which prevents the passage of many endogenous and exogenous neurotoxic agents into the brain. In contrast, the fetal brain is highly vulnerable to neurotoxic agents due to unprotected brain, especially during the first and the first half of the second trimers (Tran & Miyaki, 2017). We will briefly describe the neurotoxic effects of some of the major well-researched developmental neurotoxins, such as methylmercury, lead, polychlorinated biphenyls (PCBs), and alcohol, to link the neurotoxic effects of glyphosate, various fragrances and EDCs (Bagasra & Heggen, 2018, Semple, et al., 2013). According to the CDC the recent estimates in the United States show that about one in six, or about 15%, of children aged 3 through 17 years have one or more developmental disabilities, such as: ADHD, ASD, cerebral palsy, hearing loss, intellectual disability, learning disability, vision impairment and other developmental delays) with an estimated $80-100 Billion cost to society.

When Is the Human Fetal Brain Most Vulnerable to Environmental Agents?

An understanding of the short- and long-term adverse effects of an EA requires not only knowledge of the nature of the mechanism of action of an EA but also of the target organ or cell types at the time of insult (Costa et al., 2004, Semple et al., 2013). Over half a century of understanding of the developmental biology of human brain, mostly acquired by using experimental rodent models, we have accumulated a great deal of information on brain development. From these studies, we are able to infer the various stages of brain development in humans. Even though these are not the perfect solution since rodent brain growth rate and gestation times are very different, the overall structural similarity is very useful for gross extrapolation. Therefore, the developmental ages of rat and human embryos and fetuses are comparable when major anatomical features and histological landmarks are similar in appearance in the two species, even though their exact chronological ages are different. Different parts of the CNS develop at different stages of development; structures are built by cell proliferation, migration, and differentiation. Normal developing of a brain requires a certain number of cells in the correct location, and each cell must have the proper receptors and other features for it to differentiate and proliferate properly (Rodier, 1994; Semple et al., 2013). The neurogenesis of specific neuronal populations has been determined in rodent brain (mostly by autoradiography methods), and other primates and extrapolated to the human brain. From extensive studies it is clear that different brain areas develop at different times during gestation, and within a single brain region, subpopulations of neurons develop at different rates and at different times. For example, in the cerebellum, Purkinje cells develop early (embryonic days 13-15 in the rat, corresponding to weeks 5-7 in humans), whereas granule cells are generated much later (postnatal days 4-19 in the rat, corresponding to gestational weeks 24–40 in humans). Many EAs (i.e. many chemical, viral, and physical agents like radiation, mercury, etc.), that are known neurotoxins, impart neuromodification by interfering with cell proliferation/differentiation, and if the insult occurs during the stage of formation of a certain neuronal subpopulation, those cells will not be formed. Additionally, migration of specific types of neurons is an essential part of brain development. Migration of neurons occurs in waves and a failure in migration at precise times during neurodevelopment is either caused by direct insult to a specific neural subpopulation or indirectly by effect on neighboring cells or toxic effects on important supporting structures, such as radial glia disturbing the balance of neurodevelopment. In order for a brain to develop normally, the synaptogenesis – the process where neurons form connections so the neurotransmitters can form proper signaling pathways must remain intact. The synaptogenesis period is critical for the formation of the basic circuitry of the CNS. Furthermore, in the developing fetal and post-natal brains, neurotransmitters also play important roles other than neurotransmission to control body function. The neurotransmitters can modulate proliferation of neural stem cells, neuroblasts, and glioblasts; regulate migration; and induce differentiation. Consequently, any neurotoxin that interferes with neurotransmission during development may cause permanent defects in the CNS. We will show evidence that many of the EA, specifically fragrances, interfere with the proper development and migration of oxytocin (OXY) and Arganine-Vassopressin (AVP) receptor positive neurons or are cytotoxic to these neurons (Sealey et al., 2015; Sealey et al., 2016). In addition, any EF that interferes with apoptosis and pruning process of neurodevelopment may trigger unusual apoptotic degeneration of neurons that would not have otherwise been deleted from the developing brain, or may, in contrast, promote survival of unnecessary cells (this may explain the unusually large brain size in ~30% of ASD children) (See Figure 3) (Bagasra & Heggen, 2018). In addition to loss of neurons, pruning, defined as a loss of synapses, also occurs physiologically in the developing brain and has been documented in some ASD children. The pruning of connectomes takes much longer time than apoptosis and occurs late in childhood and adolescence (Costa et al., 2004). Any interference with this process, as has been suggested in the case of ASD, would be expected to affect the number of synaptic connections. Most of the developmental processes discussed so far have focused on neurons. Yet, it is well established that glial cells (astrocytes, oligodendrocytes, and microglia) play a pivotal role in neurodevelopment. An important period of brain development is the brain growth spurt (a transient period of growth when the brain is growing most rapidly). This occurs in the first two postnatal weeks in the rat and in the third trimester of pregnancy and early infancy in humans (Street et al., 2018). One of the general features of brain growth throughout mammalian species is that adult neuronal cell number is almost accomplished (with the exception of cerebellar granule cells and a few other neurons) before the major phase of glial multiplication begins. The brain growth spurt is essentially due to rapid proliferation of glial cells, most notably astrocytes and oligodendrocytes, which provide myelination to axons by Schwann cells-an important step in neuroconnection and transmission process. In human week 3-16 of gestation and the pre-natal and post-natal growth spur phases of neurodevelopment are the most sensitive to the toxic effects of a number of chemicals (e.g., clearly shown in mercury, alcohol, certain pesticides, and EDCs), which underlines the fact that glial cells represent an important target for neurotoxicity (Gore et al., 2015). One of the most important aspects of vulnerability of a fetal brain is the absence of a blood-brain barrier (BBB). The complete development of the BBB is a gradual process, beginning *in utero* and complete at approximately six months of age in humans (Bagasra & Heggen, 2018; Costa et al., 2004). Because the BBB restricts the passage of substances from blood to brain, in partially completed BBB, neurotoxic agents can freely enter the developing brain.

Cell-to-cell contact is also another important part of a brain development and for the proper development of a brain and the construction of complex circuits is necessary, and any interference with cell migration and cell-cell contact would spell disaster in normal brain development (Costa et al., 2004). For example, exposure to methylmercury or thiemerosal results in profound deleterious effects on the developing brain, as we describe below (Bjørklund et al., 2018).

Environmental Neuromodifying Factors and ASD

It is well documented fact that many teratogenic agents (chemicals, viral agents or physical insults) that interfere with normal fetal growth, homeostasis, development, differentiation, and behavior (Bjørklund et al 2018, Sealey et al., 2016) Teratogens are xenobiotics and other factors that cause malformations in the developing fetus. There are six basic principles of teratology that were proposed by James Wilson in 1959 and still hold to be true (Wilson, 1973). We have adapted this to neuromodifying environmental factors in the following manner:

1. Susceptibility to neuromodifying environmental factors depends on the embryo's genotype that interacts with adverse environmental factors (G x E interaction).
2. The developmental stage of the fetus at the time of neuromodifying environmental factors exposures determines the outcome.
3. Each of the neuromodifying environmental factors have specific mechanisms through which they exert their pathogenic effects.
4. The nature of the neuromodifying environmental factors (i.e., biological, chemical or heavy metals) determines its access to the developing brain and different pronator neurons.
5. The four major categories of manifestations of altered development are death, malformation, growth retardation, and functional deficits. In the case of ASD the outcome of exposures may not be apparent for several years after birth.
6. The manifestations of the altered development increase with increasing dose (i.e., ranging from no apparent effect to death and demise of a fetal brain and the fetus).

When describing teratogens, one may think of three basic characteristics of neuromodifying environmental factors:

1. A given factor may be specific to a receptor that are being expressed at the time of developmental period (i.e. like endocrine disrupting chemicals or synthetic fragrances.
2. It may be species specific meaning only certain species may express receptors for those neuromodifying environmental factors.
3. It can be dose specific meaning a very tiny dose may kill certain specific cells at certain stage of fetal development but may require much higher dose at different stage of gestation (many synthetic chemicals fall into this group). We will further explain this with regards to Oxytocin and Arginine-vasopressin positive receptors neurons (Sealey et al 2015, 2016).

Why ASD Is Primarily an Environmental and Not a Genetic Syndrome

- **Mercury-Induced Neurotoxicity:** Exposure to mercury can cause a myriad of physiologic effects including immune, sensory, neurological, motor and behavioral dysfunctions. Shown in Figure 4, the maladies caused by mercury are very similar to traits associated with ASD, and these similarities extend to neuroanatomy, neurotransmitters and biochemistry. It also affects the antioxidant system in the cell, resulting in loss of membrane integrity and finally cellular necrosis (Moneim, 2015). Mercury (Hg) is a heavy metal of known toxicity. Numerous studies have confirmed that methylmercury (or Organic Mercury, MeHg) compounds cause developmental disorders (Costa et al., 2004). Thimerosal has been one of the common preservatives in multi-dose vaccines, especially in MMR and flu vaccines. Despite its curtailment in MMR childhood vaccines in the US and EU nations, it is still in use worldwide. The current multi-dose flu vaccine also contains methylmercury. As outlined above with the six James Wilson principles, the similarities of effects of methylmercury and its resulting effects points towards the roles of EFs (i.e. synthetic fragrances, herbicides, EDCs, etc.). (Sealey et al., 2016).

Figure 3. Development of a human fetal brain from day 25 to 5 month of gestation (top). In the majority of autism cases, the problem arises during a very early stage of the fetal brain development. A few progenitor neurons, destined to mature into a specialized faculty are killed or mutated, resulting in ASD. An autistic child's brain is larger but has parts missing.

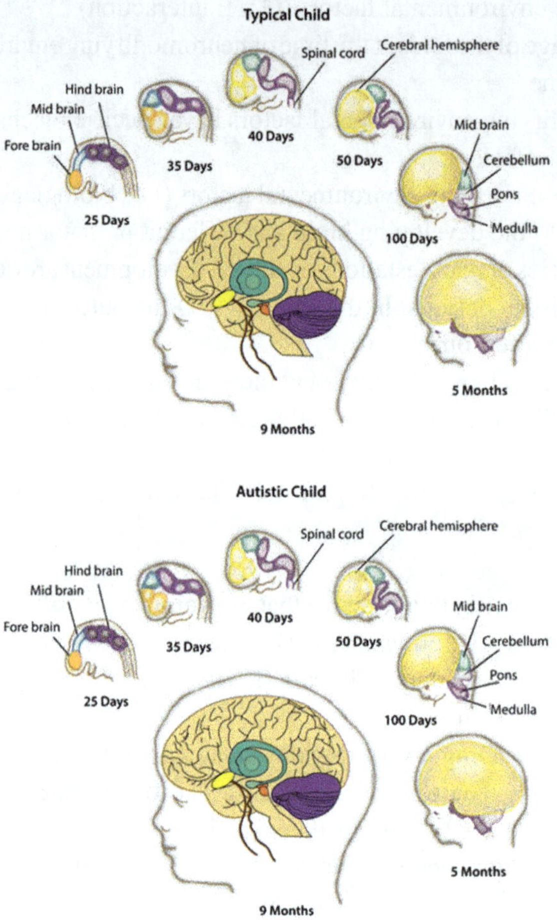

- **Lead-Induced Neurotoxicity:** Lead is a common environmental pollutant and besides reducing exposure to lead by lead-free gasoline and lead-free paint, it is still a common pollutant (Costa et al., 2004). Lead exposure during pregnancy and in young children is of particular concern because the developing nervous system is especially vulnerable to its neurotoxic effects. One of the great similarities of lead neurotoxic effects and the putative adverse effects of synthetic fragrances, EDCs and glyphosate is the subtlety of these neurotoxins. For example, epidemiological studies have associated chronic developmental lead-exposure with impairments in cognitive function and behavioral effects in young children. These effects were found despite the absence of any overt signs of neurotoxicity, and the children displayed no other apparent alterations in CNS morphology or generalized neurological function. A number of large and well-conducted longitudinal studies lend support to the claim that neurobehavioral and cognitive effects related to environmental

Figure 4. A spectrum of symptoms in mercury exposure during early post-natal period and similarities to atypical (regressive) autism
Retrieved from http://lizditz.typepad.com/i_speak_of_dreams/autism/

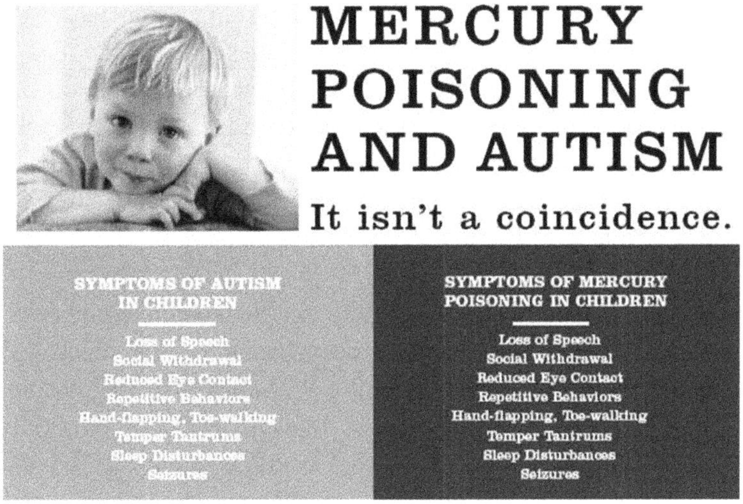
MERCURY POISONING AND AUTISM
It isn't a coincidence.
SYMPTOMS OF AUTISM IN CHILDREN
Loss of Speech
Social Withdrawal
Reduced Eye Contact
Repetitive Behaviors
Hand-flapping, Toe-walking
Temper Tantrums
Sleep Disturbances
Seizures
SYMPTOMS OF MERCURY POISONING IN CHILDREN
Loss of Speech
Social Withdrawal
Reduced Eye Contact
Repetitive Behaviors
Hand-flapping, Toe-walking
Temper Tantrums
Sleep Disturbances
Seizures

lead-exposure during neurodevelopment persist throughout childhood and adulthood. This trace degree of lead exposure points to the subtle exposure to the EFs we are investigating.

- **Fetal Alcohol Syndrome (FAS):** Ethanol is a well-documented developmental toxin causing a spectrum of physical and mental dysfunctions in children who were exposed to alcohol during gestation (reviewed in Bagasra & Heggen, 2018). This range of structural and functional abnormalities characterize a syndrome known as FAS and include pre- and postnatal growth retardation; craniofacial abnormalities (Costa et al., 2004). The most damage occurs on the CNS and results in microcephaly (in ~80% of cases), brain malformation, mental retardation and numerous behavioral abnormalities. Low dose exposure may not show obvious abnormalities but still result in a variety of neurodevelopmental disorders, including failure of certain regions of the brain to fully develop including reduced size of corpus callosum, the cerebellum, basal ganglia, and cerebral cortex and limbic system (also observed in a significant percentage of ASD cases).
- **EDCs:** The US Environment Protection Agency (EPA) defines Endocrine Disruptors as an exogenous substance interfering with synthesis, secretion, transport, binding, action or elimination of natural hormones responsible for the maintenance of normal homeostasis, interfering in reproduction, development and/or behavior. More than 800 chemicals are suspected as endocrine disruptors and the list of EDC is increasing (Gore et al., 2015; Street et al., 2018). EDC can easily pass placental layers due to their lipophilic property, which allows them to bio-accumulate in a variety of cells and tissues in a fetus. Some of the chemicals that are found in our daily lives are Eugenol, Benzyl Benzoate and Benzyl Salicylate. These EDCs are commonly found in fragrances, Musk ketone in perfume, Diethyl phthalate (DEP) in plastic products like toys, food packaging, and body lotions, Octinoxate in sunscreen (Bagasra & Pace, 2013). EDCs are well known for their estrogenic/ androgenic or anti-estrogenic and androgenic properties and evidences indicate dysregulations in the sex hormones (estrogen and androgen) can influence neurodevelopment (i.e., ASD) (Chaste et al., 2017)

Out of a chemical universe topping 80,000 agents, over 1000 have laboratory evidence of neurotoxicity but only a small fraction has been studied in humans during critical periods of development (Kalkbrenner et al., 2014). The Toxicology database has a list of these chemicals with their toxic levels. If a fetal brain is exposed to even a femtomolar concentration of certain EDCs, they can cause severe morphological changes including masculinization of female fetus and ambiguous external genitalia (Sealey et al., 2015). The subtle neurotoxic effects that we have determined *in vitro* are the changes on OXY and AVP receptor position neurons, obtained from neuroblastomas) of male and female origins but significantly worse effects on male neurons as compared to female neurons. We have examined six different EDCs: Eugenol, benzyl benzoate, benzyl salicylate, musk ketone, octinoxate and DEP. All are found in a majority of perfumes and are widely used in the fragrance and cosmetic industry.

- **Effects of Fragrances on Human Developing Brain Neurons:** Despite wide spread use of fragrances on a global scale very little work has been carried out on effects of various fragrances on fetal brains (reviewed by Bagasra & Pace, 2013; Darbre, 2018; Kamatou et al., 2012; Patel, 2017; Sarantis et al., 2010; Steiling et al., 2014; Taylor et al., 2014; Wolkoff & Nielsen, 2017). Previously, we have shown that some of the most common chemicals that we are exposed to in our everyday lives, in the form of perfumes, air fresheners, fragrances in laundry detergents, dish washing and bathroom cleaning supplies, baby lotions, and cosmetics contains highly volatile organic chemicals (VOCs), mutagenic, and neuromodulatory chemicals (Bagasra et al., 2013). These benzyl and phenolic ring compounds containing chemicals that can harm a developing fetal brain, selectively depleting the compartments of the brain that are essential for human communications (Sealey et al., 2015). Many of our daily use consumer products emit volatile organic chemical (VOCs) that spell danger to our unborn offspring and to young babies whose brain are still developing (Bang du et al., 2011; Bennike et al., 2018; Bonchak et al., 2018; kim et al., 2018; Nematollahi et al., 2018; Sowndhararajan & Kim, 2016; Steinemann, 2018). More specifically, we have shown that some of the most common ingredients in fragrances have been shown to increase human estrogen receptors including limonene, alpha-pinene, octinoxate, oxybenzone, benzo phenone-1, benzophenone-2, benzyl salicylate, benzyl benzoate, butylphenyl methylpropional, and synthetic musks (galaxolide, tonalide, and musk ketone). Of these, oxybenzone, benzophenone-1, galaxolide, and tonalide also affect androgens or androgen receptors in the fetal brains, while butylated hydroxytoluene, benzophenone-2, and octinoxate have been linked to thyroid hormone disruption (Sarantis, 2013). One may argue that if a pregnant mother is exposed to fragrances they will be expected to be diluted perhaps a million-fold and may not harm a developing fetal brain (considering an average female has 5-6 liters of blood and if VOCs enter the blood circulation via inhaling or dermal route (see section on skin-based penetration of fragrances). To explore this hypothesis, we have exposed the developing fetal brain neurons to fragrances that were diluted one to one or ten-million-fold and found that even at such low concentrations, the fetal brain neurons are still affected. Evidence suggests that even at very low concentrations, fragrances that contain these chemicals can be mutagenic and impart profound effects on developing fetal brain neurons. Most interestingly, many of the environmental chemicals exert a sex-preferred effect, generally more severe effects on male developing brain neurons than the female, at least partially explaining the male gender bias in ASD, where ASD is ~3-5 times more prevalent in males than females (Hughes et al., 2016). As shown in Figure 5, exposures to fragrances induce mutations in developing fetal brain neurons (Bagasra et al., 2013). This figure may explain why there are thousands of

Figure 5. Mutagenic/carcinogenic effects of various perfumes as assessed by Ames test. Only perfumes with high mutagenic/carcinogenic activities are shown. Briefly, 1 microL of each perfume was added into 150 mL of liquid agar containing S. typhimurium, and 1 microL of histidine, mixed well and plated on Petri dish for 48 h. The number of bacterial colonies was counted visually. Each experimental variable was performed in triplicate, and plotted as shown (Bagasra et al., 2013).

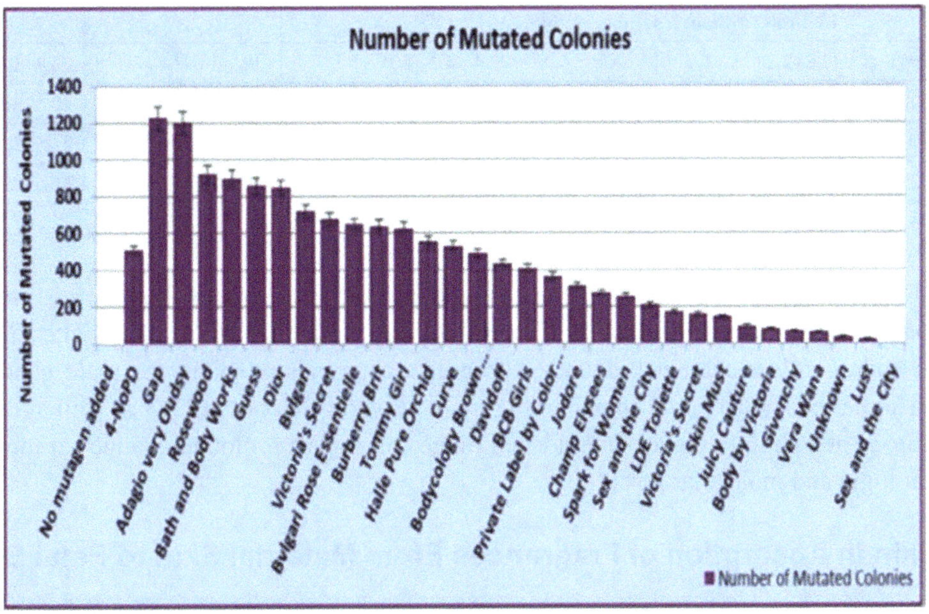

genes associated with ASD but none has been proven to cause ASD. All the fragrances we have tested so far by using Ames Test (Ames et al., 1973; Ames et al 1998) has shown mutagenic ability (Bagasra et al., 2013). Table 1 shows that exposure to even a femtomolar concentrations of three perfumes we tested, imparted a profound morphologic defect in developing neurons and depleted OXY receptors positive markers only in males but not in females suggesting a cause of gender bias in ASD s (Hughes et al., 2016).

Gender Bias and Exposure to Levels of Testosterone in a Developing Fetus

- **Extreme Male Brain Hypothesis:** In addition to the fragrances and their most common ingredients, we have also explored other hypotheses like exposure to male hormones-testosterone- during 8-24 weeks of gestation. Baron-Cohen and his team (2015) has hypothesized that the main cause of gender bias in ASD is due to high levels of testosterone found in male amniotic environment during 8-24 week of gestation and higher than normal levels translates into ASD or Asperger syndrome. This hypothesis known as "extreme male brain" (or EMB) hypothesis argues that if a female fetus is exposed to male hormones during early gestation they would exhibit more male characteristics than the female characteristics (females empathize and males systemize (Baron-Cohen, 2015). Even if one considers the high fetal testosterone levels during the early stages of gestation, this data does not explain the rising incidence of ASD, unless we take into consideration the widespread exposures to fragrances and VOCs found in perfumes that also behave

*Table 1. Statistical analysis of developing human neurons exposure to femtomolar concentrations of three fragrances (A, B, and C) and analyzed for the expressions of oxytocin receptor (OXR). The two male developing brain neuronal cell lines compared to two female developing brain cell lines. Regulation of OXR+ neurons when exposed to fragrances are represented by the average ± the standard deviation, with P values less than 0.05 reported as significance changes and designated by * sign.*

Gender	Controls (without fragrance) in percent	A	B	C
Male (CRL-2267)	42.8±2.28	24.2±1.3*	19.2±1.64*	20.8+1.79*
Female (CRL-2266)	42.0±1.58	42.4±2.7	38.4+1.79	40.6+3.05
Male (CRL-2142)	40.0+363	27.0+4.34*	18.21+2.06*	21.5+3.5*
Female (CRL-2149)	42.0+2.78	41.3+1.91	40.3+2.75	38.6+3.95

like EDCs. We know that many fragrances, and especially perfumes, contain testosterone-like hormones (Bagasra & Heggen, 2018, Clara et al., 2005; Sarantis et al., 2010). The EMB and its link to androgen-like chemicals found in fragrances may also explain the male gender bias in ASD (Hughes et al., 2016). As shown in Figure 6, we show that both EDCs as well as exposure to testosterone at a slightly higher than normal range can impart profound changes at morphologic, immunologic and molecular levels.

Role of Skin in Absorption of Fragrances From Maternal Skin to Fetal Brain

Very little attention has been paid to the key role maternal skin can play in transferring potentially harmful environmental chemicals to a developing fetus (Andrzej et al 2018; Fitzpatrick et al 1993; Slominski et al., 2012). Adult human female skin has a surface area of about 2 m^2 and constitutes approximately 6% of total bodyweight (Slominski et al., 2012; Weedon, 2010) It is the body's largest organ, and serves as the barrier between the external environment and internal milieu. Skin is akin to a plasma member of a mammalian cell that guides and determines its critical function in the preservation of the cellular homeostasis, and survival of an organism (Slominski & Wortsman, 2000; Slominski et al., 2012; 2015; 2018).

In the preceding section we have discussed some of the environmental agents that are harmful to a developing fetus including mercury, lead and several pesticides and herbicides (Sealey 2015, 2016). However, there are many safeguards in place to prevent exposures of these chemicals to pregnant women and young children. Fragrances, however, are highly ubiquitous in our daily lives and an expecting mother can be exposed to thousands of different kinds of synthetic chemicals found in fragrances without her knowledge. There are no laws to disclose the ingredients in a given perfume or fragrance. The ambiguity of the term fragrance may conceal the existence of highly harmful phenolic chemicals known to carcinogenic and interfere in normal development of human brain cells.

Perfumes and many fragrances are designed to enhance the skin penetration of chemicals. For example, a majority of perfumes contain isopropyl myristate. This and similar chemicals enhance skin penetration and absorption of many ingredients in perfumes and cosmetics (Bharati, 2004; Panigrahi, 2005). Much evidence has been obtained from studies of chemicals used for cosmetics and topical therapeutics, but the information available on compounds in perfumes is limited. The data obtained from experimental studies have confirmed that the concentration, type of vehicle, skin area, skin condition, and extent of exposure are important factors in determining the degree of skin absorption, but no general model has been developed. Furthermore, little is known about the basic chemical properties governing the rate of penetration (Grandjean, 1988; Guy, 2010). We do not to know which types of synthetic chemicals found in fragrances and perfumes enter a pregnant woman's blood circulation or via respiratory system and what concentration they reach in the amniotic fluid and subsequently reach a fetal brain. If should be noted that fragrances bind preciously "specific receptors" on neuronal surface. In adult olfactory neurons the process of olfaction is based on this precision binding (). It is not unreasonable to predict that during the process of neurogenesis hundreds if not thousands of olfactory progenitor neurons in the fetal brain would express receptors that can bind certain chemicals from fragrances that make their way into fetal brain. These progenitor neurons are expected to die similar to the olfaction neuron in the olfactory bulb that also die upon binding with chemicals that produce sense of odor. We have shown that a significant percentage of developing fetal neurons can bind progenitor neurons in vitro. Most particularly, oxytocin (OXY) and arginine-vasopressin receptors (AVPR) positive neurons. Most importantly, we have shown a significant depletion of OXYR+ and AVPR+ neurons in developing male brain neurons than the female brain neurons.

Connecting the Dots

A question that remains is why female developing neurons are relatively more protected than their male counterparts? It has been proposed by some investigators that the male bias for ASD may be partially due to under diagnosis of autism in females or the human female's ability to mask some of the symptoms of ASD (Baron-Cohen et al., 2015). Even so, these investigators agree that male bias is ~3 times more common in ASD. While in the majority of cases, the exact etiology of ASD remains unknown, novel technologies and large population-based studies have provided new insight into the risk architecture of ASD and the possible role of environmental factors in etiology (Hallmayer et al., 2011). Our studies where we have exposed fetal developing neurons to extremely miniscule concentrations of fragrances, EDCs, and testosterone have shown that one of the factors explaining why ASD is more common in boys than girls may be due to the preferential depletion of oxytocin-(OT) and arginine vasopressin (AVP)-receptor positive neurons in developing fetal brains (Sealey et al., 2015). Utilizing neuroblastoma cell lines (NBCs) derived from both genders that were exposed to femtomolar concentrations of commonly used fragrances (Table 1), we determined that both OXT and AVP-receptor positive of neurons are more significantly depleted from the male developing brain neurons as compared with female.

Role of OXT Positive Neurons in ASD

The neuropeptides oxytocin and vasopressin increasingly have been identified as modulators of human social behaviors and have been associated with neuropsychiatric disorders characterized by social dysfunction, including autism (Maud et al., 2018, Sealey et al., 2016). It has been shown that the measured volume of the olfactory bulb correlates with the functional capacity in normal individuals (e.g. larger olfactory bulbs exhibit finer olfactory discrimination). The ability to discriminate between distinct smells, which is dependent on intact functioning of the olfactory bulb, has been shown to be impaired in autism. It can be assumed, therefore, that a substantial reduction in size (or total absence) of the olfactory bulbs, as observed in some autistic children, may explain some of the symptoms. This abnormality may have impacts beyond olfactory discrimination due to utilization of the olfactory bulbs in social and emotional processing. Of note, the neuropeptide arginine vasopressin (AVP) has been hypothesized to play a role

Figure 6. Profound neuromodifications in male and female developing neurons after exposure to male hormone-testosterone and male hormone like chemical ketone musk, one of the most commonly use fragrances found in our environment. Top panel shows the effects of testosterone, white the bottom panel shows effects of ketone musk, an androgenic EDC. In each case, female (CRL-2266) and male (CRL-2267) neuroblastoma cells were exposed to three different concentrations of testosterone (i.e. 0.64 nM, 0.82 nM and 1.2 nM), each corresponding to the concentrations of androgens in the amniotic fluids of children who were later found to be either Normotypic, Autistic and Asperger children, respectively (Baron-Cohen et al., 2015 and unpublished data)

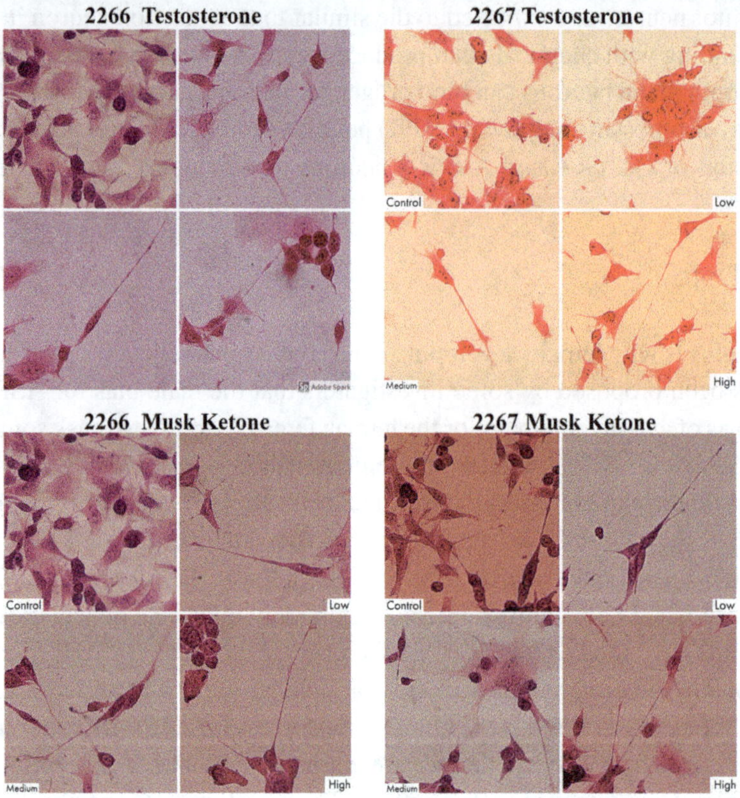

in the etiology of autism based on demonstrated involvement in social bonding and in the regulation of a variety of socially relevant behaviors in animal models. AVP regulates male social behavior not just through higher expression in males but also through steroid-sensitive brain sexual dimorphisms in AVP neurons. AVP may therefore influence sexually dimorphic social behaviors in a range of species. The role of sex hormones on AVP is of interest in the context of autism considering that the ratio of affected males with autism compared to females is markedly skewed (~5:1). This may be due to the fact that a large number of fragrances have hormone-like effects, perhaps partially explaining the underdevelopment of olfactory bulbs and male gender bias in ASD (Cataldo et al., 2018; Sealey et al., 2015, 2016). Olfactory bulbs contain a high density of oxytocin and vasopressin receptors and these neurotransmitters' actions are dependent on the proper functioning of this region of the brain. Any impairment of the olfactory bulbs during development would compromise a key mechanism of action mediating these social behaviors. As shown below, fragrances are designed to bind the smell receptors of olfactory neurons.

Therefore, the binding of any substance that may hinder or modulate normal development of fetal brains may theoretically contribute to the development of autism (Figure 7 illustrates the concept).

Produced in the hypothalamus, oxytocin (OT) is a neurotransmitter involved in social behaviors, including mammalian labor and nursing, maternal behavior, bonding, and social recognition and reward (reviewed by Maud et al., 2018, Calado et al., 2018). It binds to oxytocin receptors expressed by neurons across the brain, including in the amygdala, olfactory bulb, nucleus accumbens, brainstem, septum, and ventromedial hypothalamus. It is considered to be the key neuropeptide involved in mediating the regulation of adaptive interactions between an individual and his/her environment. Its critical role in early life sensory processing and multi-modal integration underscores its key role for normal postnatal neurodevelopment. An early alteration in the oxytocin-system may disturb its maturation and may have short-term and long-term pathological consequences such as ASD. Figure 7 shows the neurodistribution of OT and OT receptor (OTR) have been predicted to be involved in the regulation of social functioning in ASD. Studies of mice in which the oxytocin receptor gene has been deleted revealed deficits in social interaction, including spending more time alone and self-grooming, compared to their wild-type counterparts. These behaviors are similar to those of individuals with ASD, suggesting that alterations in the oxytocin receptor during fetal development may help explain some of the social deficits characteristic of individuals with ASD. In fact, decreased flow of oxytocin between mother and fetus has been associated with autistic-like characteristics in adulthood (Taurines et al., 2016). Autistic-like behavior is observed when the receptor for OT is down-regulated, thereby reducing binding of OT in the central nervous system, resulting in social interaction deficiencies that are a hallmark of ASD. Low levels of plasma OT are associated with lower social and cognitive functioning.

Although much remains to be learned about the OT-OTR system and its role in social behavior, low levels of OT have been associated with other neurodegenerative disorders, as well. In Alzheimer patients, decreased OT binding site-density in the nucleus basalis of Meynert in the brain have been observed. Similarly, individuals with Parkinson's disease have fewer neurons with oxytocin receptors in the hypothalamus (Cataldo et al., 2018).

The exact causes of OTR down regulation are not entirely clear; however, as we have shown in the preceding section that certain ingredients in fragrances act like EDCs are linked to lower levels of the receptor (Bagasra & Heggen, 2018). Sex differences have also been observed, with females often exhibiting higher levels of oxytocin than males, which may help explain ASD male bias (Grinevich et al., 2015). Environmental factors have been linked to OTR expression changes during fetal development. Increased oxytocin receptor binding in the nucleus accumbens and CA3 region of the hippocampus has been observed with exposure to nicotine and ethanol.

In healthy adult humans, OT has indeed been found to enhance social interactions by modulating the activity of a wide range on neural substrates, particularly in the temporal lobes and in the left insula (Grinevich et al., 2015). OT administration is currently proposed as a treatment for autism as well for schizophrenia. In animal models, accumulating evidence suggests that the presence of impaired social phenotypes, species difference (mouse, rat, vole), sex and dosage strongly impact on the final outcome of OT administration. For example, while acute intranasal administration increased social behavior in healthy mice and rats; however, chronic intracerebroventricular OT injection increased sociability and reduced aggression in rats. Recently Busnelli & Chini (2017), have reviewed several animal models of ASD and neurodevelopmental disorders that display defects in the OT system, indicating that very different genetic/environmental insults can ultimately target this key system.

Figure 7. Developmental trajectories of oxytocin receptor in the rat brain. (A) Schematic time course of oxytocin receptor expression in the developing brain. (B) Oxytocin receptor expression in the infant brain around prenatal period P10–P13. Regions in which a transient oxytocin receptor expression is observed are colored in red. Regions in which oxytocin receptor expression is maintained to adult life are colored in blue.
(Adapted from: Valery Grinevich et al., 2014)

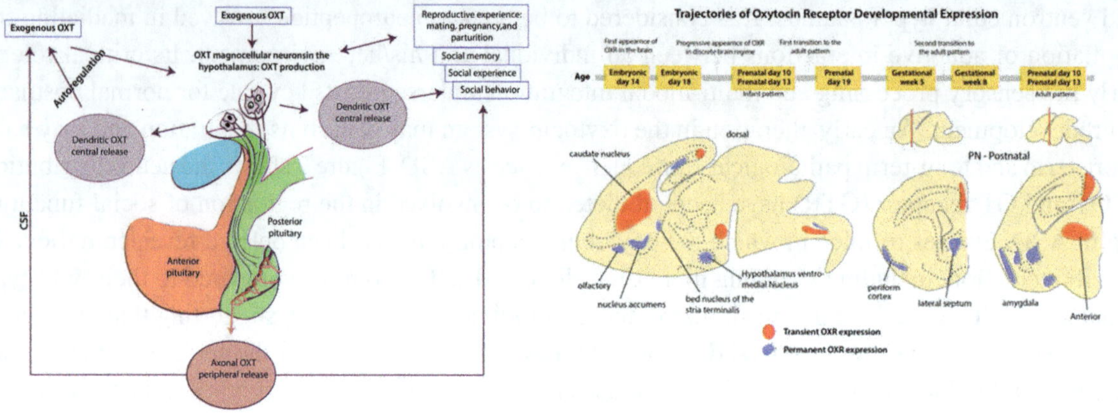

Another factor that could suppress OTR and binding is underdevelopment of olfactory bulb neurons, which has been observed in children with ASD (Bagasra & Heggen, 2018. Fragrances are known to bind to olfactory neurons in the brain and could contribute to this underdevelopment. Excessive exposure during critical periods of fetal development could overwhelm the natural system of regeneration, thereby inhibiting the normal development of the olfactory neurons. Chemical fragrance exposure may also contribute to axon thinning/elongation and increased synapses. Children with ASD are unable to eliminate excess neurons and synapses, resulting in excessive communication between different parts of the brain. The end result is inhibition of OT and AVP binding, which can result in neurodevelopmental delays and social impairment, as is observed in ASD.

FUTURE DIRECTIONS

The Major Unsolved Problems

Although advances have been made in pathogeneses of ASD, there are still certain epidemiological and clinical areas of autism that are yet to be studied. An example is the sporadic appearance and also clinical heterogeneity in some autistic members of a family and others that have "autistic traits," which suggests that autism is a complex neurodevelopmental disorder where the connections of environmental, genetic, and epigenetic influences all play a fundamental role (Tran & Miyaki, 2017). This broad spectrum in the definition of ASD suggests that the disease may be a result of exposure to certain environmental agents at different stages of fetal development, with variations in the dose of the environmental agents, and in varying combinations (Hallmayer et al., 2011, instead of primarily a genetic disorder (Bagasra & Pace, 2013).

Therefore, *in utero* exposures to TORCH microorganisms like, toxoplasmosis, measles, rubella, cytomegalovirus and herpes simplex virus, EBV, Zika virus and other microbes can manifest in a wide variety of birth defects. Similarly, such chemicals as valproic acid, thalidomide, methimazole, alcohol and numerous teratogenic agents can cause birth defects. This way all the injuries of infectious, toxic, or traumatic origin of the nerve system affecting the fetus during pregnancy, birth, or during the first years of life are susceptible to triggering the development of autism. We propose that one of the major contributors to autism is exposure to synthetic fragrances. Synthetic fragrances are an $85 billion dollar a year global industry. However, this industry is unregulated and the FDA does not require fragrance and cosmetic makers to test the ingredients found in the synthetic fragrances for any adverse effects on users or their unborn babies. Generally, a synthetic fragrance contains over 4,000 ingredients (Sarantis et al., 2010). In laboratory testing it becomes clear that many are mutagenic and contain endocrine disturbing chemicals (Bagasra et al., 2013). Compared to men, women use more synthetic fragrances. Many of these toxic and hormonal agents accumulate in women's ovaries or other fatty tissues and are released during pregnancy, reaching a fetal brain. This explains why older women are more likely to give birth to ASD children than the younger ones (Sealey et al., 2016). Most importantly, exposure of fetuses to fragrances' teratogenic, mutagenic and hormonal agents contained in synthetic fragrances would make these agents one of the primary culprits in the development ASD. All the perfumes we have analyzed by the Ames test showed mutagenic effects (Bagasra et al., 2013). This also may explain why there are thousands of genes that are associated with ASD.

CONCLUSION

Solving the Puzzle: Why There Is a Giant Spectrum in ASD

We believe that the main reason there is a spectrum in ASD is due to exposure to small doses of fragrances that are so ubiquitous in our daily lives. The synthetic chemicals that exert their effects by binding to specific receptors, in a developing fetal brain, binding specific receptors on different types of neurons, at various stages of fetal brain differentiation (i.e. OTR and AVPR). This binding can have several outcomes: i) neuronal death of those progenitors cells (Bagasra & Heggen, 2018), ii) stimulation of specific types of neurons that can disrupt the normal cell differential pathways, including cell migration (especially if during the early stages of brain development) or pruning, myelination, connectome processes, and neurotransmitters at later stages of development (Semple et al., 2013), and delaying apoptosis, that can disrupt the development process. Our preliminary data, shown in Figures 4-5 and Table 1 show that synthetic chemicals (i.e. synthetic fragrances, herbicides/pesticides and EDCs) hit specific brain progenitor cells in a developing fetus. For example, if a given chemicals enters a fetus brain and only binds to OTR positive neurons or olfactory neurons and either kills, inhibit migration, or natural process of apoptosis, those progenitor cells at very early stages of differentiation may radically change the signaling pathways of the brain, depleting or significantly reducing the repertoire of OTR+ neurons, potentially resulting in a child with impaired social communication or olfaction (smell). If we consider that in the majority of neuromodifying environmental factors we have tested so far (shown in Figures 4-5) OTR and AVPR neurons are depleted or significantly reduced in male developing brain cells as compared to female, Figure 7 A (left) shows the locations in an adult brain where OXT and AVP are secreted. Figure 7 (on the right) shows the sequences of OTR ontogenesis, therefore, in a 14 embryo OTR+ progenitors neurons are mostly clustered in caudate nucleus, olfactory area or nucleus accumbens, bed nucleus of the stria terminalis, and hypothalamus. The exposure to even a femtomolar (few molecules of synthetic chemicals) amount of chemicals that can bind OTR progenitor stem cells can partially or wholly impair the normal developments brain in these clustered areas. This is a significant point since in a majority of autism cases, the most affected area of a child are located in many of the same areas where OTR neurons are clustered (i.e. hypothalamus, caudate nucleus, nucleus accumbens, etc.). At the early stage of gestation (i.e. 5-week of gestation), there may be only few hundred to a few thousand OTR+ progenitors' neurons that would ultimately represent those faculties of communications or olfaction. The spectrum of ASD that would be observable in a 2-3 year old (at the time of diagnosis) would entirely depend on how many of OTR+ neurons were affected at 5-weeks of gestation. Now, if we consider a scenario where a fetus was exposed to the same neuromodifying chemical at a later stage of development (i.e. 8-24-week of gestation) then OTR+ neurons affected will be present in amygdala, periform cortex, and lateral septum. Interestingly, many of these areas coincide with defects that we observe in a majority of ASD children.

We hypothesize that the "spectrum" results not only from the type of the neuromodifying factors but also the dose and time and stages of fetal neurodevelopment. Therefore, if we compared the effects of a neuromodifying factor that affect OTR+ neurons at an early vs later days of gestation (i.e. 14 day embryo vs 24 week of gestation) at the same dose, then exposure at early stage of gestation would result in a much more severe form of autism as compared to the later stage of exposure, (when there would be millions of fully or partially differentiated OTR+ neuron, the effect may be less severe and a toddler would fall into close to normal range of ASD spectrum. One can think of this in the manner an oak tree grows. If one kills the seed, it will be akin to a miscarriage, if one cuts off a large branch of the tree when the oak tree is just a foot high (equitant to 15-week of fetal gestation), then the tree will be a lopsided oak (will show as a neurologic deficit of a typical autistic child). However, if one cuts multiple branches of the tree when an oak tree is one year old (32-week of gestation), the oak tree may grow almost normal but will be much bigger and those branches will regrow and a relatively small adverse effect will be observed. This will be an example of a child that exhibits what was previously referred to as High Functioning Autism (HFA) or Asperger's Disorder (Bagasra & Pace, 2013). We believe that in most of the cases one expects to see hypoconnectivity in some parts of the brain and hyperconnectivity in other areas of ASD brain. For example, Di Martino et al (Di Martino et al., 2013) used brain scans from 360 people with autism and 403 age-matched controls. They only included males in the study (since 90% of the individuals whose scans are in the database are male). They searched for abnormalities in brain function by evaluating functional connections throughout the brain, as well as in particular regions. They found a great deal of hypoconnectivity in the ASD brains, but some hyperconnectivity as well. Connectivity was weak among cortical regions, but strong between cortical regions and subcortical areas deep in the brain

We realize that all the pieces of the complex puzzle of fetal brain development are still absent and our presentation is highly simplistic. We are aware that different types of neurons grow with different rates in a developing brain and once a specific type of neuron is partially depleted (i. OTR+ neurons), other faster growing neurons take over and this may ultimately result in hyperconnectivity, not necessarily a good thing if they are not connected properly.

One of the biggest ironies of ASD is that it is considered primarily a genetic or inherited disease. We believe that this is based on incorrect assumptions and it has become part of the paradigm. We believe that classical autism results from environmental exposure to chemicals that human metabolomics is evolutionarily unfamiliar with). We lack the appropriate metabolic pathways to properly destroy 800,000 synthetic chemicals that have been introduced in the last 4 decades. No evolutionary mechanisms can evolve fast enough to adopt at a speed that can detoxify that many new chemicals. On the streets of France, where the perfumery is in vogue, every day dozens of new synthetic fragrances are introduced to fragrance industry, which are subsequently incorporated into new perfumes and in other products. The life forms on this earth have coevolved with hundreds of thousands or even millions of natural chemicals that can cause mutations if tested by the Ames test (1973). Three decades ago Ames and Gold tested thousands of natural and synthetic chemicals for their mutagenic and carcinogenic potential by using a mutant form of *Salmonella*. They catalogued potential cancer causing agents and showed that cigarette smoke was mutagenic, as was tris-BP, a flame retardant used in children's pajamas. Using that database, (the still-active Carcinogenic Potency Database), Ames and Gold showed that nearly half of the chemicals tested, whether natural or synthetic, in the Ames Test were carcinogens or mutagenic. They also determined that many plant chemicals have higher carcinogenic capacity than synthetic chemicals. However, Ames and Gold have missed one fundamental fact-co-evolution of all life forms—the life on earth have metabolic pathways—over 3,000 enzymes linked to highly complex metabolic pathways that can neutralize all-natural chemicals at a reasonable dose, neutralize adverse carcinogenic effects of the natural products-with one caveat! Doses of any chemical that may be considered tolerable can turn toxic if delivered in high doses. This is one of the fundamental principles (the 6-principles) that James Wilson established in 1956 (Ames & Gold, 1998). A simple and obvious example is sugar. Sugar, or more precisely glucose, is an essential chemical for life. Almost all the life forms on earth need glucose for survival and glycolytic and Krebs cycle are integrated cycles of life where 3,000 enzymes are linked that run like clockwork. But, if a human consumes too much sugar it will lead to diabetes, obesity and cancer. High consumption of sugar is toxic to men and women, it is harmful for the liver, it leads to insulin resistance, disturbs hormonal balance, release dopamine in the brain, and is the leading cause of obesity and cancer. It also leads to high cholesterol and increased incidence of heart attacks. High levels of blood sugar can put a person in a coma and lead to death. When a pregnant woman develops gestational diabetes during pregnancy, it can result in an overweight newborn that can develop serious illnesses after birth. Now, this is what happens when one consumes glucose-one of the most fundamental molecules of life, yet it can cause havoc when over consumed. Normally, this molecule is precisely balanced! Another, basic molecule that almost all life on earth consumes is alcohol. Here we are not referring to fermented ethanol but the molecules that results from glycolysis in our cells after glucose molecules is split into two. Our metabolic pathways efficiently consume alcohol molecules and convert them to energy. External consumption of alcohol is immediately utilized and converted into energy as long as the amount is low enough (blood alcohol content (BAC) of 0.08% or higher, can make a human neurologically impaired). This molecule is so powerful that it has open access to every cell in our body. However, exposure to this basic molecule after certain threshold results in depression of brain functions and at high enough doses can result in death. Fetal Alcohol Syndrome, a horrific disease of newborn, results from exposure of fetuses at high levels of alcohol *in utero* (Bjørklund et al., 2018). However, many of the synthetic chemicals (800,000 and counting) our metabolic system has never seen before, they have no way to detoxify them! We evolutionarily lack the metabolomics to destroy many of them. Therefore, even a minuscule amount of some of the chemicals can wreak havoc in a developing fetus. Many of them are EDCs, binding to hormone receptors in a developing fetus, distorting organogenesis and neurogenesis (Gore et al., 2015).

In summary, humans (among most of the complex organisms) lack co-evolutionary adaptation against synthetic chemicals. The majority of life forms lack the metabolic pathways to detoxify most of the synthetic chemicals. ASD is characterized by broad heterogeneity in severity as well as in intellectual and functional communication ability not only between individuals, but also within the same individual over time. In addition, a wide variety of medical and psychiatric conditions are associated with ASD, including intestinal disorders, epilepsy, and attention-deficit/hyperactivity disorder (ADHD). It is surmised that complex interactions between genes and environmental factors contribute to the broad heterogeneity observed in ASD. This complexity makes determining the underlying causes of and developing treatments for ASD very challenging. Additionally, without a clear and simplistic explanation of factors that may impact the development of ASD, it is difficult to guide pregnant women in regard to what chemicals they should avoid exposure to during stages of fetal development. We already have guidance recommending women avoid consuming larger quantities of fish during pregnancy due to potential exposure to high levels of mercury, avoiding the consumption of raw meat associated with risk of salmonella and toxoplasmosis, and avoiding any amount of alcohol. Further research and replication of the studies presented here will provide a clear picture of the role of environmental agents such as synthetic fragrances on the developing fetal brain and aid in the development of guidance for the avoidance of environmental exposure toxin exposures for pregnant women.

REFERENCES

American Psychiatric Association. (2013). DSM-5 Autism Spectrum Disorder Fact Sheet. Retrieved from https://www.psychiatry.org/.../DSM/APA_DSM-5-Autism-Spectrum-Disorder.pdf

Ames, B. N., Durston, W. E., Yamasaki, E., & Lee, F. D. (1973). Carcinogens are mutagens: A simple test system combining liver homogenates for activation and bacteria for detection. *Proceedings of the National Academy of Sciences of the United States of America*, *70*(8), 2281–2285. doi:10.1073/pnas.70.8.2281 PMID:4151811

Ames, B. N., & Gold, L. S. (1998). The causes and prevention of cancer: The role of environment. *Biotherapy (Dordrecht, Netherlands)*, *11*(2-3), 205–220. doi:10.1023/A:1007971204469 PMID:9677052

Annett, M. (2002). *Handedness and brain asymmetry: the right shift theory. East Sussex BN3 2FA*. Psychology Press.

Badzakova-Trajkov, G., Häberling, I. S., & Corballis, M. C. (2010). Cerebral asymmetries in monozygotic twins: An fMRI study. *Neuropsychologia*, *48*(10), 3086–3093. doi:10.1016/j.neuropsychologia.2010.06.020 PMID:20600189

Bagasra, O., Golkar, Z., Garcia, M., Rice, L. N., & Pace, D. G. (2013). Role of perfumes in pathogenesis of Autism. *Medical Hypotheses*, *80*(6), 795–803. doi:10.1016/j.mehy.2013.03.014 PMID:23578362

Bagasra, O., & Heggen, C. (2018). *Autism and Environmental Factors*. Wiley Blackwell Press. doi:10.1002/9781119042280

Bagasra, O., & Pace, D. G. (2013). Smell of Autism: Synthetic Fragrances and Cause for Allergies, Asthma, Cancer and Autism. OA Publishing London Reviews. *OA Autism*, *1*(2), 15. doi:10.13172/2052-7810-1-2-611

Bang du, Y., Lee, I.K. & Lee, B.M. (2011). Toxicological characterization of phthalic Acid. *Toxicological Research*, *4*, 191–203. doi:10.5487/TR.2011.27.4.191 PMID:24278572

Baron-Cohen, S., Auyeung, B., Nørgaard-Pedersen, B., Hougaard, D. M., Abdallah, M. W., Melgaard, L., ... Lombardo, M. V. (2015). Elevated fetal steroidogenic activity in autism. *Molecular Psychiatry*, *20*(3), 369–376. doi:10.1038/mp.2014.48 PMID:24888361

Bennike, N. H., Oturai, N. B., Müller, S., Kirkeby, C. S., Jørgensen, C., Christensen, A. B., ... Johansen, J. D. (2018). Fragrance contact allergens in 5588 cosmetic products identified through a novel smartphone application. *Journal of the European Academy of Dermatology and Venereology*, *1*(1), 79–85. doi:10.1111/jdv.14513 PMID:28796916

Bernier, R., Golzio, C., Xiong, B., Stessman, H. A., Coe, B. P., Penn, O., ... Eichler, E. E. (2014). Article: Disruptive CHD8 Mutations Define a Subtype of Autism Early in Development. *Cell*, *158*(2), 263–276. doi:10.1016/j.cell.2014.06.017 PMID:24998929

Bjørklund, G., Skalny, A. V., Rahman, M. M., Dadar, M., Yassa, H. A., Aaseth, J., ... Tinkov, A. A. (2018). Toxic metal(loid)-based pollutants and their possible role in autism spectrum disorder. *Environmental Research*, *166*, 234–250. doi:10.1016/j.envres.2018.05.020 PMID:29902778

Bonchak, J. G., Prouty, M. E., & de la Feld, S. F. (2018). Prevalence of Contact Allergens in Personal Care Products for Babies and Children. *Dermatitis*, *29*(2), 81–84. doi:10.1097/DER.0000000000000348 PMID:29494392

Breckpot, J., Thienpont, B., Vermeesch, J. R., Devriendt, K., Gewillig, M., & Allegaert, K. (2012). Differences in copy number variation between discordant monozygotic twins as a model for exploring chromosomal mosaicism in congenital heart defects. *Molecular Syndromology*, *2*(2), 81–87. doi:10.1159/000335284 PMID:22511896

Busnelli, M., & Chini, B. (2017). Molecular Basis of Oxytocin Receptor Signalling in the Brain: What we know and what we need to know. *Current Topics in Behavioral Neurosciences*. doi:10.1007/7854_2017_6

Cataldo, I., Azhari, A., & Esposito, G. A. (2018, February 13). Review of Oxytocin and Arginine-Vasopressin Receptors and Their Modulation of Autism Spectrum Disorder. *Frontiers in Molecular Neuroscience*, *11*, 27. doi:10.3389/fnmol.2018.00027 PMID:29487501

Centers for Disease Control and Prevention. (2014). CDC estimates 1 in 68 children has been identified with autism spectrum disease. Retrieved from https://www.cdc.gov/media/releases/2014/p0327-autism-spectrum disorder.html

Centers for Disease Control and Prevention. (2018). Autism Spectrum Disorders. Retrieved from https://www.cdc.gov/ncbddd/autism/index.html

Chaste, P., Roeder, K., & Devlin, B. (2017). The yin and yang of autism genetics: How rare de novo and common variations affect liability. *Annual Review of Genomics and Human Genetics*, *31*(18), 167–187. doi:10.1146/annurev-genom-083115-022647 PMID:28426285

Chown, N., & Hughes, L. (2016). History and first descriptions of autism: Asperger versus Kanner revisited. *Journal of Autism and Developmental Disorders*, *46*(6), 2270–2272. doi:10.100710803-016-2746-0 PMID:26883648

Christensen, D. L., Braun, K. V. N., Baio, J., Bilder, D., Charles, J., Constantino, J. N., ... Lee, L. C. (2018). Prevalence and characteristics of autism spectrum disorder among children aged 8 years—autism and developmental disabilities monitoring network, 11 sites, United States, 2012. *MMWR. Surveillance Summaries*, *65*(13). doi:10.15585/mmwr.ss6503a1

Clara, A. M., Strenn, B., Gans, O., Martinez, E., Kreuzinger, N., & Kroiss, H. (2005). Removal of selected pharmaceuticals, fragrances and endocrine disrupting compounds in a membrane bioreactor and conventional wastewater treatment plants. *Water Research*, *39*(19), 4797–4807. doi:10.1016/j.watres.2005.09.015 PMID:16242170

Colvert, E., Tick, B., McEwen, F., Stewart, C., Curran, S. R., Woodhouse, E., ... Bolton, P. (2015). Heritability of autism spectrum disorder in a UK population-based twin sample. *JAMA Psychiatry*, *72*(5), 415–423. doi:10.1001/jamapsychiatry.2014.3028 PMID:25738232

Costa, L. G., Aschner, M., Vitalone, A., Syversen, T., & Soldin, O. P. (2004). Developmental neuropathology of environmental agents. *Annual Review of Pharmacology and Toxicology*, *44*(1), 87–110. doi:10.1146/annurev.pharmtox.44.101802.121424 PMID:14744240

Darbre, P. D. (2018). Overview of air pollution and endocrine disorders. *International Journal of General Medicine*, *11*, 191–207. doi:10.2147/IJGM.S102230 PMID:29872334

Ribeiro, L. D. O. P., Vargas-Pinilla, P., Kappel, D. B., Longo, D., Ranzan, J., Becker, M. M., ... & Schuch, J. B. (2018, June 1). Evidence for Association Between OXTR Gene and ASD Clinical Phenotypes. *Journal of Molecular Neuroscience*. doi:10.100712031-018-1088-0

Fitzpatrick, T. B. E. A., Wolff, K., & Freedberg, I. M. & Austen, K.F. (1993). Dermatology in General Medicine. New York: McGraw Hill.

Hallmayer, J., Cleveland, S., Torres, A., Phillips, J., Cohen, B., Torigoe, T., ... Lotspeich, L. (2011). Genetic heritability and shared environmental factors among twin pairs with autism. *Archives of General Psychiatry*, *68*(11), 1095–1102. doi:10.1001/archgenpsychiatry.2011.76 PMID:21727249

Geschwind, D. H., & State, M. W. (2015). Series: Gene hunting in autism spectrum disorder: on the path to precision medicine. *Lancet Neurology*, *14*(11), 1109–1120. doi:10.1016/S1474-4422(15)00044-7 PMID:25891009

Gore, A. C., Chappell, V. A., Fenton, S. E., Flaws, J. A., Nadal, A., Prins, G. S., ... Zoeller, R. T. (2015). Executive Summary to EDC-2: The Endocrine Society's Second Scientific Statement on Endocrine-Disrupting Chemicals. *Endocrine Reviews*, *36*(6), 593–602. doi:10.1210/er.2015-1093 PMID:26414233

Grandjean, P., Berlin, A., Gilbert, M., & Penning, W. (1988). Preventing percutaneous absorption of industrial chemicals: The "skin" denotation. *American Journal of Industrial Medicine*, *14*(1), 97–107. doi:10.1002/ajim.4700140111 PMID:3044066

Grinevich, V., Desarménien, M. G., Chini, B., Tauber, M., & Muscatelli, F. (2015). Ontogenesis of oxytocin pathways in the mammalian brain: Late maturation and psychosocial disorders. *Frontiers in Neuroanatomy*, *20*(8), 164. doi:10.3389/fnana.2014.00164 PMID:25767437

Guy, R. H. (2010). Predicting the rate and extent of fragrance chemical absorption into and through the skin. *Chemical Research in Toxicology*, *23*(5), 864–870. doi:10.1021/tx9004105 PMID:20392076

Häberling, I. S., Badzakova-Trajkov, G., & Corballis, M. C. (2013). Asymmetries of the arcuate fasciculus in monozygotic twins: Genetic and nongenetic influences. *PLoS One*, *8*(1).

Hassall, R. (2017). How should applied psychologists conceptualise an autism spectrum disorder diagnosis and its predictive validity? *Educational and Child Psychology*, *34*(4), 20–29.

Hommer, R. E., & Swedo, S. E. (2015). Schizophrenia and autism-related disorders. *Schizophrenia Bulletin*, *41*(2), 313–314. doi:10.1093chbulbu188 PMID:25634913

Hughes, B. W., Sealey, L. A., & Bagasra, O. (2016). Mechanism of Male Gender Bias in Neuroblastoma Cell Lines Exposed to Fragrances: A Link to Autism Spectrum Disorder. *Expert Opinion on Environmental Biology*, *5*, 1–21.

Huguet, G., Benabou, M., & Bourgeron, T. (2016). The genetics of autism spectrum disorders. In *A time for metabolism and hormones* (pp. 101–129). Springer International Publishing. doi:10.1007/978-3-319-27069-2_11

Iossifov, I., O'Roak, B. J., Sanders, S. J., Ronemus, M., Krumm, N., Levy, D., ... Wigler, M. (2014). The contribution of de novo coding mutations to autism spectrum disorder. *Nature*, *515*(7526), 216–221. doi:10.1038/nature13908 PMID:25363768

Jeste, S. S., & Geschwind, D. H. (2014). Disentangling the heterogeneity of autism spectrum disorder through genetic findings. *Nature Reviews. Neurology*, *10*(2), 74–81. doi:10.1038/nrneurol.2013.278 PMID:24468882

Kalkbrenner, A. E., Schmidt, R. J., & Penlesky, A. C. (2014). Environmental chemical exposures and autism spectrum disorders: A review of the epidemiological evidence. *Current Problems in Pediatric and Adolescent Health Care*, *44*(10), 277–318. doi:10.1016/j.cppeds.2014.06.001 PMID:25199954

Kamatou, G. P., Vermaak, I., & Viljoen, A. M. (2012). Eugenol--from the remote Maluku Islands to the international market place: A review of a remarkable and versatile molecule. *Molecules (Basel, Switzerland)*, *17*(6), 6953–6981. doi:10.3390/molecules17066953 PMID:22728369

Kanner, L. (1951). The conception of wholes and parts in early infantile autism. *The American Journal of Psychiatry*, *108*(1), 23–26. doi:10.1176/ajp.108.1.23 PMID:14838158

Kim, J. H., Lee, D., Lim, H., Kim, T., Suk, K., & Seo, J. (2018). Risk assessment to human health: Consumer exposure to ingredients in air fresheners. *Regulatory Toxicology and Pharmacology*, *98*, 31–40. doi:10.1016/j.yrtph.2018.05.015 PMID:29857116

Krupp, D. R., Barnard, R. A., Duffourd, Y., Evans, S. A., Mulqueen, R. M., Bernier, R., ... O'Roak, B. J. (2017). Article: Exonic Mosaic Mutations Contribute Risk for Autism Spectrum Disorder. *American Journal of Human Genetics*, *101*(3), 369–390. doi:10.1016/j.ajhg.2017.07.016 PMID:28867142

Kuhn, T. (1939). The Structure of Scientific Revolutions. In O. Neurath (Ed.), Foundations of the unity of science (Vol. 2). Chicago, IL: University of Chicago Press.

Kulage, K., Smaldone, A., & Cohn, E. (2014). How will DSM-5 Affect Autism diagnosis? A Systematic literature review and meta-analysis. *Journal of Autism and Developmental Disorders*, *44*(8), 1918–1932. doi:10.100710803-014-2065-2 PMID:24531932

LaSalle, J. M. (2013). Epigenomic strategies at the interface of genetic and environmental risk factors for autism. *Journal of Human Genetics*, *58*(7), 396–401. doi:10.1038/jhg.2013.49 PMID:23677056

Marco, E. J., & Skuse, D. H. (2006). Autism-lessons from the X chromosome. *Social Cognitive and Affective Neuroscience*, *1*(3), 183–193. doi:10.1093can/nsl028 PMID:18985105

Maud, C., Ryan, J., McIntosh, J. E., & Olsson, C. A. (2018, May 29). The role of oxytocin receptor gene (OXTR) DNA methylation (DNAm) in human social and emotional functioning: A systematic narrative review. *BMC Psychiatry*, *18*(1), 154. doi:10.118612888-018-1740-9 PMID:29843655

McManus, I. C. (1980). Handedness in twins: A critical review. *Neuropsychologia*, *18*(3), 347–355. doi:10.1016/0028-3932(80)90130-X PMID:7191061

McPartland, J. C., Reichow, B., & Volkmar, F. R. (2012). Sensitivity and specificity of proposed DSM-5 Diagnostic criteria for autism spectrum disorder. *Journal of the American Academy of Child and Adolescent Psychiatry*, *51*(4), 368–383. doi:10.1016/j.jaac.2012.01.007 PMID:22449643

Moneim, A. E. A. (2015). Mercury-induced neurotoxicity and neuroprotective effects of berberine. *Perspective*, *10*, 881–882. PMID:26199596

Morley, W.A. & Seneff, S. (2014). Diminished brain resilience syndrome: A modern day neurological pathology of increased susceptibility to mild brain trauma, concussion, and downstream neurodegeneration. *Surgical Neurology International*, *5*, 97.

Nematollahi, N., Doronila, A., Mornane, P. J., Duan, A., Kolev, S. D., & Steinemann, A. (2018). Volatile chemical emissions from fragranced baby products. *Air Quality, Atmosphere & Health*, *11*(7), 785–790. doi:10.100711869-018-0593-1 PMID:30147808

Novarino, G., El-Fishawy, P., Kayserili, H., Meguid, N., Scott, E., Schroth, J., ... Gleeson, J. (2012). Mutations in BCKD-kinase Lead to a Potentially Treatable Form of Autism with Epilepsy. *Science*, *338*(6105), 394–397. doi:10.1126cience.1224631 PMID:22956686

O'Roak, B. J., Vives, L., Fu, W., Egertson, J. D., Stanaway, I. B., Phelps, I. G., ... Munson, J. (2012). Multiplex targeted sequencing identifies recurrently mutated genes in autism spectrum disorders. *Science*, *338*(6114), 1619–1622.

O'Roak, B. J., Vives, L., Girirajan, S., Karakoc, E., Krumm, N., Coe, B. P., ... Eichler, E. E. (2012). Sporadic autism exomes reveal a highly interconnected protein network of de novo mutations. *Nature*, *485*(7397), 246–250. doi:10.1038/nature10989 PMID:22495309

Ozonoff, S. (2012). Editorial Perspective: Autism Spectrum Disorders in DSM-5 – an historical perspective and the need for change. *Journal of Child Psychology and Psychiatry, and Allied Disciplines, 53*(10), 1092–1094. doi:10.1111/j.1469-7610.2012.02614.x PMID:22970941

Patel, S. (2017). Fragrance compounds: The wolves in sheep's clothings. *Medical Hypotheses, 102*, 106–111. doi:10.1016/j.mehy.2017.03.025 PMID:28478814

Poduri, A., & Christopher, A. (2013). Somatic Mutation, Genomic Variation, and Neurological Disease. *Science, 341*(6141), 1237758. doi:10.1126cience.1237758 PMID:23828942

Richards, C., Jones, C., Groves, L., Moss, J., & Oliver, C. (2015). Prevalence of autism spectrum disorder phenomenology in genetic disorders: A systematic review and meta-analysis. *The Lancet. Psychiatry, 2*(10), 909–916. doi:10.1016/S2215-0366(15)00376-4 PMID:26341300

Robertson, K., Stafford, T., Benedicto, J., & Hocking, N. (2013). Autism assessment: The Melton health model. *Journal of Paediatrics and Child Health, 49*(12), 1057–1062. doi:10.1111/jpc.12303 PMID:23782166

Rodier, P. M. (1994). Vulnerable periods and processes during central nervous system development. *Environmental Health Perspectives, 102*(Suppl. 2), 121–124. PMID:7925182

Sanders, J. (2009). Qualitative or quantitative differences between Asperger's disorder and Autism? Historical Considerations. *Journal of Autism and Developmental Disorders, 39*(11), 1560–1567. doi:10.100710803-009-0798-0 PMID:19548078

Sandin, S., Lichtenstein, P., Kuja-Halkola, R., Larsson, H., Hultman, C. M., & Reichenberg, A. (2014). The familial risk of autism. *Journal of the American Medical Association, 311*(17), 1770–1777. doi:10.1001/jama.2014.4144 PMID:24794370

Sarantis, H., Naidenko, O. V., Gray, S., Houlihan, J., & Malkan, S. (2010). Not so sexy: The health risks of secret chemicals in fragrance. Breast Cancer Fund, Commonwealth and Environmental Working Group. Retrieved from https://www.ewg.org/sites/default/files/report/SafeCosmetics_FragranceRpt.pdf

Schopler, E., Mesibov, G. B., & Kunce, L. (1998). *Asperger Syndrome or High-Functioning Autism? Current Issues in Autism*. Berlin, Germany: Plenum Press. doi:10.1007/978-1-4615-5369-4

Sealey, L. A., Hughes, B. W., Sriskanda, A. N., Guest, J. R., Gibson, A. D., Johnson-Williams, L., ... Bagasra, O. (2016). Environmental Factors in the Development of Autism Spectrum Disorders. *Environment International, 88*, 288–298. doi:10.1016/j.envint.2015.12.021 PMID:26826339

Sealey, L. A., Hughes, B. W., Steinemann, A., Pestaner, J. P., Pace, D. G., & Bagasra, O. (2015). Role of Environmental Factors in Autism Development and Male Bias: Neuromodifying Effects of Fragrance. *Environmental Research, 142*, 731–738. doi:10.1016/j.envres.2015.08.025 PMID:26408793

Semple, B.D., Blomgren, K., Gimlin, K. & Ferriero, D.M. (2013). Brain development in rodents and humans: Identifying benchmarks of maturation and vulnerability to injury across species. *Progress in Neurobiology, 106*, 1-16.

Silberman, S. (2016). *NeuroTribes*. New York: Avery.

Slominski, A., Majewska, M. A., Skobowiat, C., Zbytek, B., Slominski, R. M., & Steketee, J. D. (2012). Sensing the environment: Regulation of local and global homeostasis by the skin neuroendocrine system. *Advances in Anatomy, Embryology, and Cell Biology*, *212*, 1–115. doi:10.1007/978-3-642-19683-6_1 PMID:22894052

Slominski, A., & Wortsman, J. (2000). Neuroendocrinology of the skin. *Endocrine Reviews*, *21*, 457–487. PMID:11041445

Slominski, A., Zmijewski, M., Zbytek, B., Tobin, D., Tobin, D. J., Theoharides, T. C., & Rivier, J. (2013). Key Role of CRF in the Skin Stress Response System. *Endocrine Reviews*, *34*(6), 827–884. doi:10.1210/er.2012-1092 PMID:23939821

Slominski, A. T., Hardeland, R., Zmijewski, M. A., Slominski, R. M., Reiter, R. J., & Paus, R. (2018). Melatonin: A cutaneous perspective on its production, metabolism and functions. *The Journal of Investigative Dermatology*, *138*(3), 490–499. doi:10.1016/j.jid.2017.10.025 PMID:29428440

Slominski, A. T., Manna, P. R., & Tuckey, R. C. (2015). On the role of skin in the regulation of local and systemic steroidogenic activities. *Steroids*, *103*, 72–78. doi:10.1016/j.steroids.2015.04.006 PMID:25988614

Slominski, A. T., Zmijewski, A. M., Plonka, P., Szaflarski, J., & Paus, R. (2018). How ultraviolet light touches the brain and endocrine system through skin, and why. *Endocrinology*, *159*(5), 1992–2007. doi:10.1210/en.2017-03230 PMID:29546369

Slominski, A.T., Zmijewski, M.A., Skobowiat, C., Zbytek, B., Slominski, R.M., Steketee, J.D. (2012). Sensing the environment: regulation of local and global homeostasis by the skin's neuroendocrine system. *Adv Anat Embryol Cell Biol.*, *212*, 1-115.

Sowndhararajan, K., & Kim, S. (2016). Influence of Fragrances on Human Psychophysiological Activity: With Special Reference to Human Electroencephalographic Response. *Scientia Pharmaceutica*, *84*(4), 724–751. doi:10.3390cipharm84040724 PMID:27916830

Steiling, W., Bascompta, M., Carthew, P., Catalano, G., Corea, N., D'Haese, A., ... Singal, M. (2014). Principle considerations for the risk assessment of sprayed consumer products. *Toxicology Letters*, *227*(1), 41–49. doi:10.1016/j.toxlet.2014.03.005

Steinemann, A. (2018). National Prevalence and Effects of Multiple Chemical Sensitivities. *Journal of Occupational and Environmental Medicine*, *60*(3), e152–e156. doi:10.1097/JOM.0000000000001272 PMID:29329146

Street, M., Angelini, S., Bernasconi, S., Burgio, E., Cassio, A., Catellani, C., ... Gargano, G. (2018). Current knowledge on endocrine disrupting chemicals (EDCs) from animal biology to humans, from pregnancy to adulthood: Highlights from a national Italian meeting. *International Journal of Molecular Sciences*, *19*(6), 1647. doi:10.3390/ijms19061647

Taurines, R., Schwenck, R. B., Lyttwin, B., Schecklmann, M., Jans, T., Reefschlager, L., ... Romanos, M. (2016). Oxytocin plasma concentrations in children and adolescents with autism spectrum disorder: Correlation with autistic symptomatology. *Attention Deficit and Hyperactivity Disorders*, *6*(3), 231–239. doi:10.100712402-014-0145-y PMID:24989441

Taylor, K. M., Weisskopf, M., & Shine, J. (2014). Human exposure to nitro musks and the evaluation of their potential toxicity: An overview. *Environmental Health, 13*(1), 14. doi:10.1186/1476-069X-13-14 PMID:24618224

Tick, B., Bolton, P., Happé, F., Rutter, M., & Rijsdijk, F. (2016). Heritability of autism spectrum disorders: A meta-analysis of twin studies. *Journal of Child Psychology and Psychiatry, and Allied Disciplines, 57*(5), 585–595. doi:10.1111/jcpp.12499 PMID:26709141

Tran, N. V., & Miyake, K. (2017). Neurodevelopmental Disorders and Environmental Toxicants: Epigenetics as an Underlying Mechanism. *International Journal of Genomics, 7526592*. doi:10.1155/2017/7526592 PMID:28567415

Volk, H. E., Kerin, T., Lurmann, F., Hertz-Picciotto, I., McConnell, R., & Campbell, D. B. (2014). Autism spectrum disorder: Interaction of air pollution with the MET receptor tyrosine kinase gene. *Epidemiology (Cambridge, MA), 25*(1), 44–47. doi:10.1097/EDE.0000000000000030 PMID:24240654

Waterhouse, L., London, R., & Gillberg, C. (2016). ASD Validity *Rev. Journal of Autism and Developmental Disorders, 3*(4), 302–329. doi:10.100740489-016-0085-x

Weedon, D. (2010). *Weedon's skin pathology*. Churchill Livingstone Elsevier.

Wilson, J. G. (1973). *Environment and Birth Defects*. New York: Academic Press.

Wolff, S. (2004). The history of autism. *European Child & Adolescent Psychiatry, 13*(4), 201–207. doi:10.100700787-004-0363-5 PMID:15365889

Wolkoff, P., & Nielsen, G. D. (2017). Effects by inhalation of abundant fragrances in indoor air - An overview. *Environment International, 101*, 96–107. doi:10.1016/j.envint.2017.01.013 PMID:28126407

Zablotsky, B., Black, L. I., Maenner, M. J., Schieve, L. A., & Blumberg, S. J. (2015). Estimated prevalence of autism and other developmental disabilities following questionnaire changes in the 2014 National Health Interview Survey. *National Health Statistics Reports*. Retrieved from https://stacks.cdc.gov/view/cdc/38790

Chapter 4
Arsenic Exposures, Poisoning, and Threat to Human Health:
Arsenic Affecting Human Health

Arpitha Chikkanna
Indian Institute of Science, India

Luv Mehan
Indian Institute of Science, India

Sarath P. K.
Indian Institute of Science, India

Devanita Ghosh
https://orcid.org/0000-0002-6856-3868
Indian Institute of Science, India

ABSTRACT

Arsenic (As) is a naturally occurring metalloid which induces high toxicity to both human and animal health. Although As has some applications in industrial, medicinal and agricultural fields, the increasing concentrations of As in drinking water sources had made it a potential threat to living organisms. Inorganic As is naturally present in groundwater and is adsorbed by plants and crops through the irrigation system. This leads to its accumulation in crops and translocation to humans and animals through food. Increased levels of As can cause various health disorders through acute and chronic exposures such as gastrointestinal, hepatic, respiratory, cardiovascular, integumentary, renal, neurological, and reproductive disorders including stillbirth and infant mortality. Arsenic is also capable of inducing epigenetic changes, thereby causing gene mutations. This chapter focuses on the possible sources of As, leading to environmental contamination and followed by its hazardous effects which pave the way to various human health manifestations.

DOI: 10.4018/978-1-5225-7635-8.ch004

INTRODUCTION

The earth's crust is naturally comprised of approximately 4.0×10^{16} kg of arsenic (As) (Jang et al., 2016; Bhattacharya et al., 2002). In the environment, As is released either by natural processes or anthropogenic actions and once released it cannot be degraded or destroyed. Hence, it circulates in the environment and further gets easy access to plants and crops through groundwater system and finally reaches human body. Inorganic forms of As such as trivalent Arsenite [As (III)] and pentavalent Arsenate [As (V)] are the most extensive and toxic forms present in groundwater than organic As. However, the food contains both organic and inorganic As (Naujokas et al., 2013). Inorganic As (As III and As V) gets dissolved in groundwater and pumped into sub-surface soils through the irrigation system. Since, groundwater is a major source of drinking water; the population in different parts of the world are exposed to high levels of As mainly through contaminated groundwater. The most As affected places documented till now include Chile, Hungary, Mexico, U.S.A, Vietnam, Argentina, Bangladesh, and India with maximum exposure in states of West Bengal (McCarty et al., 2011; Ghosh et al., 2017; 2018a, 2018b).The increasing acute and chronic effects of As on human health have resulted in the classification of As as a class I carcinogen by the International Agency of Research on Cancer (IARC; Hong et al., 2014).

Pyrite minerals are one of the major natural sources of As in environment, whereas, anthropogenic sources include agricultural chemicals such as pesticides, insecticides, and herbicides; mining, manufacturing industries, coal burning, copper chromate arsenic-treated wood and wood preservatives (Ravenscroft et al., 2011; Naujokas et al., 2013; Jiang et al., 2013). Thus, As contamination is an equally challenging threat to both human health and sustainable farming (Brammer, 2008).

Constant usage of As-contaminated groundwater for drinking and irrigation purposes has led to several health manifestations in human body, generally termed as arsenicosis (Pimparkar & Bhave, 2010). This includes intestinal, renal, lung and bladder disorders, dermal effects and cancer in various organs. Arsenic toxicity also causes neurological dysfunction, cardiovascular diseases, and immunity-related disorders (Figure 1). Arsenic ingestion through water and food causes reproductive problems in men and women, with various maternity related issues in women such as stillbirth, early abortions, and premature birth. Notably, reports suggest that children from various As affected places may suffer from malnutrition, massive weight loss and finally death (Shankar et al., 2014; Jang et al., 2016).

This chapter aims at describing the various sources of As exposure which aids in understanding the role of human behaviour and activities in increasing global As issues. In addition, it highlights the acute and chronic health manifestations caused by As toxicity.

BACKGROUND: ARSENIC EXPOSURE

Arsenic Exposure Through Drinking Water

Water is an essential product for the sustainability of life and functioning of the global ecosystem. Ground or surface water supplies are sources of fresh water used for human activities. Other than surface water, groundwater is utilized as an important source for drinking purpose in many places around the world and As has been found in dissolved form or particulate form in many groundwater aquifers across the globe. The maximum contaminant level of As in potable water established by World Health Organisa-

Figure 1. Schematic representation of arsenic induced human health manifestations

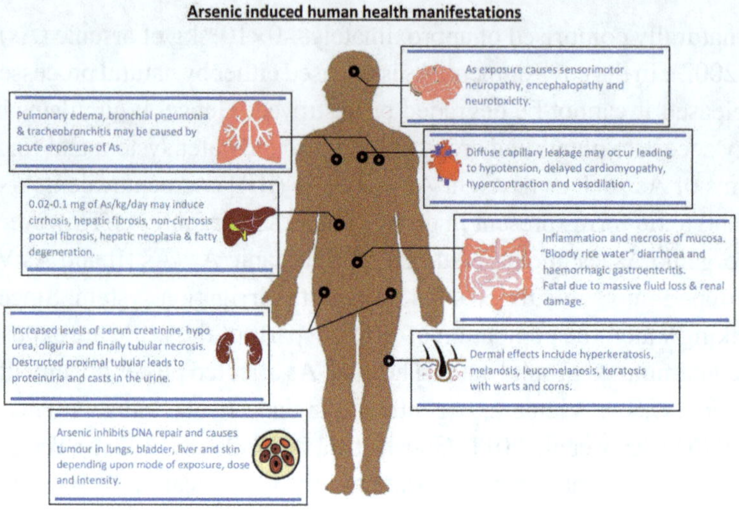

tion (WHO) is 10 μg As/l (Guidelines for drinking water quality, 2011; Smith et al., 2002).Whereas, developing countries have set their national standard values up to 0.05 mg/L (Rahman et al., 2009; Milton et al., 2012; Jang et al.,2016; Fisher et al., 2017).The present-day standard of Mexican MCL for As in drinking water is 25 μg/l which exceeds WHO guidance (Fisher et al., 2017). A large population with much of the rural communities in India and Bangladesh still rely on groundwater which is contaminated with As concentration $\geq$ 50 μg/l (Ghosh et al., 2014; 2015a; 2015b; 2018; Ghosh and Bhadury, 2018; Raessler, 2018). In India, according to Bureau of Indian Standards, required limit of As in drinking water is 0.01 mg/L with a permissible limit of 0.05 mg/L (Drinking Water- Specification, 2012). The solubility of arsenic in water depends on measurements such as pH, temperature, redox conditions and solution composition.

Arsenic Exposure Through Soil and Dietary Intake

Arsenic which is ubiquitous in the sediments can be present in concentrations of ca. 6-7 mg/kg (Sparks, 2003; Gillispie et al., 2015). Though As occurs naturally in soil environment, it is readily taken up by plants and crops through contaminated groundwater. Use of pesticides, insecticides and, herbicides rich in arsenicals is an add-on to the As pollution. Globally, As content in soil ranges from 0.01 to >600mg/kg (Hughes et al., 2011). Soil texture plays an important role during As contamination of soil. Large amounts of As accumulate in alluvial and organic soils compared to fewer amounts in sandy soils (Mandal et al., 2002; Jang et al., 2016; Ghosh et al., 2018). At neutral pH, As gets absorbed to clay particles which helps in trapping and transportation of As from soil to plants and crops (Jang et al., 2016). A range of 0.5-1 mg/kg of As in food is the limit set for consumption depending on the average ingestion of a particular agricultural product by an adult in different nations. Potato tuber and roots of sugar beets exhibit As concentration of 1.05mg/kg and 5.4 mg/kg respectively, in a study carried out in central Spain (Moyano et al., 2009). A study from Bangladesh reports the presence of As at exceeding levels in vegetables such as taro ranging between 0.09-3.99 mg/kg, potatoes with0.07-1.36 mg/kg and water spinach with0.10–1.53

mg/kg (Das et al., 2004). Since rice is an important crop grown in flooded fields with anaerobic topsoil, it is the most affected crop through As contamination. Compared to other crops such as maize, wheat, and vegetables which are grown with less water, rice irrigation requires more water which relies on groundwater resource. In one of the major As-contaminated regions, Ganga-Meghna-Brahmaputra basin, As-contaminated water for irrigation has a concentration of 0.318-0.643mg/L, whereas contamination in soil ranges from 5.7-9.7 mg/kg (Bhattacharya et al., 2010; Ghosh et al., 2014; 2015a; 2015b). Quality of agricultural products like rice, vegetable, and pulses in such areas are greatly affected. Potatoes, boro rice grain, aman rice grain, cauliflower and radish from such region exhibits As concentration of 0.654 mg/kg, 0.451 mg/kg, 0.334 mg/kg, 0.293 mg/kg and 0.344 mg/kg respectively. Though the concentrations of all these crops do not exceed the food hygiene concentration of 1 mg/kg, the limit set by WHO, daily consumption of such food products in excess leads to various health disorders which could be fatal for human and animal life (Bhattacharya et al., 2010). According to European Food Safety Authority (EFSA) the day-to-day exposure to As is contributed by dietary intake through cereal, cereal based products and dairy products with the mean concentration of 0.20 to 1.37 μg/kg b.w. per day among infants, toddlers and younger children; while the concentration ranged between 0.09 to 0.38 μg/kg b.w. per day among the adult population (EFSA, 2009; Signes-Pastor et al., 2016).

Arsenic Exposure Through Industries

Industrial arsenic exposures are mainly in the form of by-products, since, As compounds are used in processing and manufacturing of pharmaceutical products, pesticides, glass, sulphuric acid, paints, dyes, textiles, metallurgy, ammunition and wood preservative (Ravenscroft et al., 2011). A major compound of As, namely Arsenic trioxide (ATO) is the major As source produced for industries (Smith et al., 1998; Jang et al., 2016). During the 19th century, As containing pigments named Paris green and Scheele's green ($CuHAsO_3$), were being used in paints and dyes which were utilized in wallpaper, toys, clothes, and paper (Bissen & Frimmel, 2003; Hugheset al., 2011). It is widely accepted that biotransformation/methylation of As compounds present in wallpapers into arsine (AsH_3), monomethylarsine (H_2AsCH_3), dimethylarsine [HAs(CH3)2] and trimethylarsine [As(CH3)3] by the action of moulds and bacteria under anaerobic conditions was the main cause of illness to human health. A dose of 250mg/m^3 arsine with the exposure time of 30 minutes is reported fatal for human health (Bissen & Frimmel, 2003).

Alloy industries utilize As compounds like sulph-arsenide for the manufacturing of copper (Lechtman & Klein, 1999). Arsenic is added to copper and copper-based alloys to induce corrosion resistance in metals (Ishiguro, 1992). It is estimated that 62,000 tons/annum of As is emitted by nearly 80% of smelters which pollutes soil and air producing As dust and ATO vapours (Hughes et al., 2011; Bissen & Frimmel, 2003). Notably, a study reports five death cases due to intake of ATO through illicit liquor (Moonshine) poisoned with As (Gerhardt, 1980).

Another compound that is pesticidal, insecticidal, fungicidal and rodenticidal in nature known as Copper Chromated Arsenate or Chromated Copper Arsenate (CCA) was being used in the early 1940s as a wood preservative for playground structures, picnic tables, decks, fences, and walkways. Since, CCA contains 34% of inorganic As, the compound was banned by EPA in 2003. In addition, burning of CCA coated furniture is restricted as burning of such wood emits As gas which causes adverse health effects (Chen & Olsen, 2016).

Mining and Coal

Global upper crust on an average has As abundance of 6 mg/kg, whereas it is mainly associated with sulphide minerals such as orpiment (As_2S_3), loellingite ($FeAs_2$), niccolite (NiAs), realgar (AsS), mispickel (FeAsS), cobaltite (CoAsS), enargite (Cu_3AsS_4) and tennantite ($Cu_{12}As_4S_{13}$) (Bissen & Frimmel, 2003). There are possibilities of leaching of As from sulphide ores by the means of mining sludge water. Beneficiation process of metal sulphides also increases the concentration of leached out As, since ores that host As are treated with chemical pre-smelting. Mining of gold also contributes to As exposures. Soil near gold smelters can be contaminated to a concentration of 0.5-9.3g/kg (Bissen&Frimmel, 2003). Coal is an essential fossil fuel used in power plants. Since, burning of coal results in emission of As compounds, it is an add-on to As pollution. It is reported that the concentration of As in coal ranges from 2 to 82 mg As/kg, depending on the geological origin (Smith et al., 1998; Guo et al., 2004). Globally, many countries are affected by As contamination through mining with maximum exposure in places like Ghana in Africa, Nicaragua in South America, France and Portugal in Europe, South west England and Australia (Wickre et al., 2004; Fillol et al., 2010; Pearce et al., 2012; Dartey et al., 2013). Chile is one of the few countries with 12% of its total population tackling As contamination occurring mostly through mining activities (Sancha and O' Rayan, 2008).

Other Exposures: Arsenic as Medicinal Use

In the 1920s, Lewisite or Chlorovinyl dichloroarsine had been used as a chemical warfare vesicant. It is known to cause skin burns and lung irritation when in contact with even at low concentrations (Li et al., 2016). In medical sciences, ATO (As_2O_3) is used as a weapon to fight cancer as it has therapeutic efficacy for Acute Promyelocytic Leukemia (APL) with high survival chances (Hu et al., 2005). The compound is known to cause differentiation in APL cells (at low concentration dose of 0.1-0.5µmol/l) and inhibition of cell proliferation and apoptosis (with a comparatively high concentration dose of 0.5-2.0 µmol/l) (Lengfelder et al., 2012). It is reported that excess use of ATO causes differentiation of red blood cells from bone marrow with abnormalities such as irregular-size mature red cells and binuclear early erythroblasts. Other side effects include anorexia, vomiting, high chance of diarrhea, skin pigmentation and change in liver functioning (Zhang, 2017). The most utilization of As compounds in industries started in early and middle of 20th century, but with the awareness of harmful consequences, many of the uses have been banned. Applications such as in chemotherapeutic treatments, glass manufacturing, alloy industries, and mining are the sources of As exposure that are continued till now

ARSENIC POISONING AND HEALTH MANIFESTATIONS

Epigenetic Effects

Arsenic is considered as a non-mutagenic human carcinogen that induces tumours through DNA methylation leading to epigenetic changes. Epigenetics is the study of heritable changes in gene expression (Phenotype) without involving changes in DNA sequence (Genotype; fig. 2). The changes in gene expression during epigenetic include acetylation, ubiquitination, histone phosphorylation, methylation and micro RNA expression (Collotta et al., 2013; Heerboth et al., 2014; Abdul et al., 2015).

Arsenic-induced alterations in DNA methylation: Studies report DNA hypomethylation and site-specific DNA hypermethylation as the most studied As-induced epigenetic changes (Reichard & Puga, 2010; Suzuki et al., 2013; Abdul et al., 2015; Meakin et al., 2017). Arsenic induced gene methylation also causes expression of onco-genes and/or down regulation of tumour suppressor genes (Feinberg & Tycko, 2004). Several mechanisms have explained the As induced epigenetic changes in DNA methylation, however, major steps include: (Reichard & Puga, 2010; Ruiz-Hernandez et al., 2015; Meakin et al., 2017).

1. Initially, As acts on DNMT- DNA methyltransferase enzyme. Since, DNMT is an enzyme that promotes DNA methylation, As affects this mechanism by altering and reducing the activity and expression of DNMT.
2. DNMT uses S-adenosine methionine (SAM) substrate as a methyl donor to carry out CpG methylation. Since, SAM is a major co-factor for As metabolism, As decreases the availability of SAM for DNMT activity.

Arsenic-induced alterations in histone modifications: Histones are proteins which help in supercoiling of DNA. Any unspecified modifications to histones impact alterations in DNA supercoiling and hinder the formation of the nucleosome. Arsenic affects the nucleosome formation by acting on enzymes that modify histones. Mainly arsenicals act on histone methyltransferases, histone acetyltransferases (HAT), histone deacetylases (HDAC) and kinases, thereby interfering in the formation of nucleosome causing changes in phenotype (Grewal & Jia, 2007; Pournara et al., 2016; Meakin et al., 2017; fig 2).

Arsenic-induced alterations in microRNA expression: microRNA are small non-coding RNA molecules of 21-33 nucleotides that regulate gene expression by complementarily binding to 3' or 5' regions of mRNA. Arsenic compounds also interfere in microRNA expression by inducing environmentally responsive transcription factors that hinder the action of original transcription factors in microRNA mechanism. Since, transcription factors are key regulators in microRNA gene expression; any alterations in the mechanism by the action of As compounds affect microRNA expression (Arora et al., 2013; Sollome et al., 2016; Meakin et al., 2017).

Figure 2. Schematic representation of epigenetic effects due to inorganic arsenic exposure

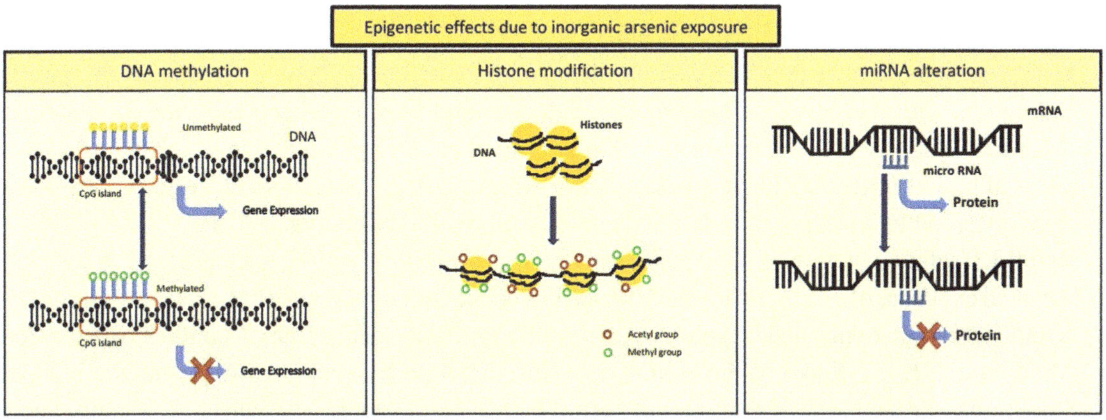

Epigenetic changes caused by As toxicity results in several diseases including cardiovascular, neurological, metabolic disorders and cancer of various types. Future research needs to focus on scientific gaps in understanding the detailed mechanism of action of As on epigenetic changes.

Clinical Effects

Arsenic exposure leads to both acute and chronic health manifestations in humans (table 1; fig. 1. Acute arsenic poisoning mostly occurs through accidental ingestion of pesticides and insecticides, and less commonly from suicidal attempts. However, long-term As exposure leads to chronic manifestations which involve multi-organ damage (Ratnaike, 2003). The clinical health manifestations include:

1. **Gastrointestinal Effects:** The As chemical when ingested, gets absorbed into the gastrointestinal system. The effects are comparatively more acute when As is ingested, than when it is inhaled or dermally absorbed. The initial symptoms include metallic taste, garlic-like taste and odour, dry mouth, burning lips and dysphagia (Saha et al., 1999; Abernathy, 2003). The manifestations that emanate because of this include nausea, vomiting, crampy abdominal pain, and diarrhoea. These manifestations are detected only above exposure levels of 0.01 mg As/kg/day (Saha et al., 1999). The absorbed As produces a high degree of damage to the submucosal capillary, which results in the inflammation and necrosis of mucosa and sub-mucosa of stomach, intestine and gut wall (Tchounwou et al., 2003). A "bloody rice water" diarrhea may also develop leading to haemorrhagic gastroenteritis (Ratnaike, 2003). Chronic exposure of As is reported to result in esophagitis, gastritis, hepatic steatosis, anorexia, malabsorption and weight loss. Finally, death occurs due to massive fluid loss, circulatory collapse and renal damage (Mandal, 2002; Tchounwou et al., 2003; Ratnaike, 2003; Abdul et al., 2015). Gastroenteritis was reported in the population of Inner Mongolian region of China which was caused due to the consumption of arsenic-contaminated drinking water (50-1860 µg/L) (Guo et al, 2007; Mazumder, 2008; Abdul et al., 2015). The dyspepsia symptoms were also reported in few individuals of West Bengal, India while screening a group of As-exposed population (Abdul et al., 2015).
2. **Hepatic Effects:** The repeated chronic exposures of As over periods of months or years results in its accumulation in the liver, leading to hepatic damage. The initial clinical symptoms reported include bleeding oesophageal varices, jaundice, enlarged tender liver, ascites, impaired mitochondrial functions and damage, and impaired porphyrin metabolism (Saha et al., 1999; Mandal& Suzuki, 2002; Abdul et al., 2015). Chronic arsenic exposure (0.02 to 0.1 mg As/kg/day) has been observed to induce cirrhosis, hepatic fibrosis, non-cirrhosis portal fibrosis, hepatic neoplasia and fatty degeneration. Elevated levels of hepatic enzymes in blood have also been reported in some cases (Mandal& Suzuki, 2002; Kapaj et al., 2006; Abdul et al., 2015). Liver expansion with increased levels of globulin, alkaline phosphatase, alanine amino-transferase and aspartate amino-transferase were observed in As-exposed individuals in West Bengal (Abdul et al., 2015).
3. **Renal Effects:** Kidneys being the major system of arsenic elimination, gets affected by long-term repeated exposure of arsenic. The renal system is also the principal site for conversion of pentavalent arsenic into more toxic and less soluble trivalent arsenic (Saha et al., 1999; Mandal& Suzuki, 2002; Abdul et al., 2015). Some of the clinical manifestations of the acute exposure include increased blood urea nitrogen, increased levels of serum creatinine, hypo urea, oliguria and finally leading to tubular necrosis (Abdul et al., 2015). Glomerular damage leads to haematuria. Proximal tubular

cells get destructed, leading to proteinuria and casts in urine. Arsine induced haemolysis is reported to cause acute tubular necrosis with partial or complete renal failure requiring haemodialysis for the removal of haemoglobin bound arsenic (Tchounwou et al., 2003).

4. **Cardiovascular Effects:** Acute and chronic exposures of increased levels of arsenic results in wide range of cardiovascular effects. Several epidemiological studies have suggested that long-term chronic arsenic exposure results in injured blood vessels, cardiovascular abnormalities, Raynaud's disease, myocardial infarction, myocardial depolarization, cardiac arrhythmias, arterial thickening especially in children (Saha et al., 1999; Mandal& Suzuki, 2002). Arsenic is also a potentially toxic element which causes peripheral vascular disease (PVD), cerebro-vascular disease (CVD) and coronary heart disease (CHD) (Hopenhayn, 2006). In acute arsenic poisoning, diffuse capillary leakage may occur leading to hypotension, delayed cardio-myopathy, hypercontracted muscle fibres, myofibrillar disruption, shock, transduction of plasma and vasodilation (Saha et al., 1999). There are recent reports of death due to cardiovascular diseases caused by high arsenic exposure of concentrations from >100µg/L to >300µg/L (Chen et al, 2011; Abdul et al., 2015). Drinking water with high levels of arsenic is also reported as a threat to the cardiovascular system (Rahaman et al, 2009; Abdul et al., 2015). Notably, few studies have reported the elevated risk of cardiovascular disease and death due to increased levels of arsenic in water, in certain places such as South-western Taiwan (Tseng et al., 2005), Utah, united states (Chen &Karagas, 2013, Lewis et al., 1999) and Bangladesh (Chen et al., 2011). The long-term arsenic exposure has a significant role in causing damage to vascular systems leading to endemic black foot disease (BFD). The early clinical symptoms of BFD include loss of circulation in hands and feet; leading to painful gangrene formation in toes and feet, arteriosclerosis and arterial occlusions. This disease was reported to be endemic in South-western Taiwan, where drinking water contained 0.17 to 0.8 ppm of arsenic (Saha et al., 1999; Mandal& Suzuki, 2002; Abdul et al., 2015; Tseng et al.,2005).
5. **Neurological Effects:** Arsenic which is being capable of crossing blood-brain barrier, targets the brain and impairs learning and concentration abilities (Mundey et al., 2013; Abdul et al., 2015). Though arsenic gets diffused all over the brain, the excessive accumulation occurs in pituitary glands. Both acute and chronic arsenic exposure causes sensorimotor neuropathy, mostly affecting the sensory nerves and long axon neurons than motor nerves and short axon neurons (Sanchez-Pena et al., 2010; Abdul et al., 2015). Acute arsenic exposures (1 mg As/kg/day) cause encephalopathy with clinical symptoms such as headache, lethargy, mental confusion, hallucination, seizures, and coma. Chronic arsenic exposure causes profuse sweating in distal lower extremities, loss of reflexes, muscle cramps, diminished memory, increased urinary urgency, paraesthesia, anxiety attacks, pain and numbness in feet (Saha et al., 1999; Vahidnia et al., 2007). Several reports have been shown that the neurotoxicity is majorly caused due to the reduced potential of the neuron to detoxify Reactive Oxygen Species (ROS) and glutathione production (Aoyama et al., 2008; Abdul et al., 2015). The extreme state involves hindering of crucial enzymes inactivation that governs the cell function and finally disorganization of cytoskeletal framework by hyperphosphorylation of proteins (Mundey et al., 2013; Abdul et al., 2015). Research on Mexican children shows that children's verbal intellectual function (IQ) and long-term memory could be decreased with increased arsenic exposure (50 µg/L) (Wasserman et al, 2004; Kapaj et al., 2006; Hong, 2014). Recent reports show that peripheral neuropathy as the principal neurological issue in patients who consumed arsenic poisoned groundwater in West Bengal, India. Also long-term arsenic exposure causes Alzheimer disease and related disorders (Mukherjee et al., 2003; O'Bryant et al., 2011; Abdul et al., 2015).

6. **Dermal Effects/ Integumentary System:** The chronic As exposure is reported to result in several dermatological diseases including hair and nail diseases. It is shown that Men are more prone to As-induced skin diseases than women (Lindberg et al., 2008; Rahman et al., 2009; Abdul et al., 2015). The clinical diagnosis includes hyperkeratosis, diffused and spotted melanosis, leucomelanosis, palmar and solar keratosis with warts and corns. Hyperkeratosis appears as dark brown spots on skin or like characteristic "rain-drops" appearance. Small areas of hypo-pigmentation are also reported on face, neck, and back. These manifestations were observed in few Inner Mongolian populations in China, who consumed arsenic (level - 50–1860 μg/L) contaminated drinking water (Saha et al., 1999; Ratnaike, 2003; Guo et al., 2007; Abdul et al., 2015). Even though long-term exposure of arsenic causes skin cancer and Bowen's disease, it is not a common manifestation in Asians due to the presence of high skin melanin and increased exposure to ultraviolet radiation. The non-melanin pigmented skin is more prone to cell carcinoma through high As exposure (Abernathy, 2003; Ratnaike, 2003). The Mee's lines are a distinct formation of white lines in fingers and toenails, which is a manifestation caused by deposition of As. Few studies report that in West Bengal, people with poor nutrition are more susceptible to hyper-pigmentation and keratosis caused by arsenic exposure. However, another study contradicts to this by stating that despite good nutrition among Atacameno people in Northern Chile, skin lesions manifested through arsenic exposure (Ratnaike, 2003; Abdul et al., 2015).
7. **Respiratory Effects:** Humans exposed to arsenic either through consumption of contaminated drinking water or occupational source are subjected to several respiratory disorders. Inhalation of As dust or fume during mining or milling of ores, smelting, industrial processing induces irritation of the mucous membrane, leading to laryngitis, tracheae bronchitis, rhinitis, and pharyngitis. The clinical symptoms observed at very high exposure are nasal congestion, perforation of nasal septum, sore throat, chronic cough, shortness of breath and rattling chest sounds(Saha et al., 1999;Parvez et al., 2010;Abdul et al., 2015). Acute exposure causes pulmonary edema, bronchial pneumonia, and trachea bronchitis; while chronic exposure causes cough, pulmonary fibrosis and lung cancer (Tchounwou et al., 2003). Notably few studies from West Bengal, India have reported that people with skin lesions prevailed with bronchiectasis compared to people without skin lesions (Ratnaike, 2003; Mazumder, 2008; Kapaj et al., 2006). Another study indicates the association of black foot disease with the occurrence of bronchitis in Taiwan patients (Ratnaike, 2003).
    a. **Reproductive and Developmental Effects:** Inorganic As is known to affect male and female reproductive organs and cause fertility issues. In males, arsenic diminishes the testosterone synthesis, apoptosis, and necrosis leading to gonad dysfunction. Since, As can readily transfer across the placenta, consumption of As-rich drinking water has been reported to cause fatal loss (Chakraborti et al., 2003; Davila-Esqueda et al., 2012; Shen et al., 2013; Abdul et al., 2015). The increased As exposure causes apoptosis, necrosis, loss of conception in uterus and death of the new-born (Chattopadhyay et al., 2002; Kapaj et al., 2006). A study reported that chronic As exposure is related to spontaneous abortion and stillbirth (Milton et al., 2005; Kapaj et al., 2006).
    b. **Carcinogenic Effects:** Arsenic is considered as a potential human carcinogen and has been classified as a group-1 carcinogen by International Agency for Research on Cancer (IARC) since 1980 (Kapaj et al., 2006; Hong et al., 2014; Abdul et al., 2015). Chronic exposure of arsenic may cause several types of cancers such as lung, bladder, liver, skin, kidney, and

leukemia. It is the only potential carcinogen which induces cancer through respiratory and gastrointestinal exposure (Centeno et al, 2006; Hong, 2014).

i. **Lung Cancer:** Arsenic exposure through theuse of pesticides and insecticides; gold mining and smelting has been observed to induce lung cancer (Saha et al, 1999). This type of cancer is shown to be dependent on dose, duration and intensity of arsenic (Smith et al., 2006; Hong et al., 2014).
ii. **Bladder Cancer:** Drinking water contaminated with As causes bladder cancer. However, studies from South Western Taiwan and Bangladesh have reported evidence of bladder cancer predominantly through high As exposure than low As exposure (Hong et al., 2014). Studies analyzed in the U.S population initially indicated no connection between As induced death for exposures below 100μg/L and bladder cancer (Lamm & Kruse, 2004; Meliker et al., 2010; Abdul et al., 2015). However, it was reported that there is a synergistic relation between high As exposure (200 μg/L) and smoking, which increases the risk of bladder cancer. This result in DNA repair inhibition and reduced levels of essential nutrients which leads to the hindrance of arsenic detoxification (Gabriel et al., 2006; Gamble et al., 2007; Hong et al., 2014; Kapaj et al., 2006).
iii. **Liver Cancer:** Arsenic in drinking waters especially the inorganic As targets liver and increases the cancer mortality. It accelerates the reducing mRNA levels and DNMT activity; and revives the partially or fully silenced genes in liver cancer cells (Liaw et al., 2008; Hong et al., 2014). A recent study on liver cancer patients in few villages of South Western Taiwan reported cancer induction through consumption of As-contaminated drinking water containing levels above 0.64 mg/L (Hong et al., 2014). Another research in Chile population indicated the occurrence of childhood liver cancer and mortality between ages 0 to 19 through As-contaminated drinking water (Guo et al., 2001; Abdul et al., 2015).
iv. **Skin Cancer:** Arsenic exposure induces skin cancer, especially the trivalent arsenite enhances the UV-induced skin cancer. The two types of non-melanoma skin cancers (NMSC) include basal cell carcinoma which is multiple and squamous cell carcinoma caused by keratinisation (Saha et al., 1999; Kapaj et al., 2006; Hong et al., 2014). The DNA methylation and DNA repair are most affected mechanisms during the As action (Kapaj et al., 2006). This type of cancer has been reported in South West Coast of Taiwan, China, Bangladesh, and India; with Taiwan population being the most affected by consumption of As-contaminated water (Guo et al., 2001; Haque et al., 2003; Abdul et al., 2015).

DETECTION TECHNIQUES FOR ARSENIC IN DIFFERENT SAMPLES

To identify and quantify arsenic species in water, it is critical to develop accurate and sensitive analytical procedures (Baig et al., 2010). The USEPA has assessed and evaluated the latest science and technologies for monitoring the arsenic content in the environment (USEPA, 2004; Komorowicz and Baralkiewicz, 2016). The approved methods include inductively coupled plasma-mass spectrometry (ICP-MS), graphite furnace atomic absorption spectrometry (GFAAS),inductively coupled plasma atomic emission spectrometry (ICP-AES), and hydride generation atomic absorption spectrometry (HGAAS), with a

Table 1. Arsenic induced human health manifestations

Organ manifestation	Acute effects	Chronic effects
Gastrointestinal effects	Nausea, vomiting, crampy abdominal pain, diarrhoea, inflammation and necrosis of mucosa and sub-mucosa	Esophagitis, gastritis, hepatic steatosis, anorexia, malabsorption, massive fluid loss, circulatory collapse, renal damage, death
Hepatic effects	Hepatic damage, jaundice, enlarged tender liver, ascites	Cirrhosis, hepatic fibrosis, non-cirrhosis portal fibrosis, hepatic neoplasia and fatty degeneration
Renal effects	Elevated blood urea nitrogen, serum creatinine, hypo urea, oliguria, tubular necrosis	Haematuria, proteinuria, cats in urine
Cardiovascular effects	Diffuse capillary leakage, hypotension, delayed cardiomyopathy, hyper-contracted muscle fibre, myofibrillar disruption, shock, transduction of plasma and vasodilation	Injured blood vessels, Raynaud's disease, myocardial infarction, myocardial depolarization, cardiac arrhythmias, arterial thickening
Neurological effects	Encephalopathy, headache, lethargy, mental confusion, hallucination, seizures, coma	Profuse sweating in distal lower extremities, loss of reflexes, muscle cramps, diminished memory, increase urinary urgency, paraesthesia, anxiety attacks, pain and numbness in feet
Dermal effects	Bowen's disease, skin lesions, Mee's lines	Hyperkeratosis diffused and spotted melanosis, leucomelanosis, palmar and solar keratosis with warts and corns
Respiratory effects	Pulmonary edema, bronchial pneumonia, trachea bronchitis	Cough, pulmonary fibrosis, laryngitis, rhinitis, pharyngitis
Reproductive effects	Apoptosis, necrosis, gonad dysfunction in men, loss of conception in the uterus in women and death of new-born	Spontaneous abortion and stillbirth

characterized method detection limits (MDL) ranging from 0.5 to 50 μg L−1 (USEPA 1999; Ma et al. 2014).A combination method of liquid chromatography with hydride generation atomic fluorescence spectrometry (LC-HG-AFS)has been designed and utilized to determine the arsenic species in freshwater samples of Southeast of Tianjin, China (Yu et al., 2014).Owing to the time consuming complex conventional methods that require laboratory-based equipment, portable smartphone-based device that utilizes aptamers, gold nano-particles and NaCl with colorimetric detection protocol has been employed in testing and optimizing As (III) content in soil, with the limit of detection (LOD) of 0.71 ppm and correlation coefficient of 0.98 (Siddiqui et al., 2018). The most sensitive atomic absorption spectrometry considered for detection of arsenic species in food samples is electrochemical atomic absorption spectrometry (ETAAS). Arsenic toxicity in rice and rice-based products are major concern of many countries and the major detection techniques employed are ETAAS, microwave-assisted dispersive liquid-liquid micro-extraction (MADLLME), cloud point extraction (CPE) and Quadrupole based ICP-QMS (Ahmadi-Jouibari and Fattahi, 2015; Costa et al., 2015; Signes-Pastor et al., 2016; Llorente-Mirandes et al., 2017).

CONCLUSION

Arsenic contamination of groundwater is a global concern as it is a major threat to human and animal health. Several biogeochemical processes such as mineral dissolution result in seepage of naturally occurring As into groundwater resources. Likewise, anthropogenic sources such as mining, industrial sources, coal burning, usage of agricultural chemicals and wood preservatives from decades added on to the release of As into environment. Both natural and anthropogenic sources of As in turn results in contamination of groundwater. Since, most of the world's population relies on groundwater resources for drinking and irrigation purposes, As toxicity results in various health manifestations in both humans and animals. Arsenic uptake and translocation in the edible crops and vegetables is potentially another toxic route to human health.

This present chapter discusses the various natural and anthropogenic sources of As in environment. Likewise, it covers most of the health manifestations caused by As contamination. Various health effects such as intestinal disorders, cardiovascular diseases, neurological, renal, respiratory, kidney, bladder, dermal and reproductive disorders; and also, several types of cancers that evolved through higher trophic levels of As contamination have been discussed. Some of the detection techniques used in determination of As in water, soil and food samples have also been discussed. It is always better to have a prevention method rather than a cure. Some of the methods of As prevention would be to utilize rain-water harvesting systems, proper disposal of the removed As, prevent pumping water for irrigation from deeper arsenic aquifers, avoid usage of pesticides and uplift farmer education.

REFERENCES

Abdul, K. S., Jayasinghe, S. S., Chandana, E. P., Jayasumana, C., & De Silva, P. M. (2015). Arsenic and human health effects: *A review. Environmental Toxicology and Pharmacology*, *40*(3), 828–846. doi:10.1016/j.etap.2015.09.016 PMID:26476885

Abernathy, C. O., Thomas, D. J., & Calderon, R. L. (2003). Health Effects and Risk Assessment of Arsenic. *The Journal of Nutrition*, *133*(5), 1536S–1538S. doi:10.1093/jn/133.5.1536S PMID:12730460

Ahmadi-Jouibari, T., & Fattahi, N. (2015). Speciation of inorganic arsenic species and total inorganic arsenic in rice using microwave-assisted dispersive liquid–liquid micro-extraction and electrothermal atomic absorption spectrometry. *Food Additives & Contaminants: Part A*, *32*(7), 1140–1147. doi:10.1080/19440049.2015.1049565 PMID:25959514

Aoyama, K., Watabe, M., & Nakaki, T. (2008). Regulation of neuronal glutathione synthesis. *Journal of Pharmacological Sciences*, *108*(3), 227–238. doi:10.1254/jphs.08R01CR PMID:19008644

Arora, S., Rana, R., Chhabra, A., Jaiswal, A., & Rani, V. (2013). miRNA-transcription factor 656 interactions: A combinatorial regulation of gene expression. *Molecular Genetics and Genomics*, *288*(3-4), 77–87. doi:10.100700438-013-0734-z PMID:23334784

Asadullah, M. N., & Chaudhury, N. (2011). Poisoning the mind: Arsenic contamination of drinking water wells and children's educational achievement in rural Bangladesh. *Economics of Education Review*, *30*(5), 873–888. doi:10.1016/j.econedurev.2011.05.001

Baig, J. A., Kazi, T. G., Shah, A. Q., Kandhro, G. A., Kandhro, G. A., Afridi, H. I., ... Jalbani, N. (2010). Speciation and evaluation of Arsenic in surface water and groundwater samples: A multivariate case study. *Ecotoxicology and Environmental Safety*, *73*(5), 914–923. doi:10.1016/j.ecoenv.2010.01.002 PMID:20363500

Bhattacharya, P., Jacks, G., Frisbie, S. H., Smith, E., Naidu, R., & Sarkar, B. (2002). Arsenic in the environment: a global perspective. In B. Sarkar (Eds.), Heavy Metals in the Environment (pp. 147-215). New York, NY: Marcel Dekker, Inc. doi:10.1201/9780203909300.ch6

Bhattacharya, P., Samal, A. C., Majumdar, A., & Santra, S. C. (2010). Arsenic Contamination in Rice, Wheat, Pulses, and Vegetables: A Study in an Arsenic Affected Area of West Bengal, India. *Water, Air, and Soil Pollution*, *213*(1-4), 3–13. doi:10.100711270-010-0361-9

Bissen, M., & Frimmel, H. F. (2003). Arsenic – a Review. Part I: Occurrence, Toxicity, Speciation, Mobility. *Clean- Soil, Air. Water (Basel)*, *31*, 9–18.

Brammer, H. (2008). Threat of Arsenic to Agriculture in India, Bangladesh and Nepal. *Economic and Political Weekly*, 43.

Centeno, J. A., Tchounwou, P. B., Patlolla, A. K., Mullick, F. G., Murakata, L., Meza, E., & Yedjou, C. G. (2006). Environmental pathology and health effects of arsenic poisoning. In *Managing Arsenic in the Environment: From Soil to Human Health* (pp. 311–327). Collingwood, Australia: Csiro Publishing.

Chakraborti, D., Mukherjee, S. C., Pati, S., Sengupta, M. K., Rahman, M. M., Chowdhury, U. K., ... Basu, G. K. (2003). Arsenic groundwater contamination in Middle Ganga Plain, Bihar, India: A future danger? *Environmental Health Perspectives*, *111*(9), 1194–1201. doi:10.1289/ehp.5966 PMID:12842773

Chattopadhyay, S., Bhaumik, S., Purkayastha, M., Basu, S., Nag Chaudhuri, A., & Das Gupta, S. (2002). Apoptosis and necrosis in developing brain cells due to arsenic toxicity and protection with antioxidants. *Toxicology Letters*, *136*(1), 65–76. doi:10.1016/S0378-4274(02)00282-5 PMID:12368058

Chen, A. Y. Y., & Olsen, T. (2016). Chromated copper arsenate–treated wood: A potential source of arsenic exposure and toxicity in dermatology. *International Journal of Women's Dermatology*, *2*(1), 28–30. doi:10.1016/j.ijwd.2016.01.002 PMID:28491998

Chen, Y., Graziano, J. H., Parvez, F., Liu, M., Slavkovich, V., Kalra, T., ... Ahsan, H. (2011). Arsenic exposure from drinking water and mortality from cardiovascular disease in Bangladesh: Prospective cohort study. *BMJ (Clinical Research Ed.)*, 342. PMID:21546419

Chen, Y., & Karagas, M. R. (2013). Arsenic and Cardiovascular Disease: New Evidence From the United States. *Annals of Internal Medicine*, *159*, 713–714. PMID:24061555

Collotta, M., Bertazzi, P. A., & Bollati, V. (2013). Epigenetics and pesticides. *Toxicology*, *307*, 35–41. doi:10.1016/j.tox.2013.01.017 PMID:23380243

Costa, B. E., Coelho, N. M., & Coelho, L. M. (2015). Determination of arsenic species in rice samples using CPE and ETAAS. *Food Chemistry*, *178*, 89–95. doi:10.1016/j.foodchem.2015.01.014 PMID:25704688

Dartey, E., Sarpong, k., Darko, G., & Acheampong-Marfo, M. (2013). Urinary arsenic and mercury levels in artisanal miners in some communities in the Obuasi Municipality of Ghana. *Journal of Environmental Chemistry and Ecotoxicology*, *55*, 113–118.

Das, H., Mitra, A., Sengupta, P., Hossain, A., Islam, F., & Rabbani, G. (2004). Arsenic concentrations in rice, vegetables, and fish in Bangladesh: A preliminary study. *Environment International*, *30*(3), 383–387. doi:10.1016/j.envint.2003.09.005 PMID:14987870

Davila-Esqueda, M. E., Jimenez-Capdeville, M. E., Delgado, J. M., De la Cruz, E., Aradillas Garcia, C., Jimenez-Suarez, V., ... Llerenas, J. R. (2012). Effects of arsenic exposure during the pre- and postnatal development on the puberty of female offspring. *Experimental and Toxicologic Pathology*, *64*(1-2), 25–30. doi:10.1016/j.etp.2010.06.001 PMID:20580540

Drinking Water–Specification (2nd Rev.). (2012). New Delhi. *Bureau of Indian Standards IS*, *10500*, 2012.

EFSA (European Food Safety Authority) Panel on Contaminants in the Food Chain. (2009). Scientific opinion on arsenic in food. *EFSA Journal*, *7*(10), 1351. doi:10.2903/j.efsa.2009.1351

Feinberg, A. P., & Tycko, B. (2004). The history of cancer epigenetics. *Nature Reviews. Cancer*, *4*(2), 143–153. doi:10.1038/nrc1279 PMID:14732866

Fillol, C., Dor, F., Labat, L., Boltz, P., Bouard, J. L., Mantey, K., ... Seta, N. (2010). Urinary arsenic concentrations and speciation in residents living in an area with naturally contaminated soils. *The Science of the Total Environment*, *408*(5), 1190–1194. doi:10.1016/j.scitotenv.2009.11.046 PMID:20004003

Fisher, A. T., López-Carrillo, L., Gamboa-Loira, B., & Cebrián, M. E. (2017). Standards for arsenic in drinking water: Implications for policy in Mexico. *Journal of Public Health Policy*, *38*(4), 395–406. doi:10.105741271-017-0087-7 PMID:28808298

Gabriel, H. E., Crott, J. W., Ghandour, H., Dallal, G. E., Choi, S. W., Keyes, M. K., ... Mason, J. B. (2006). Chronic cigarette smoking is associated with diminished folate status, altered folate form distribution, and increased genetic damage in the buccal mucosa of healthy adults. *The American Journal of Clinical Nutrition*, *83*(4), 835–841. doi:10.1093/ajcn/83.4.835 PMID:16600936

Gamble, M. V., Liu, X., Slavkovich, V., Pilsner, J. R., Ilievski, V., Factor-Litvak, P., ... Graziano, J. H. (2007). Folic acid supplementation lowers blood arsenic. *The American Journal of Clinical Nutrition*, *86*(4), 1202–1209. doi:10.1093/ajcn/86.4.1202 PMID:17921403

Gerhardt, R. E. (1980). Moonshine-related arsenic poisoning. *Archives of Internal Medicine*, *140*(2), 211–213. doi:10.1001/archinte.1980.00330140069020 PMID:7352816

Ghosh, D., & Bhadury, P. (2018). Microbial Cycling of Arsenic in the Aquifers of Bengal Delta Plains (BDP). In T. K. Adhya, B. Lal, B. Mohapatra, D. Paul, & S. Das (Eds.), *Advances in Soil Microbiology: Recent Trends and Future Prospects* (pp. 91–108). Springer Singapore. doi:10.1007/978-981-10-6178-3_5

Ghosh, D., Bhadury, P., & Routh, J. (2014). Diversity of arsenite oxidizing bacterial communities in arsenic-rich deltaic aquifers in West Bengal, India. *Frontiers in Microbiology*, *5*, 602. doi:10.3389/fmicb.2014.00602 PMID:25484877

Ghosh, D., Bhadury, P., & Routh, J. (2018). Coping with arsenic stress: Adaptations of arsenite-oxidizing bacterial membrane lipids to increasing arsenic levels. *MicrobiologyOpen*, 594. PMID:29577673

Ghosh, D., Routh, J., & Bhadury, P. (2015a). Characterization and microbial utilization of dissolved lipid organic fraction in arsenic impacted aquifers (India). *Journal of Hydrology (Amsterdam)*, *527*, 221–233. doi:10.1016/j.jhydrol.2015.04.051

Ghosh, D., Routh, J., & Bhadury, P. (2017). Sub-surface biogeochemical characteristics and its effect on arsenic cycling in the Holocene grey sand aquifers of the Lower Bengal Basin. *Frontiers in Environmental Science*, *5*, 82. doi:10.3389/fenvs.2017.00082

Ghosh, D., Routh, J., Därio, M., & Bhadury, P. (2015b). Elemental and biomarker characteristics in a Pleistocene aquifer vulnerable to arsenic contamination in the Bengal Delta Plain, India. *Applied Geochemistry*, *61*, 87–98. doi:10.1016/j.apgeochem.2015.05.007

Gillispie, E. C., Sowers, T. D., Duckworth, O. W., & Polizzotto, M. L. (2015). Soil Pollution Due to Irrigation with Arsenic-Contaminated Groundwater: Current State of Science. *Current Pollution Reports*, *1*(1), 1–12. doi:10.100740726-015-0001-5

Greber, J. F. (2003). Gallium and gallium compounds. In *Ullmann's Encyclopedia of Industrial Chemistry* (6th rev. Ed., Vol. 15, pp. 235–240). Weinheim: Wiley-VCH Verlag GmbH & Co.

Grewal, S. I., & Jia, S. (2007). Heterochromatin revisited. *Nature Reviews. Genetics*, *8*(1), 35–46. doi:10.1038/nrg2008 PMID:17173056

Guidelines for Drinking-water Quality. (2011). Geneva: WHO Press.

Guo, J. X., Hu, L., Yand, P. Z., Tanabe, K., Miyatalre, M., & Chen, Y. (2007). Chronic arsenic poisoning in drinking water in Inner Mongolia and its associated health effects. *Journal of Environmental Science and Health. Part A, Toxic/Hazardous Substances & Environmental Engineering*, *42*(12), 1853–1858. doi:10.1080/10934520701566918 PMID:17952786

Guo, X., Fujino, Y., Kaneko, S., Wu, K., Xia, Y., & Yoshimura, T. (2001). Arsenic contamination of groundwater and prevalence of arsenical dermatosis in the Hetao plain area, Inner Mongolia, China. *Molecular and Cellular Biochemistry*, *222*(1/2), 137–140. doi:10.1023/A:1017916826439 PMID:11678595

Guo, X., Zheng, C., & Xu, M. (2004). Characterization of Arsenic Emissions from a Coal-Fired Power Plant. *Energy & Fuels*, *18*(6), 1822–1826. doi:10.1021/ef049921b

Haque, R., Mazumder, D. N., Samanta, S., Ghosh, N., Kalman, D., Smith, M. M., ... Smith, A. H. (2003). Arsenic in drinking water and skin lesions: Dose-response data from West Bengal, India. *Epidemiology (Cambridge, Mass.)*, *14*(2), 174–182. doi:10.1097/01.EDE.0000040361.55051.54 PMID:12606883

Heerboth, S., Lapinska, K., Snyder, N., Leary, M., Rollinson, S., & Sarkar, S. (2014). Use of Epigenetic Drugs in Disease: An Overview. *Genetics & Epigenetics*, *6*, 9–19. doi:10.4137/GEG.S12270 PMID:25512710

Hong, Y.-S., Song, K.-H., & Chung, J.-Y. (2014). Health Effects of Chronic Arsenic Exposure. *Journal of Preventive Medicine and Public Health*, *47*(5), 245–252. doi:10.3961/jpmph.14.035 PMID:25284195

Hopenhyan, C. (2006). Arsenic in Drinking Water: Impact on Human Health. *Elements*, *2*(2), 103–107. doi:10.2113/gselements.2.2.103

Hu, J., Fang, J., Dong, Y., Chen, S. J., & Chen, Z. (2005). Arsenic in cancer therapy. *Anti-Cancer Drugs, 16*(2), 119–127. doi:10.1097/00001813-200502000-00002 PMID:15655408

Hughes, M. F., Beck, B. D., Chen, Y., Lewis, A. S., & Thomas, D. J. (2011). Arsenic Exposure and Toxicology: A Historical Perspective. *Toxicological Sciences, 123*(2), 305–332. doi:10.1093/toxsci/kfr184 PMID:21750349

Ishiguro, S. (1992). Industries using arsenic and arsenic compounds. *Applied Organometallic Chemistry, 6*(4), 323–331. doi:10.1002/aoc.590060404

Jang, Y.-C., Yashoda, S., & Hwidong, K. (2016). Source, Distribution, Toxicity and Remediation of Arsenic in the Environment – A review 2016. *International Journal of Applied Environmental Sciences, 11*, 559–581.

Jiang, J. Q., Ashekuzzaman, S. M., Jiang, A., Sharifuzzaman, S. M., & Chowdhury, S. R. (2013). Arsenic contaminated groundwater and its treatment options in Bangladesh. *International Journal of Environmental Research and Public Health, 10*(1), 18–46. doi:10.3390/ijerph10010018 PMID:23343979

Kapaj, S., Peterson, H., Liber, K., & Bhattacharya, P. (2006). Human health effects from chronic As poisoning—A review. *Journal of Environmental Science and Health, 41*(10), 2399–2428. doi:10.1080/10934520600873571 PMID:17018421

Komorowicz, I., & Barałkiewicz, D. (2016). Determination of total arsenic and arsenic species in drinking water, surface water, wastewater, and snow from Wielkopolska, Kujawy-Pomerania, and Lower Silesia provinces, Poland. *Environmental Monitoring and Assessment, 188*(9), 504. doi:10.100710661-016-5477-y PMID:27488197

Lamm, S. H., & Kruse, M. B. (2004). Arsenic Ingestion and Bladder Cancer Mortality—What Do the Dose-Response Relationships Suggest About Mechanism? *Human and Ecological Risk Assessment, 11*(2), 433–450. doi:10.1080/10807030590925678

Lechtman, H., & Klein, S. (1999). The Production of Copper–Arsenic Alloys (Arsenic Bronze) by Copper smelting: Modern Experiment, Ancient Practice. *Journal of Archaeological Science, 26*(5), 497–526. doi:10.1006/jasc.1998.0324

Lengfelder, E., Hofmann, W., & Nowak, D. (2012). Impact of arsenic trioxide in the treatment of acute promyelocytic leukemia. *Leukemia, 26*(3), 433–442. doi:10.1038/leu.2011.245 PMID:21904379

Lewis, D. R., Southwick, J. W., Ouellet-Hellstrom, R., Rench, J., & Calderon, R. L. (1999). Drinking water arsenic in Utah: A cohort mortality study. *Environmental Health Perspectives, 107*(5), 359–365. doi:10.1289/ehp.99107359 PMID:10210691

Liaw, J., Marshall, G., Yuan, Y., Ferreccio, C., Steinmaus, C., & Smith, A. H. (2008). Increased child-hood liver cancer mortality and arsenic in drinking water in northern Chile. *Cancer Epidemiology, Biomarkers & Prevention, 17*(8), 1982–1987. doi:10.1158/1055-9965.EPI-07-2816 PMID:18708388

Lindberg, A.-L., Rahman, M., Persson, L.-A., & Vahter, M. (2008). The risk of arsenic induced skin lesions in Bangladeshi men and women is affected by arsenic metabolism and the age at first exposure. *Toxicology and Applied Pharmacology, 230*(1), 9–16. doi:10.1016/j.taap.2008.02.001 PMID:18336856

Llorente-Mirandes, T., Rubio, R., & López-Sánchez, J. F. (2017). Inorganic Arsenic Determination in Food: A Review of Analytical Proposals and Quality Assessment Over the Last Six Years. *Applied Spectroscopy*, *71*(1), 25–69. doi:10.1177/0003702816652374 PMID:28033722

Ma, J., Sengupta, M. K., Yuan, D., & Dasgupta, P. K. (2014). Speciation and detection of arsenic in aqueous samples: A review of recent progress in non-atomic spectrometric methods. *Analytica Chimica Acta*, *831*, 1–23. doi:10.1016/j.aca.2014.04.029 PMID:24861967

Mandal, B. K., & Suzuki, K. T. (2002). Arsenic round the world: A review. *Talanta*, *58*(1), 201–235. doi:10.1016/S0039-9140(02)00268-0 PMID:18968746

Mazumder, G. D. N. (2008). Chronic arsenic toxicity and human health. *The Indian Journal of Medical Research*, *128*, 436–447. PMID:19106439

McCarty, K. M., Hanh, H. T., & Kim, K. W. (2011). Arsenic geochemistry and human health in South East Asia. *Reviews on Environmental Health*, *26*(1), 71–78. doi:10.1515/reveh.2011.010 PMID:21714384

Meakin, C. J., Martin, E. M., & Fry, R. C. (2017). Epigenetic mechanisms underlying arsenic-induced toxicity. *Current Opinion in Toxicology*, *6*, 1–9. doi:10.1016/j.cotox.2017.06.003

Meharg, A. A., & Rahman, M. M. (2003). Arsenic Contamination of Bangladesh Paddy Field Soils: Implications for Rice Contribution to Arsenic Consumption. *Environmental Science & Technology*, *37*(2), 229–234. doi:10.1021/es0259842 PMID:12564892

Meliker, J. R., Goovaerts, P., Jacquez, G. M., & Nriagu, J. O. (2010). Incorporating individual-level distributions of exposure error in epidemiologic analyses: An example using arsenic in drinking water and bladder cancer. *Annals of Epidemiology*, *20*(10), 750–758. doi:10.1016/j.annepidem.2010.06.012 PMID:20816314

Milton, A. H., Hore, S. K., Hossain, M. Z., & Rahman, M. (2012). Bangladesh arsenic mitigation programs: Lessons from the past. *Emerging Health Threats Journal*, 5. PMID:22558005

Milton, A. H., Smith, W., Rahman, B., Hasan, Z., Kulsum, U., Dear, K., ... Ali, A. (2005). Chronic arsenic exposure and adverse pregnancy outcomes in Bangladesh. *Epidemiology (Cambridge, Mass.)*, *16*(1), 82–86. doi:10.1097/01.ede.0000147105.94041.e6 PMID:15613949

Moyano, A., Garcia-Sanchez, A., Mayorga, P., Anawar, H. M., & Alvarez-Ayuso, E. (2009). Impact of irrigation with arsenic-rich groundwater on soils and crops. *Journal of Environmental Monitoring*, *11*(3), 498–502. doi:10.1039/B817634E PMID:19280028

Mukherjee, S. C., Rahman, M. M., Chowdhury, U. K., Sengupta, M. K., Lodh, D., Chanda, C. R., ... Chakraborti, D. (2003). Neuropathy in arsenic toxicity from groundwater arsenic contamination in West Bengal, India. *Journal of Environmental Science and Health. Part A*, *38*, 165–183. PMID:12635825

Mundey, M. K., Roy, M., Roy, S., Awasthi, M. K., & Sharma, R. (2013). Antioxidant potential of Ocimum sanctum in arsenic induced nervous tissue damage. *Brazilian Journal of Veterinary Pathology*, *6*, 95–101.

Murunga, E., & Zawada, E. (2007). Environmental and Occupational Causes of Toxic Injury to the Kidneys and Urinary Tract. In *Environmental and occupational medicine* (pp. 800–812). Lippincott Williams & Wilkins.

Naujokas, M. F., Anderson, B., Ahsan, H., Aposhian, H. V., Graziano, J. H., Thompson, C., & Suk, W. A. (2013). The broad scope of health effects from chronic arsenic exposure: Update on a worldwide public health problem. *Environmental Health Perspectives*, *121*(3), 295–302. doi:10.1289/ehp.1205875 PMID:23458756

O'Bryant, S. E., Edwards, M., Menon, C. V., Gong, G., & Barber, R. (2011). Long-term low-level arsenic exposure is associated with poorer neuropsychological functioning: A Project FRONTIER study. *International Journal of Environmental Research and Public Health*, *8*(3), 861–874. doi:10.3390/ijerph8030861 PMID:21556183

Parvez, F., Chen, Y., Brandt-Rauf, P. W., Slavkovich, V., Islam, T., Ahmed, A., ... Haque, S. E. (2010). A prospective study of respiratory symptoms associated with chronic arsenic exposure in Bangladesh: Findings from the Health Effects of Arsenic Longitudinal Study (HEALS). *Thorax*, *65*(6), 528–533. doi:10.1136/thx.2009.119347 PMID:20522851

Pearce, D. C., Dowling, K., & Sim, M. R. (2012). Cancer incidence and soil arsenic exposure in a historical gold mining area in Victoria, Australia: A geospatial analysis. *Journal of Exposure Science & Environmental Epidemiology*, *22*(3), 248–257. doi:10.1038/jes.2012.15 PMID:22434113

Pimparkar, B. D., & Bhave, A. (2010). Arsenicosis: Review of recent advances. *The Journal of the Association of Physicians of India*, *58*, 617–624. PMID:21510113

Pournara, A., Kippler, M., Holmlund, T., Ceder, R., Grafstrom, R., Vahter, M., ... Wallberg, A. E. (2016). Arsenic alters global histone modifications in lymphocytes in 616 vitro and in vivo. *Cell Biology and Toxicology*, *32*(4), 275–284. doi:10.100710565-016-9334-0 PMID:27165195

Raessler, M. (2018). The Arsenic Contamination of Drinking and Groundwaters in Bangladesh: Featuring Biogeochemical Aspects and Implications on Public Health. *Archives of Environmental Contamination and Toxicology*, *75*(1), 1–7. doi:10.100700244-018-0511-4 PMID:29520432

Rahman, M. M., Ng, J. C., & Naidu, R. (2009). Chronic exposure of arsenic via drinking water and its adverse health impacts on humans. *Environmental Geochemistry and Health*, *31*(S1), 189–200. doi:10.100710653-008-9235-0 PMID:19190988

Ratnaike, R.H. (2003). Acute and chronic arsenic toxicity. *Post Graduate Medical Journal*, *79*, 391-396.

Ravenscroft, P., Brammer, H., & Richards, K. (2011). Health Effects of Arsenic in Drinking Water and Food. In *Arsenic pollution: A global synthesis*. Chichester: Wiley-Blackwell.

Reichard, J. F., & Puga, A. (2010). Effects of arsenic exposure on DNA methylation and epigenetic gene regulation. *Epigenomics*, *2*(1), 87–104. doi:10.2217/epi.09.45 PMID:20514360

Ruiz-Hernandez, A., Kuo, C. C., Rentero-Garrido, P., Tang, W. Y., Redon, J., Ordovas, J. M., ... Tellez-Plaza, M. (2015). Environmental chemicals and DNA methylation in adults: A systematic review of the epidemiologic evidence. *Clinical Epigenetics*, *7*(1), 55. doi:10.118613148-015-0055-7 PMID:25984247

Saha, J. C., Dikshit, A. K., Bandyopadhyay, M., & Saha, K. C. (1999). A Review of Arsenic Poisoning and its Effects on Human Health. *Critical Reviews in Environmental Science and Technology*, *29*(3), 281–313. doi:10.1080/10643389991259227

Sancha, A. M., & O'Ryan, R. (2008). Managing Hazardous Pollutants in Chile: Arsenic. *Reviews of Environmental Contamination and Toxicology Reviews of Environmental Contamination and Toxicology*, *196*, 123–146. PMID:19025095

Sanchez-Pena, L. C., Petrosyan, P., Morales, M., Gonzalez, N. B., Gutierrez-Ospina, G., Del Razo, L. M., & Gonsebatt, M. E. (2010). Arsenic species, AS3MT amount, and AS3MT gene expression in different brain regions of mouse exposed to arsenite. *Environmental Research*, *110*(5), 428–434. doi:10.1016/j.envres.2010.01.007 PMID:20138265

Shankar, S., Shanker, U., & Shikha. (2014). Arsenic Contamination of Groundwater: A Review of Sources, Prevalence, Health Risks, and Strategies for Mitigation. *The Scientific World Journal*. doi:10.1155/2014/304524 PMID:25374935

Shen, H., Xu, W., Zhang, J., Chen, M., Martin, F. L., Xia, Y., ... Zhu, Y. G. (2013). Urinary metabolic biomarkers link oxidative stress indicators associated with general arsenic exposure to male infertility in a Han Chinese population. *Environmental Science & Technology*, *47*, 8843–8851. PMID:23841501

Siddiqui, M. F., Kim, S., Jeon, H., Kim, T., Joo, C., & Park, S. (2018). Miniaturized Sample Preparation and Rapid Detection of Arsenite in Contaminated Soil Using a Smartphone. *Sensors (Basel)*, *18*(3), 777. doi:10.339018030777 PMID:29510538

Signes-Pastor, A. J., Carey, M., & Meharg, A. A. (2016). Inorganic arsenic in rice-based products for infants and young children. *Food Chemistry*, *191*, 128–134. doi:10.1016/j.foodchem.2014.11.078 PMID:26258711

Singh, S. K. (2017). An analysis of the cost-effectiveness of arsenic mitigation technologies: Implications for public policy. *International Journal of Sustainable Built Environment*, *6*(2), 522–535. doi:10.1016/j.ijsbe.2017.10.004

Smith, A. (2002). Public health. Arsenic epidemiology and drinking water standards. *Science*, *296*(5576), 2145–2146. doi:10.1126cience.1072896 PMID:12077388

Smith, A. H., Marshall, G., Yuan, Y., Ferreccio, C., Liaw, J., von Ehrenstein, O., ... Selvin, S. (2006). Increased mortality from lung cancer and bronchiectasis in young adults after exposure to arsenic in utero and in early childhood. *Environmental Health Perspectives*, *114*(8), 1293–1296. doi:10.1289/ehp.8832 PMID:16882542

Smith, E., Naidu, R., & Alston, A. M. (1998). Arsenic in the soil environment: A review. *Advances in Agronomy*, 64.

Sollome, J., Martin, E., Sethupathy, P., & Fry, R. C. (2016). Environmental contaminants and microRNA regulation: Transcription factors as regulators of toxicant-altered microRNA expression. *Toxicology and Applied Pharmacology*, *312*, 61–66. doi:10.1016/j.taap.2016.06.009 PMID:27292125

Sparks, D. L. (2003). *Environmental soil chemistry*. Boston: Academic. doi:10.1016/B978-012656446-4/50001-3

Suzuki, T., Yamashita, S., Ushijima, T., Takumi, S., Sano, T., Michikawa, T., & Nohara, K. (2013). Genome-wide analysis of DNA methylation changes induced by gestational arsenic exposure in liver tumors. *Cancer Science*, *104*(12), 1575–1585. doi:10.1111/cas.12298 PMID:24118411

Tchounwou, P. B., Patlolla, A. K., & Centeno, J. A. (2003). Carcinogenic and systemic health effects associated with arsenic exposure--a critical review. *Toxicologic Pathology*, *31*, 575–588. PMID:14585726

Tseng, C. H., Huang, Y. K., Huang, Y. L., Chung, C. J., Yang, M. H., Chen, C. J., & Hsueh, Y. M. (2005). Arsenic exposure, urinary arsenic speciation, and peripheral vascular disease in black foot disease-hyperendemic villages in Taiwan. *Toxicology and Applied Pharmacology*, *206*(3), 299–308. doi:10.1016/j.taap.2004.11.022 PMID:16039941

United States Environmental Protection Agency. (1999). Analytical methods support document for arsenic in drinking water.

United States Environmental Protection Agency. (2004). Monitoring arsenic in the environment: a review of science and technologies for field measurements and sensors.

Vahidnia, A., van der Voet, G. B., & de Wolff, F. A. (2007). Arsenic neurotoxicity--a review. *Human and Experimental Toxicology*, *26*(10), 823–832. doi:10.1177/0960327107084539 PMID:18025055

Wasserman, G. A., Liu, X., Parvez, F., Ahsan, H., Factor-Litvak, P., van Geen, A., ... Hussain, I. (2004). Water arsenic exposure and children's intellectual function in Araihazar, Bangladesh. *Environmental Health Perspectives*, *112*(13), 1329–1333. doi:10.1289/ehp.6964 PMID:15345348

Wickre, J. B., Folt, C. L., Sturup, S., & Karagas, M. R. (2004). Environmental Exposure and Fingernail Analysis of Arsenic and Mercury in Children and Adults in a Nicaraguan Gold Mining Community. *Archives of Environmental Health: An International Journal*, *59*(8), 400–409. doi:10.3200/AEOH.59.8.400-409 PMID:16268116

Yu, X., Deng, T., Guo, Y., & Wang, Q. (2014). Arsenic Species Analysis in Freshwater Using Liquid Chromatography Combined to Hydride Generation Atomic Fluorescence Spectrometry. *Journal of Analytical Chemistry*, *69*(1), 88–93. doi:10.1134/S1061934814010146

Zhang, P. (2017). On arsenic trioxide in the clinical treatment of acute promyelocytic leukemia. *Leukemia Research Reports*, *7*, 29–32. doi:10.1016/j.lrr.2017.03.001 PMID:28462082

Chapter 5
Arsenic and Cancer

Arun Kumar
Mahavir Cancer Institute and Research Centre, India

Ashok Kumar Ghosh
Mahavir Cancer Institute and Research Centre, India

ABSTRACT

In the entire world, about 200 million people are exposed to arsenic poisoning in groundwater. In Bihar, India, about 50 million people are drinking arsenic contaminated water. Humans are exposed to elevated levels of inorganic arsenic mainly through the consumption of arsenic contaminated groundwater as drinking water and food crops are irrigated with high-arsenic water resources. This has caused various health-related problems in the population like skin diseases, anemia, bronchitis, gastrointestinal problems, hormonal imbalance and cancer. According to recent study, cancer risk is associated with daily consumption of 2 litres of water with inorganic arsenic 50 μg/L has been estimated to be 1/100 denotes that elevated blood arsenic levels in population can lead to cause various diseases including cancer. Skin and several types of internal cancers, including, bladder, kidney, liver, gall bladder, lung, uterus, and prostate, have been found associated with arsenic ingestion. This hospital-based study also correlates the cause of cancer due to arsenic contamination.

INTRODUCTION

Arsenic Global Scenario

Arsenic has caused various health related issues in the population worldwide. It is a naturally occurring metalloid present in air and water. Groundwater is the major source of human exposure. About 105 countries in the world have been identified where a population of > 200 million is estimated to be exposed to arsenic poisoning (IARC, 2004; WHO, 2008; Smith et al., 2000; Straif et al., 2009; Murcott, 2012; and Naujokas et al., 2013). However, arsenic concentration has been highest in La Pampa of Argentina as 5280 μg/l, the highest ever reported, 4730 μg/l in Bangladesh, 3590 μg/l in Taiwan, 3700 μg/l in South 24 Parganas of India, 2100 μg/l in Antofagasta o Chile, 1100 μg/l in Brazil respectively (Smedley et al., 2005; Chakraborti et al., 2015; Chiou et al., 2001; Chakraborti et al., 2009; Borgono

DOI: 10.4018/978-1-5225-7635-8.ch005

et al., 1977; Arminta and Segovia, 2008). Arsenic exposure causing black foot disease was for the first time coined in 1961 when there were serious health related issues in the population of southwest coast of Taiwan (Blackwell et al. 1961). In Chile, 90% population were exposed to arsenic by drinking high arsenic contaminated water in 1960's and 1970's (Byrne et al., 2010).

In Asia, after Bangladesh, India is second largest country affected from the arsenic poisoning. The most exposed populations of the countries are concentrated in Bangladesh, Cambodia, India, Nepal and Vietnam along with countries in Latin and North America, such as Argentina, Bolivia, Chile and Mexico and the USA (Figure 1). Various epidemiological studies in Taiwan, Bangladesh, Chile, India, Argentina and the USA demonstrated links between the arsenic exposure exceeding 10 µg/L in drinking water and increased all-cause mortality, linked not only to increased risk of lung, bladder and skin cancers, but also cardiovascular, neurological and respiratory diseases, and skin lesions (Ahsan et al., 2006; Argos et al., 2010; Argos et al., 2011; Argos et al., 2012; Chen et al., 2010; Chen and Ahsan, 2004; Haque et al., 2003; James et al., 2015; Wasserman et al., 2014; Yuan et al., 2010).

MAIN FOCUS

Arsenic Indian Scenario

In the Indian peninsular region, arsenic has caused severe health hazards in the population inhabiting Ganga- Meghna- Brahmaputra basin. Bangladesh and India are the most arsenic effected countries in this region. In India, West Bengal, Bihar, Uttar Pradesh and Assam are the most affected states. In the recent studies, it has been found that the Himalayan originated river plains are mostly affected from arsenic poisoning in the ground water in the Asian subcontinent. The entire Ganga- Meghna Bramhaputra (GMB) plains has high arsenic concentrations more than 10 µg/L in groundwater (Guillot and Charlet, 2007). Population residing in these plains are exposed to arsenic poisoning which has led to

Figure 1. Showing Arsenic exposed population worldwide

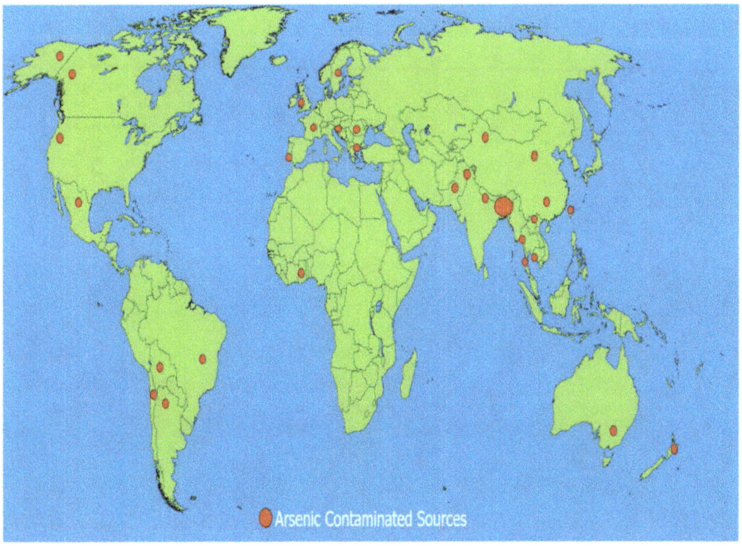

health-related problems like keratosis, melanosis and even cancer (Yunus et al., 2016; Ahamed et al., 2006; Chakraborti et al., 2002; Acharya et al., 1999). The reports of arsenic contaminated groundwater aquifers has been also reported from Punjab (Hundal et al., 2009). India's ancient and holy river is called as Ganga and among all the himalayan rivers, Ganga's river system is well known for its erosive activities throughout the evolution of himalayas. The river forms alluvial deposition around its course from its origin himalayas to its end point Bay of Bengal sea. There are various studies, which have shown that the elevated levels of arsenic in the Gangetic belt is caused due to the river's erosive and alluvial forming nature (Donselaar et al., 2013; Lenny et al., 2008) (Figure. 2).

In India, arsenic contamination in ground water was first reported in Punjab, Haryana, Himachal Pradesh and Uttar Pradesh (Datta and Kaul 1976) then after, in 1984 ground water arsenic contamination was identified in the lower Ganga plain of West Bengal (Garai et al., 1984). Furthermore, arsenic contamination in groundwater was also reported in Bangladesh (Dhar et al., 1997), in the lower Plain area (Terai) of Nepal (Shrestha et al., 2003), in Bihar (middle Ganga plain) and in Uttar Pradesh (lying in middle and upper Ganga plain) (Chakraborti et al., 2018, Chakraborti et al., 2016, Chakraborti et al., 2003, Chakraborti et al., 2002), in Jharkhand (Bhattacharjee et al., 2005) and in Assam (Chakraborti et al., 2004).

It is well known that groundwater in many districts of the West Bengal and parts of Bangladesh are enriched in arsenic enhancing a poisoning effect on humans (Acharyya et al., 1999, 2000; Charlet and Polya, 2006; Das et al., 1996; Nickson et al., 2000; Stuben et al., 2003). The arsenic content in groundwater in the Bengal delta varies from 0.05 to 3.7 mg/l with an average of 0.2 mg/l, which is 20 times higher than the limit recommended by WHO in drinking water. Although, the cartographic distribution of arsenic concentration in Ganga-Bramhaputra, Mekong and Red River fans are now relatively well modified. The primary source and its links with the paleo-hydrology remains unclear. One of the main problem in depicting of the source of arsenic is that this element is very mobile and can be easily removed from the source during alteration processes, then transported in solution in water, or in suspended particles, adsorbed onto various phases such as micas or Mn-phases, or recombined with sulfides of Fe-oxy hy-

Figure 2. Showing Ganga- Mehna- Brahmaputra plains of Indian peninsular with Arsenic contaminated regions

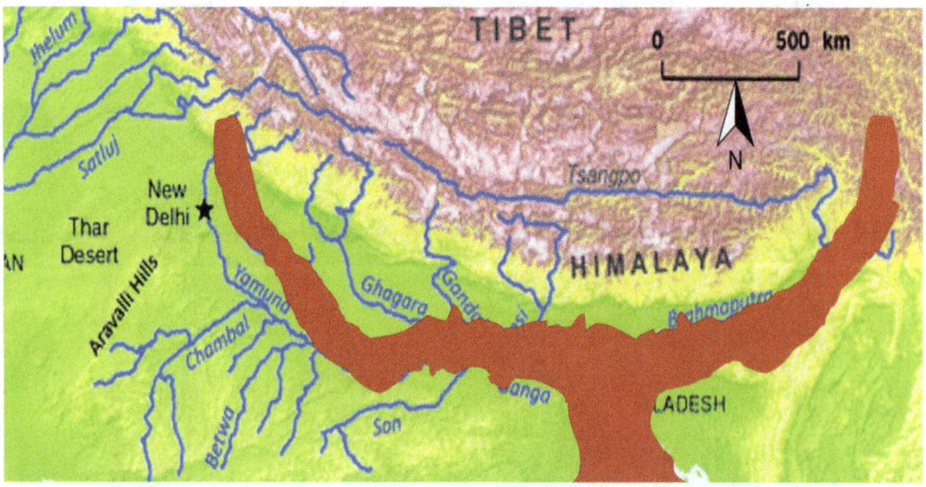

droxides, before being scavenged in reducing conditions in groundwater (Bagla and Kaiser, 1996; Dixit and Hering, 2003; Bhattacharya et al., 1997). It has been suggested that the primary geogenic sources of the arsenic in the groundwater in the Bengal basin are arsenic rich metal deposits in the Ganges basin and in the Darjeeling Himalayas, arsenic bearing pyrite coming from the Gondwana coal seams and from the Rajmahal volcanics (Ghosh and De, 1995; Chandrasekharam et al., 2001). However, as emphasized by Stuben et al. (2003) except for a few horizons with higher values of about 100 to 200 mg/l the bulk arsenic content of the aquifer sediment is comprised between 1 to 30 mg/l i.e., the normal range of the arsenic content of sedimentary rocks (Korte and Fernando, 1991). The Ganga-Brahmaputra river system mainly contributed to the buildup of the Bengal fan, which is considered as one of the largest modern deltas of the world (Milliman and Sivitsli, 1992). Ever since the Tertiary, this river system has carried enormous volumes of sediments from the Himalayan belt. Consequently, the possible source of the arsenic has probably to be searched within the Himalayan belt. It is noticeable that the average annual sediment is transported by the Ganga-Brahmaputra river system. It is estimated that about 1800 tons/km^2, with suspended load is between 540 to 1157 million tons/yr. It is the largest-river basin with the highest denudation rate on Earth (0.69 mm/yr according to Summerfield and Hulton.

Arsenic Bihar Scenario

The state Bihar also comes in the Ganga river basin system, originating from great Himalayas to the Bay of Bengal. Throughout the river course, the river Ganga carries over the silt from its origin along with its tributaries. These silts contain the compound arsenopyrite which is the major cause of arsenic contamination in the groundwater in the Gangetic basin. Bihar contributes 7 rivers originating from Himalayas as tributaries of river Ganga. These tributary river systems also add to the arsenopyrite load to river Ganga (Gulliot and Charlet 2007) (Figure 3).

Bihar along with few other states of India, is facing problem due to arsenic menace in groundwater. Groundwater is the major source of drinking water and it constitutes more than 80 percent of drinking water source in rural Bihar. The other sources of drinking water are from surface water, dug well, pond

Figure 3. Showing map of Bihar – River Ganga and its tributaries originating from Great Himalayas

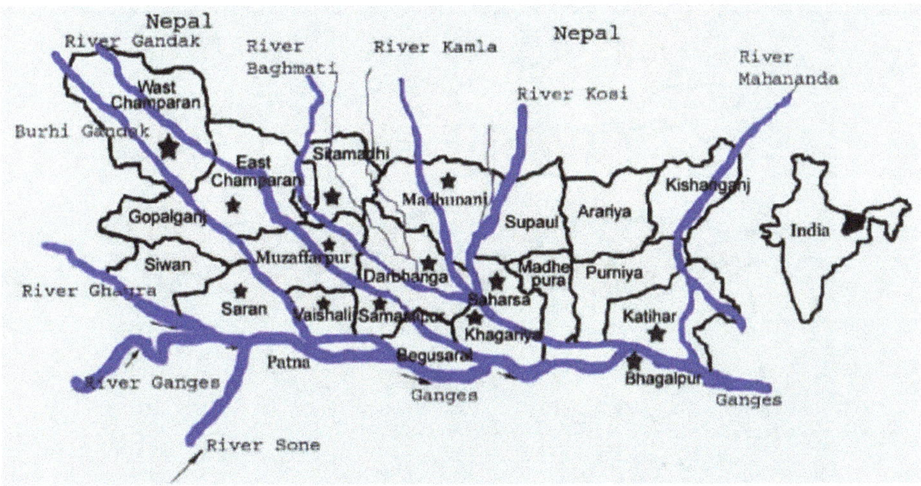

and from natural sources (lakes, rivers, etc.) and protected dug well. The groundwater sources were considered safe for drinking water once upon a time, but over the past few years, there has been arsenic contamination reporting and pollution problems in its root due to rapid urbanization, increase in population, industrialization and excess and uncontrolled extraction of groundwater for irrigation and other purposes. About 48 percent districts of Bihar have been reported with arsenic contamination in groundwater. This comprises more than 67 blocks from 18 districts (Figure 4) and covering more than 1600 habitations across the state where arsenic contamination in groundwater exceeds the Bureau of Indian Standard (BIS) limits for safe drinking water of 50 µg/L and more. If we consider the WHO limits of 10 µg/L, the coverage area will be much more and the population, which is facing the danger of arsenic hazard, will be more than the BIS standard limit. It is estimated that more than 13.85 million people could be under the threat of contamination level above 10 µg/L, out of which more than 6.96 million people could be above 50µg/L, against the total population of these area is around 50 million (Ministry of Water Resources, 2010). The actual problem of arsenic menace among the population will be more than the estimate due to increase in affected area after every new survey (Singh, 2017; Chakraborti, 2016; Singh et al., 2014; Saha, 2009). The problem of arsenic poisoning in ground water was reported for the first time in the year 2002 in village Semaria Ojhapatti in Bhojpur district of Bihar. The population in this village was highly affected from the arsenic poisoning with many visible symptoms of arsenicosis.

In a recent study, arsenic poisoning leading to health-related problems in the Buxar district of the state was studied where arsenic concentration in the ground water was reported to be highest as 1929 µg/L (Kumar et al., 2016). The most unfortunate part of this village was that in the blood samples of the subjects had arsenic concentration 664.7 µg/L which is reported to be the highest till date in the state (Kumar et al., 2016). The population residing in these areas are affected from the typical symptoms of arsenicosis like hyperkeratosis on sole and palm, hyperpigmentation and melanosis in skin of the body (Figure 5). The subjects also exhibited other diseases like diabetes, hypertension, loss of appetite, loose motions, abdominal pain, breathlessness, hormonal imbalance, mental disability and cancer etc. (Kumar et al., 2015, 2016a, 2016b, 2016c; Abhinav et al., 2016; Haque, 2003).

Figure 4. Showing map of Bihar with Arsenic affected districts

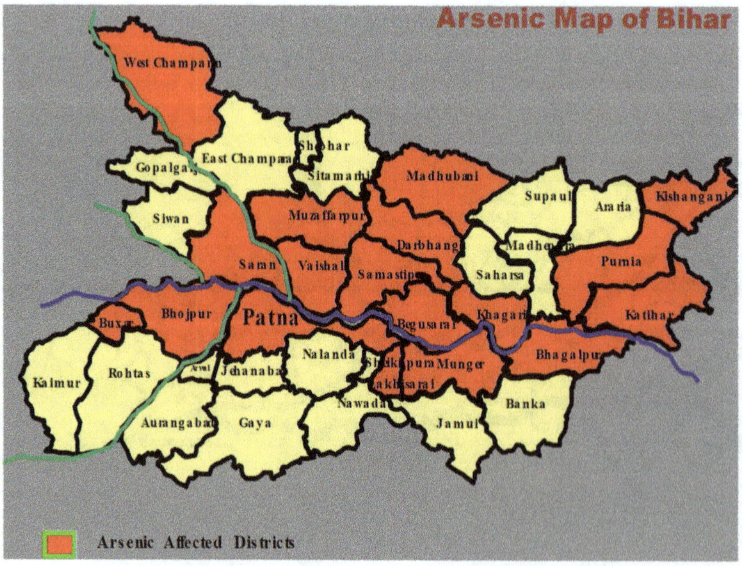

Figure 5. Showing Arsenicosis Symptoms in the subjects from Arsenic hit area of Bihar

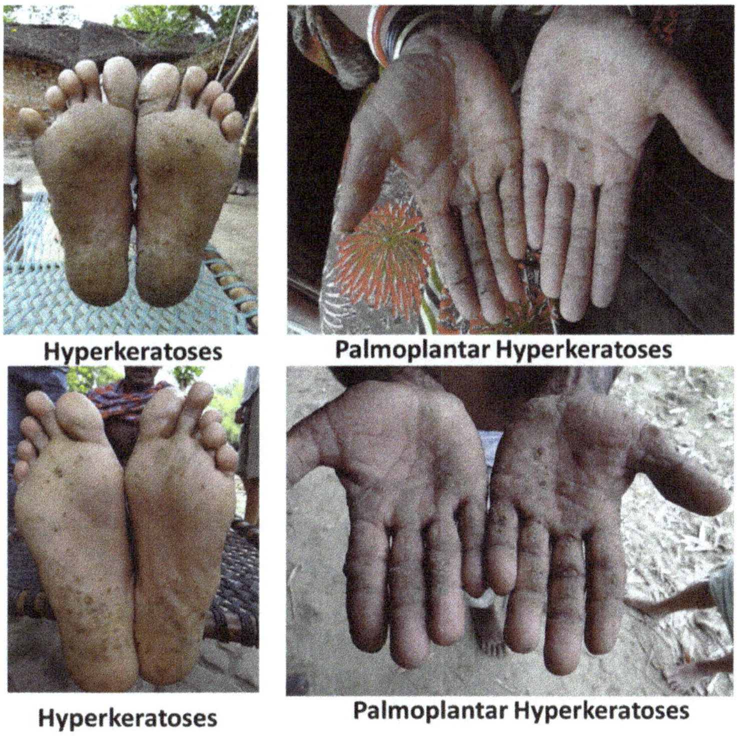

Arsenic Metabolism

After ingestion, around 95% of inorganic arsenic compounds are absorbed through the gastrointestinal tract. In humans, the ingested inorganic arsenic compound enters the blood and with a half-time of two hours, it is rapidly eliminated from the blood through the renal system. The metabolism of arsenic in human and in many other species of the animal takes place in two steps; first of all, pentavalent forms of arsenic is usually reduced to trivalent form, which is then methylated to form monomethylated and dimethylated arsenic compounds. The trivalent arsenic compounds are three to four folds more toxic than the corresponding pentavalent arsenic compounds (Sattar et al., 2016, Moe et al., 2016). The immediate acute arsenic poisoning results in vomiting, diarrhea, abdominal pain followed by the paresthesia of the extremities, muscle cramp and death in the extreme rare cases. The arsenic after long exposure in humans causes pigmentation changes in the skin leading to skin lesions followed by hard patches on the palms of the hands and soles of the feet. It also causes peripheral neuropathy, renal system effects, gastrointestinal problems, diabetes, high blood pressure, conjunctivitis, enlarged liver, bone marrow suppression, destruction of erythrocytes and cardiovascular diseases (Bates et al., 1992, Bagla and Kaiser, 1996).

The toxic inorganic arsenic is converted and utilized metabolically into organic form. It is primarily eliminated out from the human body through metabolic wastes like urine and is deposited in the hair, nails and skin of the affected ones (IPCS, 2001). Arsenic is known to be carcinogen as (Carcinogen category 1) in the form of arsenic trioxide, arsenic pentoxide, arsenous acids, arsenic acid and their salts (arsenites and arsenates) (Straif et al., 2009, Karagas et al., 2002, Valko et al., 2006, IARC, 2004). The arsenic also affects the epidermal system, the nervous system and the vascular system of humans.

Humans are exposed to elevated levels of inorganic arsenic mainly through the consumption of arsenic contaminated groundwater as drinking water. Food prepared with this contaminated water and food crops irrigated with high-arsenic water resources are the major cause of the problem. Arsenic also causes cancers of the skin, bladder, lungs, kidney, liver, and prostate (Rossman, 2003). The International Agency for Research on Cancer has classified arsenic and arsenic compounds as group I carcinogen to humans, which means that there is sufficient evidence for its carcinogenicity in humans (IARC, 2004). Most of the reproductive defects like spontaneous abortion, stillbirth and preterm birth are thought to be linked with the pregnant women who are chronically exposed to arsenic contaminated drinking water which makes their placenta vulnerable to arsenic to pass through easily. In utero and early life exposures to arsenic have been linked to the development of lung cancer and bronchiectasis later in life. The epidemiological data on human suggest an association between the arsenic exposure in drinking water and its adverse effect on reproductive system as well as outcomes (Ahmad et al., 2001).

Arsenic and Neurobehavioural Changes

Various other studies have been carried out which shows arsenic may affect the developing brain through various possible mechanisms. Arsenic as pro-oxidant causes oxidative stress in the developing brain as direct effect (Kalia, 2008; Xi et al., 2010). The second possible mode of action of arsenic is that it causes hormonal imbalance especially the estrogen and thyroid hormones and both are required for the development of the brain and arsenic disrupts the dopaminergic system. Furthermore, arsenic lowers the levels of dopamine causing neural behavioral changes like inattention, impulsivity, loss of concentration and alertness (Rodriguez et al., 2016; Hamadani et al., 2011; Concha et al., 1998). Similar studies have been observed in animal models as well (Moreno et al., 2016; Bardullas et al., 2009). Arsenic determination in urine, hair and nail are considered as most reliable indicator of exposure. Hair samples are used as a biomarker for arsenic exposure as inorganic arsenic and Dimethylarsinic acid are stored in hair root and thus reflect the past exposure (Yoshida et al., 2004). Elevated arsenic levels in hair indicates the past exposure of 6-12 months (NRC, 2001). In a study carried out in children in Mexico, it was observed that urinary arsenic concentration was inversely associated with verbal IQ and long-term memory. In addition, it was also found that long-term memory, attention and the ability to understand speech were affected in children due to exposure of arsenic with chronic malnutrition (Calderon et al. 2001; Wasserman et al. 2004; Tsai et al., 2003).Various studies have shown that in population with no arsenic exposure, the arsenic concentration in hair is generally 0.02-0.2 mg/kg (Kurttio et al., 1998; Rogers et al., 1997; Paulsen et al., 1996; Raie, 1996; Vienna et al., 1995; Wolfsperger et al., 1994; Wang et al., 1994; Koons and Peters, 1994; Takagi et al., 1988; Narang et al., 1987 and Olguin et al., 1983). The population drinking water with high arsenic concentration report with high hair arsenic contamination. In a study carried out in West Bengal, India, arsenic concentrations ranging from 3 to 10 mg/kg in hair were observed in the people drinking high arsenic contaminated water (Das et al., 1995). In a study, in Alaska, an average of 400 μg/L in drinking water corresponded to 3.3 μg/g arsenic contamination in hair (Harrington et al., 1978). In one of our studies, very high concentration of arsenic contamination was observed in the hair samples of the children. They were drinking water from three highly arsenic contaminated hand pump sources. However, they did not exhibit any arsenicosis symptoms, but, their low intelligence and memory correlates the arsenic exposure effect. In addition, the children also showed inattention, impulsivity, loss of concentration and alertness in them. Furthermore, the reporting of mental disability cases in the village is one of the major concerns in this area and is the first reporting (Figure 6).

Figure 6. Mental Disability cases in Simri Village of Buxar district

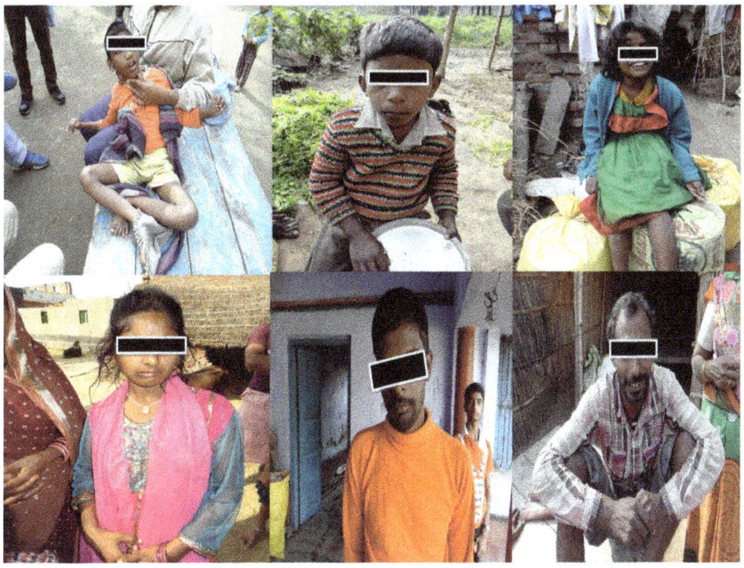

Arsenic and Cancer

The symptoms of arsenic toxicity usually first manifest in the skin by diverse cellular process in organ systems. The skin manifestations appear with hyperpigmentation, hyperkeratosis, hypermelanosis of the palms and soles (Li et al., 2011; Melkonian et al., 2012) Bowen's disease, squamous cell carcinoma and basal cell carcinoma (Yu et al., 2006; Wong et al., 1998; Ghosh et al., 2013). The arsenic exposed subjects exhibited the arsenicosis symptoms like hyperkeratosis, hyperpigmentation in the palms and soles. Their health status was very poor due to the other health related problems like gastrointestinal – gastritis and flatulence, constipation, anaemia, loss of appetite, breathlessness, mental disability, etc. The most unfortunate part was the appearance of skin cancer and breast cancer in the population. Arsenic is also responsible for causing various types other health problems in the population from acute exposure to chronic exposure effects. This includes diseases like skin manifestations, hypertension, ischemia, some peripheral vascular disorders (e.g. Black foot disease), hormonal disorders, diabetes, neuropathies, severe arteriosclerosis, hypertension and significantly many types of cancer (Chen et al., 1995; Engel et al., 1994; Kadono et al., 2002; Tseng, 1977). Various studies implicate that daily consumption of 1.6 litres of water with inorganic arsenic (50 µg/L) is associated with cancer death risk to an estimate of 21/1,000 (Bates et al., 1992).

In one of our studies, the subjects from severe arsenic hit area reported to our cancer centre with typical symptoms of arsenicosis as hyperkeratosis in sole and palm with rain drop pigmentation over his entire body. The subject had a cancerous lesion in his right palm diagnosed with squamous cell carcinoma of the skin. The patient's drinking water source was found to be 244.6 µg/L while his blood sample had arsenic concentration 48.02µg/L and hair sample as 323.32µg/L. The patient's life was saved through surgical management by amputation of his two fingers (Figure 7).

The molecular pathway behind the cause of squamous cell carcinoma of skin is that that, arsenic mediates the aberrant activation of various signal transduction pathways. Arsenic has the strong affinity

Figure 7. Showing patient with squamous cell carcinoma in his palm

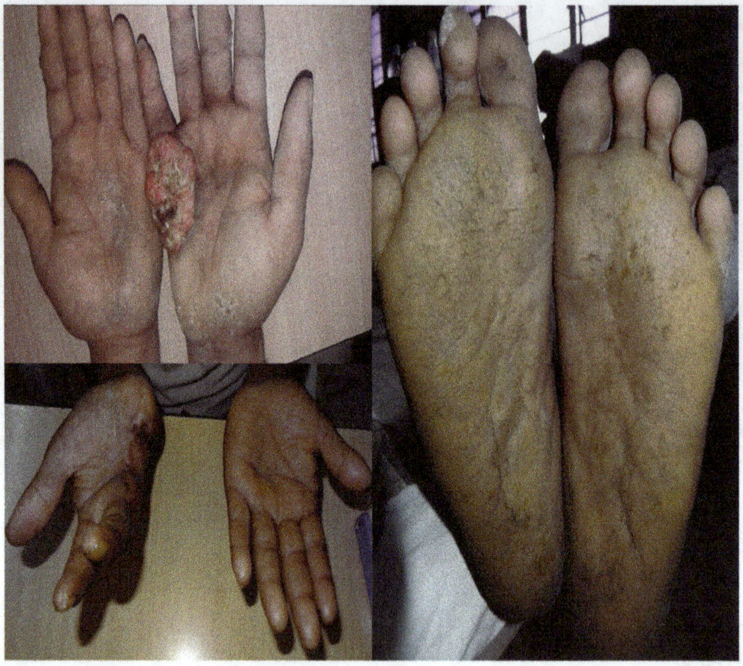

to directly bind sulfhydryl (SH) moieties and conversion of SH to S-S by free radicals (ROS) leads to cause severe toxicity at the cellular level. Although, interaction between arsenic and thiol groups may occur in 200 known human proteins (Abernathy et al., 1999). The most relevant pathways affected by arsenic may lead to the activation of oncogenes, the inhibition of tumour suppressor genes and the up-regulation of inflammatory pathways (Kumagai and Sumi, 2007; Banerjee et al., 2013; Li et al., 2013; Gilmore, 2006).

Recent study suggests that arsenic activates the canonical Hippo signalling pathway responsible for cell survival and proliferation. This pathway is responsible to cause various types of malignancies including skin cancer (Zhao et al., 2008; Halder and Johnson, 2011). Furthermore, arsenic alters Hippo signalling through upregulation of several components including STE20-like kinase ½ (Mst1), Salvador homolog 1 (Sav1), large tumour suppressor kinase 1/2 (LATS1) and Mps one binder kinase activator-like 1A (MOB1). Yes-associated protein (Yap), a known component of the Hippo signalling pathway, is a dual-function protein that serves distinctive roles depending upon its phosphorylation status. When phosphorylated, the protein regulates tight/adherens junctions of epithelium but when dephosphorylated, Yap acts as a transcription factor in the regulation of epithelial cell proliferation. Altogether, these findings demonstrate arsenic's ability to promote skin cell proliferation and survival through alteration of both Hippo signalling and Hippo-independent Yap signalling pathways (Li et al., 2013).

Related to other types of cancer another study correlates the pathway of gene p16 which is a tumour suppressor gene and arrests the cell cycle at G1/S checkpoint by inhibition of cyclin – D1/ CDK4 complex. Arsenic exposure decreases the expression of cyclin dependent kinase inhibitor 1B (p27Kip1), another inhibitor of the cyclin-D1/CDK4 complex. It promotes proliferation by altering the expression of cyclin-D1 itself leading to uncontrolled cell division (Hunt et al., 2014; Sharma et al., 2013; Tyler et al., 2003; Trouba et al., 2000). These studies provide the evidence of cause of cancer due to arsenic toxicity (Figure 8).

The association between arsenic and skin cancer has been well documented by many researchers (Armando and Angel, 1979; Zaldivar et al., 1981). The first study carried was with an increased frequency of skin cancer cases followed by the treatment with Fowler's solution (1% potassium arsenite), which was formerly used for a variety of skin and hematological disorders (Cuzick et al., 1982). Squamous cell carcinoma (SqCC) and Bowen's disease (intraepithelial carcinoma or carcinoma in situ) and basal cell carcinoma (BCC) are the most common malignancies found in the subjects with long term arsenic exposure. Merkel cell carcinoma, which is a rare and very aggressive cutaneous neoplasm has the low frequency in the population (Wong and Wang, 2010, Boonchai et al., 2000, Lien et al., 1999, Wong et al., 1998). The squamous cell carcinoma caused due to arsenic can occur from the initialization of Bowen's disease leading to malignancy of SqCC while due to skin carcinogens and exposure from UV- light from sun leads to development of BCC (Castren et al., 1998, Lee et al., 2004, Yu et al., 2001). Arsenic related Bowen's disease generally occurs after 10 years of arsenic exposure while other skin cancer types take an exposure time of 20 to 30 years (Yoshida et al., 2004). Arsenic related skin cancer and its relationship with the dose of exposure has been well described (Guo et al., 2001). There are various molecular pathways which are associated with the arsenic related skin carcinogenesis like arsenic exposure causing mutations in the normal human epidermal keratinocytes leading to abnormal exhibition of gene function. These may also add up by oxidative stress and increased transcriptional levels of keratinocyte growth factors and finally modulation of MAPK an54d NF-κB pathways (Bailey et al., 2010). The early skin manifestations or premalignant skin lesions due to arsenic exposure are often

Figure 8. Showing schematic diagram of pathway of Squamous cell Carcinoma of Skin

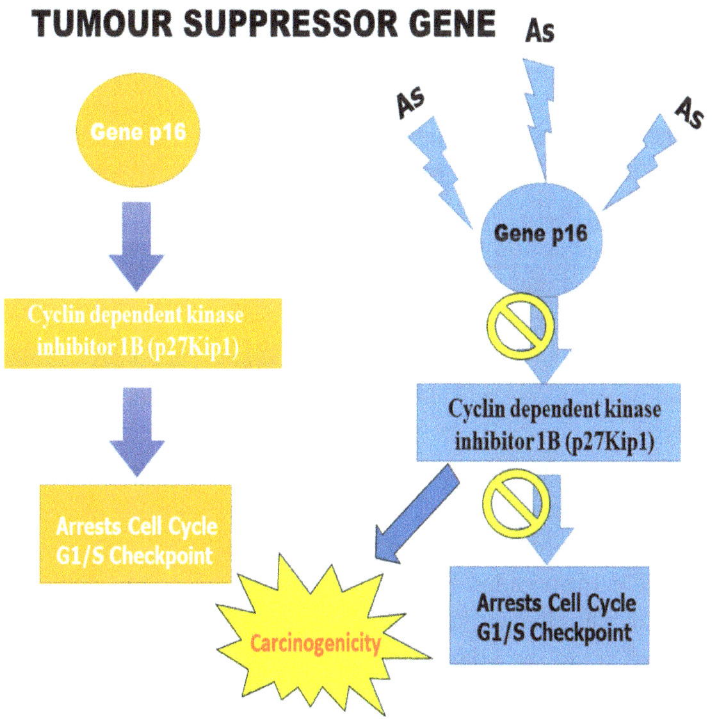

considered as the precursors of arsenic induced skin BCC and SqCC (Melkonian et al., 2011). These lesions include hyperkeratosis (skin thickening in sole or palm), rain drop pigmentation, hyperpigmentation and melanosis which are commonly found in the arsenic exposed population (Caussy, 2005). There is some possibility of association of arsenic-related skin lesions and genetic susceptibilities as this does not occur in every exposed individual (Rossman et al., 2004). Arsenic exposure causes appearance of hyperkeratosis and lesions in very short time period and most of these lesions are converted into arsenic induced skin cancer (ATSDR, 2007, Saha, 2003). Various study implicate that the skin cancer cases caused due to arsenic exposure primarily exhibited lesions caused due to hyperkeratosis, melanosis or other skin manifestations (IARC, 2012). Hence, arsenic toxicity directly induces the carcinogenic process along with the other environmental carcinogens like fertilizers, pesticides etc. Furthermore, arsenic can also act as co-carcinogen with UV light exposure leading to development of skin manifestations like hyperkeratosis finally causing skin cancer (Danaee et al., 2004; Chaudhuri et al., 2008).

Bangladesh represents largest population exposed to arsenic in the history as the groundwater used for drinking is contaminated with inorganic arsenic (Nordstrom, 2002). In the exposed population of Bangladesh, arsenic contamination in drinking water in tube wells is associated with lung cancer incidences in males with lung Squamous cell carcinoma in the areas with arsenic concentrations above 100 μg/L (Mostafa et al., 2008). The life time lung cancer mortality rate are 159.1/100 000 for males and 23.1 for females (per 100 000 population) (Chen et al., 2004). In the Southwest Taiwan, individuals exposed to arsenic are diseased with black foot disease (BFD). It is peripheral arterial disease mostly characterized by severe systemic arteriosclerosis and spontaneous gangrene leading amputation (Kadono et al., 2002). In the BFD affected areas, incidence and mortality rate for lung cancer has been well documented especially among those individuals who have been drinking arsenic contaminated water for more than 40 years (Chen et al., 1986). Smokers in these areas have a 4.1 fold higher risk for lung cancer correlation a possible relationship between arsenic and tobacco exposures causing lung tumorigenesis (Chiou et al., 1995). There are also various studies which correlate between 5 years of arsenic exposure through drinking water and elevated lung cancer risk (Tsuda et al., 1995, Hopenhayn-Rich et al., 1998, Nicolli et al., 1995, Marshall et al., 2007).

There are various genetic factors which modulate the susceptibility to arsenic-induced lung cancer. The genetic carriers like CYP1A1*2A/ GSTM1 homozygous deletion genotype showed increased odds ratio for lung cancer, especially in the smokers (Adonis et al., 2005a, 2005b). These group has furthermore stipulated that genomic aberrations in arsenic induced lung cancers exhibit distinct molecular characteristics. They used the whole genome tiling-path comparative genomic hybridization (CGH) array platform among lung SqCC cases from a Northern Chilean population chronically exposed to inorganic arsenic in drinking water. This has led to the induction of oxidative stress, alterations to DNA methylation, histone modification, and miRNA expression. (Martinez et al., 2010, Cullen et al., 1984).

Our institute has registered more than 25,000 cancer cases in year 2017. Most of the cancer cases reported were from the cities or towns which are located near the river Ganga (Figure 9). The most cancer incidences cases were from the districts - Patna, Bhojpur, Buxar, Bhagalpur, Saran, Vaishali, Darbhanga, Samastipur, Begusarai, etc. It is quite possible that drinking of arsenic contaminated groundwater had caused health related issues in the population finally leading to cancer. Our cancer epidemiological data shows that the districts which are located near the river basins emerging from the Himalayas have the more incidences in comparison to the non- river zones. The cancer cases observed were skin cancer, skin melanoma, lung cancer, bladder cancer, hepatobiliary cancer, renal cell carcinoma, breast cancer,

Figure 9. Showing cancer map of Bihar

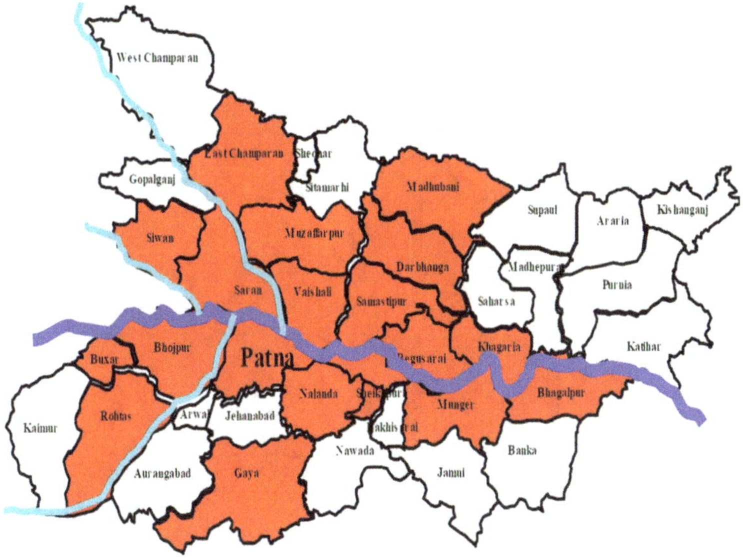

ovarian cancer, endometrium cancer etc. with typical symptoms of arsenicosis denotes that there could be some correlation with the arsenic (Figure 10).

Therefore, we conducted a random study on 400 cancer patients to know the level of arsenic concentration the blood samples of the cancer patients. We found that there were 5% cancer cases which showed normal blood arsenic levels in the patients while 95% of the cancer patients showed significant arsenic contamination levels in their blood samples which correlates the present study (Figure 11). The incidences were found maximum in female cancer patients in comparison to male cancer patients and this global phenomenon (Globocan, 2012 and Bray et al., 2018).

Arsenic Mitigation

In Tilak Rai Ka Hatta (TRKH) village of Buxar district of Bihar, India, the most unfortunate part of the study were the cases of cancer like ovarian, breast, skin melanoma, gall bladder and liver, leukemia, urinary bladder and colorectal cancer. There were 14 cancer cases reported in 2016-2017. All the cancer patients had died except the skin melanoma and colorectal cancer case patient. All the patients exhibited the typical arsenicosis symptoms (Figure 12). The patient's drinking water source was found to be 534.2μg/L while their blood sample had arsenic concentration 54.9μg/L.

A community based arsenic filter was installed in the study area in June 2017 with the help of community participation through the collaborative effort of Mahavir Cancer Institute and Research Centre, Patna, Bihar, India and Lehigh University, Pennsylvania, USA, which is based on Adsorbent Hybrid Anion Exchange Nano Resin (Figure 13). This filter is providing arsenic safe water giving good health outcomes.

Presently, this filter is providing safe drinking water to more than 100 households. People from distant villages are also coming to fetch water. Installation of arsenic filter has made drastic change in

Figure 10. Showing cancer cases with typical arsenicosis symptoms in subjects from arsenic hit area of Bihar

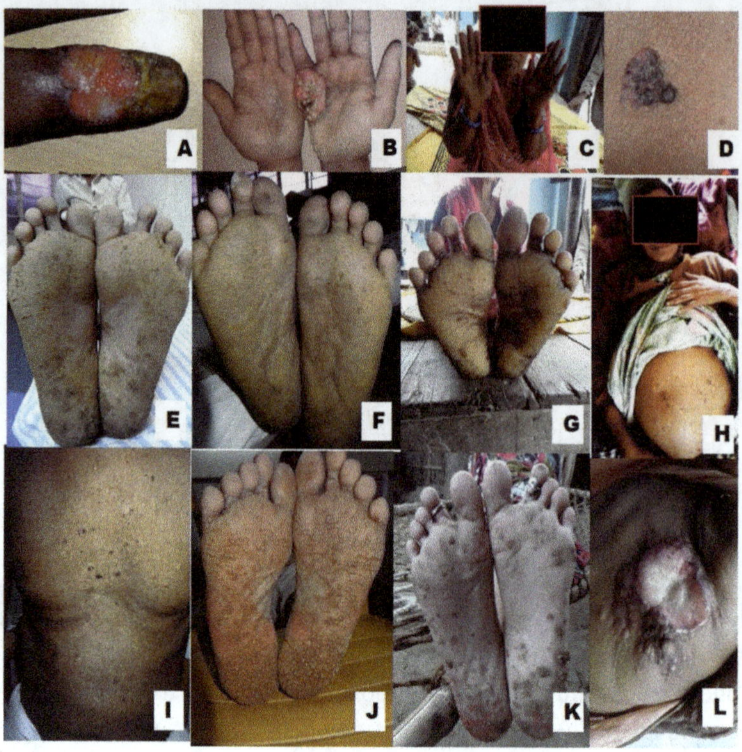

Figure 11. Showing Arsenic contamination in blood samples of cancer patients (n= 400)

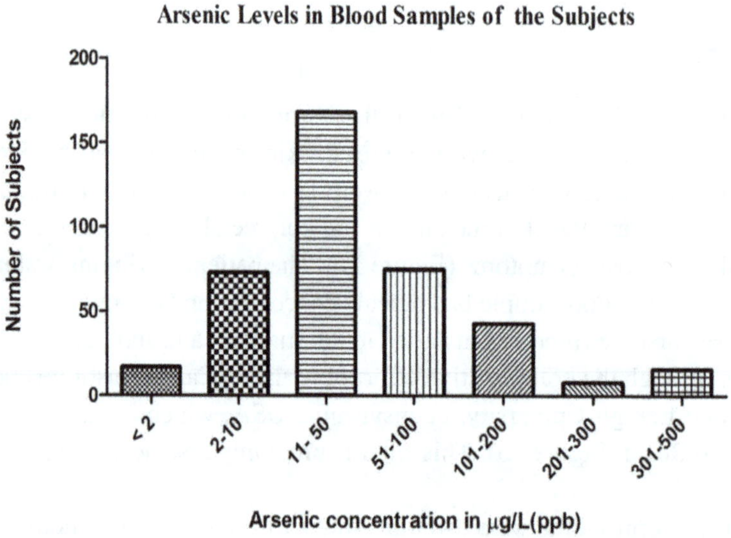

Figure 12. 1). Hyperkeratosis, melanosis, rain drop pigmentation with ovarian cancer in a 58yrs old female (As in drinking water 534.2 µg/L) 2) Hyperkeratosis, melanosis with liver cancer in 55 yr. old female (As in drinking water 624.5 µg/L) 3). Skin melanoma in a 52 yr. old female (As in drinking water 663.1 µg/L)

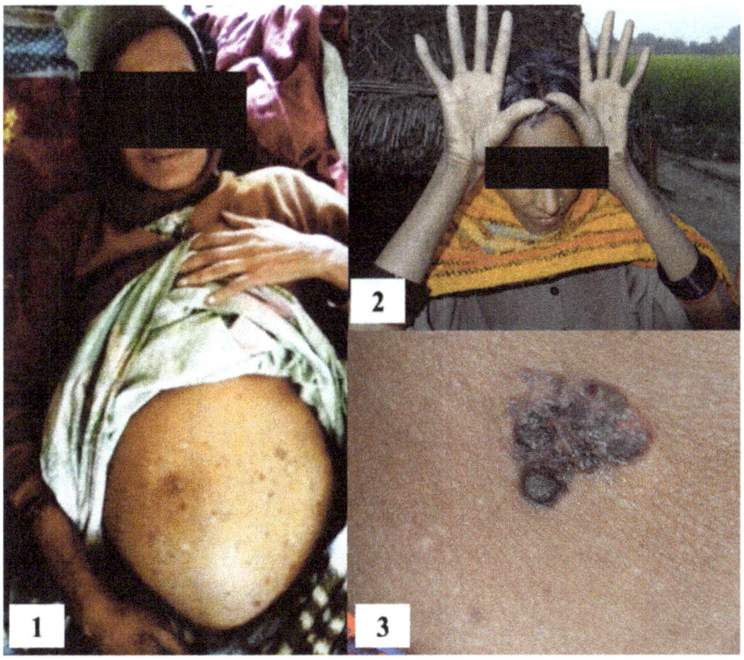

the health status of the arsenic exposed village population. Following are the changes observed in the village population after the usage of arsenic filter water:

- Decrease in the skin manifestations
- Decrease in the problems related to their gastrointestinal issues
- Decrease in the hormone related problems in the females
- Increased appetite
- Increased immunity level
- Positive changes in the neuro-behavioural activities
- No new cases of cancer reported till date
- Increased awareness in the population related to use of safe drinking water
- Village people have become more conscious about their health

CONCLUSION

Therefore, from the entire study, we conclude that arsenic contamination in drinking has become serious public health problem affecting more than 200 million people affected by it worldwide. More than a decade of exposure has led to the serious health related problems in the population like cancer. However, mitigation measures have been carried out in many arsenic exposed areas but requires managed strate-

Figure 13. Installation of arsenic filter

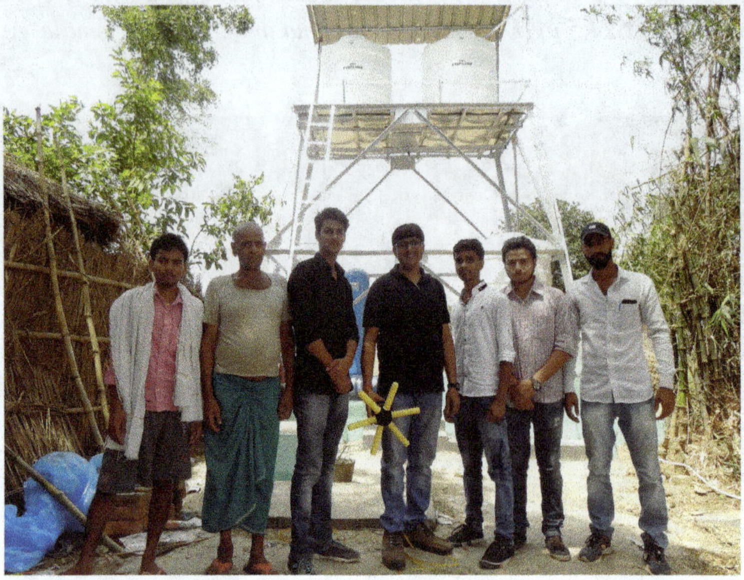

gies to combat the problem with regular surveillance and monitoring of drinking water. The entire study indicates that arsenic contamination in drinking water has exerted various deleterious health problems in the exposed population leading to skin manifestations like hyperkeratosis, melanosis, Bowen's disease leading to SqCC of skin. Furthermore, the other cancer incidences like lung cancer, bladder cancer, kidney cancer etc. has increased many folds in the population in the recent times which needs proper attention to the health department of the states. The, specific strategies for mitigation and identification of the cancer diseases will together work for the welfare of the exposed population to lower down such incidences. However, in the states like West Bengal and country like Bangladesh the incidences of cancer due to arsenic has decreased many folds. But, states like Bihar and Uttar Pradesh where huge population is presently exposed with arsenic poisoning needs the Government support. Such, cascade mitigation program along with the health department can really solve the problem in the arsenic exposed population. Finally, awareness among the affected population related to safe drinking water sources should also be the prime vision of the stakeholders working in these regions.

Conflict of Interests: The authors declare that they have no conflict of interests.

ACKNOWLEDGMENT

The authors are thankful to the institute for the entire infrastructural facilities as well as the Department of Science and Technology, (SSTP Division), Government of India for their support in the study carried out especially in Buxar district of Bihar. The authors also acknowledge Tagore-Sengupta Foundation for providing fund for installation of Arsenic filter in Tilak Rai Ka Hatta village of Buxar district of Bihar.

REFERENCES

Abernathy, C. O., Liu, Y. P., Longfellow, D., Aposhian, H. V., Beck, B., Fowler, B., ... Waalkes, M. (1999). Arsenic: Health effects, mechanisms of actions, and research issues. *Environmental Health Perspectives*, *107*(7), 593–597. doi:10.1289/ehp.99107593 PMID:10379007

Abhinav, S., Navin, S., Verma, S. K., Kumar, R., Ali, M., Kumar, A., & Ghosh, A. K. (2016): Groundwater and blood samples assessment for arsenic toxicity in rural population of Darbhanga district of Bihar, India. In *Proceedings of the 6th International congress on arsenic in the environment*, Stockholm, Sweden, June 19-23 (pp. 418-420). London, UK: Taylor & Francis group.

Acharyya, S. K., Chackraborty, P., Lahiri, S., Raymahashay, B. C., Guha, S., & Bhowmik, A. (1999). Arsenic poisoning in the Ganges delta. *Nature*, *401*(6753), 545. doi:10.1038/44052 PMID:10524619

Acharyya, S. K., Lahiri, S., Raymahashay, B. C., & Bhowmik, A. (2000). Arsenic toxicity of groundwater in parts of the Bengal basin in India and Bangladesh, the role of quaternary stratigraphy and Holocene sea-level fluctuation. *Environ. Geol.*, *39*(10), 1127–1137. doi:10.1007002540000107

Adonis, M., Martínez, V., Marín, P., Berrios, D., & Gil, L. (2005). Smoking habit and genetic factors associated with lung cancer in a population highly exposed to arsenic. *Toxicology Letters*, *159*(1), 32–37. doi:10.1016/j.toxlet.2005.04.007 PMID:16099114

Adonis, M., Martínez, V., Marín, P., & Gil, L. (2005). CYP1A1 and GSTM1 genetic polymorphisms in lung cancer populations exposed to arsenic in drinking water. *Xenobiotica*, *35*(5), 519–530. doi:10.1080/00498250500057310 PMID:16012082

Agency for Cancer Research (IARC). (2004). Some drinking-water disinfectants and contaminants including arsenic. IARC.

Agency for Toxic Substances and Disease Registry (ATSDR). (2007). *Arsenic Toxicity*. Washington, DC, USA: U.S. Department of Health and Human Services.

Ahamed, S., Kumar, S. M., Mukherjee, A., Amir, H. M., Das, B., Nayak, B., ... Chakraborti, D. (2006). Arsenic groundwater contamination and its health effects In the state of Uttar Pradesh (UP) in upper and middle Ganga plain, India: A severe danger. *The Science of the Total Environment*, *370*(2-3), 31022. doi:10.1016/j.scitotenv.2006.06.015 PMID:16899281

Ahmad, S. A., Sayed, M. H., Barua, S., Khan, M. H., Faruquee, M. H., Jalil, A., ... Talukder, H. K. (2001). Arsenic in drinking water and pregnancy outcomes. *Environmental Health Perspectives*, *109*(6), 629–631. doi:10.1289/ehp.01109629 PMID:11445518

Ahsan, H., Chen, Y., Parvez, F., Argos, M., Hussain, A. I., Momotaj, H., ... Graziano, J. (2006). Health effects of arsenic longitudinal study (heals): Description of a multidisciplinary epidemiologic investigation. *Journal of Exposure Science & Environmental Epidemiology*, *16*(2), 191–205. doi:10.1038j.jea.7500449 PMID:16160703

Argos, M., Ahsan, H., & Graziano, J. H. (2012). Arsenic and human health: Epidemiologic progress and public health implications. *Reviews on Environmental Health*, *27*(4), 191–195. doi:10.1515/reveh-2012-0021 PMID:22962196

Argos, M., Kalra, T., Pierce, B. L., Chen, Y., Parvez, F., Islam, T., ... Ahsan, H. (2011). A prospective study of arsenic exposure from drinking water and incidence of skin lesions in Bangladesh. *American Journal of Epidemiology, 174*(2), 185–194. doi:10.1093/aje/kwr062 PMID:21576319

Argos, M., Kalra, T., Rathouz, P. J., Chen, Y., Pierce, B., Parvez, F., ... Ahsan, H. (2010). Arsenic exposure from drinking water, and all-cause and chronic-disease mortalities in Bangladesh (heals): A prospective cohort study. *Lancet, 376*(9737), 252–258. doi:10.1016/S0140-6736(10)60481-3 PMID:20646756

Armando, V. L., & Angel, A. O. (1979). Chronic arsenic poisoning. *Boletín Médico del Hospital Infantil de México, 36*(5), 849–861. PMID:157141

Armienta, M. A., & Segovia, N. (2008). Arsenic and fluoride in the groundwater of Mexico. *Environmental Geochemistry and Health, 30*(4), 345–353. doi:10.100710653-008-9167-8 PMID:18335171

Bagla, P., & Kaiser, J. (1996). India's spreading health crisis draws global arsenic experts. *Science, 274*(5285), 174–175. doi:10.1126cience.274.5285.174 PMID:8927976

Bailey, K. A., Hester, S. D., Knapp, G. W., Owen, R. D., & Thai, S. F. (2010). Gene expression of normal human epidermal keratinocytes modulated by trivalent arsenicals. *Molecular Carcinogenesis, 49*(12), 981–998. doi:10.1002/mc.20677 PMID:20886546

Banerjee, N., Paul, S., Sau, T. J., Das, J. K., Bandyopadhyay, A., Banerjee, S., & Giri, A. K. (2013). Epigenetic modifications of DAPK and p16 genes contribute to arsenic-induced skin lesions and non-dermatological health effects. *Toxicological Sciences, 135*(2), 300–308. doi:10.1093/toxsci/kft163 PMID:23872714

Bardullas, U., Limo'n-Pacheco, J. H., Giordano, M., Carrizales, L., Mendoza-Trejo, M. S., & Rodrı'guez, V. M. (2009). Chronic low-level arsenic exposure causes gender-specific alterations in locomotor activity, dopaminergic systems, and thioredoxin expression in mice. *Toxicology and Applied Pharmacology, 239*(2), 169–177. doi:10.1016/j.taap.2008.12.004 PMID:19121333

Bates, M. N., Smith, A. H., & Hopenhayn-Rich, C. (1992). Arsenic Ingestion and Internal Cancers: A Review. *American Journal of Epidemiology, 135*(5), 462–476. doi:10.1093/oxfordjournals.aje.a116313 PMID:1570813

Bhattacharjee, S., Chakravarty, S., Maity, S., Dureja, V., & Gupta, K. K. (2005). Metal contents in the groundwater of Sahebgunj district, Jharkhand, India, with special reference to arsenic. *Chemosphere, 58*(9), 1203–1217. doi:10.1016/j.chemosphere.2004.09.055 PMID:15667841

Bhattacharya, P., Chatterjee, D., & Jacks, G. (1997). Occurrence of arsenic contaminated groundwater in alluvial aquifers from Delta plain, Eastern India: Options for a safe drinking water supply. *Water: Research and Development, 13*, 79–92.

Blackwell, R. Q., Yang, T. H., & Ai, I. (1961). Preliminary report on arsenic level in water and food from the endemic Blackfoot area. *Journal of the Formosan Medical Association, 60*, 1139–1140.

Boonchai, W., Green, A., Ng, J., Dicker, A., & Chenevix-Trench, G. (2000). Basal cell carcinoma in chronic arsenicism occurring in Queensland, Australia, after ingestion of an asthma medication. *Journal of the American Academy of Dermatology, 43*(4), 664–669. doi:10.1067/mjd.2000.107939 PMID:11004623

Borgoño, J. M., Vicent, P., Venturíno, H., & Infante, A. (1977). Arsenic in the drinking water of the city of Antofagasta: Epidemiological and clinical study before and after the installation of a treatment plant. [PubMed]. *Environmental Health Perspectives*, *19*, 103–105.

Bray, F., Ferlay, J., Soerjomataram, I., Siegel, R. L., Torre, L. A., & Jemal, A. (2018, November). Global cancer statistics 2018: GLOBOCAN estimates of incidence and mortality worldwide for 36 cancers in 185 countries. *CA: a Cancer Journal for Clinicians*, *68*(6), 394–424. doi:10.3322/caac.21492 PMID:30207593

Byrne, S., Amarasiriwardena, D., Bandak, B., Bartkus, L., Kane, J., Jones, J., ... Cornejo, L. (2010). Were Chinchorros exposed to arsenic? Arsenic determination in Chinchorro Mummies' hair by laser ablation inductively coupled plasma-mass spectrometry (LA-ICP-MS). *Microchemical Journal*, *94*(1), 28–35. doi:10.1016/j.microc.2009.08.006

Calderon, J., Navarro, M. E., Jimenez-Capdeville, M. E., Santos-Diaz, M. A., Golden, A., Rodriguez-Leyva, I., ... Diaz-Barriga, F. (2001). Exposure to arsenic and lead and neuropsychological development in Mexican children. *Environmental Research*, *85*(2), 69–76. doi:10.1006/enrs.2000.4106 PMID:11161656

Castren, K., Ranki, A., Welsh, J. A., & Vähäkangas, K. H. (1998). Infrequent p53 mutations in arsenic-related skin lesions. *Oncology Research*, *10*(9), 475–482. PMID:10223623

Caussy, E., & World Health Organization. (2005). A field guide for detection, management and surveillance of arsenicosis cases. World Health Organization.

Chakraborti, D., Das, B., Rahman, M. M., Chowdhury, U. K., Biswas, B., Goswami, A. B., ... Das, D. (2009). Status of groundwater arsenic contamination in the state of West Bengal, India: A 20-year study report. *Molecular Nutrition & Food Research*, *53*(5), 542–551. doi:10.1002/mnfr.200700517 PMID:19382148

Chakraborti, D., Mukherjee, S. C., Pati, S., Sengupta, M. K., Rahman, M. M., Chowdhury, U. K., ... Basu, G. K. (2003). Arsenic groundwater contamination in Middle Ganga Plain, Bihar, India: A future danger? *Environmental Health Perspectives*, *111*(9), 1194–1201. doi:10.1289/ehp.5966 PMID:12842773

Chakraborti, D., Rahman, M. M., Ahamed, S., Dutta, R. N., Pati, S., & Mukherjee, S. C. (2016). Arsenic groundwater contamination and its health effects in Patna district (capital of Bihar) in the middle Ganga plain, India. *Chemosphere*, *152*, 520–529. doi:10.1016/j.chemosphere.2016.02.119 PMID:27011321

Chakraborti, D., Rahman, M. M., & Alauddin, M. (2015). Groundwater arsenic contamination in Bangladesh - 21 years of research. *Journal of Trace Elements in Medicine and Biology*, *31*, 237–248. doi:10.1016/j.jtemb.2015.01.003 PMID:25660323

Chakraborti, D., Rahman, M. M., Chowdhury, U. K., Paul, K., Chowdhury, U. K., Sengupta, M. K., ... Mukherjee, S. C. (2002). Arsenic calamity in the Indian subcontinent: What lessons have been learned? *Talanta*, *58*(1), 3–22. doi:10.1016/S0039-9140(02)00270-9 PMID:18968730

Chakraborti, D., Sengupta, M. K., Rahman, M. M., Ahamed, S., Chowdhury, U. K., & ... . (2004). Groundwater arsenic contamination and its health effects in the Ganga– Meghna–Brahmaputra Plain. *Journal of Environmental Monitoring*, *6*, 74N–83N. PMID:15241847

Chakraborti, D., Singh, S., Rahman, M., Dutta, R., Mukherjee, S., Pati, S., & Kar, P. (2018). Groundwater arsenic contamination in the Ganga River Basin: A future health danger. *International Journal of Environmental Research and Public Health*, *15*(2), 180.

Chandrasekharam, D., Karamakar, J., Berner, J., & Stuben, D. (2001). Arsenic contamination in groundwater, Murshidabad district, West Bengal. In R. Cidu (Ed.), *Proceeding 10th International Symposium on Water Rocks Interaction*, Villasimius, Italy (Vol. 2, pp. 1051-1054).

Charlet, L., & Polya, D. (2006). Arsenic in shallow reducing ground waters in southern Asia, an environmental health disaster. *Elements*, *2*(2), 91–96. doi:10.2113/gselements.2.2.91

Chen, C. J., Chuang, Y. C., You, S. L., Lin, T. M., & Wu, H. Y. (1986). A retrospective study on malignant neoplasms of bladder, lung and liver in blackfoot disease endemic area in Taiwan. *British Journal of Cancer*, *53*(3), 399–405. doi:10.1038/bjc.1986.65 PMID:3964542

Chen, C. L., Chiou, H. Y., Hsu, L. I., Hsueh, Y. M., Wu, M. M., Wang, Y. H., & Chen, C.-J. (2010). Arsenic in drinking water and risk of urinary tract cancer: A follow-up study from north eastern Taiwan. *Cancer Epidemiology, Biomarkers & Prevention*, *19*(1), 101–110. doi:10.1158/1055-9965.EPI-09-0333 PMID:20056628

Chen, Y., & Ahsan, H. (2004). Cancer burden from arsenic in drinking water in Bangladesh. *American Journal of Public Health*, *94*(5), 741–744. doi:10.2105/AJPH.94.5.741 PMID:15117692

Chen, Y., Graziano, J. H., Parvez, F., Hussain, I., Momotaj, H., van Geen, A., ... Ahsan, H. (2006). Modification of risk of arsenic-induced skin lesions by sunlight exposure, smoking, and occupational exposures in Bangladesh. *Epidemiology (Cambridge, Mass.)*, *17*(4), 459–467. doi:10.1097/01.ede.0000220554.50837.7f PMID:16755266

Chen, Y., Graziano, J. H., Parvez, F., Liu, M., Slavkovich, V., Kalra, T., ... Ahsan, H. (2011). Arsenic exposure from drinking water and mortality from cardiovascular disease in Bangladesh: Prospective cohort study. *BMJ (Clinical Research Ed.)*, *342*(2), d2431. doi:10.1136/bmj.d2431 PMID:21546419

Chiou, H. Y., Chiou, S. T., Hsu, Y. H., Chou, Y. L., Tseng, C. H., Wei, M. L., & Chen, C. J. (2001). Incidence of transitional cell carcinoma and arsenic in drinking water: A follow-up study of 8102 residents in a arseniasis endemic area in Northeastern Taiwan. *American Journal of Epidemiology*, *153*(5), 411–418. doi:10.1093/aje/153.5.411 PMID:11226969

Chiou, H. Y., Hsueh, Y. M., Liaw, K. F., Horng, S. F., Chiang, M. H., Pu, Y. S., ... & Chen, C. J. (1995). Incidence of internal cancers and ingested inorganic arsenic: A seven-year follow-up study in Taiwan. *Cancer Research*, *55*(6), 1296–1300. PMID:7882325

Concha, G., Nermell, B., & Vahter, M. (1998). Metabolism of inorganic arsenic in children with chronic high arsenic exposure in northern Argentina. *Environmental Health Perspectives*, *106*(6), 355–359. doi:10.1289/ehp.98106355 PMID:9618352

Cullen, W. R., McBride, B. C., & Reglinski, J. (1984). The reaction of methylarsenicals with thiols: Some biological implications. *Journal of Inorganic Biochemistry*, *21*(3), 179–194. doi:10.1016/0162-0134(84)83002-0 PMID:6392480

Cuzick, J., Evans, S., Gillman, M., & Evans, D. A. P. (1982). Medicinal arsenic and internal malignancies. *British Journal of Cancer*, *45*(6), 904–911. doi:10.1038/bjc.1982.143 PMID:6212076

Danaee, H., Nelson, H. H., Liber, H., Little, J. B., & Kelsey, K. T. (2004). Low dose exposure to sodium arsenite synergistically interacts with UV radiation to induce mutations and alter DNA repair in human cells. *Mutagenesis*, *19*(2), 143–148. doi:10.1093/mutage/geh010 PMID:14981161

Das, D., Chatterjee, A., Mandal, B. K., Samanta, G., Chakraborti, D., & Chanda, B. (1995). Arsenic in groundwater in six districts of West Bengal, India: The biggest arsenic calamity in the world. Part 2. Arsenic concentration in drinking water, hair, nails, urine, skin-scale and liver tissue (biopsy) of the affected people. *Analyst (London)*, *120*(3), 917–924. doi:10.1039/an9952000917 PMID:7741255

Das, D., Samanta, G., Mandal, B. K., Chowdhury, T. R., Chanda, C. R., Chowdhury, P. P., & .... (1996). Arsenic in groundwater in six districts of West Bengal, India. *Environmental Geochemistry and Health*, *18*(1), 5–15. doi:10.1007/BF01757214 PMID:24194364

Datta, D. V., & Kaul, M. K. (1976). Arsenic content of drinking water in villages in northern India. A concept of arsenicosis. *The Journal of the Association of Physicians of India*, *24*, 599–604. PMID:1025145

De Chaudhuri, S., Kundu, M., Banerjee, M., Das, J., Majumdar, P., Basu, S., ... Giri, A. (2008). Arsenic-induced health effects and genetic damage in keratotic individuals: Involvement of p53 arginine variant and chromosomal aberrations in arsenic susceptibility. *Mutation Research*, *659*(1-2), 118–125. doi:10.1016/j.mrrev.2007.11.008 PMID:18249029

Dhar, R. K., Biswas, B. K., Samanta, G., Mandal, B. K., Chakraborti, D., Roy, S., ... & Khan, A. W. (1997). Groundwater arsenic calamity in Bangladesh. *Current Science*, *73*, 48.

Dixit, S., & Hering, J. G. (2003). Comparison of arsenic V and arsenic III sorption onto iron oxides minerals: implications for arsenic mobility: environmental science and technology. *Environmental Science & Technology*, *37*, 4182–4189. doi:10.1021/es030309t PMID:14524451

Donselaar, M. E., Bhatt, A. G., Bose, N., Bruining, J., & Ghosh, A. K. Entrapment of Arsenic Contaminated Groundwater in Point Bars: Case Study of Holocene Ganges River deposits, Bihar, India. In *Proceedings of 10th International Conference on Fluvial Sedimentology*, University of Leeds, UK.

Engel, R. R., Hopenhayn-Rich, C., Receveur, O., & Smith, A. H. (1994). Vascular effects of chronic arsenic exposure: A review. *Epidemiologic Reviews*, *16*(2), 184–209. doi:10.1093/oxfordjournals.epirev.a036150 PMID:7713176

Garai, R., Chakraborty, A. K., Dey, S. B., & Saha, K. C. (1984). Chronic arsenic poisoning from tubewell water. *Journal of the Indian Medical Association*, *82*, 34–35. PMID:6747321

Garzanti, E., Vezzoli, G., Ando, S., France-Lanord, C., Singh, S. K., & Foster, G. (2004). Sand Petrology and focused erosion in collision orogens: The Brahmaputra case. *Earth and Planetary Science Letters*, *220*(1-2), 157–174. doi:10.1016/S0012-821X(04)00035-4

Ghosh, S., & De, S. (1995). Sources of arseniferous sediments at Kauchua and Itina, Habra Block, North-24 Paragans, West Bengal, a case study. *Journal of Earth Science*, *22*, 183–189.

Ghosh, S. K., Bandyopadhyay, D., Bandyopadhyay, S. K., & Debbarma, K. (2013). Cutaneous malignant and premalignant conditions caused by chronic arsenicosis from contaminated ground water consumption: A profile of patients from eastern India. *Skinmed*, *11*(4), 211–216. PMID:24053006

Gilmore, T. D. (2006). Introduction to NF-κB: Players, pathways, perspectives. *Oncogene*, *51*(51), 6680–6684. doi:10.1038j.onc.1209954 PMID:17072321

GLOBOCAN. (2012). v1.0, cancer incidence and mortality worldwide: IARC CancerBase No. 11. International Agency for Research on Cancer Web site. Retrieved from http://globocan.iarc.fr

Guo, H. R., Yu, H. S., Hu, H., & Monson, R. R. (2001). Arsenic in drinking water and skin cancers: Cell-type specificity (Taiwan, ROC). *Cancer Causes & Control*, *12*(10), 909–916. doi:10.1023/A:1013712203455 PMID:11808710

Guriillot, S., & Charlet, L. (2007). Bengal arsenic, an archive of Himalaya orogeny and paleohydrology. *Journal of Environmental Science and Health*, *42*(12), 1785–1794. doi:10.1080/10934520701566702 PMID:17952779

Halder, G., & Johnson, R. L. (2011). Hippo signaling: Growth control and beyond. *Development.*, *138*(1), 9–22. doi:10.1242/dev.045500 PMID:21138973

Hamadani, J. D., Tofail, F., Nermell, B., Gardner, R., Shiraji, S., Bottai, M., ... Vahter, M. (2011). Critical windows of exposure for arsenic-associated impairment of cognitive function in pre-school girls and boys: A population-based cohort study. *International Journal of Epidemiology*, *40*(6), 1593–1604. doi:10.1093/ije/dyr176 PMID:22158669

Haque, R., Mazumder, D. N., Samanta, S., Ghosh, N., Kalman, D., Smith, M. M., ... Smith, A. H. (2003). Arsenic in drinking water and skin lesions: Dose-response data from West Bengal, India. *Epidemiology (Cambridge, Mass.)*, *14*(2), 174–182. doi:10.1097/01.EDE.0000040361.55051.54 PMID:12606883

Harrington, J. M., Middaugh, J. P., Morse, D. L., & Housworth, J. (1978). A survey of a population exposed to high concentrations of arsenic in well water in Fairbanks, Alaska. *American Journal of Epidemiology*, *108*(5), 377–385. doi:10.1093/oxfordjournals.aje.a112635 PMID:727207

Hopenhayn-Rich, C., Biggs, M. L., & Smith, A. H. (1998). Lung and kidney cancer mortality associated with arsenic drinking water in Ordoba, Argentina. *International Journal of Epidemiology*, *27*(4), 561–569. doi:10.1093/ije/27.4.561 PMID:9758107

Hundal, H. S., Singh, K., & Singh, D. (2009). Arsenic content in ground and canal waters of Punjab, North-West India. *Environmental Monitoring and Assessment*, *154*(1-4), 393–400. doi:10.100710661-008-0406-3 PMID:18568407

Hunt, K. M., Srivastava, R. K., Elmets, C. A., & Athar, M. (2014). The mechanistic basis of arsenicosis: Pathogenesis of skin cancer. *Cancer Letters*, *354*(2), 211–219. doi:10.1016/j.canlet.2014.08.016 PMID:25173797

International Agency for Research on Cancer (IARC). (2012). *A Review of Human Carcinogens: Arsenic, Metals, Fibres, and Dusts*.

James, K. A., Byers, T., Hokanson, J. E., Meliker, J. R., Zerbe, G. O., & Marshall, J. A. (2015). Association between lifetime exposure to inorganic arsenic in drinking water and coronary heart disease in Colorado residents. *Environmental Health Perspectives*, *123*(2), 128–134. doi:10.1289/ehp.1307839 PMID:25350952

Kadono, T., Inaoka, T., Murayama, N., Ushijima, K., Nagano, M., Nakamura, S., ... Ohtsuka, R. (2002). Skin manifestations of arsenicosis in two villages in Bangladesh. *International Journal of Dermatology*, *41*(12), 841–846. doi:10.1046/j.1365-4362.2002.01668.x PMID:12492966

Kalia, M. (2008). Brain development: Anatomy, connectivity, adaptive plasticity, and toxicity. *Metabolism: Clinical and Experimental*, *57*, S2–S5. doi:10.1016/j.metabol.2008.07.009 PMID:18803960

Karagas, M. R., Stukel, T. A., & Tosteson, T. D. (2002). Assessment of cancer risk and environmental levels of arsenic in New Hampshire. *International Journal of Hygiene and Environmental Health*, *205*(1-2), 85–94. doi:10.1078/1438-4639-00133 PMID:12018020

Koons, R. D., & Peters, C. A. (1994). Axial distribution of arsenic in individual human hairs by solid sampling graphite furnace AAS. *Journal of Analytical Toxicology*, *18*(1), 36–40. doi:10.1093/jat/18.1.36 PMID:8127082

Korte, E., & Fernando, Q. (1991). A review of arsenic (III) in groundwater. *Critical Reviews in Environmental Control*, *21*(1), 1–39. doi:10.1080/10643389109388408

Kumagai, Y., & Sumi, D. (2007). Arsenic: Signal transduction, transcription factor, and biotransformation involved in cellular response and toxicity. *Annual Review of Pharmacology and Toxicology*, *47*(1), 243–262. doi:10.1146/annurev.pharmtox.47.120505.105144 PMID:17002598

Kumar, A., Ali, M., Rahman, S. M., Iqubal, A. M., Anand, G., Niraj, P. K., ... & Kumar, R. (2015). Ground Water Arsenic Poisoning in "Tilak Rai Ka Hatta" Village of Buxar District, Bihar, India Causing Severe Health Hazards and Hormonal Imbalance. *Journal of Environmental & Analytical Toxicology*, *5*, 290.

Kumar, A., Ghosh, A. K., & Singh, N. (2016c). Arsenic on drinking water: An emerging human right challenge in India. In N. Singh (Ed.), The Human Right to water – From concept to reality (Ch. 4). Springer International Publishing Switzerland.

Kumar, A., Kumar, R., Ali, M., Gahlot, V., & Ghosh, A. K. (2016b). Groundwater Arsenic poisoning in Buxar district of Bihar. In *Proceedings of the 6th International congress on arsenic in the environment*, Stockholm, Sweden, June 19-23 (pp. 378-379). London, UK: Taylor & Francis group.

Kumar, A., Rahman, M. S., Iqubal, M. A., Ali, M., Niraj, P. K., Anand, G., & Kumar, P. (2016a). Ground water arsenic contamination: A local survey in India. *International Journal of Preventive Medicine*, 7.

Kurttio, P., Komulainen, H., Hakala, E., Kahelin, H., & Pekkanen, J. (1998). Urinary excretion of arsenic species after exposure to arsenic present in drinking water. *Archives of Environmental Contamination and Toxicology*, *34*(3), 297–305. doi:10.1007002449900321 PMID:9504979

Lee, C. H., Yu, C. L., Liao, W. T., Kao, Y. H., Chai, C. Y., Chen, G. S., & Yu, H. S. (2004). Effects and interactions of low doses of arsenic and UVB on keratinocyte apoptosis. *Chemical Research in Toxicology*, *17*(9), 1199–1205.

Li, C., Srivastava, R. K., Elmets, C. A., Afaq, F., & Athar, M. (2013). Arsenic-induced cutaneous hyperplastic lesions are associated with the dysregulation of Yap, a Hippo signaling-related protein. *Biochemical and Biophysical Research Communications*, *438*(4), 607–612. doi:10.1016/j.bbrc.2013.08.008 PMID:23942117

Li, C., Xu, J., Li, F., Chaudhary, S. C., Weng, Z., Wen, J., ... Athar, M. (2011). Unfolded protein response signaling and MAP kinase pathways underlie pathogenesis of arsenic-induced cutaneous inflammation. *Cancer Prevention Research*, *4*(12), 2101–2109. doi:10.1158/1940-6207.CAPR-11-0343 PMID:21911445

Lien, H. C., Tsai, T. F., Lee, Y. Y., & Hsiao, C. H. (1999). Merkel cell carcinoma and chronic arsenicism. *Journal of the American Academy of Dermatology*, *41*(4), 641–643. PMID:10495389

Marshall, G., Ferreccio, C., Yuan, Y., Bates, M. N., Steinmaus, C., Selvin, S., ... Smith, A. H. (2007). Fifty-Year study of lung and bladder cancer mortality in Chile related to arsenic in drinking water. *Journal of the National Cancer Institute*, *99*(12), 920–928. doi:10.1093/jnci/djm004 PMID:17565158

Martinez, V. D., Buys, T. P. H., Adonis, M., Benítez, H., Gallegos, I., Lam, S., ... Gil, L. (2010). Arsenic-related DNA copy-number alterations in lung squamous cell carcinomas. *British Journal of Cancer*, *103*(8), 1277–1283. doi:10.1038j.bjc.6605879 PMID:20842114

Melkonian, S., Argos, M., Chen, Y., Parvez, F., Pierce, B., Ahmed, A., ... Ahsan, H. (2012). Intakes of several nutrients are associated with incidence of arsenic-related keratotic skin lesions in Bangladesh. *The Journal of Nutrition*, *142*(12), 2128–2134. doi:10.3945/jn.112.165720 PMID:23077185

Melkonian, S., Argos, M., Pierce, B. L., Chen, Y., Islam, T., Ahmed, A., ... Ahsan, H. (2011). A prospective study of the synergistic effects of arsenic exposure and smoking, sun exposure, fertilizer use, and pesticide use on risk of premalignant skin lesions in Bangladeshi men. *American Journal of Epidemiology*, *173*(2), 183–191. doi:10.1093/aje/kwq357 PMID:21098630

Milliman, J. D., & Sivitsli, J. P. M. (1992). Geomorphic/tectonic control of sediment discharge to the ocean: The importance of small mountainous rivers. *The Journal of Geology*, *100*(5), 525–544. doi:10.1086/629606

Ministry of Water Resources, Government of India. (2010). *Groundwater quality in shallow aquifers of India.* Central Groundwater Board: Faridabad, India.

Moe, B., Peng, H., Lu, X., Chen, B., Chen, L. W., Gabos, S., ... Le, X. C. (2016). Comparative cytotoxicity of fourteen trivalent and pentavalent arsenic species determined using real-time cell sensing. *Journal of Environmental Sciences (China)*, *49*, 113–124. doi:10.1016/j.jes.2016.10.004 PMID:28007166

Moreno Ávila, C. L., Limón-Pacheco, J. H., Giordano, M., & Rodríguez, V. M. (2016). Chronic exposure to arsenic in drinking water causes alterations in locomotor activity and decreases striatal mRNA for the D2 dopamine receptor in CD1 male mice. *Journal of Toxicology*.

Mostafa, M. G., McDonald, J. C., & Cherry, N. M. (2008). Lung cancer and exposure to arsenic in rural Bangladesh. *Occupational and Environmental Medicine*, *65*(11), 765–768. doi:10.1136/oem.2007.037895 PMID:18417558

Murcott, S. (2012). *Arsenic Contamination in the World: an International Sourcebook 2012*. IWA Publishing.

Narang, A. P. S., Chawla, L. S., & Khurana, S. B. (1987). Levels of arsenic in Indian opium eaters. *Drug and Alcohol Dependence*, *20*(2), 149–153. doi:10.1016/0376-8716(87)90064-0 PMID:2824159

Naujokas, M. F., Anderson, B., Ahsan, H., Aposhian, H. V., Graziano, J., Thompson, C., & Suk, W. A. (2013). The broad scope of health effects from chronic arsenic exposure: Update on a worldwide public health problem. *Environmental Health Perspectives*, *121*(3), 295–302. doi:10.1289/ehp.1205875 PMID:23458756

Nickson, R., McArthur, J., Ravenscroft, P., Burgess, W., & Ahmed, I. K. M. (2000). Mechanism of arsenic poisoning of groundwater in Bangladesh and West Bengal. *Applied Geochemistry*, *15*(4), 403–413. doi:10.1016/S0883-2927(99)00086-4

Nicolli, H. B., O'Connor, T. E., & Suriano, J. M. (1985). Geoquimica del arsenico y de otros oligoelementos en aguas subterraneas de la llanura Sudoriental de la provinda de Cordoba. *Miscelanea*, *71*, 1–112.

Nordstrom, D. K. (2002). Public health. Worldwide occurrences of arsenic in ground water. *Science*, *296*(5576), 2143–2145. doi:10.1126cience.1072375 PMID:12077387

NRC. (2001). *Arsenic in drinking water: 2001 update.* Washington, DC: The National academies press.

Olguin, A., Jauge, P., Cebrián, M., & Albores, A. (1983). Arsenic levels in blood, urine, hair, and nails from a chronically exposed human population. *Proceedings of the Western Pharmacology Society*, *26*, 175–177. PMID:6889337

Paulsen, F., Mai, S., Zellmer, U., & Alsen-Hinrichs, C. (1996). Blood and hair arsenic, lead and cadmium analysis of adults and correlation analysis with special reference to eating habits and other behavioral influences. *Gesundheitswesen (Bundesverband der Arzte des Offentlichen Gesundheitsdienstes (Germany))*, *58*, 459–464. (in German) PubMed PMID:9011262

Raie, R. M. (1996). Regional variation in As, Cu, Hg, and Se and interaction between them. *Ecotoxicology and Environmental Safety*, *35*(3), 248–252. doi:10.1006/eesa.1996.0107 PMID:9007001

Rodriguez-Barranco, M., Gil, F., Hernández, A. F., Alguacil, J., Lorca, A., Mendoza, R., ... Lacasaña, M. (2016). Postnatal arsenic exposure and attention impairment in school children. *Cortex*, *74*, 370–382. doi:10.1016/j.cortex.2014.12.018 PMID:25682472

Rogers, C. E., Tomita, A. V., Trowbridge, P. R., Gone, J. K., Chen, J., Zeeb, P., ... Durant, J. L. (1997). Hair analysis does not support hypothesized arsenic and chromium exposure from drinking water in Woburn, Massachusetts. *Environmental Health Perspectives*, *105*(10), 1090–1097. doi:10.1289/ehp.971051090 PMID:9349834

Rossman, T. G. (2003). Mechanism of arsenic carcinogenesis: An integrated approach. *Mutation Research*, *533*(1-2), 37–65. doi:10.1016/j.mrfmmm.2003.07.009 PMID:14643412

Rossman, T. G., Uddin, A. N., & Burns, F. J. (2004). Evidence that arsenite acts as a cocarcinogen in skin cancer. *Toxicology and Applied Pharmacology*, *198*(3), 394–404. doi:10.1016/j.taap.2003.10.016 PMID:15276419

Saha, D. (2009). Arsenic groundwater contamination in parts of middle Ganga plain, Bihar. *Current Science, 97*(6), 753–755.

Saha, K. C. (2003). Diagnosis of arsenicosis. *Journal of Environmental Science and Health Part A, 38*(1), 255–272. doi:10.1081/ESE-120016893 PMID:12635831

Sattar, A., Xie, S., Hafeez, M. A., Wang, X., Hussain, H. I., Iqbal, Z., ... Yuan, Z. (2016). Metabolism and toxicity of arsenicals in mammals. *Environmental Toxicology and Pharmacology, 48*, 214–224. doi:10.1016/j.etap.2016.10.020 PMID:27829199

Sharma, M., Sharma, S., Arora, M., & Kaul, D. (2013). Regulation of cellular Cyclin D1 gene by arsenic is mediated through miR-2909. *Gene, 522*(1), 60–64. doi:10.1016/j.gene.2013.03.058 PMID:23562784

Shrestha, R. R., Shrestha, M. P., Upadhyay, N. P., Pradhan, R., Khadka, R., Maskey, A., ... Shrestha, K. (2003). Groundwater arsenic contamination, its health impact and mitigation program in Nepal. *Journal of Environmental Science and Health. Part A, 38*(1), 185–200.

Singh, S. K. (2017). Groundwater arsenic contamination in Bihar: Causes, issues, and challenges. *International Journal of Current Research, 9*(08), 56787–56790.

Singh, S. K., Ghosh, A. K., Kumar, A., Kislay, K., Kumar, C., Tiwari, R. R., ... Imam, M. D. (2014). Groundwater Arsenic contamination and associated health risks in Bihar, India. *International Journal of Environmental of Research, 8*(1), 49–60.

Smedley, P. L., Kinniburgh, D. G., Macdonald, D. M. J., Nicolli, H. B., Barros, A. J., Tullio, J. O., ... Alonso, M. S. (2005). Arsenic associations in sediments from the loess aquifer of La Pampa, Argentina. *Applied Geochemistry, 20*(5), 989–1016. doi:10.1016/j.apgeochem.2004.10.005

Smith, A. H., Lingas, E. O., & Rahman, M. (2000). Contamination of drinking-water by arsenic in Bangladesh: A public health emergency. *Bulletin of the World Health Organization, 78*(9), 1093–1103. PMID:11019458

Straif, K., Benbrahim-Tallaa, L., Baan, R., Grosse, Y., Secretan, B., El Ghissassi, F., ... Cogliano, V. (2009). A review of human carcinogens–part C: Metals, arsenic, dusts, and fibres. *The Lancet Oncology, 10*(5), 453–454. doi:10.1016/S1470-2045(09)70134-2 PMID:19418618

Stuben, D., Berner, Z., Chandrasekharam, D., & Karamakar, J. (2003). Arsenic enrichment in groundwater of west Bengal, India: Geochemical evidence for mobilization of As under reducing conditions. *Applied Geochemistry, 18*(9), 1417–1434. doi:10.1016/S0883-2927(03)00060-X

Takagi, Y., Matsuda, S., Imai, S., Ohmori, Y., Masuda, T., Vinson, J. A., ... Kaniewski, A. (1988). Survey of trace elements in human nails: An international comparison. *Bulletin of Environmental Contamination and Toxicology, 41*(4-6), 690–695. doi:10.1007/BF02021020 PMID:3233368

Trouba, K. J., Wauson, E. M., & Vorce, R. L. (2000). Sodium arsenite-induced dysregulation of proteins involved in proliferative signaling. *Toxicology and Applied Pharmacology, 164*(2), 161–170. doi:10.1006/taap.1999.8873 PMID:10764629

Tsai, S. Y., Chou, H. Y., The, H.-W., Chen, C.-M., & Chen, C.-J. (2003). The HW, Chen CM, Chen CJ.The effects of chronic arsenic exposure from drinking water on the neuro behavioral development in adolescence. *Neurotoxicology*, *24*(4–5), 747–753. doi:10.1016/S0161-813X(03)00029-9 PMID:12900089

Tseng, W. P. (1977). Effects and dose response relationships of skin cancer and blackfoot disease with arsenic. *Environmental Health Perspectives*, *19*, 109–119. doi:10.1289/ehp.7719109 PMID:908285

Tsuda, T., Babazono, A., Yamamoto, E., Kurumatani, N., Mino, Y., Ogawa, T., ... Aoyama, H. (1995). Ingested arsenic and internal cancer: A historical cohort study followed for 33 years. *American Journal of Epidemiology*, *141*(3), 198–209. doi:10.1093/oxfordjournals.aje.a117421 PMID:7840093

Tyler, L. N., Ai, L., Zuo, C., Fan, C. Y., & Smoller, B. R. (2003). Analysis of promoter hypermethylation of death associated protein kinase and p16 tumor suppressor genes in actinic keratoses and squamous cell carcinomas of the skin. *Modern Pathology*, *16*(7), 660–664. doi:10.1097/01.MP.0000077516.90063.7D PMID:12861061

Valko, M., Rhodes, C. J., Moncol, J., Izakovic, M., & Mazur, M. (2006). Free radicals, metals and antioxidants in oxidative stress induced cancer. *Chemico-Biological Interactions*, *160*(1), 1–40. doi:10.1016/j.cbi.2005.12.009 PMID:16430879

Vienna, A., Capucci, E., Wolfsperger, M., & Hauser, G. (1995). Heavy metals in hair of students in Rome. *Anthropologischer Anzeiger*, *53*, 27–32. PMID:7755371

Wang, C. T., Chang, W. T., Huang, C. W., Chou, S. S., Lin, C. T., Liau, S. J., & Wang, R. T. (1994). Studies on the concentrations of arsenic, selenium, copper, zinc, and iron in the hair of blackfoot disease patients in different clinical stages. *European Journal of Clinical Chemistry and Clinical Biochemistry*, *32*(3), 107–111. PMID:8031959

Wasserman, G. A., Liu, X., Loiacono, N. J., Kline, J., Factor-Litvak, P., van Geen, A., ... Graziano, J. H. (2014). A cross-sectional study of well water arsenic and child IQ in Maine school children. *Environmental Health*, *13*(1), 23. doi:10.1186/1476-069X-13-23 PMID:24684736

Wasserman, G. A., Liu, X., Parvez, F., Ahsan, H., Factor-Litvak, P., van Geen, A., ... Graziano, J. H. (2004). Water arsenic exposure and children's intellectual function in Araihazar Bangladesh. *Environmental Health Perspectives*, *112*(13), 1329–1333. doi:10.1289/ehp.6964 PMID:15345348

WHO. (2008). Guidelines for drinking-water quality (3rd ed., Vol. 1). Geneva, World Health Organization.

Winkel, L., Berg, M., Amini, M., Hug, S. J., & Annette Johnson, C. (2008). Predicting groundwater arsenic contamination in Southeast Asia from surface parameters. *Nature Geoscience*, *1*(8), 536–542. doi:10.1038/ngeo254

Wolfsperger, M., Hauser, G., Gössler, W., & Schlagenhaufen, C. (1994). Heavy metals in human hair samples from Austria and Italy: Influence of sex and smoking habits. *The Science of the Total Environment*, *156*(3), 235–242. doi:10.1016/0048-9697(94)90190-2 PMID:7801110

Wong, H. H., & Wang, J. (2010). Merkel cell carcinoma. *Archives of Pathology & Laboratory Medicine*, *134*(11), 1711–1716. PMID:21043828

Wong S. S., Tan K. C., and Goh C. L. (1998). Cutaneous manifestations of chronic arsenicism: review of seventeen cases. *Journal of the American Academy of Dermatology*, *38*(2), 179-185.

World Health Organization. (2001). *Arsenic and arsenic compounds* (2nd ed.). Geneva, International Programme on Chemical Safety.

Xi, S., Guo, L., Qi, R., Sun, W., Jin, Y., & Sun, G. (2010). Prenatal and early life arsenic exposure induced oxidative damage and altered activities and mRNA expressions of neurotransmitter metabolic enzymes in offspring rat brain. *Journal of Biochemical and Molecular Toxicology*, *24*(6), 368–378. doi:10.1002/jbt.20349 PMID:20376865

Yoshida, T., Yamauchi, H., & Sun, G. F. (2004). Chronic health effects in people exposed to arsenic via the drinking water: Dose-response relationships in review. *Toxicology and Applied Pharmacology*, *198*(3), 243–252. doi:10.1016/j.taap.2003.10.022 PMID:15276403

Yu, H. S., Lee, C. H., Jee, S. H., Ho, C. K., & Guo, Y. L. (2001). Environmental and occupational skin diseases in Taiwan. *The Journal of Dermatology*, *28*(11), 628–631. doi:10.1111/j.1346-8138.2001.tb00049.x PMID:11770720

Yu, H. S., Liao, W. T., & Chai, C. Y. (2006). Arsenic carcinogenesis in the skin. *Journal of Biomedical Science*, *13*(5), 657–666. doi:10.100711373-006-9092-8 PMID:16807664

Yuan, Y., Marshall, G., Ferreccio, C., Steinmaus, C., Liaw, J., Bates, M., & Smith, A. H. (2010). Kidney cancer mortality: Fifty-year latency patterns related to arsenic exposure. *Epidemiology (Cambridge, Mass.)*, *21*(1), 103–108. doi:10.1097/EDE.0b013e3181c21e46 PMID:20010213

Yunus, F. M., Khan, S., Chowdhury, P., Milton, A. H., Hussain, S., & Rahman, M. (2016). A Review of Groundwater Arsenic Contamination in Bangladesh: The Millennium Development Goal Era and Beyond. International Journal of Environmental Research and Public Health, 13(2).

Zaldivar, R., Prunes, L., & Ghai, G. L. (1981). Arsenic dose in patients with cutaneous carcinomata and hepatic haemangio-endothelioma after environmental and occupational exposure. *Archives ofToxicology*, *47*(2), 145–154. doi:10.1007/BF00332356 PMID:7271443

Zhao, B., Ye, X., Yu, J., Li, L., Li, W., Li, S., ... Guan, K. L. (2008). TEAD mediates YAP- dependent gene induction and growth control. *Genes & Development*, *22*(14), 1962–1971. doi:10.1101/gad.1664408 PMID:18579750

Chapter 6
A Review on Chemsensors:
A Versatile Tool to Detect Environmentally Toxic Metal Ions

Richa Saxena
ITM University, India

Shweta Saxena
KRG College, India

ABSTRACT

Chemsensors have been playing a crucial role in various aspects of biomedical science, analytical and environmental chemistry. The toxic metal ions like Zn, Cd, Cu, Pb and Hg have increased gradually but now have reached an alarming situation, crossing the threshold value. Due to high toxicity of these heavy metals there is an obvious need for a sensor system to detect their presence. Chemsensors including surface acoustic wave sensors, enzymes, carbon nanotubes, nanoparticles, and chromophore-based sensors have attracted increasing attention over the last few years. Chemsensors prove very promising as the system is rapid, selective, sensible, low-cost, easy-to-use, and has the ability to provide real-time signals. However, recently, considerable effort has been devoted to the synthesis of sterically encumbered selenium containing species reported to display strong affinities with Hg2+ or Ag2+. This chapter reviews the basic principles involved in the design of chemsensors, their variety and applications in various established and emerging fields.

INTRODUCTION

Till today a great variety of sensors has been synthesized by man, few of which are those that allows us to detect chemical species, this particular type is called a chemical sensor, and is defined by IUPAC as, a device that transforms chemical information, ranging from the concentration of a specific sample component to total composition analysis, into an analytically useful signal (Seyma, Fueki, Shiokawa et al., 1983). This device can be either macroscopic (e.g. a pH measuring electrode) or microscopic, it

DOI: 10.4018/978-1-5225-7635-8.ch006

refers to those molecule (or an assembled supra-molecular unit) that could selectively bind the target analyte and furnish information about this binding, therefore acting as a microscopic chemical sensor.

Molecular recognition and signal transduction are the two different processes that take place in chemical sensing through analyte detection. A chemsensor usually constitute three parts: A receptor (which is responsible for the selective analyte binding), an active unit (whose properties should change upon the aforementioned binding) and, in few cases, a spacer that is able to modify the geometry of the system and tune the electronic interaction between the two other components (White, 1996).

Actually, chemsensors are sensory receptors that transduce a chemical signal into an action and have vast potential as detecting units and thus, are continuously emerging as a tool for industrial, research, scientific, and pharmaceutical markets. In this series coordination compounds are also emerging as a potent tool in which chalcogen (O, S, Se and Te) containing compounds plays a significant role. Selenium is one of the elements from chalcogen series which is a naturally occurring element considered a link between metals and non-metals. It is found in nature in small concentration in rocks, plants, coal and fossil fuels (Shapira, 1973). One of such sterically encumbered selenium compound, tetrakis(iso-propyl seleno methyl benzene) on complexation with Hg^{2+}, Ag^{2+}, Pb^{2+}& Cd^{2+} showed selectivity towards Hg^{2+} ions though coordination to selenium is not an exclusive feature for mercury. As confirmed by physico-chemical data the presence of multiple soft selenium donor, the flexibility of the arms, steric bulk and open exterior geometry make these molecules potent tool for trapping Hg (II) selectively. Thus, there is a great potential in designing of sterically hindered organoselenium molecule to bind environmentally toxic metal ion selectively. Hence such tailored ligand and complexes could serve a great potential for trapping environmentally toxic metal ion and thus has application as sensors.

BACKGROUND

Large number of solid-state sensor devices based on various principles and materials are known which detect gaseous components for example semiconductor gas sensors which uses metal oxides, which detect the presence of inflammable gases in air such as CH_4, LPG and H_2 are therefore are used in large scale as gas leakage alarms domestically (Yamazoe & Miura, 1992). Sensors have also become increasingly

Figure 1. Working of a Chemsensor
Source: White, 1996

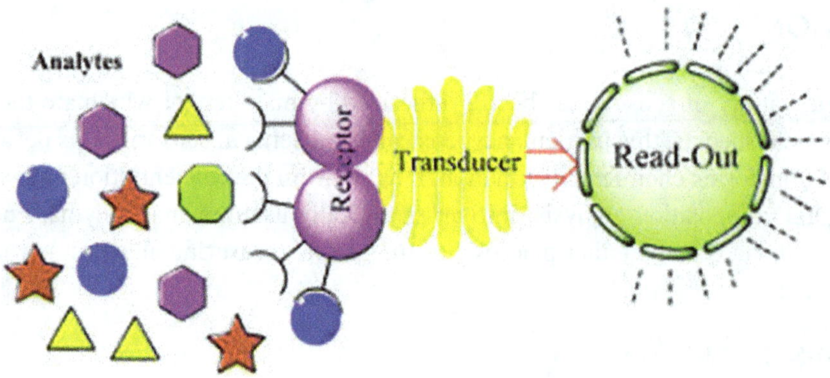

Figure 2. Structure of magnetic silica yolk–shell nanoparticle, and its color change with Hg^{2+}
Source: Yao & Shen, 2014

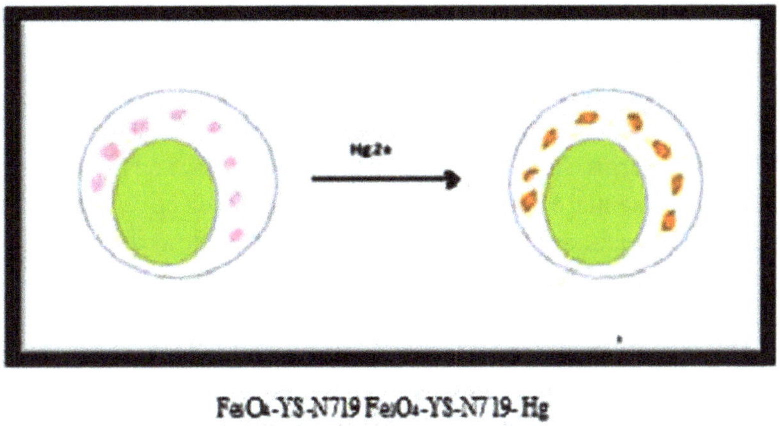

important in food industries for the detection of various volatile gases or smells generated from food or food materials. However, the most burning issue today is of energy and environment are increasing the necessity of those sensors which can detect air pollutants in environment like SO_X, NO_X, etc., as well as can be applied for control systems of combustion exhaust from stationary facilities and automobiles.

Enzymatic sensors, based on the inhibition of a selected enzyme, are the most extended biosensors used for the determination of these compounds. Based on the inhibition of acetyl cholinesterase (AChE) and colin oxidase, various biosensors have been developed for the detection of organophosphorous and carbamate pesticides (Cesarino, Moraes, Lanza et al., 2012; Singh & Agarwal, 1983). Although there are number of commercial successes, but most successful biosensor to date is the glucose biosensor which measures the concentration of glucose in diabetic patients (Toghill & Richard, 2010). In modern world, heavy metal ions are resulting in a serious environmental problem due to their high toxicity these heavy metal ions are determined by typical detection methods such as atomic absorption spectrometry and inductively coupled plasma mass spectrometry (Jackson & Chen, 1996). Electrochemical methods are able to selectively detect heavy metal ions with less complex instrumentation. The techniques developed so far include ion selective electrodes, polarography and other voltametric methods (Anderson, Bowden & Pickup, 1996). However cold vapor atomic absorption spectrometry and coupled mass spectrometry are conventional analytical techniques which suffers from disadvantage of high cost and requirement of trained personnel.

Yao et al. (Yao, Shen, Cao et al., 2014) have shown the construction of magnetic silica yolk–shell structure nanoparticles (Figure 2). Filling of N719 endowed the nanocomposites with detecting and eliminating functions towards mercury ions. This probe response to mercury ions within 1 minute and eliminate more than 97% of Hg^{2+} ions therefore acting as excellent sensor.

Several groups have designed organoselenium based polynucleating centres in which the open co-ordinating site of selenium is restricted sterically by incorporating allied organic groups (Milton, Singh & Butcher, 2004). The specific orientation of a donor selenium sites in a polynuclear species may also be controlled by a large number of weaker interactions, available due to heteroatoms present in allied organic groups and therefore the organochalcogens may exhibit more diverse behaviour than generally expected (Mansfield, Grundy, Coles et al., 2006).

The incorporation of selenium atoms substituted at the 1,2,4,5 positions of the central benzene ring leads to architectures which an act as suitable bridging bidentate chelating ligands towards M^{2+} ions. Addition of a solution of Ag(I), Pb(II) and Cd(II) ions to solution of newly synthesized selenium ligands, did not induce any change in the UV-Vis spectra. The complexation process caused notable changes in the absorption spectrum, upon addition of an increasing amount of Hg^{2+} ions. Since, coordination to selenium is not an exclusive feature of mercury, the non-reactivity of species with other metal ions is strange. The flexibility of the arms, steric bulk, open exterior geometry and multiple soft selenium donor sites make these molecules potential candidates for trapping Hg(II) selectively. Both 1:1 complex and 2:1 complex (metal-ligand) were successively formed, which is in complete agreement with physicochemical data. The effects in terms of metal ion, substrate specific response, of the coordinating ligand has been studied by potentiometric and spectrofluorometric measurement.

Mercury being a heavy-metal with environmental and physiological toxicities that are recognizable even at very low concentrations. Thus, mercury is widely studied in terms of its bioavailability, bioaccumulation, and cellular toxicity. Long-term exposure to this metal leads to permanent deterioration of the central nervous and endocrine system in the human body because mercury passes easily through biological membranes, such as skin, respiratory, and gastrointestinal tissues. As is well known that, effective metal responsive groups are crucial in defining the sensitivity and selectivity of fluorescent probes. Therefore, fluorescent probes for metal ion has been an area of research. Up to now, several types of small organic molecules, oligonucleotides, proteins, DNA and DNAzyme platforms have been examined for potential as Hg^{2+}-responsive groups in fluorescent probes. However, most of these probes shows quenched emission, required the involvement of an organic solvent, and also had limitations on selectivity and sensitivity. Therefore, not all the reported fluorescent probes could successfully detect Hg^{2+} ions in biological samples, only a few probes based on small organic molecules have achieved this goal and give fluorescence images of biological samples. Bo Tang et al have also reported seleno fluorescent probe, an organoselenium fluorescent probe (FSe-1) for mercury, based on the irreversible deselenation mechanism. Here FSe-1 exhibits an ultrahigh selectivity and sensitivity for Hg^{2+} detection due to the strong affinity between Se and Hg. Furthermore, the new probe has been successfully used for imaging mercury ions in RAW 264.7 cells (a mouse macrophage cell line). The experimental results proved that FSe-1 was selective for Hg^{2+} ions over other relevant metal ions and bioanalytes, and also showed an enhancement in sensitivity of up to 1.0 nM, which is lower than the current EPA standard for drinking water (Tang, Ding, Xu et al., 2009).

Analysis of Heavy Metal Ions

Heavy metal poisoning due to various contamination is a matter of serious concern all around the globe. Sample collection and their laboratory analysis is the traditional approach to detect toxic metal ion which suffers from various disadvantages for it being expensive, inconvenient, time consuming and also prone to errors during sample collection, transportation and handling. However today number of portable devices like x-ray fluoroscence, voltammetry, etc., are there which could help in such detection but again they are not widely used because of technical and other limitations. In developing country like India there has been an urgent need of low cost, easy to use and reliable device which could be used in medical diagnostics, environmental monitoring of heavy metal poisoning.

Anode stripping voltametry (Wang, 1990) and surface plasmon resonance spectroscopy (Homola, Yee & Gsuglitz, 1999; Myszka, 1999) are two of the established technologies for sensitive and selective detection of metal ions and other electrochemically active substances

CHEMSENSORS FOR HEAVY METALS

Fluorescent Chemsensors for Cations

There are a number of metal ions that play a vital role in our daily physiological life. Few of them are sodium (Na^+) potassium (K^+), calcium (Ca^{2+}), copper (Cu^+ and Cu^{2+}) and zinc (Zn^{2+}), among others. However, some metal ions such as lead (Pb^{2+}), cadmium (Cd^{2+}) and mercury (Hg^{2+}) are highly toxic and may cause serious health and environmental problems.

Fluorescent Chemosensors for Detection of Alkali and Alkaline Earth Metal Ions

The first fluorescent chemsensor for cations was recorded in the year 1867, when Goppelsröder reported that morin forms a strongly fluorescent chelate with Al^{3+}. Initially, most fluorescent chemsensors for cations were based on the coordination interactions between the hosts and the guests. However later supramolecular chemistry was used in chemsensor designing, Sousa et al. (1977) reported two naphthalene based chemsensors 1 and 2 for the detection of alkali metal ions (Figure 3) using supramolecular chemistry in fluorescent chemsensor design (Sousa & Larson et al., 1977). Interestingly, these closely related chemsensors exhibit dichotomous behavior. Chemsensor 1 displayed a decrease in fluorescence quantum yield, also an increase in phosphorescence quantum yield, and a slight decrease in phosphorescence lifetime when it formed a complex with alkali metal chloride salts in 95% ethanol glass at 77 K. On the contrary, complexation of chemsensor 2 with potassium (K^+), rubidium (Rb^+), or caesium (Cs^+) chloride salts caused a noticeable increase in fluorescence quantum yield, also a decrease in phosphorescence quantum yield, and a substantial decrease in phosphorescence lifetime. These observed changes can be attributed to the heavy atom effect (for Rb^+ and Cs^+) and/or a complexation induced change in triplet energy relative to the ground and excited singlet state energies as well as rigidification and conformational effects.

Calcium ion is the most abundant element in the human body and it plays important roles in many biological processes. The monitoring of the intracellular free Ca^{2+} is important since imbalances of Ca^{2+} are related to a number of diseases such as neurodegeneration, heart disease and skeletal muscle defects. The already reported fluorescent chemsensors for Ca^{2+} suffered several problems such as

1. Low selectivity towards competing cations and in particularly H^+ and Mg^{2+}
2. Complex stoichiometry with Ca^{2+}
3. Inflexibility of molecular design, etc. (Tsien, 1980). These chemsensors show good selectivity and sensitivity towards Ca^{2+} over Mg^{2+}, and their application *in vivo* opened up a new area and understanding of cellular function and indeed revolutionized our understanding of biochemical processes within cells.

Figure 3. Structures of the fluorescent Chemsensors 1–3
Source: Sousa, 1977

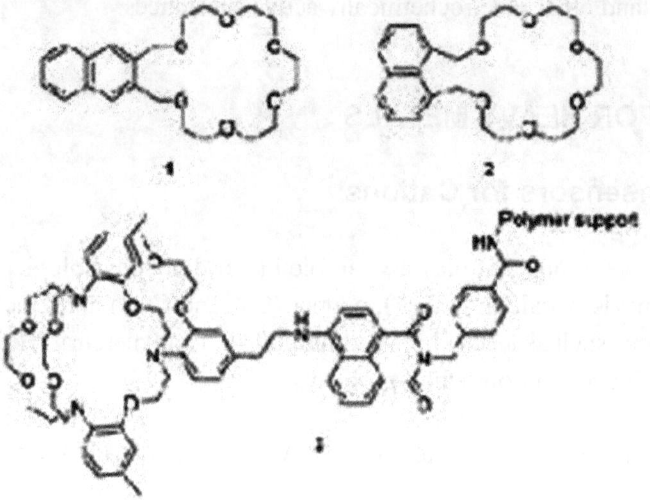

Along with the development of the field of fluorescence dyes and the advancement in microscopic imaging technologies, a series of BAPTA and derived fluorescent chemsensors for Ca^{2+} have been reported. In 2010, Kim, Cho and coworkers described a two photon (TP) fluorescent chemsensor, in which 2-(2′-morpholino-2′-oxoethoxy)-*N*, *N*-bis(hydroxycarbonylmethyl) aniline (MOBHA) was used as the Ca^{2+} receptor and 6-(benzo[*d*]oxazol-2′-yl)-2-(*N*, *N*-dimethylamino) naphthalene was used as the fluorophore (Kim, Han, Kim et al., 2010).

Fluorescent Chemsensors for D-Block Metal Ions

Apart from the above-mentioned fluorescent chemsensors for alkali and alkaline earth metal ions, which are all based on coordination interaction there are other set of transition metal ion based fluorescent chemsensors in which chemical reaction is the main basis since these metal ions have the tendency to trigger specific reactions. As known copper (Cu) is the third most abundant and essential transition metal in the human body, as it is involved in various physiological and pathological processes. Loss of copper homeostasis is linked with diseases such as Menkes (copper deficiency), Wilson's (copper overload), Alzheimer's disease, prion disorders, neurodegeneration and cancer. The structure, mechanism and applications of fluorescent chemsensors for Cu^{2+} has been successfully studied by Shuo Liu et al. (2017). However earlier in 1997, Czarnik and co-workers have reported pioneering work on a rhodamine-B derivative and its ring-opening reaction for sensing copper ion (Cu^{2+}) (Liu, Wang & Han, 2017). Mercury (Hg) is one of the most prevalent deadly toxins on earth, which arises from many sources such as gold production, coal plants, thermometers, barometers and mercury lamps etc. Since earlier times, a huge number of fluorescent chemsensors have been developed for the detection of Hg^{2+}. Initially, the fluorescent chemsensors (Dujols, Ford & Czarnik, 1997) being non-fluorescent due to the PET process, however the addition of Hg^{2+} induces an enhancement in fluorescence, whereas other metal ions except for Ag^{+} caused no interference. Selvan et al. (Chae & Czarnik, 1992) have recently developed an ON/OFF dual fluorescent chemsensor based on a naphthalene diamine β-diketone derivative LH for the selective detection of Fe^{2+} and Cu^{2+} ions. The fluorescence emission intensity of LH was remarkably high after the addition of Fe^{2+} ion, and quenching was observed after the addition of Cu^{2+} ion. The compound LH binds to both the metal ions in a 1:2 stoichiometry.

Fluorescent Chemosensors for Anions

In contrast to the previously described sensing devices, the field of anion sensing is a relatively mature science. Anion plays an important role in biological and industrial processes as well as the presence of anionic pollutants in the environment has driven the need to produce such sensors. Recently, Zhang and coworkers (Zhang, Kim, Lin et al., 2015) reported two anion induced supramolecular assemblies of expanded porphyrins 4 and 5 (Figure 4). Porphyrins 4 and 5 can form supramolecular polymers with several diacids, which can be used as chemsensors for both anions and organic solvents.

Coumarin-Based Fluorescent Chemsensors

Such sensors have received increasing interest in recent years (Su, Chen, Guo et al., 2010; Kim, Kim, Kim, et al., 2009; Chen, Shang, Li et al., 2018) due to their low toxicity, excellent photophysical properties and ease of modification. Direct interaction with the carbonyl group of coumarin is frequently exploited as a good model for chemsensor design, because their spectroscopic response is fast and are efficient in the presence of other metals ions.

Fluorescent Chemsensors for Biomacromolecules

Biomacromolecules are vital for the function of living biological systems. The fluorescence imaging techniques provides us a powerful tool for studying these biomacromolecules and to completely understand their purpose in these complex biological systems due to excellent spatial and temporal resolution and high molecular specificity. Czarnik carried out pioneering work on anthrylpolyamines to sense polyanions such as heparin, poly-L-glutamate, ds DNA and ss DNA in water (Van Arman & Czarnik, 1990).

Figure 4. Structures of fluorescent chemsensors 4 & 5 and the schematic illustrates the construction of supramolecular assemblies using 4, 5, and diacids as the building blocks
Source: Zhang, Kim, Lin et al., 2015

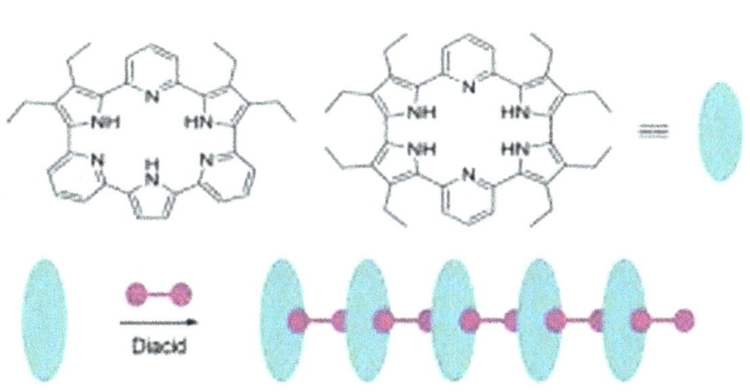

Luminescent Chemsensors

Luminescent chemsensors for transition metal ions has been recently studied by Bargossi et al. (Bargossi, Fiorini, Montalti et al., 2000) in which various systems active units and receptors are different, as are the target ions: Zn^{2+}, Ni^{2+}, Cd^{2+}, Hg^{2+}, Co^{2+}, Ag^{+} and Cu^{2+}. In solution a good selectivity and affinity was observed and the binding is signalled in all cases by pronounced changes in the photophysical properties such as emission wavelength, intensity, and excited state lifetime of the inserted luminophore. The mechanism for signal transduction depends strongly on the chosen receptor and luminophore moieties, and has been investigated in detail by means of steady state and time resolved spectroscopy (Bargossi, Fiorini, Montalti et al., 2000). Luminescent zinc complexes as chemsensors for adenine detection are well known.

Optical Chemsensors

Variety of optical chemsensors are known till now. Recently highly sensitive optical chemsensors have been reported, which implement bragg grating structures which though insensitive to chemicals, is made sensitised by effective etching (Zhan, Chen, Lin et al., 2006). As known silica nanoparticles, silica gel and mesoporous silica are used as supporting platforms to fabricate optical chemsensors because of certain properties like high porosity and expectant adsorption capacity etc., similarly, silica-based optical chemsensors are good alternatives to classical instrumental methods for detecting and adsorbing metal ions, due to their effect and lower price. Chromogenic type and fluorogenic type optical probes, such as azobenzene, naphthalimide and rhodamine, are grafted to the surface of silica-based materials by sol–gel reaction, the limit of detection, response time and selective properties of optical sensors are improved sequentially (Huang, Yan, Fu et al., 2017).

Congugate Sensors

Alternatively known as photoinduced electron transfer (PET) sensors. In such sensors there is a nitrogenous ligand or chelator which has sufficiently selective for the targeted analyte and then covalently tether this to a fluorophore. When the amine nitrogen of the ligand chelator is free they will quench the fluorescence in the solution via photoinduced electron transfer, sometimes up to 1000-fold. However, when the amine electrons are involved in interactions with metal ions or H-bonding with the analyte, quenching does not take place and the original fluorescence of the parent fluorophore is restored so the analyte is signalled by an increase in the fluorescence intensity without any spectral shift, which is considered as a major drawback but some advantages of conjugate probes are also known. Fluoroscence of azacrown squaraine as well as water soluble squaraine is studied along with the ion sensing of squaraine-based chemsensors in water (Das, Thomas, Thomas et al., 1994).

APPLICATIONS

Chemsensors have been playing a crucial role in the field of bio-medicinal science, analytical and environmental chemistry by being a molecule that can selectively bind the target analyte and furnish information about this binding. A Highly selective and sensitive detection of inorganic phosphate in aqueous solution and living cells by fluorescent chemsensor is also studied (Meng, Wang, Yang et al., 2015).

Few of the sensors are designed especially for the detection and volumetric analysis for a wide spectrum of chemicals and gases in real time. High concentration of NO_2 gas could be detected by resistive low-temperature sensor based on the SiO_2ZrO_2 film (Myasoedova, Mikhailova, Yalovega et al., 2018). The sensors have added benefit of continually monitoring large volume of liquid or air for the presence and quantity of target substances. Adulteration, inconsistencies and contamination in food products and beverage samples are detected fast but accurate through chemsensors. Chemsensor (gas chromatograph-mass coupled with chemometric analysis software) as an early discrimination tool of Iberian pig ejaculates according to their freezability (Gómez-Fernández, Tomás, Carrasco et al., 2015). Chemical sensors also have space applications for biomedical experimentation, monitoring of water and air recycling processes on space station freedom and later long-term space missions (Bonting, 1992). Use of chemsensors for the detection of pollutants such as heavy metals or radionuclide are among the main targets since their detection and removal could be envisioned at very low concentrations because of their ability to display specific and strong complexing abilities. Wearable chemsensors in the healthcare system focused on sweat-based, saliva-based and tear-based analysis (Qian & Long, 2017) makes them a convenient tool for the detection and long-term monitoring of the chemical, biological, and physical status of the human body in real time.

CONCLUSION

The field of chemsensors has developed significantly over 150 years. The present chapter highlights few of the important chemsensors used in the area of heavy metal ion detection and there are advantages in terms of its easy production, low cost, ease of operation, reliability and good sensor to sensor reproducibility, etc. However, operating a chemsensor in a natural environment poses substantial challenges in terms of ruggedness, long-term stability and calibration. Today, we are witnessing the explosive development in this field of chemsensors, their applications have covered almost all of the fields. However, biggest truth, that we will always need "new" chemsensors for yet unknown analytes. Also, the biological and environmental analysis has increasingly stringent requirements imposed by regulatory bodies, so while a current chemsensor may work it may fall short of the required selectivity or sensitivity required for use in a specific practical application in future or so. To meet the upcoming challenges of present and future world we need, and will continue to need an increasing number of chemsensors.

REFERENCES

Anderson, J. L., Bowden, E. F., & Pickup, P. G. (1996). Dynamic electrochemistry: Methodology and application. *Analytical Chemistry, 68*(12), R379–R444. doi:10.1021/a1960015y PMID:11008788

Bargossi, C., Fiorini, M. C., Montalti, M., Prodi, L., & Zaccheroni, N. (2000). Recent developments in transition metal ion detection by luminescent chemosensors. *Coordination Chemistry Reviews, 208*(1), 17–32. doi:10.1016/S0010-8545(00)00252-6

Bonting, S. L. (1992). Chemical sensors for space applications. Advances in Space Biology and Medicine. *Advances in Space Biology and Medicine, 2*, 263–293. doi:10.1016/S1569-2574(08)60024-6 PMID:1342247

Cesarino, I., Moraes, F. C., Lanza, M. R. V., & Machado, S. A. S. (2012). Electrochemical detection of carbamate pesticides in fruit and vegetables with a biosensor based on acetylcholinesterase immobilised on a composite of polyaniline–carbon nanotubes. *Food Chemistry, 135*(3), 873–879. doi:10.1016/j.foodchem.2012.04.147 PMID:22953799

Chae, M.-Y., & Czarnik, A. W. (1992). Fluorometric chemodosimetry. Mercury(II) and silver(I) indication in water via enhanced fluorescence signalling. *Journal of the American Chemical Society, 114*(24), 9704–9705. doi:10.1021/ja00050a085

Chen, Y., Shang, X., Li, C., Xue, Z., Chen, H., Wu, H., & Wang, T. (2018). The synthesis, crystal, hydrogen sulfide detection and cell assement of novel chemsensors based on coumarin derivatives. *Scientific Reports, 8*(1), 16159. doi:10.103841598-018-34331-9 PMID:30385799

Das, S., Thomas, K. G., Thomas, K. J., Kamat, P. V., & George, M. V. (1994). Photochemistry of squaraine dyes. Photophysical properties of crown ether squaraine fluorophore and their metal ion complexes. *Journal of Physical Chemistry, 98*(37), 9291–9296. doi:10.1021/j100088a033

Dujols, V., Ford, F., & Czarnik, A. W. (1997). A Long-Wavelength Fluorescent Chemodosimeter Selective for Cu(II) Ion in Water. *Journal of the American Chemical Society, 119*(31), 7386–7387. doi:10.1021/ja971221g

Gómez-Fernández, J., Tomás, C., Carrasco, J. A., Sánchez-Sánchez, R., González-Bulnes, A., Gómez-Izquierdo, E., & de Mercado, E. (2015). Use of "ChemSensor" as an early discrimination tool of Iberian pig semen according to their freezability. *ITEA, 111*(1), 34–49.

Homola, J., Yee, S. S., & Gsuglitz, G. (1999). Surface Plasmon Resonance Sensors: Review. Sensors and Actuators B: Chemical. *Sensors and Actuators. B, Chemical, 54*(1-2), 3–15. doi:10.1016/S0925-4005(98)00321-9

Huang, Y., Yan, F., Fu, M., & Zhang, R. (2017). Silica-based optical chemosensors for detection and removal of metal ions. *Journal of the Indian Chemical Society, 14*(1), 157–176.

Jackson, K. W., & Chen, G. (1996). Atomic Absorption, Atomic Emission, and Flame Emission Spectrometry. *Analytical Chemistry, 68*(12), 231–256. doi:10.1021/a1960012l PMID:8092468

Kim, H. J., Han, J. H., Kim, M. K., Lim, C. S., Kim, H. M., & Cho, B. R. (2010). Dual-Color Imaging of Sodium/Calcium Ion Activities with Two-Photon Fluorescent Probes. *Angewandte Chemie International Edition*, *49*(38), 6786–6789. doi:10.1002/anie.201002907 PMID:20715036

Kim, J. H., Kim, H. J., Kim, S. H., Lee, J. H., Do, J. H., Kim, H.-J., ... Kim, J. S. (2009). Fluorescent coumarinyl dithiane as a selective chemodosimeter for mercury (II) ion in aqueous solution. *Tetrahedron Letters*, *50*(43), 5958–5961. doi:10.1016/j.tetlet.2009.08.045

Liu, S., Wang, Y.-M., & Han, J. (2017). Fluorescent chemosensors for copper(II) ion: Structure, mechanism and application. *Journal of Photochemistry and Photobiology C, Photochemistry Reviews*, *32*, 78–103. doi:10.1016/j.jphotochemrev.2017.06.002

Mansfield, N. E., Grundy, J., Coles, M. P., Avent, A. G., & Hitchcock, P. B. (2006, October). A Conformational Study of Phospha(III)- and Phospha(V)-guanidine Compounds. *Journal of the American Chemical Society*, *128*(42), 13879–13893. doi:10.1021/ja064212t

Meng, Q., Wang, Y., Yang, M., Zhang, R., Wang, R., & Zhang, Z. (2015). A new fluorescent chemosensor for highly selective and sensitive detection of inorganic phosphate (Pi) in aqueous solution and living cells. *RSC Advances*, *5*(66), 53189–53197. doi:10.1039/C5RA08712K

Milton, M. D., Singh, J. D., & Butcher, R. J. (2004). Synthesis of b-ketoenamine donors having O, N, Se/Te donor functionalities and their reaction chemistry with Pd(II) and Pt(II) metal ions. *Tetrahedron Letters*, *45*(36), 6745–6747. doi:10.1016/j.tetlet.2004.07.057

Myasoedova, T. N., Mikhailova, T. S., Yalovega, G. E., & Plugotarenko, N. K. (2018). Resistive Low-Temperature Sensor Based on the SiO_2ZrO_2 Film for Detection of High Concentrations of NO_2 Gas. *Chemosensors*, *6*(4), 67. doi:10.3390/chemosensors6040067

Myszka, D. G. (1999). Improving Biosensor analysis. *Journal of Molecular Recognition*, *12*, 390–408. doi:10.1002/(SICI)1099-1352(199911/12)12:6<390::AID-JMR482>3.0.CO;2-8 PMID:10556875

Qian, R. C., & Long, Y. T. (2017). Wearable Chemosensors: A Review of Recent Progress. *ChemistryOpen*. doi:10.1002/o00pen.2017159 PMID:29435397

Seyma, T., Fueki, K., Shiokawa, J., & Suzuki, S. (Eds.). (1983). *Proceedings of the International Meeting on Chemical Sensors*, Fukuoka, Japan, September 19-22. Tokyo, Japan: Elsevier-Kodanscha.

Shapira, J. R. (1973). In D.L. Klayman & W.H. Gunther (Eds.), Organic selenium compounds: Their Chemistry and Biology. John Wiley & Sons Inc.

Singh, D. K., & Agarwal, R. A. (1983). Inhibition kinetics of certain organophosphorus and carbamate pesticides on acetylcholinesterase from the snail Lymnaeaacuminate. *Toxicology Letters*, *19*(3), 313–319. doi:10.1016/0378-4274(83)90136-4 PMID:6658844

Sousa, L. R., & Larson, J. M. (1977). Crown ether model systems for the study of photoexcited state response to geometrically oriented perturbers. The effect of alkali metal ions on emission from naphthalene derivatives. *Journal of the American Chemical Society*, *99*(1), 307–310. doi:10.1021/ja00443a084

Su, Z., Chen, K., Guo, Y., Qi, H., Yang, X. F., & Zhao, M. (2010). A coumarin-based fluorescent chemosensor for Zn 2+ in aqueous ethanol media. *Journal of Fluorescence*, *20*(4), 851–856.

Tamil Selvan, G., Varadaraju, C., Tamil Selvan, R., Enoch, I. V., & Mosae Selvakumar, P. (2018). On/off fluorescent chemosensor for selective detection of divalent iron and copper ions: Molecular logic operation and protein binding. *ACS Omega*, *3*(7), 7985–7992.

Tang, B., Ding, B., Xu, K., & Tong, L. (2009). Use of selenium to detect mercury in water and cells: An enhancement of the sensitivity and specificity of a seleno fluorescent probe. *Chemistry*, *15*(13), 3147–3151. doi:10.1002/chem.200802165 PMID:19204963

Toghill, K. E., & Richard, G. (2010). Compton Electrochemical Non-enzymatic Glucose Sensors: A Perspective and an Evaluation. *International Journal of Electrochemical Science*, *5*, 1246–1301.

Tsien, R. Y. (1980). New calcium indicators and buffers with high selectivity against magnesium and protons: Design, synthesis, and properties of prototype structures. *Biochemistry*, *19*(11), 2396–2404. doi:10.1021/bi00552a018 PMID:6770893

Van Arman, S. A., & Czarnik, A. W. (1990). A general fluorescence assay for enzyme catalyzed polyanion hydrolysis based on template directed excimer formation. Application to heparin and polyglutamate. *Journal of the American Chemical Society*, *112*(13), 5376–5377. doi:10.1021/ja00169a070

Wang, J. (1990). *New Approaches to metal speciation in natural waters Based on Modified and Microvoltametric Electrodes*. La Cruces, NM: Department of Chemistry, New Mexico State University.

White, N. J. (1996). The treatment of malaria. *The New England Journal of Medicine*, *335*(11), 800–806. doi:10.1056/NEJM199609123351107 PMID:8703186

Yamazoe, N., & Miura, N. (1992). New Approaches in the Design of Gas Sensors. In G. Sberveglieri (Ed.), *Gas Sensors*. Dordrecht: Springer. doi:10.1007/978-94-011-2737-0_1

Yao, L., Shen, B., Cao, C., Feng, W., & Li, F. (2014). Chemodosimeter functionalized magnetic silica yolk–shell nanocomposite for sensing and removal of Hg^{2+}. *RSC Advances*, *4*(39), 20252–20255. doi:10.1039/c4ra02410a

Zhan, K., Chen, X., Lin, Z., & Bennian, I. (2006). Implementation of optical chemsensors based on HF etched fibre bragg grating structures. *Measurement Science & Technology*, *5*, 17.

Zhang, Z., Kim, D. S., Lin, C. Y., Zhang, H., Lammer, A. D., Lynch, V. M., ... Sessler, J. L. (2015). Expanded porphyrin-anion supramolecular assemblies: Environmentally responsive sensors for organic solvents and anions. *Journal of the American Chemical Society*, *137*(24), 7769–7774. doi:10.1021/jacs.5b03131

KEY TERMS AND DEFINITIONS

Atomic Absorption Spectroscopy (AAS): It is a spectroanalytical procedure for the quantitative determination of chemical elements using the absorption of optical radiation (light) by free atoms in the gaseous state.

Biomacromolecules: Are the biomolecules which have molecular weights higher than 1000 daltons (Da) approximately and found in the acid soluble pool in the chemical analysis of the living tissue. For e.g. proteins, nucleic acids etc.

Cold Vapor Atomic Absorption Spectroscopy or CVAAS: Is one of the primary techniques for mercury analysis. It has a peristaltic pump that transports sample and stannous chloride into a Gas Liquid Separator (GLS) where a stream of pure, dry gas (typically argon) is introduced to the liquid mixture to release mercury vapor.

Coumarin: It is a fragrant organic chemical compound in benzopyrone chemical class may also be seen as subclass of lactone.

Fluoroscence Quantum Yield: Ratio of number of photons emitted by the fluorophore to the number absorbed. The possible values are between 0 and 1.

Fluoroscent Probes: These are molecules that absorb light of a specific wavelength and emit light of a different, typically longer, wavelength (a process known as fluorescence).

Glucose Biosensor: Are devices that measure the concentration of glucose in diabetic patients by means of sensitive protein that relays the concentration by means of fluorescence, an alternative to amperometric sension of glucose.

Heteroatom: This term is used to indicate that non-carbon atoms have replaced carbon in the backbone of the molecular structure. Typical heteroatoms are nitrogen, oxygen, sulphur, phosphorus, chlorine, bromine and iodine.

Inductively Coupled Plasma Mass Spectrometry or ICP-MS: Is an analytical technique used for elemental determinations. It combines a high-temperature ICP (Inductively Coupled Plasma) source with a mass spectrometer.

Organochalcogen Compound: Is a compound containing at least one carbon-chalcogen bond.

Phosphorescence: It is a process in which energy absorbed by a substance is released relatively slowly in the form of light. This is in some cases the mechanism used for "glow-in-the-dark" materials which are "charged" by exposure to light. In phosphorescence, the electron which absorb the photon (energy) undergoes an unusual intersystem crossing into an energy state of higher *spin multiplicity* usually a triplet state from singlet state, which then returns to the ground state.

Physicochemical Data: Relating to both physical and chemical properties of any sample or substance.

Polarography: A method of analysis in which a sample is subjected to electrolysis using a special electrode and a range of applied voltages, a plot of current against voltage showing steps corresponding to particular chemical species and proportional to their concentration.

Spectrofluorometer: An instrument which takes advantage of fluorescent properties of compounds in order to provide information regarding their concentration and chemical environment in a sample. A certain excitation wavelength is selected, and the emission is observed either at a single wavelength, or a scan is performed to record the intensity versus wavelength, also called an emission spectra.

APPENDIX

List of Abbreviations

ASV: Anode stripping voltametry.

BAPTA: (1,2-bis(*o*-aminophenoxy)ethane-*N, N, N′, N′*-tetraacetic acid), is a calcium-specific aminopolycarboxylic acid.

DNA: Deoxyribonucleic acid.

dsDNA and ssDNA: Double stranded and Single stranded DNA.

EPA: Environmental Protection agency.

LH: Luteinizing hormone.

N719: Di-tetrabutylammonium cis-bis(isothiocyanato)bis(2,2′-bipyridyl-4,4′-dicarboxylato) ruthenium (II); Synonym N719 standard Dye.

PET Process: Photoelectron transfer.

SPR: Surface Plasmon resonance spectroscopy.

SOx, NOx: Oxides of Sulphur & Nitrogen (SO_2, SO_3, NO, NO_2).

Chapter 7
Environmental and Occupational Epidemiology Principles

Emmanouil G. Velonakis
National and Kapodistrian University of Athens, Greece

ABSTRACT

Occupational epidemiology studies the distribution of health events and health related determinants and its relation to the working environment. Environmental epidemiology focuses on the involuntary exposure to physical and chemical factors in the indoor or outdoor environment that may affect health patterns. Occupational and environmental epidemiology use similar methodology although the conditions differ. The environmental epidemiology studies beyond the health effect of exposure to specific environmental factors and must consider the long-term impact of the ecosystems to nearby populations. Molecular technologies allow the detection of effects at the molecular level originated by very low levels of exposure. The concept of an exposome is a kind of database with information concerning environmental exposure measurements in a life time and corresponding biomarkers concentrations in different biospeciments, considering internal individual genetic characteristics.

INTRODUCTION

Any adverse health effect related to genetic and external factors is linked to the conditions of life. Nutrition, smoking, alcohol consumption, physical activity are the most studied risks. The physical and social environment at the workplace may cause accidents, occupational diseases and it contributes to common diseases occurrence. The natural and artificial environment have a permanent influence. Eventual harmful factors in the environment are produced either physically like cosmic or ultra violet radiations, radon exposure from the ground, volcano activities, or by human activities like traffic and industrial pollution, war attacks, noisy events, etc. Humans are exposed to hazards mostly either by inhalation or orally by food and water consumption. Other ways of exposure are through the skin like radiation or by dermal absorption of chemicals. The noise may be harmful by audition under circumstances (Sherwin,

DOI: 10.4018/978-1-5225-7635-8.ch007

1983; Shepherd et al., 2016). Epidemiology studies the distribution of health events and health related determinants in defined populations, it is therefore applied to the modification of risk factors for reducing the morbidity and mortality and improving the quality of life. This chapter discusses how epidemiology explores the association between occupational and environmental factors and health outcomes and what the limits and the prospectives are.

BACKGROUND

Occupational epidemiology focuses on the working environment where people spend one third of their life, and where they are exposed to physical or chemical risks. Environmental epidemiology focuses on physical and chemical factors from the indoor or outdoor environment that may affect health patterns. The exposure to these factors is involuntary. Biological factors are part of the environment; however, this field is claimed by infectious diseases epidemiology (Rothman, 1993). The conditions in which people are born, grow, live, work and age are considered as social determinants, that may have either a direct effect to health or influence the exposure to the specific harmful factors. Due to the dynamic nature and complexity of public health evidence, traditional epidemiological study designs are often insufficient to make conclusions informing policy or practice at the population level, for improving population health. Environmental epidemiology faces problems with correlated exposures and small relative risks. Occupational epidemiology must estimate risks related to the changing working conditions and its emerging psycho social effects. Molecular biology and ecosystems studies offer new challenges.

OCCUPATIONAL / ENVIRONMENTAL FACTORS AND HEALTH OUTCOMES: METHODS USED AND CHALLENGES

Occupational and environmental epidemiology associate exposure to health effects. They need therefore data related to health effects and data related to exposure to potential hazards. Health effects concern exposed population and their descendants. They also concern no exposed populations to examine the extent to which observed rates differ significantly between exposed and no exposed.

Health Data

Health data, referring to events by time, place and person, are (CDC, 2012):

- Incidence of diseases: Rate of new cases to the population during a period. It is interpreted as the risk for a new outcome.
- Prevalence of diseases: Rate of existing cases to the population at a moment of time. It describes the probability of an existing outcome in a population at a point in time
- General mortality and mortality by specific causes as indirect indices of diseases incidence.
- Birth outcomes, including fertility and infertility, premature birth, perinatal mortality, birthweight, sex ratio.
- Biological indices that may show either even minor health effect or indicate that the exposure exceeds allowed levels.

Some of the above rates, like mortality are retrieved from civil registries. They also may be retrieved from specific registries for example cancer, infectious diseases registries, or by the health surveillance of a population at risk. The biological indices come from the health surveillance of the population and relevant monitoring (Solomon et al., 1991; Public Health Information Systems, 2017).

Exposure Data

Qualitative Approach

The evaluation of the exposure may be qualitative or quantitative. The qualitative evaluation is a dichotomous approach: yes-no. This approach is more applicable to occupational epidemiology studies based on job description, however same jobs may have totally different exposures at different periods or under different production processes. The qualitative approach in the environmental studies is limited exclusively to populations exposed to hazards like after a major industrial accident. It can be also applied to compare the health data between populations living in different ecosystems associated with different exposures and life conditions.

Quantitative Approach

Obviously, the quantitative estimation of exposure is more reliable. Any quantitative approach is related to the magnitude of the harmful factor like its concentration in the respirable air or in the drinking water and the duration of exposure to it. The exposure assessment is complex. The difficulties are related to simultaneous exposure to more than one harmful factor with possible synergistic effect, to varying levels of exposure at different time periods, to exposure at low levels with borderline effects.

In the occupational epidemiology studies, the concentration is estimated using the industrial hygienist's measurements and previous employment history. The dose of individual occupational exposure is attempted through respective adjustment, considering differences among jobs in the same industry and seasonal declines. In occupational epidemiology, exposure time considered to be the working time (hours per day, days and years of exposure). (Loomis and Kromhout, 2004).

In the environmental epidemiology studies, exposure is best characterized using a combination of information sources. The exposure depends on the pollution magnitude and the distance from the pollution's source. People's mobility and activities differentiate the burden of exposure even in the same day. Long term effects must estimate the different exposures at different home addresses during a person's years of life and the difference of exposure between home and workplace. The exposure assessment is mainly based on questionnaires concerning the current and past locations of the respondents' homes and workplaces, their distance from the sources of pollution, as well as how the living conditions may reduce the exposure (for example the orientation, the level of the floor, the door and windows framing). The meteorological conditions are also considered to adjust the exposure levels among peoples at the same distance from the source of the pollution but with different orientation. Retrospectively for the assessment of the pollution a historical approach concerning industrial accidents, implementation of new technologies or other measures for the reduction of the pollution is also considered. Beyond appropriate questionnaires, systematic monitoring of pollution like records of traffic or industrial pollution by local authorities and of patterns of human activities can approximate the exposure considering the above limitations. Geographical information systems and elaborated models are used for this purpose (Nuckols et al., 2004; Nieuwenhuijsen, 2015).

Exposure and Exposure's Effects

Environmental studies mostly concern low dose exposures to a complex array of factors with long latency periods to express any health effect. Air pollutants are a mixture of different chemicals, each one with specific toxicology and very often with synergistic action. Same concentrations of pollutants in the air may lead to different uptake according the air flow, the humidity, the temperature, and the size of particles. The toxicity and irritability of the particles after inhalation depends on their chemical composition and the specific properties of each compound. Independently to it, an additional irritating effect on the respiratory tract is related to the physical characteristics of the particles and mainly their size. Particles below 10μ are inhaled and as their size is small, they affect the lower respiratory tract. It is therefore evident that the indicated technique and the indicated duration for the estimation of the exposure must consider the kind of pollution and the characteristics of the pollutants (Richard and Thomas, 2013). More accurate estimates of uptake are based on biological measures of pollutants or related biomarkers. Biomarkers are traceable substances that reflect adverse biological responses towards environmental toxins, even at low exposure levels. As an example, biomarkers may be deposits of heavy metals in tissues, enzymes alterations, oxidative stress and DNA damage indicators. Different biomarkers are used for different chemical factors. (Kaviraj et al., 2014).

Beyond the assessment of the exposure and the recognition of related adverse health effects the epidemiologist must consider how physical and chemical factors may affect human health. Most have only a deterministic, no stochastic, effect, which is generated above a threshold dose. This means that an adverse effect after exposure to a factor with only deterministic effect may be induced if it is over the threshold level. The effect may be irritating or toxic, or it may be a consequence of a short time exposure as an acute effect or of a long-term exposure as a chronic effect. The severity of such effects depends on the exposure dose over the threshold level. Some factors may have also a stochastic effect. Stochastic effects are those that may be harmful to genes and cause cancer or a hereditable genetic effect. These effects occur at random; there is not a safe threshold level of exposure. The higher the dose and the duration of the exposure, the more probable is the harmful genetic effect. The effect appears to the exposed or to their descendants years after the exposure (Leenhouts and Chadwick, 1989). Some individuals react with hypersensitivity to some compounds. Sensitivity may be generated at very low doses in some individuals and may be absent in others. Some compounds act frequently as sensitizers (Dotson et al., 2015).

Exposure Through Drinking Water

A potential source of environmental exposure is drinking water. The exposure assessment to hazards by drinking water requires the measurement of their concentration in the water. Usual hazards of interest in the water are heavy metals, chlorinated compounds, nitrates etc. Drinking water supplies of a community, presumes that it affects equally all consumers. Such approach may underestimate the risk since part of the population use alternative sources like bottled water. The measurement of this alternative consumption obviously meets difficulties (White et al., 2008).

Methodology to Explore Relationship

To set up any relationship between exposure and health effects the occupational and environmental epidemiological studies follow various methodological approaches. Both they use similar methodology to explore exposure – health effects relationship, although the conditions differ, since in the working environment the exposure is usually more intensive, limited to space and time and the surveillance of the population easier. Both Accordingly, they are classified into two types descriptive and analytic.

Descriptive Studies

Descriptive studies may induce hypothesis, but never lead to causal association. They include:

1. Cases report, concerning individuals or small groups. These reports may be useful for rare diseases related to a single risk factor, like mesothelioma related to asbestos exposure and lever sarcoma related to vinyl chloride. Both examples concern work environments where the exposure was high and the frequency of appearance of such rare malignancies in a small population was unusually high. Environmental exposure may lead to cases reporting if it is severe like after a major pollution episode. Cases are reported by primary health authorities, if they consider that there is clustering of an infrequent disease in a population with specific common characteristics. Such a cluster must be submitted to further analysis in order for the researcher to investigate statistical difference from the expected incidence (Wartenberg, 1994).
2. Ecological studies compare health outcomes between a group exposed to a factor and a not exposed, or between groups with estimated different exposure or for the same group between periods with different exposure status (Coggon et al., 1989). These studies do not consider individual differences in the duration and the extent of the exposure. Statistical evidence leads to a causal hypothesis generation. Further documentation of causality hypothesis needs analytic studies of the same or similar populations. Such studies consider the mortality and hospital admissions for respiratory and or cardiovascular diseases, during or after peaks of traffic air pollution or the acute not stochastic health effects after a nuclear accident. The diachronic reduction of children's asthma is supposed to be related with passive smoking reduction, while the reduction of stomach cancer is supposed to be related to the improvement of food sanitation and nutritional habits (Millett et al., 2013). The observed decrease in children's blood lead concentration seems to be related to the replacement of lead mixtures in gasoline (Tsoi et al., 2016). The comparison between different populations or between different periods must consider not only environmental differences, but also differences of nutritional habits, social and economic conditions.
3. Cross-sectional studies look for a health outcome of interest after exposure to a risk factor at a specific point of time. The exposure may be also measured. These are prevalence studies, comparing the prevalence of the outcome between exposed or not exposed populations or in a single population before and after the exposure. They allow simultaneously the study of multiple outcomes. They contribute to generate hypothesis of causality.
4. Longitudinal studies make repeated observations of concerned outcome for a more or less long period of time. Epidemiological surveillance allows a continuous and systematic collection and analysis of health data. Such a surveillance system may focus on the respiratory health problems related to air

pollution episodes or any adverse health effect related to chronic exposure. These systems estimate the occurrence of diseases and allow comparisons among populations with different exposure levels or between exposed and not exposed individuals. Systematic surveillance provides exposure and illness data necessary for analytical studies (Teutsch and Churchil, 2000). Syndromic surveillance is a daily registration of cases with a similar clinical syndrome, i.e. common symptoms related to different clinical entities. If there is an evident increase of the occurrence of a syndrome in an area, this signals the need for a more sophisticated research that will investigate what is the clinical entity behind it. Syndromic surveillances allow the early detection of an outbreak related to biological factors, chemical or physical pollutants. A syndromic surveillance is indicated after a physical or technological disaster for the early detection of health problems related to the degradation of the water supply, the sanitary infrastructure, and the living conditions or to the direct exposure to a liberated harmful agent after technological accident or terrorist attack (Henning, 2004; Buehler et al., 2003).

Analytic Studies

Analytic studies include: Cohort studies and case control studies. Cohort studies estimate the health outcome occurrence at a population with a common exposure for a long period and they compare this with those of the general population. The population of individuals with common exposure, but different level and duration of exposure for each one is a cohort group. Cohort studies are longitudinal studies; however, all longitudinal studies are not cohort studies since they may include people not exposed to the studied factor. These studies estimate the relative risk of the incidence of an outcome in the cohort group dividing the incidence of this outcome in the cohort to this of the general population. As an example, the relative risk of lung cancer for passive smokers is 1.5. This means that the ratio of the incidence of lung cancer among passive smokers to those of non-exposed to passive smoking is 1.5, or in other words, exposed people have 50% more probability to develop lung cancer. It also correlates with the fact that the 30% of lung cancer cases among exposed people are attributed to passive smoking. Environmental risk factors are associated with low levels of relative risk in comparison to occupational exposures and to habits like smoking. For example, the relative risk for lung cancer is about 10 for smokers and 1,26-1,46 for indoor exposure to radon (Garzillo et al., 2017). Occupational exposure to asbestos is related to lung cancer with a relative risk varying between twofold and tenfold (Nynas et al., 2017). Occupational cohort studies compare the incidence rate of an outcome between the cohort group and the expected incidence of the general population, however the *a priori* incidence of the cohort is likely to differ from the general population. Employed persons are on average healthier than the general population encompassing vulnerable unemployed individuals. This is the health worker effect bias (Arrighi and Herz-Picciotto, 1994).

Cohort studies may be prospective or retrospective. Prospective studies collect individual exposure data and health effects on a real-time basis. Retrospective studies estimate exposure and health data using available records. Although a cohort group is defined by exposure to the same factor, the duration and extent of exposure varies among the members of a group. The members of the cohort are therefore sub-grouped according to the years and the magnitude of exposure. To compare the occurrence of a disease among peoples with similar exposure levels but different duration a new variable is created: "person-years" of exposure. Person-years of exposure are the product of the number of peoples by the duration of exposure. Both the chronic health effect and the stochastic effect are related to the long-life exposure burden. Since the exposure levels vary for different life periods, the total burden is estimated as the total of sub products at different time segments. A comparison of health effects among different exposure groups reveals the relative risk not only between exposure and not exposure, but also according to the exposure level. Other determinants of health like smoking, nutritional habits, racial characteristics, job conditions must be considered for everyone. In case of a major pollution effect, like after a major industrial accident, the investigation of future health effects in the exposed population is effective prospectively, by the registration of the morbidity and mortality of the individuals of this population according to the duration and the estimated dose of exposure. Case- control studies estimate the exposure rate at a hazard among individuals (cases) with a health outcome (a clearly defined adverse health effect) and they compare this with the exposure to the same hazard among individuals without the outcome (healthy controls). The comparison metric is the odds ratio (OR). The OR represents the odds that the health effect occurs given an exposure to a putative factor, compared to the odds of the same effect occurring if that exposure does not exist. If the OR is 1 the odds of the health effect is not affected by the exposure. If it is higher than 1, the exposure is associated with a higher outcome of the health effect. If it is less than 1, the exposure seems to have a protective role. Any result must be statistically significant. Case- control studies must include for cases and controls, the analysis of all eventual determinants, for example environmental factors should not be analyzed without considering smoking. We always must think if an association between exposure to a putative factor and outcome is affected by a third variable, which is independently associated with the same outcome it is also associated with the exposure (Szklo and Nieto, 2007). This is a confounding factor. For example, the hypothesis that a health outcome is related to poor environmental conditions should analyze the role of the socioeconomic level, since low level socioeconomic conditions may affect directly the health outcome and from the other hand peoples with lower socioeconomic level live in areas with poor environmental conditions. In case- control studies the health effect concerning the study and the criteria of its diagnosis must be concrete. The health data are therefore accurate. The exposure is mainly based to questionnaires concerning the exposure to the putative factor like the home address, current and previous employments, the estimated exposure's duration and any variable that should be analyzed as determinant or confounder. Since in case-control studies the exposure is estimated retrospectively, the cases (patients) remember exposure better than the controls (healthy individuals). The exposure is underestimated for controls and overestimated for cases. This is a systematic error, referred as differential recall bias leading to an overestimation of the odds ratio. Statistical techniques allow the assessment of this phenomenon by further adjustment (Teschke et al., 2002). The controls must have a similar expected risk to manifest the adverse health effect. It is therefore suggested to match cases with controls in terms of age, gender and race. Matching variables cannot be analyzed as risk factors. Over-matching must be avoided because it may cover the role of some determinants. However, for diseases where a risk factor has a known very strong relationship, if we look for the effect of another minor determinant, we can limit the study to cases and controls without exposure to this factor. For example, smoking is strongly related to lung cancer; to study the relation of air pollution to lung cancer, we can exclude smokers from cases and controls (Pearce, 2016).

FUTURE RESEARCH DIRECTIONS

The classical occupational and environmental epidemiology contributed to the recognition of risk factors by providing enough arguments for effective protection measures. The environmental epidemiology studies concern the impact of specific risk factors on individuals; however, it is important to consider the long-term impact of the ecosystems on populations. The increased life expectancy and the improvement of life conditions are related to enormous technological developments; however, the global climate change poses new threats to public health, affecting the safety of water bodies and food, facilitating the transmission of infectious diseases and causing natural disasters (Barrett et al., 2015). The long-term consequences of ozone depletion, the massive urbanization, and the increasing demands for nature resources are yet less evident. Occupational epidemiology meets also new challenges as the nature and the location of work change. Technological improvements reduce exposure to traditional risks and increase work safety; however, there is an emerging interest in the impact of social and psychological factors at the work place. With high migration movements and ageing societies in industrialized countries, the employment of immigrants, vulnerable people and older workers is a new field of research for occupational epidemiology.

Genetic research showed that the nucleotide polymorphisms include genes with a different metabolism of environmental expressions. It means that some people are more susceptible to an environmental exposure to a specific factor than others. This phenomenon also explains why some people will develop an adverse health effect while others exposed to the same factors will not. Obviously, this differential response is related to genetic differences. Environmental exposures and genetic variations must be reliably measured to detect these differences. Microarray technology and new omics technologies are much promising in relation to this challenge. Genetic research also permits the detection of proteins (metabonomics) and DNA adducts (adductomics). These are alterations generated by exposure to specific mutagens.

They serve as a biomarker for exposure to carcinogens. The association of polymorphisms for enzymes metabolizing environmental mutagens and adduct levels may help develop preventive strategies for the protection of more susceptible individuals. Although molecular technologies allow detecting effects at the molecular level originated by very low levels of exposure, the clinical significance of such effects and their impact in the public health in terms of quality and perspective of life remain unclear (Davis and Milner, 2004).

In 2005, the concept of exposome - enclosing the totality of human environmental exposures - it was first proposed (Wild, 2005). The exposome is a kind of a database with information concerning environmental exposure measurements in a person's life time and corresponding biomarkers concentrations in different biospecimens. Population characteristics are also considered. The individual's exposure begins before birth. The biomarkers are mostly related to dietary, occupational and other pollutant exposures. Exposomics is the study of the correlation of measurements of environmental exposures and of biomarkers' concentrations to the disease occurrence and reproducibility, considering internal individual genetic characteristics. It is expected to develop hypothesis for diseases etiology and genetic promptness. The International Agency for Research on Cancer (IARC) developed such an Exposure- Explorer data basis (Steyner et al., 2017). The pregnancy period has a high potential lifetime impact. Recent environmental studies assess the effects of the multiple exposures during pregnancy on child development (Robinson and Vrijheid, 2015). The concept of the human exposome created the "urban exposome" defined as a permanent qualitative and quantitative monitoring of internal or external factors that affect the quality of life and the health of the residents of a city. These data are related to routinely collected health indicators (Andrianou and Makris, 2018).

CONCLUSION

Environmental and occupational epidemiology studies, despite the above constraints, contributed to the implementation of impressive measures for the protection of public health like the restriction of passive smoking; the banning of asbestos, of chlorinated pesticides, of lead in the gasoline and home paints; the abatement of industrial and car exhausts; the implementation of new waste management technologies etc. Epidemiologists are called to meet a challenge: using accurate methodology, they are called to address, with evidence-based arguments, public concerns related to new environmental threats.

REFERENCES

Andrianou, X., & Makris, K. (2018). The framework pf urban exposome: Application of exposome concept in urban health studies. *The Science of the Total Environment*, *636*, 963–967. doi:10.1016/j.scitotenv.2018.04.329 PMID:29729514

Armstrong, B. K., White, E., & Saracci, R. (1992). Principles of exposure measurement in epidemiology. *Monographs in Epidemiology and Biostatistics, 1*(21).

Arrighi, M., & Herz-Picciotto, I. (1994). The evolving concept of the healthy worker survivor effect. *Epidemiology*, *5*(2), 189–195. doi:10.1097/00001648-199403000-00009 PMID:8172994

Barrett, B., Charles, J. W., & Temte, J. L. (2015, January). Climate change, human health, and epidemiological transition. *Preventive Medicine*, *70*, 69–75. doi:10.1016/j.ypmed.2014.11.013 PMID:25434735

Buehler, J. W., Berkelman, R. L., Hartley, D. M., & Peters, C. J. (2003). Syndromic surveillance and bioterrorism-related epidemics. *Emerging Infectious Diseases*, *9*(10), 1197–1204. doi:10.3201/eid0910.030231 PMID:14609452

CDC. (2012): Principles of epidemiology in public health practice (3rd ed.). CDC USA.

Coggon, D., Barker, D. J., Cole, R. B., & Nelson, M. (1989). Stomach cancer and food storage. *Journal of the National Cancer Institute*, *81*(15), 1178–1182. doi:10.1093/jnci/81.15.1178 PMID:2746670

Davis, C. D., & Milner, J. (2004). Frontiers in nutrigenomics, proteomics, metabolomics and cancer prevention. *Mutation Research*, *551*(1-2), 51–64. doi:10.1016/j.mrfmmm.2004.01.012 PMID:15225581

Dotson, G. S., Maier, A., Siegel, P. D., Anderson, S. E., Green, B. J., Stefaniak, A. B., ... Kimber, I. (2015). Setting occupational exposure limits for chemical allergens—Understanding the challenges. *Journal of Occupational and Environmental Hygiene*, *12*(Suppl. 1), S82–S98.

Dotson, G. S., Maier, A., Siegel, P. D., Anderson, S. E., Green, B. J., Stefaniak, A. B., ... Kimber, I. (2015). Setting occupational exposure limits for chemical allergens—Understanding the challenges. *Journal of Occupational and Environmental Hygiene, 12*(supl), S82-S98. doi:10.1093/acprof:oso/9780198509851.001.0001

Garzillo, C., Pugliese, M., Loffredo, F., & Quarto, M. (2017). Indoor radon exposure and lung cancer risk: A meta-analysis of case-control studies. *Translational Cancer Research*, *6*(Supplement 5), S934–S943. doi:10.21037/tcr.2017.05.42

Henning, K. J. (2004). What is syndromic surveillance. *Morbidity and Mortality Weekly Report*, *53*(Supplement), 7–11.

Kaviraj A., Unlu E., Gupta A., Nemr A. (2014). Biomarkers of environmental pollutants. *BioMed Research International*. doi:. doi:10.155/2014/806598

Leenhouts, H. P., & Chadwick, K. H. (1989). The molecular basis of stochastic and nonstochastic effects. *Health Physics*, *57*(Suppl. 1), 343–348. doi:10.1097/00004032-198907001-00048 PMID:2606691

Loomis, D., & Kromhout, H. (2004). Exposure variability: Concepts and applications in occupational epidemiology. American journal of industrial medicine, 45(1), 113-122. doi:10.1002/ajim.10324 PMID:14691975

Millett, C., Lee, J. T., Laverty, A. A., Glantz, S. A., & Majeed, A. (2013). Hospital admissions for childhood asthma after smoke-free legislation in England. *Pediatrics*, *131*(2), 495–501. doi:10.1542/peds.2012-2592 PMID:23339216

Neveu, V., Moussy, A., Rouaix, H., Wedekind, R., Pon, A., Knox, C., ... Scalbert, A. (2017). Exposome-Explorer: A manually-curated database on biomarkers of exposure to dietary and environmental factors. *Nucleic Acids Research*, *45*(D1), 979–984. doi:10.1093/nar/gkw980 PMID:27924041

Nieuwenhuijsen, I. M. (2015). *Exposure Assessment in Environmental Epidemiology* (2nd ed.). Oxford University Press. doi:10.1093/med/9780199378784.001.0001

Nuckols, J. R., Ward, M. H., & Jarup, L. (2004). Using Geographic Information Systems for Exposure Assessment in Environmental Epidemiology Studies. *Environmental Health Perspectives*, *112*(9), 1007–1015. doi:10.1289/ehp.6738 PMID:15198921

Nynas, P., Pukkala, E., Vainio, H., & Oksa, P. (2017). Cancer incidence in asbestos- exposed workers: An ubdate on four Finnish cohorts. *Safety and Health at Work*, *8*(20), 169–174. doi:10.1016/j.shaw.2016.11.003 PMID:28593073

Pearce, N. (2016). *Analysis of matched case-control studies*. Academic Press.

Public Health Information Systems. (2017). *Registries - Routine and Public*. Retrieved from www.coursera.org/learn/epidemiology-public-health/lecture/pYnBq/public-health-information-systems-July-24

Richard, J., & Thomas, R. J. (2013). Particle size and pathogenicity in the respiratory tract. *Virulence*, *4*(8), 847–858. doi:10.4161/viru.27172 PMID:24225380

Robinson, O., & Vrijheid, M. (2015). The Pregnancy Exposome. *Current Environmental Health Reports*, *2*(2), 204–213. doi:10.100740572-015-0043-2 PMID:26231368

Rothman, K. J. (1993). Methodologic frontiers in environmental epidemiology. *Environmental Health Perspectives*, *101*(suppl. 4), 19–21.

Shepherd, D., Dirks, K., Welch, D., Dride, D., & Landon, J. (2016). The covariance between air pollution annoyance and noise annoyance, and its relationship with health-related quality of life. *International Journal of Environmental Research and Public Health, 13*(8), 792. doi:10.3390/ijerph13080792 PMID:27509512

Sherwin, R. P. (1983). What is an adverse health effect? *Environmental Health Perspectives, 52*, 177–182. PMID:6653520

Solomon, D. J., Henry, R. C., Hogan, J. G., Van Amburg, G. H., & Taylor, J. (1991). Evaluation and implementation of public health registries. *Public Health Reports (Washington, D.C.), 106*(2), 142–150. PMID:1902306

Stayner, L., Collins, J., Guo, Y., Heederik, D., Kogevinas, M., Steenland, K., ... Demers, P. (2017). Challenges and Opportunities for Occupational Epidemiology in the Twenty-first Century. *Current Environmental Health Reports, 3*(3), 319–324. doi:10.100740572-017-0154-z PMID:28803393

Szklo, M., & Nieto, F. J. (2007). *Epidemiology beyond the Basics* (2nd ed.). Boston, MA: Jones and Bartlett Publishers.

Teschke, K., Olshan, A., Daniels, J., De Roos, A., Parks, C., Schulz, M., & Vaughan, T. (2002). Occupational exposure in case-control studies: Opportunities for improvement. *Occupational and Environmental Medicine, 59*(9), 575–594. doi:10.1136/oem.59.9.575 PMID:12205230

Teutsch, S., & Churchil, E. (2000). *Principles and practice of public health surveillance* (2nd ed.). Oxford University Press.

Tsoi, M. F., Cheung, C. L., Cheung, T. T., & Cheung, B. M. Y. (2016). Continual decrease in blood lead level in Americans: United States National Health Nutrition and Examination Survey 1999-2014. *The American Journal of Medicine, 129*(11), 1213–1218. doi:10.1016/j.amjmed.2016.05.042 PMID:27341956

Wartenberg, D. (1994). *When is a Cluster Really a Cluster? The competing agendas of science, society and social programs. Environmental Epidemiology: Science for society or science in society?* Hamilton, Canada: McMaster University.

Wild, C. P. (2005). Complementing the genome with an "exposome": The outstanding challenge of environmental exposure measurement in molecular epidemiology. *Cancer Epidemiology, Biomarkers & Prevention, 14*(8), 1847–1850. doi:10.1158/1055-9965.EPI-05-0456 PMID:16103423

Chapter 8
Lifelong Consumption of Plant-Based GM Foods:
Is It Safe?

Matthew Chidozie Ogwu
https://orcid.org/0000-0001-6054-1667
Seoul National University, South Korea

ABSTRACT

Genetically modified (GM) crops are cultivated in over 30 countries with their products and by-products imported by over 60 countries. This chapter seeks to highlight general concerns and potential lifelong effects of consuming GM plant-based food. The consumption of GM plant-based food is as risky as consuming conventional plant-based food. However, the alien genes in these products may be unstable leading to antinutritional and unintended short-term consequences. Due to the paucity of research, no long-term effects have been attributed to the lifelong consumption of these products. Nonetheless, possible lifelong health and socioeconomic effects may result from outcrossing of genes, increasing antibiotic resistance, development of new diseases, as well as potential effects on the environment and biodiversity. Biotechnology companies need to invest more in interdisciplinary research addressing the potential lifelong effects of these products. Although GM foods are safe for consumption, clarification of current risks and lifelong effects are required.

INTRODUCTION

Plants remain the central food resources for humans and other animals. However, there is increasing pressure on the resources to fulfil this basic need. Population growth, particularly in countries with developing economies, will result in a need to overexploit plant resources to increase food production (Ogwu et al., 2014; Delaney, 2015). Climate change might make economic crops unsuitable for cultivation in their centre of origins and diversity as these areas become increasingly threatened by drought, floods, spread of plant diseases and altered weather patterns (Thompson, 2017). More so, lifestyle changes continue to influence plant use patterns across the globe. For instance, Łuczaj et al. (2012), reported

DOI: 10.4018/978-1-5225-7635-8.ch008

significant changes in the contemporary use of wild food plants in parts of Europe due to the decline of plant knowledge, the disappearance of traditional methods of plant use, reduced availability of plants due to ecosystem changes, land access rights for foragers and intoxication hazards. Hence, even though global agricultural productivity has significantly improved, issues related to food security persist because of multidirectional issues (Lamichhane, 2014).

This chapter seeks to highlight general concerns pertaining to the consumption of genetically modified (GM) plant-based food products. The chapter will address it from an environment and health perspective. Short-term effects of consuming GM plant-based food are easily discernible but not the long-term effects, which may take years, decades or even a lifetime to appear (Murnaghan, 2018). The need to be vigilant and assess the potential risks of such unpredictable occurrences cannot be ignored (Butler and Reichhardt, 1999). GM plants and plant-based products are here to stay regardless of conflicting standpoints. In the sustainable future, which is a long-term global goal, these products might become indispensable. Therefore, so much needs to be done from the different players to make GM products more acceptable. The objective of this chapter is to promote the knowledge of GM plants and plant-based products, their lifelong health and environmental effects as well as to proffer salient recommendations to address pertinent issues. Through these contributions, this chapter will reduce existing fears as well as increase the knowledge, understanding and highlight practical gaps concerning the production and consumption of GM plants and plant-based products.

PUBLIC PERCEPTION OF THE NEEDS AND BENEFITS OF GM PLANTS

The need to achieve food security has led to the intensification of agriculture, which naturally interferes with natural ecological cycles. The agricultural sector contributes to the emission of environmentally dangerous chemicals like ammonia, methane, and nitrates (Zhu et al., 2006). GM plants held under cultivation has long been considered as a sustainable alternative to attain food self-sufficiency and sovereignty albeit controversial. The three pathways by which GM crops contribute to food security include increasing food production and availability, influencing food safety and quality as well as enhancing the economic and social situation of farmers, thereby influencing food accessibility (Qaim and Kouser, 2013). Hunger is a major threat to humanity and it affects an estimated more than 1 billion people many of whom live in developing countries (Delaney, 2015; Hefferon, 2016). It remains our moral obligation to feed the hungry billions. To this end, the GM crop movement has overseen enormous good but also presented significant adverse consequences and prompted controversies (Schlett and Beke, 2015).

GM is the application of gene technology to alter an organism's genome by combining genes from different organisms through recombinant DNA technology to produce a new or modified organism, which may be described as 'GM', 'genetically engineered' or 'transgenic' (Bawa and Anilakumar, 2013). This technology exploits gene variations, expressions and modifications to produce outstanding crops for human benefits. It is distinct from the production of clones, which culminates in genetically identical copies. This technology-based manipulation of living things began with microorganisms and then economic plants but have since expanded to include other organisms from diverse taxa. Insertion of defined foreign genes into the genome of bacteria, moulds, yeast, etc., has resulted in the creation of genetically modified organisms (GMOs). These GMOs or their by-products are primarily used for human food productions as well as in different industrial processes including the production of pharmaceuticals (Lisowska, 2011). Therefore, most GM foods stem mostly from plants, which have been GM to improve their yield, through the introduction of one or several resistant-components against plant pests, disease prevention or increased tolerance of herbicides and environmental extremes (Domingo, 2016).

The original aim of producing GM plants was to produce plant varieties that are fast-growing, disease and drought resistance, more nutritious and can out-compete weeds to maximize plant resources for food security. However, the pressure to feed the ever-increasing human population continues to drive the expansion of the limits of GM companies and GMOs. The potentials of this technology is limitless because of the possible manipulation of the processes and outcomes to serve other contemporary societal challenges besides food security with adverse implications on plant diversity and the environment. For instance, bananas that produce human vaccines against infectious diseases such as hepatitis B, fruit and nut trees that yield years earlier and plants that produce new plastics with unique properties (Bawa and Anilakumar, 2013). All these have succeeded in exacerbating the consequences of GM technology and public concerns. According to Frewer and Shepher (1995), these are manifested as an overall rejection of specific aspects of the technology, where public attitudes may be defined by a complex set of perceptions incorporating risk, benefit, control, and ethical concerns. Underlying this concern is that a large proportion of the public remains unaware of what a GM plant and plant-based product actually are or what advantages and disadvantages the technology has to offer (Key et al., 2008). This stem from the persistence of concerns related to environmental quality and human health risks since the introduction of the technology. As suggested by Qaim and Kouser (2013), GM products may have impacts on food quality, quantity, availability, nutrient composition, and household income. All of which may potentially lead to diverse psychological effects at the personal, family and community levels. In spite of the increase in available information on the potential toxic effects of GM foods and plants, concerns about their environment and health risks persist (Domingo, 2000; Domingo and Gomez, 2000; Domingo, 2007; Domingo, 2011; Domingo and Bordonaba, 2011; Domingo, 2016).

Recent concerns regarding the safety of GM plant-based foods from diverse groups including consumers and environmental non-governmental organizations (NGO) have led to social and political debates on the potential negative impacts of transgenic plants, with suggestions that all the related products should be subjected to long-term studies before approval for human consumption (Domingo and Bordonaba, 2011; Domingo, 2016). More than 20 years have passed since the approval of genetic modifications in food and the world is yet to fully come to terms with their success albeit increasing number of products. In the same vein, the declaration by the World Health Organization's (WHO) that these products should be subjected to risk assessments for human nutrition and health have not been systematically performed (Domingo, 2007; Magaña-Gómez and de la Barca, 2009). However, with an increasingly less productive environment affecting the yields of most major crops, the future is very promising for GM technologies to meet the future global needs for food, feed and fibre in a sustainable and responsible way (Oliver, 2014). GM plants for food use has the potential to offer benefits in agricultural practice, food quality, nutrition and health, but several aspects of GM technology still require further clarifications (The Royal Society, 2002) including areas under cultivation, risk assessment, and the level of uncertainty and unpredictability associated with each GM crop (Tsatsakis et al., 2017). In addition, the public is often uninformed or misinformed about most GMOs and their potential side effects (Twardowski and Małyska. 2015).

GM PLANTS AND GM PLANT-BASED FOOD AND PRODUCTS

There is a heavy burden on the world to eliminate food insecurity in all regions and technology seem to be the most plausible option. Plant breeders desire to develop plant varieties that express good agronomic qualities but through conventional breeding, there is little to no guarantee of obtaining any particular gene combination from millions of test crosses in search of desirable characters (Lamichhane, 2014). This shortcoming can be overcome through genetic engineering, which allows the direct transfer of one or just a few genes of interest between seemingly related or unrelated organisms to obtain the desired agronomic traits. Modern biotechnology has the potential to be a significant tool in fighting hunger as it is well positioned to address agricultural problems such as yield loss from insect infestation, competition with weeds, drought, etc. (Delaney, 2015). Hence, through modern biotechnology, GM plant and plant-based products are asexually and artificially produced when two or more alien genetic materials are added to the recombinant DNA technology or genetic engineering process to solve specific agricultural challenge.

Historically, the technology became popular in the twentieth century when the bacteria *Escherichia coli* was used to produce insulin in human diabetic patients. However, it was only after the discovery of Polymerase Chain Reaction technique, which allowed the amplification of target nucleic acid fragments, thus making it possible to copy or change DNA sequence that the technology could take on wider applications. Moreover, novel applications of recombinant DNA technology evolved alongside the development of genetic processes and biological variations, which made the production of important products possible (Shivanand and Noopur, 2010). In addition, there has been a generational trend aimed at making necessary techniques simpler and easier to perform. At that pace, plants with recognizable economic value became the subject of genetic modification with little to no consideration of their ethnobotany, diversity or environmental implications. The first attempts to genetically modify crops were undertaken in the 1980s on tobacco. However, the first GM food crops were FLAVR SAVR™ tomato that was engineered for delayed ripening and were subsequently commercialized in 1994 in the USA (Kok and Kuiper, 2003; Lisowska, 2011). The FLAVR SAVR™ tomato contained a foreign gene that prevented the breakdown of cell walls as the fruit ripened as well as for the fruits to remain firm after extended shipping and storage period (Schneider et al., 2017). Worldwide, over 148 million hectares of GM crops were cultivated in 2010 (ISAAA 2010). ISAAA (2012) reported that in 2012, GM crops were planted in 28 countries with developing countries accounting for a majority of the total GM harvest. From 1996 to 2014, 357 GM crops were approved and the global value of the GM crop market reached 35% of the global commercial seed market in 2014 albeit with different controversies (Lin and Pan, 2016). Each year the EU imports about 30 million tons of grain, soybeans, and maize, most of which are transgenic (Twardowski and Małyska. 2015).

In summary, GM crops are produced after identifying a trait of interest (in the same or different plant species), isolating that trait through comparative analysis (or via deletion, knock down, seed chipping process), inserting that trait into the genome of the test crop using gene gun or microorganism (commonly used ones are the bacteria *Agrobacterium tumefaciens* and *Bacillus thuringiensis*), and then propagating the GM crop (Figure 1). The newly produced plants containing genes from another organism are called "transgenic plant", "GM crop", "genetically engineered plants," or, more broadly, "genetically modified organisms" (Wieczorek, 2013, Magaña-Gómez and Calderón de la Barca, 2009).

Production of GM plant involves targeting the best genotypes based on phenotype for regeneration in tissue culture by exploiting the DNA transfer mechanisms of organisms like bacteria (Southgate et al., 1995; Powell, 2015; Bawa and Anilakumar, 2013). The main limiting steps are locating genes for

Figure 1. An overview of how GM crops are produced
Source: Pighin, 2003.

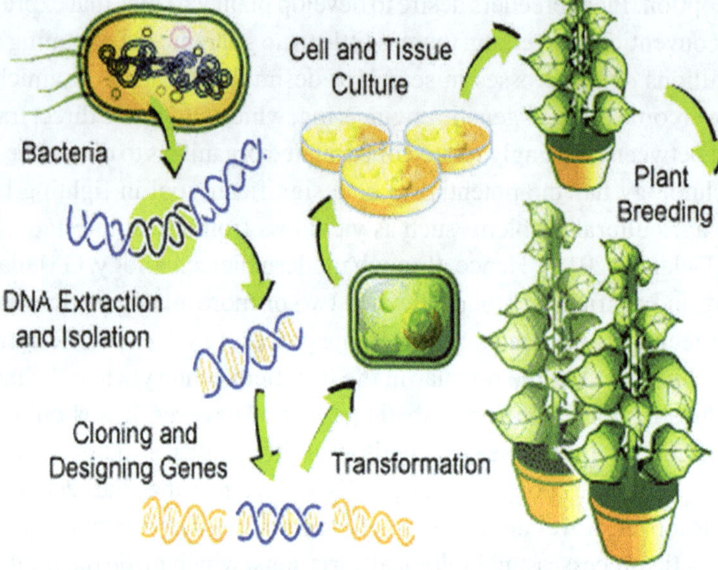

important traits (Bawa and Anilakumar, 2013). According to Schneider et al. (2017), GM plants are the outcome of moving genes from one organism to another causing the transferees' genetic makeup to be altered and the expression of hitherto unexpressed attributes like delayed-ripening in tomatoes, pest-resistant in squash and potato, herbicide-tolerance in cotton and soybean, etc. Through this process, major transgenic economic plants have been produced including tobacco, tomato, canola, alfalfa, cantaloupe, radicchio, papaya, flax, plum, wheat, apple, creeping bentgrass, sugar beet, maize, cotton, soybean, potato, squash, eggplants, strawberry, lettuce, rice, carrots, etc.

This procedure has raised health concerns through the use of selectable markers to identify transformed cells, transfer of extraneous DNA into the plant genome and the increased mutations in GM plants compared to non-GM counterparts due to tissue culture processes used in their production and the rearrangement of DNA around the insertion site of foreign genes (Key et al., 2008). Other considerations include antibiotic resistance, disease resistance, extreme weather resistance, early or delayed ripening, modified composition and herbicide resistance. Nonetheless, these crops find their way to our dining table, pharmaceutical and departmental stores through major biotechnology companies and their subsidiaries like Calgene, Monsanto, Asgrow, Zeneca and Peto. Different bodies like the Food and Drug Administration (in the USA) and European Food Safety Authority (of the European Union) regulate the production of GMO and their food or other products. Testing on GMOs in plant food can be done using molecular techniques like DNA microarrays or qPCR to screen for genetic elements like p35S, tNos, pat, or bar or event specific markers for the official GMOs like Mon810, Bt11, or GT73 (Bawa and Anilakumar, 2013). Hundreds of millions of people have knowingly or unknowingly used products derived from GM crops across the world for more than 15 years (Key et al., 2008).

When GM plants become mature, they are harvested either wholly or in parts and from it a variety of products (domestic and/or industrial) can be derived. Ready-to-eat plant-based food and/or food ingredients (materials) derived from plants whose genome has been modified through an artificial process is referred to as GM plant-based foods and GM plant-based products respectively. Some of these products include omega-3 supplements (Usher, 2017), vaccines (Phillips, 2008), industrial vegetable oil (European Chemicals Agency, 2012), fattening feed for farm animals (Grant, 2017), etc. The labelling of products with ingredients sourced from GM plant enables the identification of GM plant-based products (Wong, 2003; Carter and Gruere, 2003; Byrne et al., 2014). The review by Domingo and Bordonaba (2011) suggest that a huge research void exists for certain GM crops (especially cucumber, peas or tomatoes) while reporting that many research studies on certain GM crops (like maize and soybeans) implicate that they are as safe and nutritious as the respective conventional non-GM plant. Over 90% of biotechnology crops produced worldwide include just four plants: soybean, maize, rape and cotton (Lisowska, 2011). Most GM crops are commonly engineered to be resistant to the herbicide glyphosate that enables farmers to increase efficiency in eliminating weeds without harming their crops or with a natural insecticide to protect the yields of these crops against insect infestation, which is more environmentally friendly than using toxic sprays (Thompson, 2017). Most plants naturally perceive foreign organisms capable of causing infections but efficiency varies within and between species. Therefore, the proteins that identify an infection and activate defences can be moved between and within species using genetic modification to enable previously vulnerable crops to turn on their innate resistance mechanisms (Thompson, 2017). Recent advances in gene editing technology using CRISPR-Cas9 have also made it possible to rewrite plant genes so that they work for different sensing function.

Fernandez-Cornejo and Caswell (2006); Magaña-Gómez and Calderón de la Barca (2009); Lin and Pan (2016); Schneider et al. (2017) classified GM plants into one of four generations based on the objective of the introduced traits;

1. First-generation i.e. crops enhanced through the input of single traits to increase production, such as herbicide tolerance, better insect resistance, and tolerance to environmental stress. Most first-generation GM crops contain common transgene elements such as the cauliflower mosaic virus (CaMV), 35S promoter (CaMV35S-P), aminoglycoside 30 -phosphotransferase gene (nptII), phosphinothricin acetyltransferase gene (pat/bar), 5-enolpyruvylshikimate 3-phosphate (CP4-epsp) gene, nopaline synthase promoter (nos-P), and terminator (nos-T) (Lin and Pan, 2016).
2. Second-generation i.e. crops with added-value output through hybrid crosses between commercialized first-generation GM crops to increase consumer benefits, such as nutrient enhancement for animal feed.
3. Third-generation i.e. crops with increased resistant to abiotic stress with industrial roles including pharmaceuticals and biofuels. They are also called near-intragenic, or GM crops where the inserted transgenic.
4. The fourth generation i.e. these are true intragenic and cisgenic, which genuine host genes. Thus, fourth-generation GM crops/foods cannot be distinguished via their transgenic elements and can be identified by inspecting the specific order and insertion loci of its transgenes (Lin and Pan, 2016).

Seed producers are required to submit applications to USDA APHIS (United States Department of Agriculture Animal and Plant Health Inspection Service) for field-testing (Fernandez-Cornejo and Caswell 2006). Approvals are not easily granted but crops with most approvals include corn, cotton, tomatoes, soybeans, rapeseed/canola, potatoes, sugar beets, papaya, rice, squash, alfalfa, plum, rose, tobacco, flax, and chicory (USDA 2014). The percentage of products available in the market that contains at least one GM product is high. Approximately 60 – 70% of processed foods in the United States contain GM components (Ahmed 2002; Dahl, 2012; Schneider et al. 2017). More so, the use of GM plants has increased. For instance, Fernandez-Cornejo (2012) reported that the use of *Bacillus thuringiensis* corn has increased dramatically from its introduction in 1996 to about 15 per cent of total corn acreage in 2012, although those numbers have varied dramatically depending on the year. Recently, Bushey et al. (2014) opined that GM crops may contain newly expressed proteins that are described as ''intractable', which have properties that make it extremely difficult or impossible with current methods to express in heterologous systems; isolate, purify, or concentrate; quantify (due to low levels); demonstrate biological activity; or prove equivalency with plant proteins. Bushey et al concluded that their use and subsequent expression does not present any risk and gave the five classes of these intractable proteins as membrane proteins, signalling proteins, transcription factors, N-glycosylated proteins, and resistance proteins (R-proteins, plant pathogen recognition proteins that activate innate immune responses). Some of the contributions of GM crops and plant-based product include an increase in global agricultural production and farmer's income, reduced application of insecticides, herbicides and fertilizers, increased investment in agriculture, land management, and reduced GHG emission

LIFELONG EFFECTS OF CONSUMING GM PLANTS AND PLANT-BASED PRODUCTS

Lifelong experiences associated with the consumption of GM plants and plant-based products may be expressed in human (or animal) health as well as through lasting environmental changes. Although the issue remains unattractive to scientists and large GMO-based companies probably because of the potential outcomes. Whereas the possibility of short-term side effects of consuming GM crops has attracted attention from both scientific and public groups (Kok and Kuiper, 2003). Healthwise, these lifelong effects may include diseases or genetic predispositions with environment-specific interactions, which may result in physiological adaptations or disruptions with lifelong outcomes in learning, behaviour, as well as in emotional, physical and mental well-being. This is because constant experiences are built into our bodies, creating biological memories that shape development, for better or for worse. For instance, the elderly are most susceptible to new dietary experiences because they have an accumulated burden of chemical exposure over their lifetime hence, some of their body processes are shutting down as well as hormonal disruptions (Swanson, 2013). Moreover, Fontes et al. (2002) suggested some accumulated experience related to exposure of insect-resistant transgenic crops. In addition, the introduction of non-native GM plants in the ecosystems also pose potential long-term risks to the environment whose consequences may be difficult to predict from diverse standpoints (Tsatsakis et al., 2017). Kuiper et al (2001) argued that the consumption of non-GM crops might also result in similar side effects as those from GM crops. Nonetheless, it is worrisome that many potential short and long-term side effects remain undetected due to analysing focussed only on specific compounds or intermediates especially in relation to important nutritional and anti-nutritional pathways. Thereby giving rise to likely undetected lifelong effects.

The subsequent sections will focus on potential health and environmental lifelong effects from the consumption of GM plants and plant-based products.

1. Potential Lifelong Health Effects of Consuming Plant-Based GM Products

The safety of plant-based GM foods for consumption has remained a hot topic and the rarity of research data in this regard may be a contributory factor. Health risks associated with GM foods fall into three main categories: toxins, allergens, and genetic hazards (Conner and Jacobs, 1999). The Royal Society (2002) without considering gene expression products, suggested that there is no evidence of intact gene transfer to humans (and animals) either from vector organisms used in GM plants in the gut or from foodstuffs, despite daily consumption of GM food. Thereby emphasizing that the risks associated with food and food products derived from this recombinant biotechnology are only similar to those for conventional foods (ISAAA, 2009). However, risks exist and may not have been properly defined neither are the consumers always made aware of whatever level of risk exist. Potential transfer of genes from GM plant-based foods are capable of inducing insertional mutagenesis resulting from gene integration due to the inserted genes and their expression products, secondary and pleiotropic effects of gene expression (Bawa and Anilakumar, 2013). More so, the proteins produced by the transgene may be toxic, which can result in additional allergic reactions and/or on the other hand, the production of complex multimeric proteins such as antibodies, which are not readily expressed by microbial systems (Key et al., 2008). These potential transgene protein activities were also acknowledged by USDA (2013) cited in Arya (2015) and could occur because the traits that are introduced into a particular plant are new to that plant but are often found naturally in other plants. The Royal Society (2002) supports this when they reported that the introduction of a new gene into a plant or a change in the expression of an existing gene might cause it to become allergenic, although, in principle, these might not be greater than those posed by conventionally derived crops. Swanson (2013) presented another scenario, wherein, the bacteria (vector) genes are not only potentially toxic but as in some cases, the transgenic herbicide-resistant plants are sprayed and absorb the poisons, which are later consumed and could cause infertility, birth defects, organ diseases as well as neurological, intestinal and immune-diseases. Although the author pointed out that correlation does not necessarily imply causation and there are now a host of other chemicals in our food and our environment.

Generally, food-related issues are known to have lifelong health and socio-psychological effects. For instance, because of food poisoning from microorganisms, kidney failure, chronic arthritis, gastrointestinal infections, Crohn's disease, brain and nerve damage, rheumatism, and death have developed. The safety of the vector used in producing GM plant-based food is a potential source of lifelong effects — such as the *Agrobacterium tumefaciens* vector (Butler and Reichhardt, 1999). Rats fed GM corn over a period of 90 days developed problems with their liver, kidneys, heart, blood cells, spleen and adrenal glands in a sex- and dose-dependent manner (de Vendômois et al., 2009). The authors also showed that rats fed with GM corn over a long period became increasingly infertile as well as developed mammary gland tumours and suggested that it may be due to the new pesticides specific to each GM corn. In the same way, broad unintended direct or indirect metabolic consequences of genetic modification cannot be excluded. Bawa and Anilakumar (2013) opined that many transgenes encode enzymes capable of altering biochemical pathways causing an increase or decrease in certain biochemical or enzyme substrate and a subsequent build-up of the enzymatic product that supports the latter point.

Furthermore, technological advancement in GM crop production have enabled the modification of traits that can affect the functional properties of the final product like the long-ripening tomatoes with favourable post-harvest characteristics suitable for processing the tomato into paste and oilseed crops with modified oil composition such as high oleic acid (more stable during frying) (Kok and Kuiper, 2003).

Kok and Kuiper suggested that these modifications might be used to alleviate nutritional deficiencies such as vitamin A deficiency and/or anaemia in through consumption of 'Golden Rice' fortified with provitamin A and iron-fortified GM rice. Food allergies and severe allergic reactions (anaphylaxis) are caused by allergens, which are mostly proteins. The protein components of GM plants may be implicated in their functional properties because the introduction of a new gene into a plant, or a change in the expression of an existing gene, may cause that plant to become allergenic even though no evidence exists at present that GM foods cause any clinical manifestations of allergenicity (The Royal Society, 2002). The persistence of pesticide residues in GM food is a hot topic in Europe. A popular notion highlighted in Kok and Kuiper (2003) is that traditional crop plant varieties on which our livelihood depends are not elaborately tested for safety prior to their popular use, therefore this history of safe use can be used as a baseline for the safety assessment of new GM plant varieties derived from established plant lines. Although GM and conventional sources induce similar nutritional performance and growth, adverse microscopic and molecular effects of some GM foods in different organs or tissues have been reported to a certain extent (Magaña-Gómez and de la Barca, 2009; Domingo and Bordonaba, 2011). The norm is to *ab initio* compare GM outputs with cultivars but this approach is not sustainable. The principle of substantial equivalence is based on the notion that, "if a new food is found to be substantially equivalent in composition and nutritional characteristics to an existing food, it can be regarded as being as safe as the conventional food" (SOT, 2003). The application of the concept is not a safety assessment per se; rather it enables the identification of potential differences between the existing food and the new product, which should then be further investigated with respect to their toxicological impacts (Domingo and Bordonaba, 2011). Moreover, the concept of substantial equivalence was introduced with the aim of establishing a scientifically sound approach that would meet global acceptance but it emphasizes compositional analysis as a requirement for toxicological and nutritional studies (Kook and Kuiper, 2003). Such comparative analysis ignores the contribution of natural and artificial abiotic components that influence the expression of certain genes in both lines capable of causing lifelong or long-term health effects. More so, it is common knowledge that the principle fulfils local and national interest more than global considerations. New approaches have since evolved for food safety assessments of GM plant-based food like the European Thematic Network, Entransfood. The focus of Entransfood is on the different levels of the safety evaluation of GM food crops including:

- **DNA Level:** Based on sequence analysis of the insertion point of the gene fragment to identify any potential side effects through the interruption of regulatory or gene sequences.
- **Gene Expression Level:** Using microarrays techniques to monitor large-scale gene expression simultaneously.
- **Protein Level:** By monitoring shifts in protein levels using proteomic analysis of the tissues of interest.
- **Metabolite Level:** Direct analysis of secondary metabolites using gas and liquid chromatography (GC/LC) in combination with MS or nuclear magnetic resonance.

Kleter et al. (2005); Arya (2015) highlighted the possibility of horizontal gene transfer due to the absorption of DNA fragments by gut microflora or somatic cells lining the intestinal cell since the DNA from ingested food is not completely degraded by digestion and small fragments of DNA from GM foods have been found in different parts of the gastrointestinal tract. A comprehensive scientific evaluation of this problem is a colossal task because only about 1% of the naturally existing bacteria can be cultured and thus analysed. Already, GM crops with glyphosate have been implicated in different gastrointestinal disorders including irritable bowel syndrome, Celiac diseases and chronic constipation through interference with gut microflora and immune systems (Group, 2016). However, it is generally hypothesized that the uptake of GM DNA into the cells of the gastrointestinal tract will not have any biological consequences because they may be degraded in the cells. Recently, outcrossing have also been observed of genes from GM plants to traditional plants, related species and unrelated species. The insertion of a new gene may lead to an increase in the existing levels of anti-nutrients as well as interfere with the utilization of nutrients. Although humans have been ingesting CaMV and its 35S promoter in high amounts, no disease has been associated with it neither has it recombined with other viruses (Arya, 2015).

2. Potential Long-Term Environmental Effects of Plant-Based GM Products

Conventional agriculture and food production systems are environmentally costly, as it requires certain levels of environmental modification. Although GM plant production remains a possible pathway for humanity to achieve food security, it is a significant contributor to genetic erosion and reduction of plant gene pool and genetic diversity. The production of GM crops is not environmentally neutral rather it may have positive or negative impacts on the environment in the long and short-term albeit their detection remains challenging to measure economically and otherwise. Generally, the negative environmental impacts of GM crops result from their impacts on non-target species, increased weediness (combination of traits that make them as competitive as natural weeds), increase in soil toxin levels, exchange of genetic materials and selection for resistance among populations of the target pests (Fontes et al., 2002). Osawaru and Ogwu (2014) reported that global plant diversity and their ecological importance has not been sufficiently studied. Therefore, reducing this diversity through GM plant production may result in unpredictable environmental consequences including heightened vulnerability to climate change.

Environmental challenges of GM plant production only began to attract research attention long after the process has been established because it was earlier perceived to only pose ethical, health, biotechnology and bioengineering-related challenges. However, possible long-term environmental implications of GM plant production are expressed through direct impacts, indirect impacts and in science and governance (Figure 2) with evolutionary, ecological, epidemiological and environmental perspectives (Tsatsakis et al., 2017).

Gene transfer, trait effects on target and non-target species, wild plant changes through targeted and non-targeted invasiveness and genetic recombination of free DNA are considered as the direct environmental impacts whereas undesirable side-effects, evolution of new pests, diseases and weeds, environmental contamination and the global decline of biodiversity are indirect environmental impacts (Tutelyan, 2013; Tsatsakis et al., 2017). These broad challenges may be responsible for public anxiety, political activity, and regulations that have frustrated the resulting GM products (Regal, 1986). The dynamic requirement to establish societal policies and regulations make up the science and politics effects. According to Tsatsakis et al. (2017) the rapid expansion of GM-based technology and their applications, have led to altered agricultural, and food production practices posing multidimensional direct and indirect environmental implications through biodiversity and ecosystem gene flow and genetic recombination processes, function and services as well as evolution i.e. development of resistance in micro and macro-organisms. The science and politics dimension also include operational legal frameworks and environmental risk assessments of plant-based GM products. GM products environmental risk assessment deals with the potential long-term adverse effects resulting from interactions of GM components with populations,

Figure 2. Dimensionality of the environmental implications of GM crops and plant-based products
Source. Adapted from Tsatsakis et al. (2017)

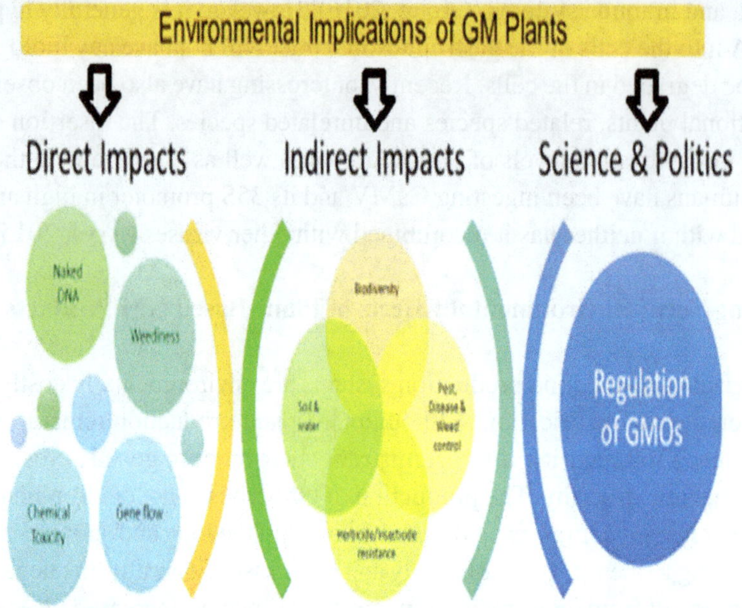

community, ecosystems and ecological resources. It does not focus on individuals rather it describes living and non-living groups by exposure potentials and characterizes the potential for adverse effects to define uncertainties, generates response options to deal with the risks (Iyyanki and Manickam, 2017). The assessment has the assumption that with no risk on individual's life-history traits (i.e., feeding, survival, growth, reproduction) there will no environmental or ecosystem effects (Jager, 2016). With this approach, the lifelong environmental impact of plant-based GM products can be modelled. Risk assessments of the impacts of GM plants on the environment are conducted before they are approved for commercial use, as a core requirement of the biosafety regulatory frameworks (Fontes et al., 2002).

The lifelong risks from GM plant-based food and products have economic, environmental, social, ethical, and political dimensions. GM foods may reduce production costs and environmental degradation from pesticides and fertilizers but these costs are in turn passed on to the consumer through many other ways (Schneider et al., 2017). In addition, the toxic chemicals produced by GM crops result in a long-term challenge to the environment, non-target species as well as to the generation of the inherited plants with the potential of undesirable effects (Tsatsakis et al., 2017). The perceived benefits of this genetic engineering process include increased and sustainable crop production, natural resource conservation, to decrease nutrient runoff in the rivers, and to help meet the increasing world food demands using a limited amount of land (USDA, 2013; Arya, 2015' Tsatsakis et al., 2017).

Over thousands of years, farmers developed commercially viable plants with desirable traits, such as increased resistance to disease, larger fruit, and greater nutritional content with and without elaborate technological processes (Arya, 2015). The process was less environmentally costly compared to GM plant-based agricultural breeding but not sustainable enough to meet food needs. Post introduction of recombinant technology in the field of agriculture is synonymous with increased interest in the environmental impacts of food production practices. Traditional agricultural methods involve modification of plant genes to develop desirable traits but scientific breeders' selects for genes indirectly by selecting parent plants with the desirable traits; there is no direct control at the DNA level because the reorganization of the genetic material occurs in a random fashion (Arya, 2015). Moreover, recombinant DNA technology is used to change the plant's genome using the desired genetic trait that was identified, extracted and inserted in the plant. Lifelong environmental complication through the evolution of resistant pests and weeds termed superbugs and superweeds is a problem (Bawa and Anilakumar, 2013). Using the case of insect-resistant GM plants, Fontes et al. (2002) outlined the following environmental impacts, effects on individual natural enemies that may be beneficial to the environment and community, effects on non-target insect species that are directly susceptible to *Bt* toxin including bees, and persistence of insecticidal toxins produced by the plant in the soil environment. These environmental impacts persist beyond the growing season of the GM plant.

RECOMMENDATIONS AND CONCLUSION

Plant-based GM foods and products are leading the global fight to alleviate global food insecurity but questions about their long-term health and environmental suitability remains a militating factor. The use of fewer inputs including synthetic pesticides and herbicides to increase yield is an environmental gain that is clouded by the loss of biodiversity. Therefore, this paper joins voice with the call for more research to make GM plant-based products more acceptable through greater understanding of their long-term effects. Despite present gains and perceived safety of GM plant-based food products, the full range of economic, ecologic, environmental and epidemiologic potential can be reached after serious consideration is given to lifelong consequences of consuming the products. Although it is difficult to identify hazards that are fundamentally different from those that can occur in the short-term, in most cases, the long-term and cumulative hazards are the same as the short-term ones (Henry et al., 2006). Modelling potential long-term concerns after short and long-term consequences of consuming conventional (non-GM) plant food is a good starting point.

Scientists and biotechnology companies must engage with the public to ensure that potential concerns are debated rationally (Key et al., 2008). It is important to note that there is no epidemiological studies of the human population nor lifelong monitoring of farm animals and domestic pets in an attempt to correlate any ill health observed with the consumption of GM crops (Seralini et al., 2014). Lifelong studies of laboratory animals consuming GM plant-based feeds should be performed in contrast to what is currently obtainable from as little as two-year long tests. These life-long studies should be correlated with transgenerational, reproductive and endocrine research (Krimsky, 2015) as well as with environmental studies and impact assessments. However, with lifelong health effects, it is difficult to assess whether a single GM plant-based food is entirely responsible for observed effects. Therefore, this calls for a multidimensional and interdisciplinary approach. This can shape the future of businesses related to GM plant from product design to sale and eventual consumption. The popularity of a GM crop is commensurate with research investment regardless of clear policy regulations (Sánchez and León, 2016).

In addition, the global adoption of a standardized comparative safety risk assessment strategy and other toxicological and nutritional evaluations pertaining to GM technology, market, etc. is necessary (Kok and Kuiper, 2003). This may help allay some of the challenges associated with the current global imbalance in the acceptance of GM plant-based food and food product. Controversies should not be avoided rather they should be addressed with a resolve to innovate solutions where necessary. This could be in the form of an extended GM food safety evaluation based on the guidelines of OECD (1993; 1996), the European Scientific Committee on Foodstuffs (1997), the United Nations Food and Agriculture Organisation [FAO]/WHO (1996; 2000; 2001; 2002), and Kuiper et al. (2001) summarized herein as comprising:

1. Molecular characterization of introduced genetic fragments especially those capable of producing new proteins and/or metabolites
2. Compositional analysis of plant parts correlated with key nutrients and anti-nutrients
3. Gene transfer potential
4. Allergenicity and toxicity assessment of the transgenes and their products
5. Estimated safety intake levels of the newly introduced proteins and their final products, including any altered constituent
6. Risk assessment of the transgene on the environment (especially on soil and biodiversity)

Also important is the adoption of a clear regulatory and assessment framework through environmental risk assessment, feed and feed approvals, product labelling, biosafety regulation and legislation, and research support in line with the recommendations of Sánchez and León (2016), which can be achieved through element-specific, construct-specific, and event-specific comprehensive detection of GM crops (Lin and Pan, 2016). The reason for existing gaps between public opinion and scientific evidence also needs to be clarified and balanced (Blancke et al., 2015).

According to the results of Entine and Wendel (2000) on the safety and environmental impacts of GM-foods, there is no short-term harm to humans or animals. This is a good basis for key players to support long-term studies. Biotechnology companies, international, national, regional and non-governmental organizations, should support and participate in the long-term investigations of the effects of GM plant-based foods. However, no country should be forced to adopt any GM plant-based food and food products without evidential support about their long-term health and environmental suitability.

Developing countries may be the future of sustainable market and development of GM products because they are the most stricken by food insecurities. However, the number of studies focused on the safety of GM plant-based food is limited, which may be responsible for their non-widespread acceptance in developing countries (Domingo and Bordonaba, 2011). In the same way, the existence of either financial or professional conflicts of interest is significantly associated with studies' showing favourable results for the GM foods (Diels et al., 2011), which does more harm than good to the reputation of GM plant-based food. Although strong public opposition to GMOs persists with resulting impacts on the development of national and international policies, GM crops continue to make valuable contributions towards the development of a sustainable type of agriculture (Blancke et al., 2015) by substantially increase productivity, quality, environmental sustainability and the nutritional content of crops (Sánchez and León, 2016).

Finally, labelling is an important tool, and knowing the ingredients of a product helps to decipher their risks and benefits. Hence, the European Union mandatory labelling of GMOs and GM products should be adopted globally.

REFERENCES

Ahmed, F. E. (2002). Detection of Genetically Modified Organisms in Foods. *Trends in Biotechnology*, *20*(5), 215–223. doi:10.1016/S0167-7799(01)01920-5 PMID:11943377

Arya, D. (2015). *Genetically Modified Foods Benefits and Risks*. Massachusetts Medical Society. http://www.massmed.org/Patient-Care/Health-Topics/Nutrition-and-Physical-Activity/Genetically-Modified-Foods-(pdf)/

Bawa, A. S., & Anilakumar, K. R. (2013). Genetically modified foods: Safety, risks and public concerns - a review. *Journal of Food Science and Technology*, *50*(6), 1035–1046. doi:10.100713197-012-0899-1 PMID:24426015

Blancke, S., Van Breusegem, F., De Jaeger, G., Braeckman, J., & Van Montagu, M. (2015). Fatal attraction: The intuitive appeal of GMO opposition. *Trends in Plant Science*, *20*(7), 414–418. doi:10.1016/j.tplants.2015.03.011 PMID:25868652

Bushey, D. F., Bannon, G. A., Delaney, B. F., Graser, G., Hefford, M., Jiang, X., ... Harper, M. S. (2014). Characteristics and safety assessment of intractable proteins in genetically modified crops. *Regulatory Toxicology and Pharmacology*, *69*(2), 154–170. doi:10.1016/j.yrtph.2014.03.003 PMID:24662477

Butler, D., & Reichhardt, T. (1999). Long-term effect of GM crops serves up food for thought. *Nature*, *398*(6729), 651–653. doi:10.1038/19381 PMID:10227281

Byrne, P., Pendell, D., & Graff, G. (2014). *Labeling of Genetically Modified Foods. Food and Nutrition Series (Health). Colorado State University Extension.* Retrieved from https://extension.colostate.edu/docs/pubs/foodnut/09371.pdf

Carter, C.A., &. Gruere, G.P. (2003). Mandatory labeling of genetically modified foods: does it really provide consumer choice? *AgBioForum, 6*(1 and 2), 68 – 70.

Conner, A. J., & Jacobs, J. M. E. (1999). Genetic engineering of crops as potential source of genetic hazard in the human diet. *Mutation Research/Genetic Toxicology and Environmental Mutagenesis*, *443*(1-2), 223–234. doi:10.1016/S1383-5742(99)00020-4 PMID:10415441

Dahl, R. (2012). To Label or Not to Label, Environmental Health Perspectives. *Environmental Health Perspectives*, *120*(9), 359–361. Retrieved from http://ehp.niehs.nih.gov/wp-content/uploads/2012/09/ehp.120-a358.pdf PMID:23487845

de Vendômois, J. S., Roullier, F., Cellier, D., & Séralini, G. E. (2009). A Comparison of the Effects of Three GM Corn Varieties on Mammalian Health. *International Journal of Biological Sciences*, *5*(7), 706–726. doi:10.7150/ijbs.5.706 PMID:20011136

Delaney, B. (2015). Safety assessment of foods from genetically modified crops in countries with developing economies. *Food and Chemical Toxicology*, *86*, 132–143. doi:10.1016/j.fct.2015.10.001 PMID:26456807

Diels, J., Cunha, M., Manaia, C., Sabugosa-Madeira, B., & Silva, M. (2011). Association of financial or professional conflict of interest to research outcomes on health risks or nutritional assessment studies of genetically modified products. *Food Policy*, *36*(2), 197–203. doi:10.1016/j.foodpol.2010.11.016

Domingo, J. L. (2000). Health risks of GM foods: Many opinions but few data. *Science*, *288*(5472), 1748–1749. doi:10.1126cience.288.5472.1748 PMID:10877692

Domingo, J. L. (2007). Toxicity studies of genetically modified plants: A review of the published literature. *Critical Reviews in Food Science and Nutrition*, *47*(8), 721–733. doi:10.1080/10408390601177670 PMID:17987446

Domingo, J. L. (2011). Human health effects of genetically modified (GM) plants: Risk and perception. *Human and Ecological Risk Assessment*, *17*(3), 535–537. doi:10.1080/10807039.2011.571065

Domingo, J. L. (2016). Safety assessment of GM plants: An updated review of the scientific literature. *Food and Chemical Toxicology*, *95*, 12–18. doi:10.1016/j.fct.2016.06.013 PMID:27317828

Domingo, J. L., & Bordonaba, J. G. (2011). A literature review on the safety assessment of genetically modified plants. *Environment International*, *37*(4), 734–742. doi:10.1016/j.envint.2011.01.003 PMID:21296423

Domingo, J. L., & Gomez, M. (2000). Health risks of genetically modified foods: A literature review. *Revista Espanola de Salud Publica*, *74*, 255–261. PMID:10918812

Entine, J., & Wendel, J. (2013). 2000+ Reasons Why GMOs Are Safe to Eat and Environmentally Sustainable. *Forbes*. Retrieved from http://www.forbes.com/sites/jonentine/2013/10/14/2000-reasons-why-gmos-are-safe-to-eat-and-environmentally-sustainable

European Chemicals Agency. (2012). *The status of industrial vegetable oils from genetically modified plants*. Retrieved from https://echa.europa.eu/documents/10162/22816103/the_status_of_industrial_vegetable_oils_from_genetically_modified_plants_expert_report_en.pdf/e6b0de1b-c9d5-4e07-8fc6-8f4dae318c55

European Union. (1997). EU 97/618/EC. Commission Recommendations 29 July 1997 concerning the scientific aspects and the presentation of information necessary to support applications for the placing on the market of novel foods and novel food ingredients and the preparation of initial assessment reports under Regulation EC 259/97 of the European Parliament and of the Council. *Official Journal of the European Communities*.

FAO/WHO. (1996). *Biotechnology and Food Safety. Report of a Joint*. FAO/WHO consultation, Rome, Italy, 1996. Retrieved from ftp://ftp.fao.org/es/esn/food/biotechnology.pdf

FAO/WHO. (2000). *Safety Aspects of Genetically Modified Foods of Plant Origin*. Report of a Joint FAO/WHO Expert Consultation on Foods Derived from Biotechnology, Geneva, Switzerland, 2000, Food and Agriculture Organisation of the United Nations, Rome. Retrieved from ftp://ftp.fao.org/es/esn/food/gmreport.pdf

FAO/WHO. (2001). *Allergenicity of Genetically Modified Foods. Report of a Joint FAO/WHO Expert Consultation on Foods Derived from Biotechnology.* Rome, 2001, Food and Agriculture Organisation of the United Nations, Rome. Retrieved from http://www.who.int/fsf/Documents/Biotech_Consult_Jan2001/report20.pdf

FAO/WHO. (2002). *Report of the Third Session of the Codex Ad Hoc Intergovernmental Task Force on Foods Derived from Biotechnology (ALINORM 01/34).* Codex Ad Hoc Intergovernmental Task Force on Foods Derived from Biotechnology, Food and Agriculture Organisation of the United Nations, Rome. Retrieved from ftp://ftp.fao.org/codex/alinorm03/Al03_34e.pdf

Fernandez-Cornejo, J., & Caswell, M. (2006). The first Decade of Genetically Engineered Crops in the United States. *USDA ERS Economic Bulletin.* Retrieved from http://www.ers.usda.gov/publications/eib11/eib11.pdf

Fontes, E. M. G., Pires, C. S. S., Sujii, E. R., & Panizzi, A. R. (2002). The environmental effects of genetically modified crops resistant to insects. *Neotropical Entomology, 31*(4), 497–513. doi:10.1590/S1519-566X2002000400001

Frewer, L. J., & Shepherd, R. (1995). Ethical concerns and risk perceptions associated with different applications of genetic engineering: Interrelationships with the perceived need for regulation of the technology. *Agriculture and Human Values, 12*(1), 48–57. doi:10.1007/BF02218074

Grant, J. (2017). List of foods containing GMOs. *Live Strong.* Retrieved from https://www.livestrong.com/article/314824-list-of-foods-containing-gmos/

Group, E. (2016). GMO foods cause gut damage. *Global Healing Center.* Retrieved from https://www.globalhealingcenter.com/natural-health/gmo-foods-cause-gut-damage/

Hefferon, K.L. (2016). *Food Security of Genetically Modified Foods.* doi:10.1016/B978-0-08-100596-5.03532-0

Henry, C., Hugo, S., & Blackburn, J. (2006). Cumulative long-term effects of genetically modified (GM) crops on human/animal health and the environment: risk assessment methodologies. *European Union.* Retrieved from https://ec.europa.eu/food/sites/food/files/plant/docs/gmo_rep-stud_2006_report_lt-effects.pdf

International Service for the Acquisition of Agri-Biotech Applications. (2010). *Global Status of Commercialized Biotech/ GM crops: 2010. ISAAA Brief 42-2010: Executive Summary.* Retrieved from http://www.isaaa.org/resources/publications/briefs/42/executivesummary/default. asp

ISAAA. (2009). Pocket K No. 3: Are the food derived from GM crops safe? Retrieved from http://www.isaaa.org/resources/publications/pocketk/3/default.asp

ISAAA. (2012). *Annual report Executive Summary.* International Service for the Acquisition of Agribiotech Applications.

Iyyanki, V. M., & Manickam, V. (2017). Chapter Eight – Environmental Risk Assessment. In V. M. Iyyanki & V. Manickam (Eds.), *Environmental Management: Science and Engineering for Industry* (pp. 135–152). India: BS Publications. doi:10.1016/B978-0-12-811989-1.00008-7

Jager, T. (2016). Dynamic Modeling for Uptake and Effects of Chemicals. In J. Blasco, P. M. Chapman, O. Campana, & M. Hampel (Eds.), *Marine Ecotoxicology: Current Knowledge and Future Uses* (pp. 718–798). Academic Press. doi:10.1016/B978-0-12-803371-5.00003-5

Key, S., Ma, J. K. C., & Drake, P. M. W. (2008). Genetically modified plants and human health. *Journal of the Royal Society of Medicine*, *101*(6), 290–298. doi:10.1258/jrsm.2008.070372 PMID:18515776

Kleter, G. A., Peijnenburg, A. A. C. M., & Aarts, H. J. M. (2005). Health Considerations Regarding Horizontal Transfer of Microbial Transgenes Present in Genetically Modified Crops. *Journal of Biomedicine & Biotechnology*, *2005*(4), 326–352. doi:10.1155/JBB.2005.326 PMID:16489267

Kok, E. J., & Kuiper, H. A. (2003). Comparative safety assessment for biotech crops. *Trends in Biotechnology*, *21*(10), 439–444. doi:10.1016/j.tibtech.2003.08.003 PMID:14512230

Krimsky, S. (2015). An illusory consensus behind GMO health assessment. *Science, Technology & Human Values*, *1*, 32. doi:10.1177/0162243915598381

Kuiper, H. A., Kleter, G. A., Noteborn, H. P. J. M., & Kok, E. J. (2001). Assessment of the food safety issues related to genetically modified foods. *The Plant Journal*, *27*(6), 503–528. doi:10.1046/j.1365-313X.2001.01119.x PMID:11576435

Lamichhane, S. A. (2014). Genetically Modified Foods-Solution for Food Security. *International Journal of Genetic Engineering and Biotechnology*, *5*(1), 43–48.

Lin, C.-H., & Pan, T.-M. (2016). Perspectives on genetically modified crops and food detection. *Journal of Food and Drug Analysis*, *24*(1), 1–8. doi:10.1016/j.jfda.2015.06.011 PMID:28911391

Lisowska, K. (2011). Genetically modified crops and food: Pros and cons. *Chemik*, *65*, 1193–1203.

Łuczaj, L., Pieroni, A., Tardío, J., Pardo-de-Santayana, M., Sõukand, R., Svanberg, I., & Kalle, R. (2012). Wild food plant use in 21st century Europe: The disappearance of old traditions and the search for new cuisines involving wild edibles. *Acta Societatis Botanicorum Poloniae*, *81*(4), 359–370. doi:10.5586/asbp.2012.031

Magaña-Gómez, J. A., & de la Barca, A. M. (2009). Risk assessment of genetically modified crops for nutrition and health. *Nutrition Reviews*, *67*(1), 1–16. doi:10.1111/j.1753-4887.2008.00130.x PMID:19146501

Murnaghan, I. (2018). *The long-term effects of GM foods*. Retrieved from www.geneticallymodifiedfoods.co.uk/longterm-effects-gm-foods.html

OECD. (1993). *Safety Evaluation of Foods Derived by Modern Biotechnology: Concepts and Principles*. Organisation for Economic Co-operation and Development. Retrieved from http://www.oecd.org/pdf/M00034000/M00034525.pdf

OECD. (1996). *Food Safety Evaluation*. Paris: Organization for Economic Cooperation and Development.

Ogwu, M. C., Osawaru, M. E., & Ahana, C. M. (2014). Challenges in conserving and utilizing plant genetic resources (PGR). *International Journal of Genetics and Molecular Biology*, *6*(2), 16–22. doi:10.5897/IJGMB2013.0083

Oliver, M. (2014). Why we need GMO crops in agriculture. *Missouri Medicine*, *111*, 492–507. PMID:25665234

Osawaru, M. E., & Ogwu, M. C. (2014). Conservation and Utilization of Plant Genetic Resources. In: K. Omokhafe, & J. Odewale (Eds), *Proceedings of 38th Annual Conference of the Genetics Society of Nigeria*. (pp 105 -119). Nigeria: Empress Prints Nigeria Ltd.

Phillips, T. (2008). Genetically modified organisms (GMOs): Transgenic crops and recombinant DNA technology. *Nature Education*, *1*(1), 213.

Pighin, J. (2003). Transgenic crops: how genetics is providing new ways to envision agriculture. *The Science Creative Quarterly*. Retrieved from http://www.scq.ubc.ca/transgenic-crops-how-genetics-is-providing-new-ways-to- envision-agriculture/

Powell, C. (2015). How to make a GMO. Retrieved from http://sitn.hms.harvard.edu/flash/2015/how-to-make-a-gmo/

Qaim, M., & Kouser, S. (2013). Genetically Modified Crops and Food Security. *PLoS One*, *8*(6), e64879. doi:10.1371/journal.pone.0064879 PMID:23755155

Regal, P. J. (1986). Models of genetically engineered organisms and their ecological impact. In H. A. Mooney & J. K. Drake (Eds.), *Ecology of Biological Invasions of North America and Hawaii* (pp. 111–129). New York: Springer. doi:10.1007/978-1-4612-4988-7_7

Sánchez, M. A., & León, G. (2016). Status of market, regulation and research of genetically modified crops in Chile. *New Biotechnology*, *33*(6), 815–823. doi:10.1016/j.nbt.2016.07.017 PMID:27474111

Schlett, A. & Beke, J. (2015). Food security and GMOS. *Studia Mundi – Economica, 2*(1), 94-102. doi:. doi:10.18531/Studia.Mundi.2015.02.01

Schneider, K. R., Schneider, R. G., & Richardson, S. (2017). *Genetically Modified Food. FSHN02-2 series Food Science and Human Nutrition Department*. UF/IFAS Extension.

Seralini, G. E., Mesnage, R., Defarge, N., & Spiroux de Vendômois, J. (2014). Conclusiveness of Toxicity Data and Double Standards. *Food and Chemical Toxicology*, *69*(7), 357–359. doi:10.1016/j.fct.2014.04.018 PMID:24747919

Shivanand, P., & Noopur, S. (2010). Recombinant DNA technology: Applications in the field of biotechnology and crime sciences. *International Journal of Pharmaceutical Sciences Review and Research*, *1*(1), 43–49.

SOT (Society of Toxicology). (2003). The safety of genetically modified foods produced through biotechnology. *Toxicological Sciences*, *71*(1), 2–8. doi:10.1093/toxsci/71.1.2 PMID:12520069

Southgate, E. M., Davey, M. R., Power, J. B., & Merchant, R. (1995). Factors affecting the genetic engineering of plants by microprojectile bombardment. *Biotechnology Advances*, *13*(4), 631–657. doi:10.1016/0734-9750(95)02008-X PMID:14536367

Swanson, N. L. (2013). *Genetically modified organisms and the deterioration of health in the United States*. Retrieved from https://people.csail.mit.edu/seneff/glyphosate/NancySwanson.pdf

The Royal Society. (2002). Genetically modified plants for food use and human health— an update. Policy document 4/02. Retrieved from https://royalsociety.org/~/media/royal_society_content/policy/publications/2002/9 960.pdf

Thompson, S. (2017). How GM crops can help us feed a fast-growing world. *The Conversation*. Retrieved from http://theconversation.com/how-gm-crops-can-help-us-to-feed-a-fast-growing-world-71112

Tsatsakis, A. M., Nawaz, M. A., Kouretas, D., Balias, G., Savolainen, K., Tutelyan, V. A., ... Chung, G. (2017). Environmental impacts of genetically modified plants: A review. *Environmental Research, 156*, 818–833. doi:10.1016/j.envres.2017.03.011 PMID:28347490

Tutelyan, V. A. (2013). *Safety Assessment and Control* (1st ed.). Academic Press. doi:10.1016/C2011-0-08818-X

Twardowski, T., & Małyska, A. (2015). Uninformed and disinformed society and the GMO market. *Trends in Biotechnology*, *33*(1), 1–3. doi:10.1016/j.tibtech.2014.11.006 PMID:25528967

United States Department of Agriculture (USDA). (2014). *Genetically Engineered Crops in the United States, February 2014.*

USDA. (2013). *Biotechnology Frequently Asked Questions*. Retrieved from http://www.usda.gov/wps/portal/usda/usdahome?navid=AGRICULTURE&contentid=BiotechnologyFAQs.xml

Usher, S., Han, L., Haslam, R. P., Michaelson, L. V., Sturtevant, D., Aziz, M., ... Napier, J. A. (2017). Tailoring seed oil composition in the real world: Optimising omega-3 long chain polyunsaturated fatty acid accumulation in transgenic *Camelina sativa. Scientific Reports*, *7*(1), 6570. doi:10.103841598-017-06838-0 PMID:28747792

Wieczorek, A. (2013). History of Agricultural Biotechnology: How Crop Development has Evolved. *Nature*. Retrieved from http://www.nature.com/scitable/knowledge/library/history-of-agricultural-biotechnology-how-crop-development-25885295

Wong, D. (2003). *Genetically Modified Food Labelling*. Hong Kong: Research and Library Services Division Legislative Council Secretariat. Retrieved from http://www.legco.gov.hk/yr02-03/english/sec/library/0203rp05e.pdf

Zhu, X., Van Wesenbeeck, L., & Van Ierland, E. C. (2006). Impacts of Novel Protein Foods on Sustainable Food Production and Consumption: Lifestyle Change and Environmental Policy. *Environmental and Resource Economics*, *35*(1), 59–87. doi:10.100710640-006-9006-2

Chapter 9
Dairy:
Environmental Concerns, Health, and Alternatives

Danielle McKain
Beaver Area School District, USA

ABSTRACT

In many parts of the world, dairy is consumed daily, while in other parts, dairy consumption is uncommon. Regardless, the impact dairy has on sustainability and health raises many questions. There are a growing number of options to dairy milk, including many nut and grain milks. Many of these options are new, so research is limited on their consumption and impact on sustainability and health. This chapter provides an overview of milk consumption around the world, sustainability, health concerns, and dairy milk alternatives. In addition, advantages and disadvantages are discussed, as individuals are often faced with choosing the option that best meets their individual needs.

INTRODUCTION

Dairy milk consumption varies significantly around the world. An estimated two-thirds of the world's population is lactose intolerant (Renub Research, 2018), yet the dairy industry was the third largest market in the global food and beverages market in 2017 (Global Dairy Market Briefing, 2018). Dairy production and consumption are connected to many environmental and health concerns. A few of the challenges include land, water, antibiotic use, feed, equipment, animal treatment, and sanitation. There is growing debate over human dairy consumption. As more milk alternatives become available and popular, this chapter will concentrate on the arguments for and against dairy milk consumption, as well as the environmental impact of the dairy industry across the world.

The purpose of this chapter is to present research on dairy consumption, sustainability, and human health. Specifically, the chapter will present research on the arguments surrounding dairy consumption around the world relating to, (1) sustainability (2) health and (3) alternatives.

DOI: 10.4018/978-1-5225-7635-8.ch009

The objectives of this chapter include:

1. Dairy Milk Consumption Around the World: Providing a brief history of milk consumption around the world.
2. Dairy Milk Consumption and Sustainability: Providing an overview of dairy milk production.
3. Dairy Milk Consumption and Health Concerns: Providing an overview of the various health concerns and complications with dairy milk consumption.
4. Alternatives to Dairy Milk: Providing an overview of the growing number of dairy milk alternatives.
5. Limitations of Current Research: Providing limitations of current research.

BACKGROUND: DAIRY MILK CONSUMPTION AROUND THE WORLD

Historical studies show that fluid dairy consumption was rare in the Netherlands, Sweden, Scotland, Hungary, Germany, and in other parts of Europe; the buttermilk and whey that resulted from making butter was often used to feed livestock (Dupuis, 2002). Milk became more commonly used as a breast milk substitute in the mid-1800s as the United States became more urban, although it was often dangerous due to limited sanitation (Dupuis, 2002).

Dupuis (2002) explains the story of how milk became viewed as a perfect food in the United States and how and is part of social relationships. She points out that drinking fluid milk is not an ancient custom, but rather new to modern times and that northern European countries typically consumed preserved or fermented forms of cheese, sour milk, and yogurt, rather than the fluid form. Furthermore, Americans had very limited amounts of milk from colonial times to the mid-nineteenth century. On family farms, the little milk provided would typically be used to make butter and cheese. Dupuis goes on to explain that drinking milk became more common in the 1940s. Americans were drinking over a pint per day as it became a staple of the American diet and for most of the twentieth century, the majority of Americans drank milk in large quantities (Dupuis, 2002).

Hooijdonk and Hettinga (2015) provide an estimated food consumption per capita for major commodities in developed versus developing countries. As of 2005, the average milk consumption per person per year in developed countries was approximately 200 kg, and in developing countries, it was approximately 50 kg. Milk consumption is estimated to increase by approximately 25 kg per person per year in both developed and developing countries (Alexandratos & Bruinsma, 2012).

Dairy products can provide valuable nutrients and may reduce the risk of chronic diseases especially to those living in poverty (Hooijdonk & Hettinga, 2015). In the countries that dairy products are a major resource of nutrients, demand increases with population growth. The estimated increase in food demand in the world is an average of 1.1% per year (Hooijdonk & Hettinga, 2015). By 2050, it is estimated that in parts of the world like Africa, the undernourished population will be over 300 million. In other countries, it is estimated that overeating will significantly increase obesity (Hooijdonk & Hettinga, 2015).

The United States Department of Agriculture has been recommending milk and dairy in food guidelines since 1916. As of 2017, the USDA ChooseMyPlate.gov through the United States Department of Agriculture recommends the amount of food that should be eaten from the Dairy Group depends on age and gender. Children 2-3 years old are recommended to have 2 cups while those 4-8 years old are recommended to have 2.5 cups. Ages 9-18 are recommended to have 3 cups. Both males and females ages 19 and older are recommended to have 3 cups. The site explains that 1 cup could be milk, yogurt, or soy milk, 1.5 oz of natural cheese, or 2 oz of processed cheese (USDA ChooseMyPLate.gov, n.d.).

The U.S. Dairy Export Council presents the daily dairy intake recommendations for countries around the world (Role of Dairy in the Diet, 2018). Australia and Canada are similar to the United States with servings based on age. Australia and Canada both recommend 2 cups at the age of 19 compared to the United States recommendation of 3 cups (in Canada the recommendation does go up to 3 cups after age 51). China recommends 3 cups, France 3 servings, Japan 2 servings, Korea 2 cups, and Spain 2 servings. The World Health Organization (WHO) provided a healthy diet fact sheet in 2015. On this fact sheet there was no dairy recommendation (Healthy Diet, 2015). They did, however, recommend that children breastfeed until the age of 2.

DAIRY MILK CONSUMPTION AND SUSTAINABILITY

Industrial animal agriculture raises a lot of environmental concerns. The World Wildlife Fund explains that the global demand for dairy is increasing due to population growth, rising incomes, westernized diets, and urbanization (Dairy Sustainable Agriculture, 2018). Thus, there is pressure for natural resources, like water and soil. With approximately 270 million dairy cows worldwide, the impact on the environment depends on the farming methods (Dairy Sustainable Agriculture, 2018). Alberta Milk dairy farm explains the issues they face with soil degradation, managing manure, quality of water, and greenhouse gas (Alberta Milk, 2018). Greenhouse gases produced from cows contribute to climate change, and manure and fertilizers can have an impact on water resources (Dairy Sustainable Agriculture, 2018). Each cow produces 250 to 500 liters of methane (Milk Life?, 2018).

One Green Planet explains how much water is used in dairy production (Milk Life?, 2018). Systems for cleaning manure can use up to 150 gallons of water per day per cow. Additionally, each cow can drink 23 gallons of water per day. Furthermore, additional water is used for cow feed. Grossman (2014) writes that a farm with 2,000 dairy cows creates approximately 240,000 pounds of manure each day.

Environmental, animal, and human health concerns are reflected in the amount of milk cows produce per year varies significantly with 9682 kg per cow in the United States to 2538 kg per cow in China (Hooijdonk & Hettinga, 2015). Public and environmental health are a concern in countries with growing populations such as the Netherlands, India, Ethiopia, and Uganda (Groot & Hooft, 2016). In these countries there is increasing concern for human resistance to antibiotics from the indirect consumption of antibiotics through dairy, multi-resistant microbes, and antimicrobial resistant (AMR) infections (Groot & Hooft, 2016). Residue in dairy products is also a concern in these countries.

Baskaran, Cullen, and Colombo (2009) estimate the environmental impacts of dairy farming in New Zealand, as the country is the largest exporter of dairy products and faces many environmental challenges due to dairy production. Streams and rivers are contaminated with nitrates; there are greenhouse gas emissions, ground and surface water irrigation, and landscapes transformed. DairyNZ is a site dedicated to the dairy industry in New Zealand and the steps that are taken for climate change, waterways, water use, effluent systems, land management, nutrient management, waste management, and responsible conversions (DairyNZ, n.d.).

Pesticide use is another component to sustainable dairy farming. Greger (2015) cites a study of eighteen countries testing thousands of food samples and found PCB contamination was highest in fish and fish oil, then eggs, dairy, and other meats. Another pesticide, hexachlorobenzene, could also be found in dairy and meat. Another study that Greger cites involved over 300,000 participants and found Parkinson's disease was associated with dairy consumption. He goes on to explain that this could be due to elevated levels of pesticides. Cohen (1998) also raises concern over the pesticides and bacteria that could be in milk.

Fuhrman (2011) explains that animal products like dairy contain the residue of toxic pesticides due to the tainted feed that cows consume. Dangerous chemicals and pesticides such as dioxin have been found in dairy. Dioxin has been linked to different cancers. According to the Physicians Committee for Responsible Medicine, dairy accounts for up to half of the dioxins that humans consume. Dioxins can build up in the human body and cause immune, central nervous system, and reproductive problems (Health Concerns about Dairy Products, 2016). Oski (1996) reports that the Consumers Union found 84% of milk samples tested contained a traceable amount of the pesticide chlorinated hydrocarbon. This pesticide is thought to accumulate in the human body and mutations can lead to birth defects and cancer.

Fuhrman (2015, p. 19) states "a diet centered on milk, cheese, pasta, bread, fried foods, and sugar-filled snacks and drinks leads to obesity, cancer, heart disease, diabetes, and autoimmune illnesses." Fuhrman calls this the standard American diet (SAD). Furthermore, he cites multiple studies that explain how dairy consumption increases IGF-1 levels and that although IGF-1 levels are important for growth in infants and children, in adults, higher levels promote aging and the duplication of cells that can lead to cancer (Fuhrman, 2015).

DAIRY MILK CONSUMPTION AND HEALTH CONCERNS

Dairy products are said to promote overall bone health in adults (Role of Dairy in the Diet, 2018). Also, they may reduce the risk of high blood pressure, and risk of cardiovascular disease, coronary heart disease, and stroke; dairy is also linked to a reduced risk of type 2 diabetes (Role of Dairy in the Diet, 2018). The proteins in dairy are supposed to promote muscle repair and recovery, help maintain a healthy weight, build lean muscle, and reduce hunger. There are, however, many concerns over dairy including lactose intolerance, hormones, cardiovascular disease, cancer, diabetes, protein, vitamin D, and calcium. The Physicians Committee for Responsible Medicine suggests bone health, fat content, cardiovascular disease, cancer, contaminants, diabetes, and allergies are all concerns about dairy consumption (Health Concerns about Dairy Products, 2016).

The World Health Organization's report *Diet, Nutrition and the Prevention of Chronic Diseases* states that studies of the dietary factors of fat, meat, dairy, fruits, and vegetables are inconclusive (Diet, nutrition and the prevention of chronic diseases, 2003). They do however recommend using milk and dairy products that are low in fat and salt. The Cancer Council of Australia explains that dairy has shown positive and negative effects (Dairy food and cancer, 2015). Although milk has been shown to protect against colorectal cancer, cheese could increase the risk (Dairy food and cancer, 2015). In a meta-analysis of 29 cohort studies, a neutral association was found between dairy products and cardiovascular mortality (Guo et al., 2017). Other research suggests dairy increases the risk of prostate cancer. The Nutrition Ecology International Center Panel 5 report, *Milk and Dairy in Human Nutrition* explains that milk lacks fiber and phytochemicals and does not provide anything unique nutritionally (Muehlhoff, Bennett, & McMahon, 2013).

The domestication of animals is very recent on an evolutionary time scale, and dairy could have a role in modern heart disease, ulcers, insulin resistance, acne, asthma, cataracts, and osteoporosis (Cordain, 2012). Oski (1996) suggests that the progesterone hormone in cow milk turns into androgens that can contribute to acne. McDougall and McDougall (1983) designated dairy as a harmful food group focusing on high fat, protein, environmental contaminants, lack of fiber, and carbohydrates. Dairy is prominent in affluent societies and can cause food allergies; dairy is poorly digested by most and can cause diarrhea, gas, and stomach cramps (McDougall & McDougall, 1983).

The gastrointestinal reactions that McDougall and McDougall (1983) contribute to dairy include canker sores, vomiting, colic, stomach cramps, abdominal distention, intestinal obstruction, bloody stools, colitis, malabsorption, loss of appetite, growth retardation, diarrhea, constipation, painful defecation, irritation of tongue, lips, and mouth. The respiratory reactions that McDougall and McDougall (1983) contribute to dairy include nasal stuffiness, runny nose, otitis media (inner ear trouble), sinusitis, asthma, and pulmonary infiltrates. The skin reactions that McDougall and McDougall (1983) contribute to dairy include rashes, atopic dermatitis, eczema, seborrhea, and hives. The behavioral reactions that McDougall and McDougall (1983) contribute to dairy include irritability, restlessness, hyperactivity, headache, lethargy, fatigue, allergic-tension fatigue syndrome, muscle pain, mental depression, and enuresis (bed wetting). The blood reactions that McDougall and McDougall (1983) contribute to dairy include abnormal blood clotting, iron deficiency anemia, low-serum proteins, thrombocytopenia, and eosinophilia. Other reactions that McDougall and McDougall (1983) contribute to dairy include anaphylactic shock and death, cancer, multiple sclerosis and sudden infant death syndrome.

Schmid and Fallon (2003) cite numerous occasions of pasteurized milk causing illnesses. Goff and Griffiths (2006) explain that there have been many advancements in dairy production since the 1980s, but foodborne diseases still occur. Zhang and Kesteloot (2005) report that milk consumption is strongly correlated with prostate cancer and breast cancer. Oski (1996) explains that consuming cow milk is linked to iron-deficiency anemia in children, cramps, diarrhea, allergies, atherosclerosis, and heart attacks. Cohen (1998) explains that milk contains pus from cows with mastitis. The mastitis is then treated with antibiotics and can cause antibiotic resistance in humans. *What the Health* reports that 80% of pharmaceutical antibiotics are used on animals in the United States (Anderson & Kuhn, 2017).

Lactose Intolerance

Humans are the only species to drink milk from another species (Walia, 2014). The Physicians Committee for Responsible Medicine reports that lactose intolerance is the inability to digest lactose, the sugar found in milk, due to a lack of lactase enzymes that are used to break lactose down into glucose and galactose (Health Concerns about Dairy Products, 2016). Oski (1996) explains that lactose is made of the monosaccharides, glucose and galactose that form disaccharide lactose. Lactose must be broken down by the lactase (B-galactosidase) enzyme during digestion to be absorbed into the bloodstream (Oski, 1996). Infants and children have lactase enzymes, but lactase decreases in adults and varies by ethnic group. There is typically a decrease of lactase production in mammals after weaning (Walia, 2014). The body produces D-galactose as it breaks down lactose. Animal studies have found that D-galactose can cause oxidative stress damage and chronic inflammation (Michaëlsson et al., 2014). Michaëlsson et al. also found that D-galactose is used as an injection to promote aging (2014).

Cow milk contains approximately 45 grams of lactose per quart, while human milk contains approximately 75 grams per quart (Oski, 1996). Lack of lactase can cause gastrointestinal problems including flatulence, bloating, cramps, and diarrhea when trying to digest lactose. An estimated 90% of Asian Americans, 70% of African Americans, 74% of Native Americans, 53% of Mexican Americans, and 25% of Americans are lactose intolerant (Health Concerns about Dairy Products, 2016). Oski (1996) references the prevalence of lactase deficiency by population group with Bantus, Thais, Filipinos, Greek Cypriots, Japanese, Taiwanese, Greenland Eskimos, Arabs, Ashkenazic Jews, Peruvians, American blacks, Israeli Jews, and Indians all having a deficiency of 50% or higher while Finns, American whites, Swiss, and Danes have a lactase deficiency of less than 20%.

Through evolution, the populations in geographic areas that consume dairy milk have adapted genes that digest lactose through adulthood (Walia, 2014). The ability to digest milk is often referred to as lactase persistent since in many parts of the world the ability of humans to digest dairy is more uncommon (Health Concerns about Dairy Products, 2016). While many people are lactose intolerant, some can tolerate yogurt and cheese, due to the breakdown of lactose during fermentation (Oski, 1996). Milk products are often easier to digest when the lactase enzyme is present, but this enzyme is lost during pasteurization; many people who cannot tolerate pasteurized milk can tolerate raw milk (Schmid & Fallon, 2003).

Hormones rBGH, rBST

Recombinant bovine growth hormone (rBGH) is also known as recombinant bovine somatotropin (rBST). In 1993 the U.S. Food and Drug Administration (FDA) approved the man-made growth hormone rBGH to increase milk production in cows (Recombinant Bovine Growth Hormone, 2018). At that time, the growth hormone was not approved in Europe, Canada, and other countries. In humans, the natural hormone is called somatotropin, and in cattle, it is known as bovine somatotropin. Both the natural and recombinant hormones cause milk production by interacting with the insulin-like growth factor (IGF-1) hormone (Recombinant Bovine Growth Hormone, 2018). According to the American Cancer Society, concerns with cows treated with the artificial hormones were increased IGF-1 growth in humans possibly linked to cancer and an increase in mastitis, udder infections, leading to more antibiotic use and possibly bacteria becoming antibiotic resistant in humans (Recombinant Bovine Growth Hormone, 2018). Despite the controversy, the Food and Drug Administration assured that it was safe for cows and humans and banned companies from labeling products as rBGH or rBST free. It was not until 2010 that companies were allowed to label milk as not coming from cows treated with rBGH or rBST. Even without artificial hormone use, the natural hormones that occur in cow milk affect human hormones (Health Concerns about Dairy Products, 2016).

Cancer

In the *China Study*, Campbell and Campbell (2004), found the casein in cow milk was capable of turning cancer on and off in animal studies. The protein, casein, accounts for 87% of the protein in cow milk and consistently promoted cancer in the *China Study* (Campbell & Campbell, 2004). In the study, rats who ate a diet with higher casein content had increased cancer growth. The casein found in human breast milk is 2.7 g/liter, while cow milk contains 26g/liter. Campbell and Campbell (2004) also site a Harvard research review that found a positive association between dairy products and prostate cancer.

The link between dairy and prostate cancer is contributed to the increase in IGF-1 levels. The insulin-like growth factor occurs naturally in cow milk. Those with increased IGF-1 levels are at a higher risk for prostate cancer (Health Concerns about Dairy Products, 2016). In addition, increased IGF-1 levels affect the reproductive system and may increase the risk of breast and ovarian cancer due to the estrogen content (Health Concerns about Dairy Products, 2016).

Diabetes

Cow milk consumption is also associated with diabetes in different countries. Campbell and Campbell (2004) show the countries with the lowest milk consumption have the lowest rate of type 1 diabetes, while the countries with the highest milk consumption have the highest rate of type 1 diabetes. Infants who are fed cow milk in the first three months of life have an increased risk of type 1 diabetes (Health Concerns about Dairy Products, 2016).

Protein, Vitamin D, Calcium

Dairy milk is known to provide protein, vitamin D, and calcium. Although dairy is often advertised for the calcium content, the protein in dairy inhibits calcium absorption (Cohen, 1998). The Physicians Committee for Responsible Medicine reports that calcium loss is often due to consumption of animal protein as it leaches calcium from the bones (Health Concerns about Dairy Products, 2016). A study published in the British Medical Journal concluded that drinking milk does not lower the risk of bone fractures. On the contrary, it could create a higher risk of bone fractures and be associated with a higher rate of death (Michaëlsson et al., 2014). According to Oski (1996), human milk contains 300 milligrams of calcium per quart and cow milk contains 1,200 milligrams per quart; however, the body absorbs more calcium from human milk. Furthermore, vitamin D is necessary for the human body to absorb calcium. Natural vitamin D in milk is lost during pasteurization and replaced with artificial vitamin D (Cohen, 1998). McDougall & McDougall (1983) contribute many food allergies to the protein in dairy products, suggesting gastrointestinal, respiratory, skin, behavioral, and blood reactions can be from consuming the protein in dairy. Cohen (1998) explains that it is possible that when Americans started drinking more low or non-fat milk the amount of protein consumed increased and could have led to the increase in asthma deaths. Casein protein creates casomorphins that could be linked to sudden infant death syndrome and autism (Anderson & Kuhn, 2017).

ALTERNATIVES TO DAIRY MILK CONSUMPTION

The U.S. Dairy Milk Market Report by Mintel reported that dairy milk sales decreased 7% in 2015 and are predicted to decrease an additional 11% by 2020 (Chiorando, 2018). Flavored dairy milk sales, however, did increase and are predicted to continue to grow. Meanwhile, non-dairy milk alternatives grew 9% in 2015 and are predicted to continue to grow (Chiorando, 2018). Mintel also reported that nearly half of Americans consume non-dairy milk and that reasons include heart health and diet (Chiorando, 2018). Plant-based milks have the potential to greatly impact the health food market (Sethi et al., 2016).

Petherick (2016) cited the first quantitative global estimates of milk consumption; the results correlated milk consumption with national per capita income and found the global average of calcium consumption is significantly below the recommended amount. Additionally, it revealed that those older adults consume more milk than younger adults who seem to consume more sugary drinks, such as fruit juice and sodas. There is a lot of research concerning sugary drinks and obesity. In the 1950s liquid dairy product consumption decreased as soft drink consumption increased significantly in the United States (Heaney, 2013). Concern continues to grow over sugar-sweetened beverage (SSB) consumption, obesity, and chronic disease (Welsh, Lundeen, & Stein, 2013).

In 2017, 6% of Americans identified as vegan, compared to 1% in 2014; globally, the numbers are similar (TopTrends, 2017). There are a growing number of dairy alternatives. Sethi, Tyagi, and Anurag (2016) describe plant-based milk as water-soluble extracts of legumes, oilseeds, cereals, or pseudocereals that appear similar to cow milk and are often used to replace cow milk for medical or lifestyle reasons. These alternatives are popular due to low cholesterol content and no lactose. The production of these milk substitutes consists of extracting the plant material in water, removing solids, homogenizing and treating with heat.

Plant-based milks are produced by breaking down the plant, extracting water, and homogenizing fluids to a consistency and appearance similar to cow milk (Sethi et al., 2016). There are many types of non-dairy milk alternatives. Soy, almond, cashew, coconut, and rice seem to be the most common, but there are a growing number of additional options such as flax, hemp, oat, hazelnut, macadamia, pea, and quinoa. Research and information are very limited for these additional options. There is not a stated definition or classification for plant-based milk, but Sethi et al (2016) provides five categories, cereal-based (oat, rice, corn, spelt), legume-based (soy, peanut, lupin, cowpea), nut-based (almond, coconut, hazelnut, pistachio, walnut), seed-based (sesame, flax, hemp, sunflower), and pseudocereal based (quinoa, teff, amaranth). Many brands offer additional products such as ice cream and coffee creamers. Additionally, many stores offer their own brand of non-dairy products.

There is growing debate over non-dairy milk being called milk and the labeling of plant-based milks. In Europe legislation prohibits the use of the word milk in labeling of products not made from mammary secretions except almond and coconut (Sethi et al., 2016). The Food and Drug Administration in the United States identifies plant-based milk as imitation milk; although they have similar tastes, flavors, textures, and appearance, since the nutritional values differ, imitation milk is required to be separated from dairy milk in store displays (Sethi et al., 2016).

Silk makes soymilk, almond milk, coconut milk, cashew milk blends, creamer products, and yogurt alternatives. They offer protein nut milk in original, vanilla, and chocolate, as well as, omega-3 ALA almond and cashew milk and prebiotics almond and cashew milk (Silk, 2018). *Silk* products are advertised as dairy-free, lactose-free, casein-free, and gluten-free. They are vegan with no animal by-products or derivatives. The products are pasteurized using ultra-high temperature (UHT) to ensure the products are free from harmful microorganisms. The calcium used is derived from natural limestone, and all other vitamins and live cultures used for fortification are vegetable-based. *Silk* products are also certified Kosher OU-D. *Silk* products are not intended to be used as infant formula.

So Nice is a Canadian company that offers organic soy milk and organic almond milk. The *So Nice Soy* beverages are fortified with 14 essential nutrients, including calcium and vitamin D. The So Nice web site explains that soy is a high quality, complete protein, meaning it contains all the amino acids that are necessary for the body to fully utilize the benefits of the protein (So Nice, 2014). Additionally, the benefits of almonds include vitamins and minerals, fiber protein, and unsaturated fat. The advantages of organic include free of pesticides and herbicides, better for the environment, and non-GMO. So Nice is committed to sustainability through a partnership with Evergreen, a national not-for-profit that works to restore the connection between Canada's cities and natural environments.

A brief overview of plant-based dairy alternatives will be provided including information on Soy, Almond, Coconut, Cashew, Rice, Flax, Hemp, Oat, Hazelnut, Macadamia, Pea, and Quinoa.

Example brands and ingredients are provided.

Soy

Silk uses whole non-GMO soybeans to produce soymilk. The beans are pressed in filtered water, the insoluble fiber (okara) is removed, preserving soy protein, and vitamins and minerals are added. *Silk* explains that soymilk originated in Asia over 2,000 years ago (Silk, 2018).

Silk Soymilk is free of dairy, lactose, gluten, casein, egg, and MSG. Soymilk is offered in a variety of flavors: vanilla, original, chocolate, very vanilla, DHA omega-3, light vanilla, light original, light chocolate, organic vanilla, and organic unsweetened. The soybeans used are grown in North America. *Silk* Organic unsweetened soymilk ingredients: organic soymilk (filtered water, soybeans), contains 2% or less of: vitamin and mineral blend (calcium carbonate, vitamin a palmitate, vitamin D2, riboflavin (B2), vitamin B12), sea salt, natural flavor, gellan gum.

So Good Soy beverages based in Canada claim to be the most complete alternative to milk (So Good, 2018). The products are high in protein, calcium, and provide 14 vitamins and minerals. So Good soy milk is available in original, fat-free, vanilla, and chocolate. So Good Original soymilk ingredients: filtered water, soy protein (isolate, whole soybeans), cane sugar, canola oil, natural flavor, gellan gum, sea salt, locust bean gum, sodium bicarbonate, vitamin and minerals (tricalcium phosphate, potassium citrate, dipotassium phosphate, magnesium phosphate, vitamin c, niacin, pantothenate, riboflavin, vitamin a, thiamine, vitamin b6, folacin, vitamin d2, vitamin B12, zinc gluconate).

Frequent soy milk consumption was associated with a decreased risk of prostate cancer in men (Jacobsen, Knutsen, & Fraser, 1998). Soy milk was also found to lower blood pressure in men and women in a study by Rivas et al. (2002). Smedman, Lindmark-Mansson, Drewnowski, and Edman (2010) found that the carbon footprint for soy to be lower than dairy. Soy milk provides monounsaturated and polyunsaturated fatty acids, isoflavones, phytochemicals, and protein (Sethi et al., 2016). Soy milk was the first plant-based milk and typically had a bean flavor; however, advances in technology remove the strong bean flavor, provide a longer shelf life, and maximize nutrients (Sethi et al., 2016). Other brands of soy milk are Vitasoy in Hong Kong, and Alpro and Tesco in the United Kingdom.

Soy production also comes with many environmental concerns as it puts many forests and ecosystems at risk. However, in a project report by Birgersson, Karlsson, and Söderlund (2009) soy milk was found to have less of an impact on land use, fossil energy use, eutrophication, acidification, and climate change when compared to dairy. The Worldwide Fund for Nature explains how soy was one of the first domesticated food crops almost 6,000 years ago in China and is now the second most consumed oil worldwide (Soy facts & data, 2017). Soy is also often the primary source of feed for many animals including chickens, pigs, and cows.

Almond

Almonds provide calcium, copper, magnesium, phosphorus, potassium, selenium, vitamin E, zinc, and provide prebiotic properties (Sethi et al., 2016). Almond milk typically has fewer calories than cow milk. Unsweetened almond milk usually has 30 calories per cup, while sweetened almond milk usually has 90 calories per cup. Almond milk is high in vitamin E and riboflavin. *Blue Diamond* Almonds, *Almond Breeze* almond milk is a company based in Sacramento, California. Using *Blue Diamond* almonds grown in California, they produce a variety of Almond Milk products and blends including original, unsweetened original, reduced sugar original, chocolate, unsweetened chocolate, vanilla, unsweetened vanilla, reduced sugar vanilla, hint of honey, hint of honey vanilla, almond coconut original, almond coconut unsweetened original, almond coconut unsweetened vanilla, almond cashew original, almond cashew unsweetened original, almond cashew vanilla, and almond cashew unsweetened vanilla (Blue Diamond, 2018). The original Almond milk is lactose-free, soy free, and calcium enriched.

Blue Diamond Almond Breeze Original Almond milk ingredients: Almond milk (Filtered water, almonds), Cane sugar, Calcium Carbonate, Sea Salt, Potassium Citrate, Sunflower Lecithin, Gellan Gum, Vitamin A Palmitate, Vitamin D2, D-Alpha-Tocopherol (Natural Vitamin E).

Blue Diamond Almond Breeze unsweetened Almond milk ingredients: Almond milk (Filtered water, almonds), Calcium Carbonate, Sea Salt, Potassium Citrate, Sunflower Lecithin, Gellan Gum, Vitamin A Palmitate, Vitamin D2, D-Alpha-Tocopherol (Natural Vitamin E).

Silk also makes a brand of Almond milk which has a mild nutty flavor. The history of almond dates back to the fifth century in ancient Spain and Eastern Asia (Silk, 2018). Almond milk does not have any cholesterol or saturated fat and provides vitamin E. *Silk* Almond milk almonds are produced in North America and are non-GMO. The products are free of dairy, soy, lactose, gluten, casein, egg and MSG. *Silk* Almond milk is available in a variety of flavors: vanilla, original, organic original, dark chocolate, unsweetened vanilla, unsweetened, light vanilla, light original, almond and coconut blend, and unsweetened almond and coconut blend. Other brands of Almond milk include Alpro in the United Kingdom, Hiland and 365 in the United States, and Pure harvest in Australia (Sethi et al., 2016).

Coconut

Coconuts are a fruit that grow on trees in warm sunny climates. A single tree can produce 75 coconuts a year (Silk, 2018). *Silk* coconut milk is offered in vanilla, original, and unsweetened. Coconuts are husked, halved, and pressed to squeeze the milk, then blended with filtered water, vitamins, minerals and natural flavors. Coconut milk is high in fat and a good source of fiber, both uncommon to most plant-based milks. Coconut milk contains calcium, magnesium, potassium, vitamins C and E, and zinc and is known to have anti-carcinogenic, anti-microbial, anti-bacterial, and anti-viral benefits (Sethi et al., 2016).

Silk Coconut milk is produced with non-GMO coconuts from Indonesia and Thailand. It is free of dairy, soy, lactose, gluten, casein, egg and MSG.

So Delicious is another coconut milk brand. *So Delicious* also produces dairy-free products including shreds, frozen desserts and toppings, yogurt alternatives, creamers, and beverages (So Delicious, n.d.). *So Delicious* Original Coconutmilk ingredients: Coconutmilk (Filtered water, Organic Coconut Cream), Cane Sugar, Contains 2% or less of: Vitamin and Mineral Blend (Calcium Phosphate, magnesium phosphate, L-Selenomethionine [selenium], Vitamin A Acetate, Vitamin D2, Zinc Oxide, Vitamin B12), Sea Salt, Organic Sunflower Lecithin, Organic Locust Bean Gum, Gellan Gum.

So Delicious unsweetened Coconutmilk ingredients: Coconutmilk (Filtered water, organic Coconut Cream), Contains 2% or less of: Vitamin and Mineral Blend (Calcium Phosphate, magnesium phosphate, L-Selenomethionine [selenium], Vitamin A Acetate, Vitamin D2, Zinc oxide, Vitamin B12), Sea Salt, Organic Sunflower Lecithin, organic Locust Bean Gum, Gellan Gum.

Cashew

The cashew tree was commonly used for wood, cashew balm, and cashew apples. The cashew nut became popular at the beginning of the 20th century (Silk, 2018). *Silk* roasts and grinds cashews into a butter that is used to make cashew milk. Cashews have a low-fat content and provide monounsaturated fats. Cashew milk provides a creamy texture, and provides 50% more calcium than dairy milk (Silk, 2018). It is also free of dairy, soy, lactose, gluten, casein, egg and MSG. *Silk* cashew milk is offered in original, unsweetened, unsweetened vanilla, and chocolate.

Silk Original cashew milk ingredients: Cashewmilk (Filtered water, cashews), Cane sugar, Contains 2% or less of: Almond butter, Vitamin and Mineral Blend (Calcium Carbonate, Vitamin E Acetate, Vitamin A Palmitate, Vitamin D2), Sea Salt, Natural Flavor, Sunflower Lecithin, Locust Bean Gum, Gellan Gum, Ascorbic Acid.

Silk Unsweetened cashew milk ingredients: Cashewmilk (Filtered water, cashews), Contains 2% or less of: Almond butter, Vitamin and Mineral Blend (Calcium Carbonate, Vitamin E Acetate, Vitamin A Palmitate, Vitamin D2), Sea Salt, Natural Flavor, Sunflower Lecithin, Locust Bean Gum, Gellan Gum, Ascorbic Acid.

Rice

Dream rice milk is non-GMO, certified organic, free of lactose, dairy, and cholesterol. *Dream* rice original rice drink ingredients: Filtered water, Organic brown rice (partially milled), Organic expeller Pressed canola oil and/or organic safflower oil and/or organic sunflower oil, Sea salt (Dream, 2018).

Dream rice original enriched unsweetened rice drink ingredients: Organic rice base (Filtered water, organic rice), Organic expeller pressed canola oil and/or organic safflower oil and/or organic sunflower oil, Tapioca tarch, Tricalcium phosphate, Carrageenan, Natural flavors, Sea salt, Xanthan gum, Vitamin A, Palmitate, Vitamin D2, Vitamin B12.

Flax

Good Karma Foods produces flax milk and describes it as a major allergen-free, non-dairy milk alternative with a smooth and creamy texture and delicious taste that is produced with high-quality cold-pressed flaxseed oil and contains 1200 mg of Omega-3s per serving (Good Karma, 2016). Flax milk has a smooth and creamy texture and is made in original, unsweetened, vanilla, unsweetened with protein, and unsweetened vanilla with protein. *Good Karma* also makes dairy-free yogurts. The products are dairy-free, gluten-free, vegan, major-allergen free, Non-GMO certified, and Kosher certified by Orthodox Union (circle U). They use steam infused UHT pasteurization.

Original flax milk ingredients: Flaxmilk (filtered water, cold pressed flax oil), cane sugar, tricalcium phosphate, vanilla extract, sunflower lecithin, natural flavors, sea salt, gellan gum, xanthan gum, vitamin a palmitate, vitamin d2, vitamin b12.

Unsweetened flax milk ingredients: Flaxmilk (filtered water, cold pressed flax oil), tapioca starch, tricalcium phosphate, sunflower lecithin, natural flavors, sea salt, vanilla extract, gellan gum, xanthan gum, vitamin a palmitate, vitamin d2, vitamin b12.

Hemp

Hemp milk is made from the cannabis sativa L plant, the same plant used to make marijuana. Unlike marijuana, the seeds do not contain any THC delta-9 tetrahydrocannabinol. The seeds provide a rich, nutty flavor similar to sunflower seeds. The milk is made by pulverizing the seeds, mixing them with water, then straining them (High on Hemp Milk, 2016). Hemp milk provides omega-6 and omega-3 essential fatty acids in a three to one ratio. The omega-3 provides alpha-linolenic acid and could be linked to improved cognitive performance (5 Proven Benefits of Hemp Milk, 2018). The milk also provides magnesium, phytosterols, ascorbic acid, beta-carotene, calcium, fiber, iron, potassium, phosphorus, riboflavin, niacin, and thiamin.

Hemp milk provides the ten essential amino acids which is desirable for vegetarians (5 Proven Benefits of Hemp Milk, 2018). Hemp protein does not contain phytates (enzyme inhibitors that can interfere with the assimilation of essential minerals) or oligosaccharides (complex sugars that can cause flatulence when not adequately broken down during digestion) (High on Hemp Milk?, 2016). Hemp seeds do not pose the same allergy risk as tree nuts do for many people. Hemp milk is high in vitamins E and A which possibly benefit the skin as antioxidant compounds that reduce oxidative stress that can cause wrinkles and inflammation. Hemp milk may boost immunity, improve bone density with calcium, magnesium, zinc, potassium, and iron.

Living Harvest Foods produces Tempt Hempmilk. Hemp seeds are used to make a creamy non-dairy beverage that provides vitamins, minerals, and all ten essential amino acids, as well as, omega-3 and omega-6 fats. Hemp seeds provide a balance of omega-3s with SDA and Omega-6s with GLA. They have no known allergens and provide protein, magnesium, phosphorus, vitamin E, iron, and zinc. Living Harvest also makes hemp ice cream that is said to be creamier and thicker than other dairy alternatives. Other hemp products include cereals, waffles, and snack bars (Living Harvest, n.d.). Living Harvest Foods considers hemp an environmentally friendly renewable resource that does not require pesticides or herbicides. The milk is free of dairy, soy, peanut, tree-nut, cholesterol, gluten, GMOs, and trans fats. It is offered in original, unsweetened, vanilla, unsweetened vanilla, and chocolate.

Original Tempt Hemp milk ingredients: Hemp Nut bBase (filtered water, whole hemp nut [shelled hemp seed]), brown rice syrup, organic evaporated cane juice, tricalcium phosphate, carrageenan, sea salt, vitamin a palmitate, vitamin d2, riboflavin, vitamin B12.

Unsweetened Tempt Hemp milk ingredients: hemp nut base (filtered water, hemp nut [shelled hemp seed]), vanilla extract, sunflower lecithin, tricalcium phosphate, gellan gum, sea salt, vitamin a palmitate, vitamin d2, riboflavin, vitamin b12.

Oat

The benefits of oats include hypocholesterolemic and anti-cancerous properties, dietary fiber content, and protein and amino acid balance (Sethi et al., 2016). *Pacific Natural* foods organic oat non-dairy beverages are free of carrageenan, added sugar, lactose, cholesterol, and soy (Pacific Foods, 2018). They are vegan and kosher and offered in original and vanilla. Other brands of oat milk include Pureharvest in Australia, Simpli in Finland, Vitasoy in Hong Kong, Bioavena drink in Italy, Alpro in the United Kingdom, and Pacific in the United States (Sethi et al., 2016).

Original Pacific Natural oat milk ingredients: Water, Oats, Oat Bran, Tricalcium Phosphate, Sea Salt, Gellan Gum, Vitamin D2, Riboflavin (B2), Vitamin A Palmitate.

Hazelnut

Pacific Natural Foods produces a hazelnut non-dairy beverage as an alternative to dairy. Hazelnut milk is described as smooth and creamy with a subtle flavor. It is sweetened with brown rice and provides calcium, vitamin D, riboflavin, vitamin A and vitamin E. It is lactose, soy, gluten, and cholesterol-free (Pacific Foods, 2018.). It is available in original and chocolate and is kosher, vegan and non-GMO.

Pacific Natural Hazelnut milk ingredients: Roasted Hazelnut Base (water, ground roasted hazelnuts), Brown Rice Sweetener (water, brown rice), Tricalcium Phosphate, Gellan Gum, Sea Salt, Carrageenan, Vitamin D2, Riboflavin, (B2), Vitamin A Palmitate.

Macadamia

Milkadamia uses macadamia nuts for their macadamia milk. This non-GMO, vegan, dairy-free drink is made from nuts grown on family farms in Australia with low impact farming methods. *Milkadamia* is advertised as free of dairy, soy, GMOs, and gluten. It is sustainably farmed in Australia and comes in original, unsweetened, unsweetened vanilla, and latte da barista (Milkadamia, n.d.).

Original Macadamia milk ingredients: macadamia milk (filtered water, macadamias), cane sugar, calcium phosphate, pea protein, natural flavors, locust bean gum, sea salt, sunflower lecithin, gellan gum, vitamin a palmitate, vitamin d2, vitamin b12.

Unsweetened Macadamia milk ingredients: macadamia milk (filtered water, macadamias), calcium phosphate, pea protein, natural flavors, locust bean gum, sea salt, sunflower lecithin, gellan gum, vitamin a palmitate, vitamin d2, vitamin b12.

Pea

Ripple produces a lactose-free, pea milk. Built on the idea that small actions can have big impacts, they see a world where everything is connected and strive to offer simple choices for plant-based foods (Ripple Foods, 2017). The pea milk is offered in original, vanilla, and chocolate.

Ripple Original plant protein pea milk ingredients: water, pea protein, organic cane sugar, sunflower oil. contains less than 0.5% of organic vanilla extract, vitamin a palmitate, vitamin d2, DHA algal oil, calcium phosphate, potassium phosphate, sunflower lecithin, natural flavors, sea salt, organic guar gum, gellan gum.

Quinoa

Suzie's Quinoa milk is dairy-free, gluten-free, and vegan. It is offered in unsweetened, unsweetened vanilla, and vanilla (Good Groceries Company, n.d.). Unsweetened quinoa milk ingredients: quinoamilk (filtered water, quinoa), calcium carbonate, gellan gum, sea salt, vitamin a palmitate, vitamin d2, d-alpha tocopherol (Vitamin E).

Dairy Alternatives Comparison

When comparing both the sweetened and unsweetened dairy alternatives to dairy, almost all varieties are lower in calories, sodium, carbohydrates, sugar, protein, and cholesterol. When comparing the vitamin and mineral content of dairy alternatives to dairy, all varieties have the same 10% of the daily recommended amount of vitamin A as dairy. Most varieties have the same 25% of vitamin D as dairy. The calcium content in dairy is 30%, all alternative varieties have 30% or higher except coconut and rice. Dairy milk does not contain iron, while more dairy alternatives contain 2% or more. Soy, hemp, hazelnut, and oat milks have 25% or higher of Riboflavin (B2), while coconut, flax, hemp, rice, and flax have 25% or higher of vitamin B12. Soy, almond, coconut, hemp, and quinoa all contain 4% or more of magnesium. Almond, cashew, and quinoa all have 20% or more vitamin E, while 10% or more phosphorus can be found in rice, flax, and hemp. Soy contains vitamins B6 and B3 and selenium can be found in coconut milk. It is important to consider if these vitamins and minerals occur naturally or are added. Future research is necessary to determine the value of natural versus added vitamins and minerals in both dairy and dairy alternatives.

Original Sweetened Comparison

Of the sweetened non-dairy milk types presented, flax milk contains the fewest calories with 50 per cup, while hazelnut has the highest calorie content of 110 per cup. Almond, rice, and flax all have the lowest fat content of 2.5 grams per cup, while hemp is the highest at 6 grams per cup, followed by coconut and pea with 4.5 grams per cup. All the varieties have 1 gram or less of saturated fat, except coconut milk having 4 grams per cup. None of these milks contain cholesterol except for flax milk with 80 mg per cup. Sodium is lowest in coconut milk with 30 mg and highest in cashew milk with 170 mg per cup. Carbohydrates range from 6 grams per cup of pea milk to 23 grams per cup of rice milk. Soy and pea milk have the highest protein with 7 and 8 grams respectively, while most other varieties contain 2 grams or less.

Unsweetened Comparison

Of the unsweetened non-dairy milk types presented, cashew and flax milk have the lowest calories with 25 per cup, while oat has the highest calorie content of 130 per cup. Quinoa has the lowest fat content of 1 gram per cup, while hemp is the highest at 6 grams per cup, followed by coconut with 4.5 grams per cup. All the varieties have 1 gram or less of saturated fat, except coconut milk having 4 grams per cup. None of the milks contain cholesterol except for flax milk with 80 mg per cup. Sodium is lowest in coconut milk with 25 mg and highest cashew milk with 160 mg per cup. Almond, coconut, cashew, flax, hemp, and macadamia all have 1 gram of carbohydrates per cup, while rice, quinoa, and oat are higher with 11, 12, and 24 grams per cup respectively. Soy has the highest protein with 7 grams per cup, while most other varieties contain 2 grams or less.

LIMITATIONS OF CURRENT RESEARCH

Research on dairy as it relates to health is complicated and shows conflicting results. The World Health Organization and the Cancer Council of Australia results were inconclusive (Dairy food and cancer, 2015; Diet, nutrition and the prevention of chronic diseases, 2003). Plant-based diets consistently suggest health benefits (Campbell & Campbell, 2004; Fuhrman, 2011; Greger, 2015; Health Concerns about Dairy Products, 2016). Research on dairy alternatives is limited since many non-dairy milk options are new to the market. There are insufficient studies on the health and environmental advantages and disadvantages of these milk alternatives. The plant-based milk market is growing so rapidly that it is difficult to conduct research, but there is existing research on soy and rice milks since they have been in production longer. The other limiting factor is the number of variables that must be considered. It is overwhelming to interpret all the information for all the varieties of milk.

Those living in developed countries are looking for dairy alternatives, while those living in developing countries are seeking milk for nutrients. As the developed countries seek alternatives, dairy milk is often labeled as the best option. Dairy milk is a key part of the U.S. government subsidized school lunch program and food supplement program and is also a major component of food guideline in many countries (Oski, 1996).

SOLUTIONS AND RECOMMENDATIONS

There is not a simple solution to dairy consumption, sustainability, health concerns, or alternatives. Dairy consumption varies around the world and as countries develop and adapt consumption could increase or decrease based on desire, availability, and options. The impact dairy has on the environment has evolved. Family farms have changed from a single cow to dairy farms with thousands of cows, in order to meet the demand for dairy in developed countries. Health concerns are just as complicated as many seek dairy products for nutrients, others stay away due to the fat and cholesterol content. Currently, the number of dairy alternatives to choose from is complicated and lacks research.

The number of variables must be reduced to get a better understanding of the nutritional and environmental aspects of dairy and dairy alternatives. One or two milk varieties could be focused on, and one or two components studied. Individuals need to be educated and informed so that they can choose the best way to improve their health and wellbeing. As more options become available, one must consider the advantages and disadvantages as they relate to sustainability and the environment.

FUTURE RESEARCH DIRECTIONS

As concerns grow over sustainability and human health, many questions are directed at the dairy industry. Advances in technology will potentially lower plant-based milk costs and increase availability (Sethi et al., 2016). Future research must concentrate on the potential health and environmental benefits of these products. Additional research could also include organic dairy and dairy alternatives as it relates to health and sustainability, fermented dairy compared to non-fermented, and raw compared to pasteurized as it relates to lactose intolerance.

Future research should also build on current research concerning dairy and dairy alternatives, specifically as it relates to infants and children. Dairy concerns consistently relate to children and infants, but most dairy alternatives advise not to use as infant formula. The Physicians Committee for Responsible Medicine links type 1 diabetes to infants who are fed cow milk in the first three months of life (Health Concerns about Dairy Products, 2016). Mothers who breastfeed are more likely to have colicky babies if they consume cow milk (Cohen, 1998; Health Concerns about Dairy Products, 2016; McDougall & McDougall, 1983). Dairy has also been linked to sudden infant death syndrome (Anderson & Kuhn, 2017; McDougall & McDougall, 1983). The World Health Organization made a recent recommendation to restrict marketing milk and dairy products for children and infants. This recommendation has been challenged by the International Dairy Foods Association (IDFA Calls on HHS to Challenge WHO Policies at World Health Assembly, 2018).

More research related to cardiovascular disease, the leading cause of death worldwide, is also needed. Although smoking, poor diet, and lack of exercise are often cited as the main contributing factors to cardiovascular disease, the connection between cardiovascular health and dairy consumptions is a controversial issue (Guo et al., 2017). According to the Physicians Committee for Responsible Medicine, exercise combined with a low-fat plant-based diet can potentially prevent and reverse heart disease (Health Concerns about Dairy Products, 2016).

CONCLUSION

In the 2015 Nielsen report, *We Are What We Eat*, nearly half of worldwide respondents reported being overweight (Nielsen Report, 2015). While diabetes and heart disease are becoming more common, the Nielson report revealed that consumers are seeking fresh, natural and minimally processed foods and that younger consumers are willing to pay a premium for health benefits. The report provided a global average of 75% (also broken down by region: Asia-Pacific, Europe, Middle East/Africa, Latin America, and North America) of respondents reported changing diet as a way to lose weight. A study on dairy consumption in Switzerland (Chollet et al., 2014) revealed that over 25% of participants had reduced milk or dairy consumption due to fat or cholesterol.

The non-dairy milk industry is growing as consumers around the world are reaching for these products for various, health, environmental, and ethical concerns. These dairy alternatives have mixed reviews as dairy replacements. Research shows that many people who consume milk alternatives also include dairy milk in their diet (Chiorando, 2018). Dairy & Dairy Alternative Beverage Trends in the U.S., 4th edition (2017) looks into the reduction of dairy milk consumption and the rise in plant-based milk for health and animal welfare concerns. The Top Trends in Prepared Foods 2017 identified six trends as impacting innovation in prepared foods as (1) Go Meat-Free (2) Premium Junk Food (3) Healthy Swaps (4) Inspiration Borrowers (5) Fresh and Easy (6) Ethical Eating (Top Trends in Prepared Foods, 2017).

While people around the world try to make healthy choices, it is often difficult. When there is data demonstrating the benefits of something, there seems to be just as much data against it. This chapter is not to be used for or against milk dairy or plant-based dairy, but rather a resource for existing information so that individuals can make more educated decisions based on their situation and needs. What is recommended one day, can be the opposite the next. More research is crucial in this area.

REFERENCES

AlexandratosN.BruinsmaJ. (2012). World agriculture towards 2030/2050: the 2012 revision. Food and Agriculture Organization. Rome, Italy: Retrieved from http://www.fao.org/fileadmin/templates/esa/Global_persepctives/world_ag_2030_50_2012_rev.pdf

Anderson, K., & Kuhn, K. (2017). *What the Health*. United States: A.U.M Films & Media.

Baskaran, R., Cullen, R., & Colombo, S. (2009). Estimating values of environmental impacts of dairy farming in New Zealand. *New Zealand Journal of Agricultural Research, 52*(4), 377–389. Retrieved from https://www.tandfonline.com/doi/pdf/10.1080/00288230909510520?needAccess=true doi:10.1080/00288230909510520

Birgersson, S., Karlsson, B. S., & Söderlund, L. (2009). *Soy milk – an attributional Life Cycle Assessment examining the potential environmental impact of soy milk*. Stockholm, Sweden: KTH Royal Institute of Technology.

Blue Diamond Launches "Almond Breeze" as Thailand's Brand Leader for the Dairy-Free Almond Milk Global Trend [Press release]. (2017, June 30). Retrieved from https://assets.ctfassets.net/99ef2wobcp71/6RHDBpFaSWMKMwsSSsm40G/7db7b31f9f185a3018715283541ddb84/Press_Release_Blue_Diamond_Almond_Milk_launch_En_Final_0617.pdf

Campbell, T. C., & Campbell, T. M. (2004). *The China study: The most comprehensive study of nutrition ever conducted and the startling implications for diet, weight loss and long-term health*. Dallas, TX: BenBella Books.

Chiorando, M. (2018). US Dairy Sales to Drop 11% by 2020. *Plant Based News*. Retrieved from https://www.plantbasednews.org/post/us-dairy-sales-drop-11-2020-other-positive-vegan-stats

Chollet, M., Gille, D., Piccinali, P., Bütikofer, U., Schmid, A., Stoffers, H., ... Walther, B. (2014). Short communication: Dairy consumption among middle-aged and elderly adults in Switzerland. *Journal of Dairy Science, 97*(9), 5387–5392. doi:10.3168/jds.2014-8193 PMID:24997665

Cohen, R. (1998). *Milk the deadly poison*. New Jersey: Argus.

Cordain, L. (2012). *The Paleo Answer: 7 days to lose weight, feel great, stay young*. Hoboken, NJ: JohnWiley & Sons.

Dairy, N. Z. (n.d.). Dairy NZ. Retrieved from https://www.dairynz.co.nz/

Dairy and Dairy Alternative Beverage Trends in the U.S. (2017). 4th ed.). Retrieved from https://www.packagedfacts.com/Dairy-Alternative-Beverage-Trends-Edition-11000293/

Dairy foods and cancer. (2015). Cancer Council NSW. Retrieved from https://www.cancercouncil.com.au/1958/cancer-prevention/diet-exercise/nutrition-diet/fruit-vegetables/dairy-foods-and-cancer/

Dairy Sustainable Agriculture. (2018). World Wildlife Fund. Retrieved from https://www.worldwildlife.org/industries/dairy

Delicious, S. (n.d.). So Delicious. Retrieved from http://sodeliciousdairyfree.com/

Blue Diamond. (2018). Almond Breeze. Retrieved from https://www.bluediamond.com/brand/almond-breeze

Diet, nutrition and the prevention of chronic diseases. (2003). World Health Organization. Retrieved from http://www.who.int/dietphysicalactivity/publications/trs916/en/

Dream. (2018). Rice Dream. Retrieved from http://www.dreamplantbased.com/product/rice-dream-classic-original-organic-rice-drink/

DuPuis, E. M. (2002). Natures perfect food: How milk became Americas drink. New York: New York University Press.

Ripple Foods. (2017). Ripple Foods. Retrieved from https://www.ripplefoods.com/

Pacific Foods. (2018). Pacific Foods. Retrieved from https://www.pacificfoods.com/

Fuhrman, J. (2011). *Eat to live: The amazing nutrient-rich program for fast and sustained weight loss*. Little and Brown.

Fuhrman, J. (2015). *The end of dieting: How to live for life*. HarperOne.

Global Dairy Market Briefing 2018 - Milk and Butter, Cheese, Dry, Condensed, and Evaporated Dairy Product, Ice Cream and Frozen Dessert. (2018, January 22). *Business Wire*. Retrieved from https://www.businesswire.com/news/home/20180122006338/en/Global-Dairy-Market-Briefing-2018---Milk

Goff, H., & Griffiths, M. (2006). Major advances in fresh milk and milk products: Fluid milk products and frozen desserts. *Journal of Dairy Science*, *89*(4), 1163–1173. doi:10.3168/jds.S0022-0302(06)72185-3 PMID:16537949

So Good Beverage. (2018). So Good. Retrieved from https://sogoodbeverage.com/

Good Groceries Company. (n.d.) Suzie's Quinoa Milk. Retrieved from http://www.goodgroceries.com/quinoa-milk/

Greger, M. S. (2015). *How not to die: Discover the foods scientifically proven to prevent and reverse disease*. PAN Books.

Groot, M. J., & Hooft, K. E. (2016). The hidden effects of dairy farming on public and environmental health in the Netherlands, India, Ethiopia, and Uganda, Considering the use of antibiotics and other agro-chemicals. *Frontiers in Public Health*, *4*. doi:10.3389/fpubh.2016.00012 PMID:26942171

Grossman, E. (2014, May 27). As Dairy Farms Grow Bigger, New Concerns About Pollution. Retrieved from https://e360.yale.edu/features/as_dairy_farms_grow_bigger_new_concerns_about_pollution

Guo, J., Astrup, A., Lovegrove, J. A., Gijsbers, L., Givens, D. I., & Soedamah-Muthu, S. S. (2017). Milk and dairy consumption and risk of cardiovascular diseases and all-cause mortality: Dose–response meta-analysis of prospective cohort studies. [PubMed]. *European Journal of Epidemiology*, *32*(4), 269–287. doi:10.100710654-017-0243-1

Harvest, L. (n.d.). Living Harvest. Retrieved from https://livingharvest.com

Health Concerns about Dairy Products. (2016, January 26). Physicians Committee for Responsible Medicine. Retrieved from http://www.pcrm.org/health/diets/vegdiets/health-concerns-about-dairy-products

Healthy Diet. (2015). World Health Organization. Retrieved from http://www.who.int/mediacentre/factsheets/fs394/en/

Heaney, R. P. (2013). Dairy intake, dietary adequacy, and lactose intolerance. *Advances in Nutrition*, *4*(2), 151–156. doi:10.3945/an.112.003368 PMID:23493531

High on Hemp Milk? Dr. Weil. (2016, December 01). Retrieved from https://www.drweil.com/diet-nutrition/nutrition/high-on-hemp-milk/

Hooijdonk, T. V., & Hettinga, K. (2015). Dairy in a sustainable diet: A question of balance. *Nutrition Reviews*, *73*(Suppl 1), 48–54. doi:10.1093/nutrit/nuv040 PMID:26175490

IDFA Calls on HHS to Challenge WHO Policies at World Health Assembly. (2018). Retrieved from https://www.idfa.org/news-views/headline-news/article/2018/05/16/idfa-calls-on-hhs-to-challenge-who-policies-at-world-health-assembly

Jacobsen, B. K., Knutsen, S. F., & Fraser, G. E. (1998, December). Does high soy milk intake reduce prostate cancer incidence? The Adventist Health Study (United States). *NCBI*. Retrieved from https://www.ncbi.nlm.nih.gov/pubmed/10189040

Karma, G. (2016). Good Karma. Retrieved from http://goodkarmafoods.com/products/?gclid=EAIaIQobChMIu4aLqarg2wIVyAOGCh1lqQYIEAAYASAAEgLF0_D_BwE

McDougall, J. A., & McDougall, M. A. (1983). *The McDougall plan*. Clinton, NJ: New Win Pub.

Michaëlsson, K., Wolk, A., Langenskiöld, S., Basu, S., Lemming, E. W., Melhus, H., & Byberg, L. (2014). Milk intake and risk of mortality and fractures in women and men: Cohort studies. *BMJ (Clinical Research Ed.)*, *349*. Retrieved from https://www.bmj.com/Content/349/bmj.g6015 PMID:25352269

Milk, A. (2018). Alberta Milk. Retrieved from https://albertamilk.com/

Milk Life? How About Milk Destruction: The Shocking Truth About the Dairy Industry and the Environment. (2018, April 13). *OnegreenPlanet*. Retrieved from http://www.onegreenplanet.org/animalsandnature/the-dairy-industry-and-the-environment

Milkadamia. (n.d.) Milkadamia. Retrieved from http://www.milkadamia.com/#products

Muehlhoff, E., Bennett, A., & McMahon, D. (2013). *Milk and dairy products in human nutrition*. Rome: Food and Agriculture Organization of the United Nations.

SoNice. (2014). So Nice. Retrieved from https://sonice.ca/

Oski, F. A. (1996). *Don't drink your milk!: The frightening new medical facts about the worlds most overrated nutrient*. Ringgold, GA: TEACH Services.

Petherick, A. (2016). Milk consumption around the world. *Splash! Milk science update. International Milk Genomics Consortium.* Retrieved from http://milkgenomics.org/wp-content/uploads/2016/01/January-2016-SPLASH.pdf

Organic Facts. (2018, April 265 Proven Benefits of Hemp Milk. Retrieved from https://www.organicfacts.net/hemp-milk.html

Recombinant Bovine Growth Hormone. (2018). American Cancer Society. Retrieved from https://www.cancer.org/cancer/cancer-causes/recombinant-bovine-growth-hormone.html

Renub Research. (2018). Global Dairy Alternatives Market to cross US $34 Billion by the year 2024. Retrieved from https://www.renub.com/global-dairy-alternatives-market-nd.php

Nielson Report. (2015). We are what we eat: Healthy eating trends around the world. Retrieved from https://www.nielsen.com/content/dam/nielsenglobal/eu/nielseninsights/pdfs/Nielsen%20Global%20Health%20and%20Wellness%20Report%20-%20January%202015.pdf

Rivas, M., Garay, R. P., Escanero, J. F., Cia, J. R., Cia, P., & Alda, J. O. (2002, July). Soy milk lowers blood pressure in men and women with mild to moderate essential hypertension. NCBI. Retrieved from https://www.ncbi.nlm.nih.gov/pubmed/12097666

Role of Dairy in the Diet. (2018). Think USA dairy by the U.S. Dairy Export Council. Retrieved from http://www.thinkusadairy.org/health-and-wellness/role-of-dairy-in-the-diet

Schmid, R. F., & Fallon, S. (2003). *The untold story of milk: Green pastures, contented cows and raw dairy foods*. Washington, DC: New Trends Pub.

Sethi, S., Tyagi, S. K., & Anurag, R. K. (2016). Plant-based milk alternatives an emerging segment of functional beverages: A review. [PubMed]. *Journal of Food Science and Technology*, *53*(9), 3408–3423. doi:10.100713197-016-2328-3

Silk. (2018). Silk. Retrieved from https://www.silk.com/

Smedman, A., Lindmark-Månsson, H., Drewnowski, A., & Edman, A. M. (2010). Nutrient density of beverages in relation to climate impact. *Food & Nutrition Research*, *54*(1), 5170. doi:10.3402/fnr.v54i0.5170

Soy facts & data. (2017). Worldwide Fund for Nature. Retrieved from http://wwf.panda.org/our_work/food/agriculture/soy/facts/

Top Trends in Prepared Foods 2017: Exploring trends in meat, fish and seafood; pasta, noodles and rice; prepared meals; savory deli food; soup; and meat substitutes. (2017). Retrieved from https://www.reportbuyer.com/product/4959853/top-trends-in-prepared-foods-2017-exploring-trends-in-meat-fish-and-seafood-pasta-noodles-and-rice-prepared-meals-savory-deli-food-soup-and-meat-substitutes.html

USDA ChooseMyPlate.gov. (n.d.). Choose My Plate. Retrieved from https://www.choosemyplate.gov/food-groups/dairy-amount.html

Walia, A. (2014, October 30). Most Human Beings Are Lactose Intolerant: Here's Why. Collective-evolution. Retrieved from http://www.collective-evolution.com/2013/04/03/over-75-of-earths-population-is-lactose-intolerant-for-a-reason-dairy-is-harmful/

We Are What We Eat. (2015). Nielsen Report. Retrieved from http://www.nielsen.com/us/en/insights/reports/2015/we-are-what-we-eat.html

Welsh, J. A., Lundeen, E. A., & Stein, A. D. (2013). The sugar-sweetened beverage wars. *Current*Opinion in Endocrinology & Diabetes and Obesity, 20(5), 401-406. PMID:23974767

Zhang, J., & Kesteloot, H. (2005). Milk consumption in relation to incidence of prostate, breast, colon, and rectal cancers: Is there an independent effect? *Nutrition and Cancer*, *53*(1), 65–72. doi:10.120715327914nc5301_8 PMID:16351508

ADDITIONAL READING

Campbell, T. C., & Jacobson, H. (2014). *Whole: Rethinking the science of nutrition*. Dallas, TX: Benbella Books.

Esselstyn, C. B. (2011). *Prevent and reverse heart disease: The revolutionary, scientifically proven, nutrition-based cure*. Auckland, New Zealand: Royal New Zealand Foundation of the Blind.

Fuhrman, J. (2012). *Nutritarian handbook and ANDI food scoring guide*. Flemington, NJ: Gift of Health Press.

Fuhrman, J. M. (2008). *Eat for health: The mind makeover*. Nutritional Excellence.

Hartwig, D., & Hartwig, M. (2014). *It starts with food*. Las Vegas, NV: Victory Belt.

Junger, A. (2015). *Clean Gut: The breakthrough plan for eliminating the root cause of disease and revolutionizing your health*. New York: HarperCollins.

Lipman, F., & Doyle, M. (2012). *Revive: Stop feeling spent and start living again*. New York: Pocket Books.

Oosterveer, P., & Sonnenfeld, D. A. (2012). *Food, globalization and sustainability*. London, UK: Earthscan.

Sumner, J. (2016). *Learning, food, and sustainability: Sites for resistance and change*. New York: Palgrave Macmillan. doi:10.1057/978-1-137-53904-5

KEY TERMS AND DEFINITIONS

Disaccharide: A water soluble sugar that is found in lactose formed from two monosaccharides joined by glycosidic.

Galactose: A monosaccharide that when combined with glucose results in disaccharide lactose.

Lactase: The enzyme required to digest lactose, that catalyzes the hydrolysis of lactose to glucose and galactose.

Lactose: The natural sugar in dairy milk.

Lactose Intolerant: The inability to digest lactose.

Non-Dairy: Plant, grain, or nut-based milk.

Plant-Based: Non-dairy milk.

Sweetened: Milk alternatives containing added sugar.

Unsweetened: Milk alternatives that do not contain added sugar.

Chapter 10
Cotton Textiles and Human Health Challenges

Radostina A. Angelova
Technical University of Sofia, Bulgaria

ABSTRACT

Cotton is the most used natural fiber in the world for the production of textiles and apparel. Nowadays, there are three different possibilities for cotton growth in the world: production of conventional, organic, or genetically modified cotton. Their influence on human health, due to the application of pesticides, is discussed. The influence of the pesticides on the environment, which, in turns, affects the human health through the water, soil, and food chain, is also discussed. The preferable cotton sector is presented, giving a chance to the customers of cotton textiles and apparel, and to assess the positive influence of the existing initiatives in the cotton field on the human health and the environment.

INTRODUCTION

Cotton textiles are the most widely used textiles in the world. The production of cotton occupies the first place among the natural textile fibers and the second place among all textile fibers after the polyester fibers (Textile Exchange, 2017). It takes about half a year from planting the cotton seeds to harvesting the cotton. The cotton fibers have to be separated from the cotton seeds, so gins are applied after the harvest. During the process of separation, the thin wax coating of the cotton fibers that protects them from humidity is also removed. Finally, the raw cotton is pressed into bales, which are sent to the spinning mills to produce cotton yarns. Spinning is the first stage of the cotton textiles production chain, which will finish with garments (apparel, interior textiles, floor coverings, protective clothing, etc.)

The use of pesticides in cotton growth has attracted several studies, and both reports and research papers provide a lot of data for the effect of the cotton pesticide (over)use on the environment and human health. Depending on the year (weather and season) the pests and crop disease change, which require selection of the most effective pesticides. However, this is in most cases far beyond the abilities of the smallholders, and they frequently react with overuse of the known pesticides. Large-scale cotton farms are more

DOI: 10.4018/978-1-5225-7635-8.ch010

likely to adopt technologies and management that are environmentally friendly (Cameron, 2007). The observations in Northern Greece show that young farmers would care more about the pesticides related hazards and the use of personal protective equipment than the older farmers (Damalas and Hashemi, 2010). In any case, information, knowledge of new technologies is one of the ways to tackle the effects of pesticide use in cotton growing. The low level of knowledge is correlated with overuse of pesticides in small-scale farms. The use of the foliar application, for example, is more effective than the spraying (Kumar et al., 2012), but spraying continues to be the most widely used way for pesticide application in the cotton fields. The effect of GMO technologies on the use of cotton pesticides was remarkable at the beginning, but later the cotton pesticide use increased again and today in China is even higher than it was in 1997 (Jin et al., 2015).

The chapter aims to give the reader an overview on the relationship between the production of cotton crops for textiles and the use of pesticides in the cotton fields in the light of the human health and the effects on the environment, which, in turns, affect once again the human health. The differences in the three types of cotton, used in the textile and clothing industries nowadays: conventional, organic, and genetically modified cotton, are discussed. An overview of the cotton production in the world is presented regarding the production volume, leading cotton producers and leading exporting/importing countries, to underline the global problem of the environmental pollution due to cotton crop cultivation. The health problems, arising from the application of pesticides on the cotton fields are discussed for both occupational and non-occupational exposure. Special attention is given to the effect of cotton pesticides on children's health and production of cottonseeds oil. Environmental problems, related to wildlife and cattle poisoning, as well as water and soil poisoning due to the application of pesticides in cotton fields, are also considered. An analysis on the preferred cotton textile segment, namely Fair Trade Cotton, CmiA initiative, Better Cotton Initiative, Cleaner Cotton™, REEL Cotton and e³ Cotton is made. The last gives a chance to the reader, which is a customer of cotton textiles and apparel, to assess the possible influence of the nowadays initiatives in the cotton industry on the human health and the environment.

THE COTTON IN THE COTTON FIELDS

Three types of cotton are used nowadays for the production of cotton textiles and clothing:

- Non-Organic cotton: the conventional plant, grown since millenniums
- Organic cotton: cultivated nowadays without the application of pesticides
- Genetically modified cotton

Conventional (Non-Organic) Cotton

The man had grown cotton for about 5,000 years. Until the 1950s no hazardous chemicals were used, and soil treatment practices controlled the cotton pests. Agricultural management considered the pest cycles and used annual crop rotation. Cotton plants were grown at a sufficient distance to reduce the damage from the pest population. In fact, cotton growth was based on organic agriculture practices.

The development of the chemical industry after World War II has led to significant advances in the discovery of neurotoxic chemicals. DDT was the first chemical applied to limit the pests in the cotton fields. The growth of the pesticides caused cotton farmers to change their agricultural management habits, and the traditional methods of pest control were gradually being abandoned and even forgotten. In developing countries, this process was slower than in industrialized countries, but still existing: in 1983, in Punjab (Pakistan), up to 10% of the cotton was grown with pesticides, whereas in 1991, this share rose to 95-98% (Action, 2007).

Nowadays 16% of the total amount of pesticides, used in the world, is applied on the conventional (non-organic) cotton, making it the most pesticide-intensive crop in the world (Striepe, 2011). The major part of pesticides used in cotton growing - nearly 60% - are targeted at insect pests. They affect insects' nervous and reproductive systems, which is of particular danger, as these systems are similar to most animals on the Earth, including humans.

Organic Cotton

The organic cotton is an alternative of the conventional cotton regarding the production system. The organic cotton possesses the same properties and characteristics as the conventional one. There are no differences in the use, the technological processes applied for production of the textiles (spinning, weaving, knitting) or the properties of the textiles in terms of structural, geometric or other characteristics, including the hand of the fabric, comfort, etc. The difference lies in the production of the crop, which is entirely different in organic agriculture. As a result, the cultivation of organic cotton is completely dissimilar regarding its effect on people and nature, compared to conventional cotton.

The production of organic cotton is the only farming way for cotton growth entirely free of pesticides and, as a consequence, entirely risk-free for human health. Instead of hazardous chemicals, the farmers use crop rotation on their land and count for the natural predators to kill the insects on the cotton plants.

Given the increasing demand for organic cotton textiles, it is surprising that the share of organic cotton fibers remains limited to 0.2% -1% of the world production (van Duijn & Maas, 2017). There are signs of a certain decrease in organic cotton production: if in 2013/2014 there was a 10% growth in the sector, in 2016/2017 there was a decline of 3.8%. The example of India, the largest organic cotton producer in the world, where organic cotton production declined by more than 62% from 2009/10, clearly points to the issues affecting the sector (Textiles Exchange, 2016).

Four main threats to the development of organic cotton could be emphasized (van Duijn & Maas, 2017):

- Weak business. Organic cotton farmers' businesses are often weak, especially when compared to conventional or genetically modified cotton. Organic cotton yields are lower, compared to the conventional cotton, and farmers need special, higher prices for their production. The lack of purchasing contracts along with the uncertainty in the market demand often makes the farmers sell their organic cotton as a conventional one. Several difficulties also exist in finding good quality organic seeds due to the dominance of genetically modified cotton seeds on the market.
- Lack of transparency along the chain. Due to the length of the chain from the cotton farms to the shopping galleries, the connection between the farmers and the textile and apparel brands is very weak, despite the desire of both the producers to grow organic cotton and the brands to sell it. The farmers rarely receive the promised premiums for their organic cotton production, even where the price difference has been paid downstream (Gruere and Plastina, 2010). Textile and apparel brands, on the other hand, are unsure about the regular supplies and where exactly go the premiums they pay. As a result, both sides lose certainty about the environmental and social effects of organic cotton cultivation and use.

- Lack of organization. The sector, which deals with the organic cotton production, processing of the cotton fiber into yarns and fabrics and sales of organic cotton textiles and apparel is too segmented. There is no single standard of production as well as traceability and proof of the cotton origin throughout all stages of cotton fiber processing.
- Risk of reputation damage. There is already media criticism about the environmental impact and economic benefits of growing organic cotton, which in the long run may change the attitude of the end-users to it. Unfortunately, there is no such a visible discussion on the absolute benefits of the organic cotton growth for the health of both the farmers and all people living in the cotton production regions.

Genetically Modified Cotton

There is another "type" of cotton, which nowadays exists in the fields and stock exchanges: the genetically modified cotton.

The cultivation of cotton involves serious measures against pests, which most often involve the use of pesticides. Unfortunately, over the last 40 years, much of the pest has developed resistance to pesticides. There are two ways of addressing the problem at present: development of more and more hazardous pesticides, or application of the methods of genetic engineering.

There genetically modified cotton is engineered with one of two possible features:

- Resistance to glyphosate-based herbicides (Monsanto's Roundup)
- Production of a toxin that kills the bollworm, one of the cotton's primary pests

The second type of genetically modified cotton is most used. The plant is modified to produce an own toxin through a process called *Agrobacterium-Mediated Transfer (AMT):* a gene from the bacteria Bacillus Thurengiensis that produces the insecticidal protein is integrated into the genes of the cotton plant. Thus, instead of relying on the bacteria to produce the protein that kills the bollworm (A. Lepidoptera), the cotton makes this protein by its own. Because of the name of the bacteria, the "new" cotton plant is called "Bt cotton."

There are three types of crops of global importance for humanity and which are genetically modified with Bt toxin: cotton, potatoes, and corn.

Bt toxin is similar to other pesticides but has a less harmful effect on the environment (soil, water) and non-target organisms such as mammals, fish, birds. The caterpillars that are trying to feed the leaves of Bt cotton become lethargic, less mobile and cause less damage to the plant.

Invented to make the cotton plant more resistant to pests, especially insects, the Bt cotton occupies an intermediate place between organic cotton and conventional cotton concerning the necessary use of pesticides. The Bt cotton still needs pesticide application, but spraying is limited (approx. twice per season), as opposed to conventional cotton, which requires over ten spraying per season.

THE COTTON PRODUCTION IN THE WORLD

Figure 1 represents the volume of the global cotton production from 1990 to 2017, expressed in thousands of 480-pound cotton bales (data from Statista, 2018a). The trend in the global average price of cotton is shown in Fig. 2 (data from Statista, 2018b). The cotton price pick from 2011 was due to the floods in

Figure 1. Global cotton production from 1990 to 2017
(data from Statista, 2018a)

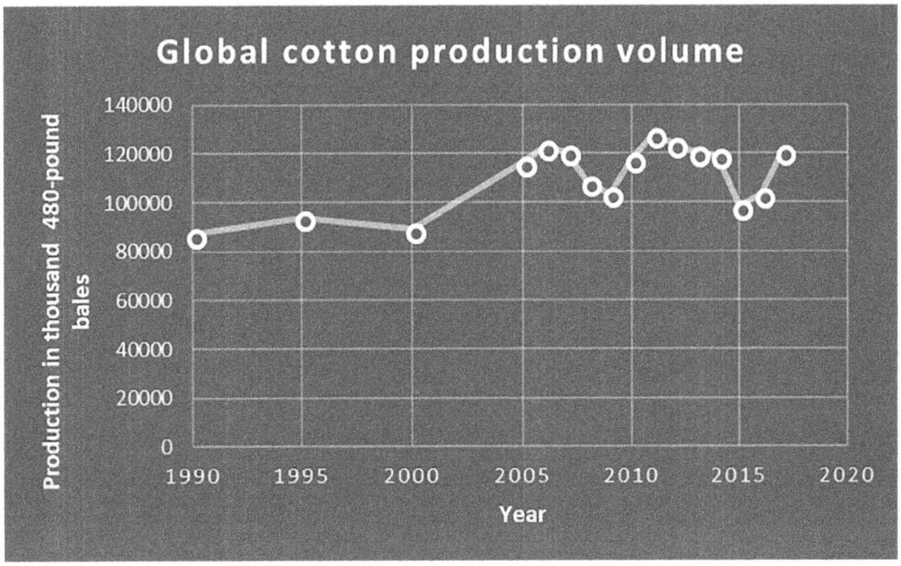

Figure 2. Global average price of cotton from 1990 to 2017
(data from Statista, 2018b)

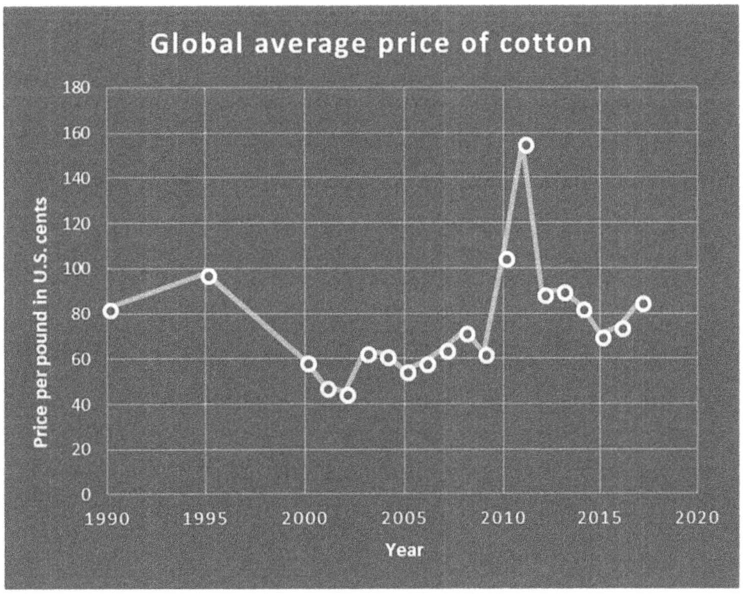

China, Pakistan, and Australia, which affected the major cotton-producing farms in a period, while the demand from China, the biggest producer of cotton textiles, was soaring.

The three countries hit hard by the floods in 2011 are among the top 10 cotton producers in the world. Figure 3 represents the biggest cotton producers in 2017/2018 (data from Statista, 2018c)

It can be seen that India, China, and the United States have a significant lead over the other cotton manufacturers, producing 2.5-3.5 times more cotton than Brazil and Pakistan (on the fourth and fifth places respectively) and a lot more than the other five countries in the Top 10.

The three countries represent three different cases that can be analyzed if the produced cotton volume (Fig. 3) is compared with the leading cotton exporting countries in 2017/2018 in Fig. 4 (data from Statista, 2018d) and the largest importers of cotton in Figure 5 (data from Statista, 2018e) for 2017-2018. India, the top cotton producer in the world, had overproduction and had exported 15.8% of the cotton harvest. At the same time, the United States exported 74.1% of the produced cotton fiber, which means that most of the cotton farmers in the country export their harvest and depend on the world markets. China, the second largest cotton producer worldwide, cannot afford the necessary cotton volume for its textile industry, so the country has imported additional quantity of 18.5% (compared to the volume of the cotton fiber, produced in the country).

PESTICIDES IN THE NON-ORGANIC COTTON GROWTH AND HUMAN HEALTH

This section discusses the effect of the most dangerous pesticides, used in the fields for both conventional and genetically modified cotton, on the human health: Aldicarb, Parathion, Methamidophos, and Monocrotophos. Poisoning due to occupational and non-occupational exposure is presented together with the consequences on children's health and use of cottonseeds oil.

Figure 3. Top 10 cotton producers in the world in 2017/2018 season
(data from Statista, 2018c)

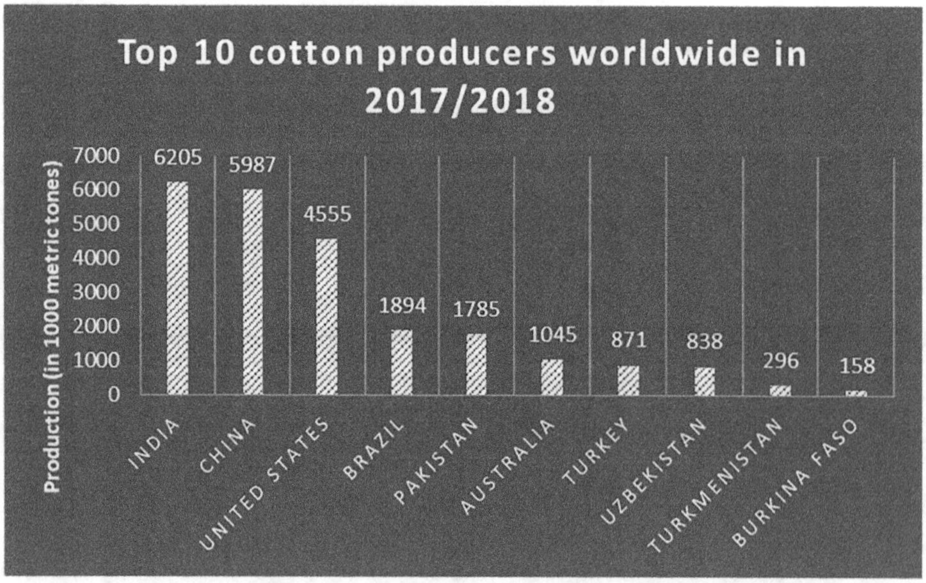

Figure 4. Leading cotton exporting countries in the world in 2017/2018 season (data from Statista, 2018d)

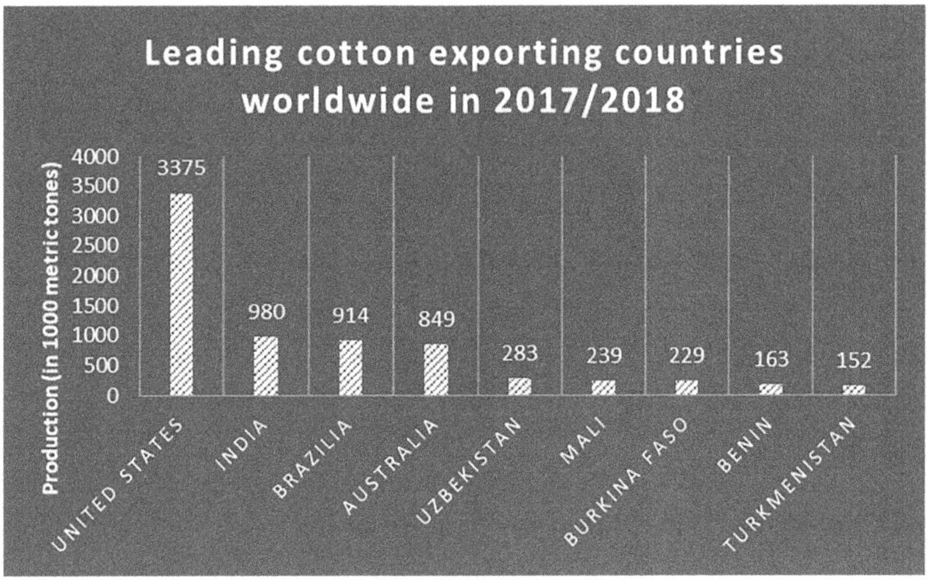

Figure 5. Leading cotton importing countries in the world in 2017/2018 season (data from Statista, 2018e)

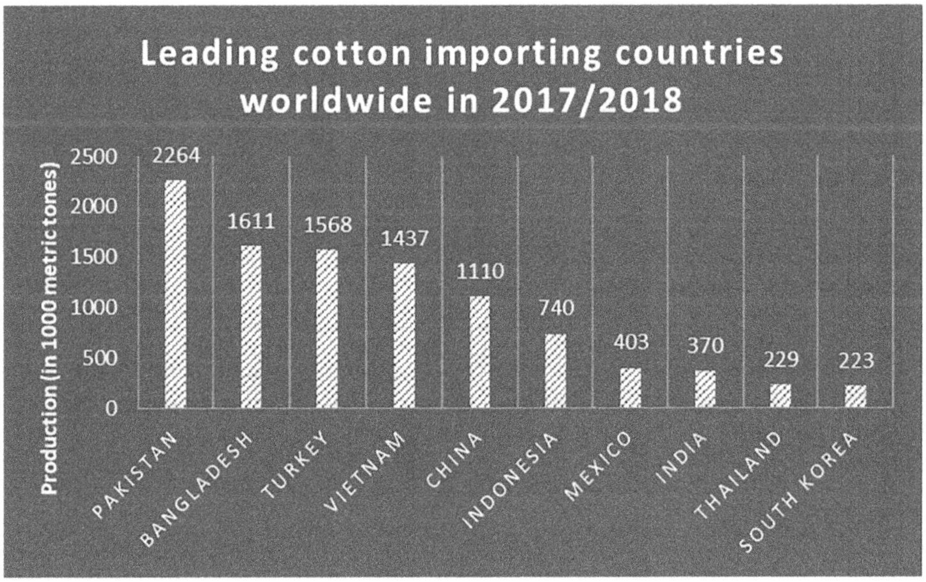

Figure 6. Major hazardous pesticides in cotton by their hazardous category (WHO category)

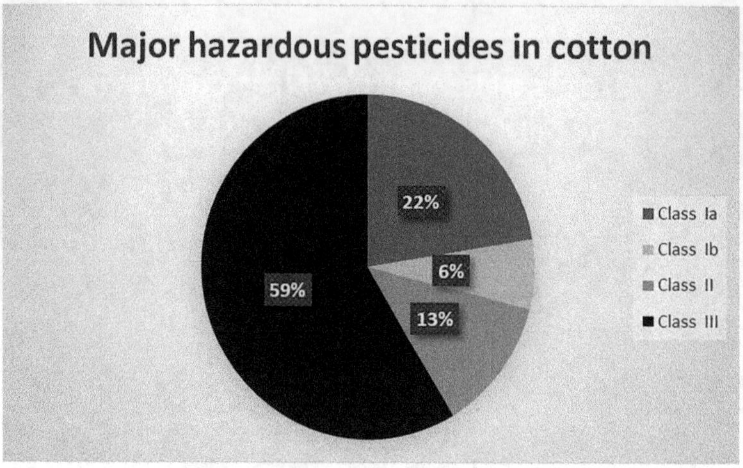

Pesticide Classification According to Their Toxicity

Insecticides (insect-directed chemicals) are the most hazardous for human health types of cotton pesticides. Of 201 agrochemicals classified by the World Health Organization (WHO) as extremely, highly or moderately dangerous for human health, insecticides represent 52%, herbicides (15%), fungicides (14%) and rodenticides chemicals are 10%.

The World Health Organization classifies the pesticides according to their toxicity, using the Lethal Dose 50% (LD50) benchmark. LD50 represents the amount of a pesticide substance, required to mortify 50% of an exposed population of laboratory rats.

There are four categories of pesticides:

- **WHO Class Ia:** Extremely hazardous chemicals
- **WHO Class Ib:** Highly hazardous chemicals
- **WHO Class II:** Moderately hazardous chemicals
- **WHO Class III:** Slightly hazardous chemicals

The analysis of the data in Action (2007), where 17 hazardous pesticides and their volume are cited, shows that 22% (7275 tones) from the worldwide used chemicals in cotton farms belong to Class Ia, 6% (2100 tones) to Class Ib, 13% (4083 tones) to Class II, and 59% (19023 tones) to Class III.

Pesticide Poisoning

28% of the used cotton pesticides are extremely or highly dangerous. These are the insecticides Aldicarb and Parathion (Class Ia) and Methamidophos and Monocrotophos (Class Ib). The risk for human health comes from the action of these chemicals: they inhibit the enzyme acetylcholinesterase, which is essential for the proper functioning of the nervous system either of insects or humans. The disabled communication between the nerve cells and impaired nervous coordination lead to a set of different symptoms, starting with nausea, and tremor and ending with paralysis and death (Townsend, 1997). The exposure to pesticides, disrupting the acetylcholinesterase enzyme, has been associated to the impaired neurological development of infants and fetus, Parkinson's disease, and syndrome of chronic fatigue (MacDonald and Vollrath, 2005). There is also an evident association between the application of pesticides in agriculture and different types of cancer diseases (Nanda et al., 2016, Ali et al., 2018): prostate cancer (Dich & Wiklund, 1998; Alavanja et al. 2003), lung cancer (Pesatori et al., 1994; Alavanja et al. 2003), bladder cancer (Webster, McKenzie, & Moriarty, 2002), breast cancer (Cohn, Wolff, Cirillo & Sholtz, 2007; Niehoff et al., 2016), etc. Cancer cases among children have also been largely reported (Garry, 2004; Infante-Rivard & Weichenthal, 2007; Bouchard et al., 2011, Lehmann et al., 2018).

Aldicarb (Class Ia) is a carbamate insecticide, the second most used pesticide in the cotton fields. It was introduced in agriculture over 40 years ago (Baron, 1994). A drop of Aldicarb, absorbed by the skin, is enough to kill an adult (Clay, 2013). Therefore, it is produced in a granular form, applied in the soil. Aldicarb dominates the cotton production in Argentina and the United States. In 2003, due to the application of almost 1,000 tones of Aldicarb, the groundwater of 16 states was contaminated (United States Department of Agriculture, 2004). Nowadays several countries restrict the use of Aldicarb, and it is banned in the European Union. However, many cotton farms continue to apply it.

Aldicarb can penetrate the human body orally, through the skin or be inhaled. Its targets are both the central nervous system and reproductive system. The poison is metabolized quickly and in the next 24 hours is excreted through the urine.

Occupational exposure is among the main reasons for Aldicarb poisoning. Another way is consumption of contaminated water or food. The symptoms of the Aldicarb poisoning start from 15 minutes to 3 hours after the contamination. As a cholinesterase inhibitor, the insecticide provokes headaches, blurred vision, lethargy, tearing, nausea, sweating, and tremors. High dose exposures or long-term exposures can initiate vomiting, diarrhea, abdominal cramps, seizures, cardio-respiratory difficulty, hypertension, dyspnea, bronchospasms and even pulmonary edema (Baron, 1994; Yarsan, Tanyuksel, Celik, & Aydin, 1999).

Parathion or Methyl Parathion (Class Ia) is an organophosphorus insecticide used on cotton among other crops. It is extremely dangerous for human health. Humans can be exposed to Parathion during occupational activities, related to agricultural tasks or in the workplace during the manufacture of the pesticide. Being liquid chemical, which is sprayed on the crop, Parathion can be a reason for poisoning due to spray drift adjacent to the cotton fields areas. Individuals may also be exposed to the chemical by ingesting food containing its residues (Rubin et al., 2002).

The acute exposure to Parathion affects the central nervous system, blood circulation, eyes, respiratory system, and skin. The chemical provokes nausea, vomiting, diarrhea, excessive salivation, headache, abdominal cramps, weakness, breathing difficulty, blurring or dimness of vision, convulsions, paralysis, central nervous system depression, coma, and respiratory failure (Budavari, 1989). The poison effects can be felt from a few minutes to 12 hours after the exposure. The chronic exposure has been observed to provoke nausea, headaches and depressed red blood cell cholinesterase activity (Eyer et al., 2003). The ingestion of Parathion has also provoked depressed plasma and red blood cell cholinesterase activity (De Bleecker, Willems, Van Den Neucker, De Reuck, and Vogelaers, 1992).

Methamidophos (Class Ib) is a neurotoxin that impairs the action of essential enzymes, essential for the correct transmission of nerve impulses. It is the fourth most significant cotton pesticide, used worldwide (Action, 2007). Residues of Methamidophos have been found in cottonseeds and their derivatives, which are potentially hazardous to humans and mammals that consume cottonseed oil or its by-pass products (Zia, Khan, Qasim, and Rehman, 2009).

Symptoms of Methamidophos poisoning include blurred vision, confusion, shakiness, tightness in the chest, convulsions, changes in heart rate, coma, cessation of breathing, and paralysis (Extension Toxicology Network, 2003).

Monocrotophos (Class Ib) is an organophosphate insecticide, which has been banned in the European Union and the United States but is still used in countries in Asia and South America. Monocrotophos is the most applied pesticide in cotton fields in India (Santhakumar & Balaji, 2000).

Symptoms of Monocrotophos poisoning may be a muscular weakness, confusion, blurred vision, profuse perspiration, pain, vomiting, pain, and narrow pupils (Extension Toxicology Network, 2003). The possible respiratory failure, provoked by the chemical, leads to death.

The most used herbicide worldwide is glyphosate (or Roundup), especially applied to genetically modified crops, including cotton (Benbrook, 2016). Two recent studies on the effects of glyphosate on human health reported contrary opinions. The study of IARC found that the herbicide is a "probable human carcinogen" (Class IIa) (International Agency for Research on Cancer, 2015). At the same time, the peer review of EFS) concluded the lack of evidence of carcinogenic hazard (European Food Safety Authority, 2015). These conflicting results have produced regulatory uncertainty that needs clarification (Landrigan & Belpoggi, 2018).

Human Poisoning Due to Occupational Exposure

99% of the cotton farmers worldwide live in the developing countries, where pesticides are widely used with lower levels of safety awareness, compared to the farms in the United States, for example (Action, 2007). The lack of personal protective clothing and devices, insufficient safeguards, inadequate labeling of chemicals, combined with illiteracy of the workers and low living standards precondition the vast number of accidents with pesticides in the cotton fields.

In the world, 1-3% of the workers in the cotton fields suffer from pesticide poisoning (Chemicals Program of the UN Environment Programme, 2004). The acute forms of poisoning require hospitalization and the effects of the pesticides on human health are more visible. But the chronic poisoning due to regular exposure to smaller doses of cotton pesticides can be hardly seen and often it is not part of the medical statistics. Impaired memory, reduced concentration, severe depression, disorientation, and confusion are among the symptoms of chronic exposure to pesticides in the cotton fields.

Human Poisoning Due to Non-Occupational Exposure

While the workers in the cotton fields are close to the hazardous pesticides and might be affected by the occupational exposure, the effect of the chemicals applied to cotton goes far beyond the persons, who are in direct contact with the cotton crop treatment. Individuals can be subject to poisoning via contact with pesticides, stored inappropriately. Glin et al. (2006) reported that 86% of the farmers in the investigated region of West Africa stored the pesticides in their bedroom. A way for accidental exposure to toxic chemicals is the contact with contaminated equipment, which is related again to the improper storage or non-compliance with occupational hygiene rules. Empty containers of cotton pesticides are often used for carrying drinking water or other household activities (Dewan et al. 2004). The study of Dewan et al. (2004) has found accidental poisoning of wheat and wheat flour, which are the primary food in the investigated farms; however, the exact way of contamination of the food could not be determined. Last but not list the toxic exposure to cotton pesticides can be due to drift from spray application in neighbor fields.

The Effect of Cotton Pesticides on Children's Health

Children are more susceptible to cotton pesticides than the adults due to their smaller body size, increased metabolism and faster blood circulation, as well as their unripe organ and systems, which cannot oppose to the poison as effective as the body of an adult. Children in the cotton farms in the developing countries are at an elevated risk due to the intentional or accidental contact with the hazardous chemicals.

In the context of cotton farming poisoning of children can occur in diverse ways. The participation of children in agricultural work is the prime source for children's acute or chronical poisoning. There are data about the use of children for pesticide spray in cotton fields or work in the fields soon after the chemicals' application when the poisoning risk is still too high because of the pesticide residues (Mancini, Van Bruggen, Jiggins, Ambatipudi, & Murphy, 2005; Athreya, 2006). Another way for the hazardous impact of the cotton pesticides on the children's health is the scenario when the kids follow their parents in the fields during the pesticide spraying. All other ways for poisoning from non-occupational exposure, are equal for both adults and children.

Specific condition for toxic impact on children's health is the work of pregnant women in the cotton fields during or a brief time after the pesticide application, which could affect the health of the fetus negatively (Rother, 2000). However, the evidence of children's poisoning due to cotton pesticides use is often poorly documented (Bennett, Buthelezi, Ismael, & Morse, 2003).

The study of Dewan et al. (2004) has summarized the differences between the pesticide poisoning of children and that of adults:

- The toxic effect (or illness) of the pesticide exposure is first manifested in children;
- At the time of hospitalization children have more severe symptoms of poisoning than the adults;
- Fatalities occur mainly among children;
- Electroencephalography (EEG) abnormalities can be seen only in children, though the levels of poisoning are the same for the children and the adults.

The Hidden Danger in the Cottonseeds

Around 34 million tons of cottonseed are produced annually as an additional product of the cotton growth (Action 2007). Cottonseed oil used as a cooking product accounts for approx. 2.4% (in 2016/17) to 3.05% (in 2013/14) of the world's vegetable oil consumption – see Table 1. Data compiled by WHO shows the potential of both cottonseed oil for humans and cottonseed derivatives for animals to be contaminated by the pesticides, applied in the cotton fields.

ENVIRONMENTAL PROBLEMS RELATED TO NON-ORGANIC COTTON GROWTH AND THEIR EFFECTS ON HUMAN HEALTH

In fact, there is no pure "environmental" effect of the application of pesticides in the cotton fields, as the poisoning of wild animals, cattle, water, and soil affects sooner or later the human body. This section discusses the particular effect of the most dangerous pesticides, already presented in the previous section, on the wildlife, water, and soil resources, as well as on cattle breeding.

Table 1. Consumption of vegetable oils worldwide from 2013/14 to 2017/2018 (data from Statista, 2018f)

Consumption of vegetable oils worldwide from 2013/14 to 2017/2018 (in a million metric tones)					
Year	2013/14	2014/15	2015/16	2016/17	2017/18
Palm oil	57,52	58,69	59,28	59,97	62,92
Soybean oil	45,27	47,83	52,15	53,62	55,99
Sunflower seed oil	14,14	14,11	15,18	16,52	16,79
Palm Kernel oil	6,58	7,22	6,81	7,02	7,21
Peanut oil	5,68	5,51	5,44	5,77	5,99
Cottonseed oil	5,09	5,06	4,4	4,38	4,93
Coconut oil	3,34	3,29	3,26	3,17	3,22
Olive oil	2,97	2,64	2,81	2,63	2,64
Rapeseed oil	26,17	27,29	28,18	29,22	29,35
Total vegetable oils	166,76	171,64	177,51	182,3	189,04

Pesticide Poisoning

Aldicarb (Class Ia) is nonvolatile, but highly water-soluble (approximately 6000 ppm) (Baron, 1994). It is easily degraded under alkaline conditions and relatively stable under the action of acids. Aldicarb contaminants water and soil and is acutely toxic to mammals, birds, fishes and aquatic invertebrates (Dowling, Costella, & Lemley, 2018). The chemical is absorbed by the roots, stems, and leaves of the plants; therefore, it is allowed to be used only for farming of some crops, including cotton. It is not allowed Aldicarb to be used in most fruits, especially after the case of human poisoning after consumption of watermelons, which soil was treated with Aldicarb (D'Haenens et al., 2013).

Parathion (Class Ia) is moderately toxic to mammals and highly toxic for aquatic invertebrates (Pesticide Action Network UK, 2000). The insecticide has been implicated in the deaths of birds, including waterfowl, as well as severe poisoning or deaths of fish, cattle, and wild animals. In 1995 heavy rainfalls washed the pesticide from the cotton fields and through the rivers led to the death of over 240,000 fish in Alabama (Clay, 2013).

Methamidophos (Class Ib) is toxic to insects, birds, and aquatic organisms. In water, the chemical has a half-life of up to 309 days (Action, 2007). In laboratory experiments, eggs and milk of hens and goats showed traces of the pesticide, after feeding the animals with contaminated food (Leeman, Van Den Berg, and Houben, 2007).

Monocrotophos (Class Ib) is used as a bird poison, as it is extremely toxic to birds. It has been found to be highly toxic to bees and very dangerous to mammals (Extension Toxicology Network, 2003).

Water Poisoning

Several studies undertaken in major cotton producing countries have reported detectable levels of cotton pesticides in local water resources (Thurman, Zimmerman, Scribner, and Coupe, 1998; Tariq, Afzal, and Hussain, 2004; Tariq, Afzal, and Hussain, 2006; Ntow, 2005; Pazou et al., 2006; Musa, Gichuki, Raburu, and Mul, 2011; Yadav et al., 2015). The water poisoning undoubtedly occurs despite the economic status of the investigated country. However, in the developing countries, the water is nor frequently or not enough treated, and the monitoring of these processes is often missing. At the same time, the pesticide contamination of the groundwater is of vital importance, as a significant part of the population (not only in the cotton farms) use groundwater aquifers as a primary source of drinking water (Yadav et al., 2015).

The study of Ntow (2005) investigated the water contamination by pesticides, used mainly in the cotton fields of Lake Volta: the chemicals Lindane and Endosulfan (Class II) were found in 22.7% and 18% of the water samples respectively. Yadav et al. (2015) reported that more than 90% of the fish and water samples, taken within their study on pesticides residues in India, showed a presence of one or more pesticides. Due to the mobility of pesticides in soil, groundwater is very susceptible to chemical contamination. On the contrary, Lari, Khan, Gandhi, Meshram, and Thacker (2014) found out that the surface water was more contaminated with pesticides than the groundwater.

Cattle Poisoning

Every year approximately 23 million tons of cottonseeds or their derivatives (hulls and meal) are fed to domestic animals (Action, 2007). Together with the beneficial ingredients like protein, minerals, and fibers, this food is also known to contain pesticide residues (Blasi and Drouillard, 2002). The levels of poisoning are significantly higher than those, measured in the cottonseed oil.

There is convincing evidence that cotton pesticide residues consumed by animals can affect food products, meant to humans. Laboratory experiments (Joint Meeting on Pesticide Residues, 2004) showed that the cotton pesticides Parathion (Class Ia) and Methamidophos (Class Ib) shifted from the hens' food to their eggs. Similarly, fodder, containing Parathion and Aldicarb (Class Ia), as well as Methamidophos (Class Ib), given to cows, was the reason to find residues of the same pesticides in the milk. The study of Pastor Ciscato, Gebara, and de Souza Spinosa (2002) has found traces of Endosulfan (Class II) in 10% of the samples of cows' milk in Brazil, where this pesticide is largely used in the cotton farms. The same conclusions were made in the studies of Zapata, Santamaría, Alvarez, Salazar, and Müller (1996) for Nicaragua and Waliszewski et al. (1997) for Mexico.

Thus, the cottonseeds and the residuals from the production of cottonseed oil can effectively damage the human health, being part of the animals' food and entering the human food chain.

Soil Poisoning

The most dangerous effect of the pesticides, which enter the soil, on the human health, is related with the pesticides' transportation to the groundwater, especially in regions, where the groundwater is the only source for drinking water. The main factors, which influence the process of water poisoning via the contaminated soil, are (Jabbar, Masud, Parveen, and Ali, 1993):

- Volatilization (and subsequent diffusion)
- Decomposition
- Contingent retention by the soil

The process of decomposition of the pesticides, used in cotton fields is different, but some of them can be destroyed by the sunlight (Samsonov and Pokrovskii, 2001). However, runoff from heavy rainfalls can not only facilitate the penetration of the pesticides to the groundwater but also spreads the chemicals through the ground, leading to further soil damage

The replacement of conventional cotton by Bt cotton decreases the pesticides in the fields, but the genetically modified crop damages the soil enzymes and microorganisms. In fact, the soil in which the cotton was grown is virtually dead by the time of the cotton harvest. The study of Chen et al. (2016) has found that the Bt cotton disrupts the mycorrhizal fungi in the soil and the broader ecosystem of the soil, which, consequently, may be a reason for the low yields and poor pest resistance among Bt cotton crops.

THE PREFERRED COTTON TEXTILE SEGMENT: WHAT TO KNOW

Preferred cotton is defined as ecologically and/or socially progressive because it offers greater sustainability in comparison to other conventional options. Cotton, currently defined by Textile Exchange (2017) as "preferred cotton," includes several types of cotton: recycled, organic, CmiA, Fair Trade, BCI, Cleaner Cotton, REEL, and e3cotton. They are shortly discussed below.

The consumers of cotton textiles and apparel may be confused by the different names, acronyms, projects, and platforms, mentioned in Textile Exchange (2017). The reason is that, in general, the end-users can make some difference between conventional cotton and organic cotton products, being long-term trained by the textile and apparel brands through the special labels for organic cotton. However, all other types of cotton, which are part of the Preferred cotton (Textile Exchange, 2017), can be confused with the organic cotton, without being organic. The customers of cotton textiles and apparel need the knowledge to make an informed choice, which cotton products to support and how their purchase would affect the human health and the environment.

Fair Trade Cotton

This is cotton, certified by a fair-trade organization, e.g., Fairtrade Labelling Organizations International (FLO) (Pay, 2009). FLO is the largest organization for certification of fair-trade cotton, which serves as an umbrella group for smaller organizations.

The certificate for fair trade cotton means that the cotton producers receive a fair price for their cotton yield. The cotton producers from Burkina Faso, Cameroon, Egypt, India, Mali, and Senegal are the target group for the FLO certificates. Only the raw cotton can be certified, not the textile products made of it. However, the fair-trade cotton has quite small to do with the effects of the cotton growth on the human health and the environment: this is not necessarily organic cotton. FLO requires the farmers, applying for a certificate, to limit the amount of the pesticides used in the cotton fields. FLO encourages the organic cotton cultivation, offering higher prices to organic cotton producers.

CmiA

CmiA is the acronym for "Cotton Made in Africa," an initiative, started in 2005 by the Aid by Trade Foundation. The mission of this foundation is to improve the living conditions in the developing countries in Africa through sustainable development while promoting environmental protection.

The cotton harvested in Sub-Saharan Africa counts for about 8% of the world traded cotton. The cotton growth is favored by the high temperatures and the alternation of the wet and dry seasons. Smallholder farmers produce the cotton following the CmiA standard criteria. Natural rainfall is used for irrigation. Crop rotation is used, which decreases leaching of soil and occurrence of cotton pests, thus decreasing the application of pesticides.

The cotton, having the label of CmiA, is not pesticide free. However, all pesticides ranked by WHO as Class Ia and Class Ib may not be used in the CmiA fields (Rüchardt, 2017). The criteria of CmiA does not allow pregnant or nursing women, sick people, untrained or inexperienced persons and children to work with pesticides. The child labor is strictly prohibited.

Though encouraged, organic cotton production is still too expensive for the African farmers. An alternative is the Bt cotton, which is only grown by smallholder farmers in South Africa, Burkina Faso, and Sudan. According to the criteria of CmiA genetically modified cotton seeds (e.g., Bt cotton) are not allowed to be used under the initiative (Rüchardt, 2017).

BCI

The Better Cotton Initiative (BCI) aims to transform the production of cotton into a better occupation for people, better influence on the environment and the agricultural sector's future. The Better Cotton principles and criteria were developed in 2010, having the input of regional working groups in India, Pakistan, Brazil and countries from Central and West Africa (Better Cotton Principles and Criteria, 2018).

BCI involves different stakeholders in the cotton and cotton textiles production chains, aiming to sustainably improve the conditions in the cotton crop cultivation concerning the environment and farming communities. The revised Better Cotton Standard launched in Mart 2018 (Better Cotton Principles and Criteria, 2018) restricts the highly hazardous pesticides and banns the pesticides Class Ia and Ib. Besides, BCI requires the use of minimum personal protective equipment for people, working with pesticides.

BCI is "technology neutral" (Better Cotton Principles and Criteria, 2018) to Bt cotton: it neither encourage its production, nor restricts it. Instead, the focus is on the informed choices of the farmers regarding the availability of modern technologies, and their proper applications. BCI encourages all practices that work for improved outcomes – environmentally, economically, and socially.

It has to be mentioned that BCI discusses the quality of the cotton fibers. The initiative supports, among other activities, the farmers that preserve the cotton fibers characteristics and work on increasing or maintaining the cotton quality.

Cleaner Cotton™

Cleaner Cotton™ is a supply chain within the Sustainable Cotton Project (SCP), based in California. The main aim of the program is to change the way cotton is produced and marketed. SCP has started in 1996 and supports the sustainability in farming of domestic cotton (Sustainable Cotton Project, 2018).

It works with the farmers to eliminate the most toxic pesticides from the cotton fields, providing information about sustainable cotton growth and pest management. On the other hand, SCP connects cotton producers, cotton textiles manufacturers, and various brands to create a working Cleaner Cotton™ supply chain. The program is dedicated to the education of students, professionals from the textile industry and fashion as well as the society about the importance of reducing the toxic chemicals, used in fiber and food production.

Cleaner Cotton™ is not concerned with the production of organic cotton. The reason is that the cost of organic cotton production in California is much higher than the producers of cotton textiles are willing to pay. The yield of organic cotton is approx. 40% less than the conventional (non-organic cotton) and the producers would not like to risk their financial return (Sustainable Cotton Project, 2018). At the same time producers calculate that organic cotton farming costs five times more compared to conventional cotton. Though the growers have tried to produce organic cotton for years, the organic cotton fields in California are less than 200 acres a year (Sustainable Cotton Project, 2018). 98% of the organic cotton is produced outside the United States.

The policy of Cleaner Cotton™, dedicated to achieving the chemical reduction in cotton growth, takes that the decrement of pesticides in the production of conventional cotton has a more significant potential for the total reduction of the pesticides in California than the farming of organic cotton.

Cleaner Cotton™ does not involve Bt cotton. The SCP project aims to ensure the demand for non-genetically modified cotton seeds. At present, approx. 80% of the cotton, grown in the United States is BT cotton, as the general belief is that it ensures maximum cotton yield (Sustainable Cotton Project, 2018). A targeted objective of SCP is to demonstrate that integrated pest management and historical and cultural practices are adequate for high crop yields without using genetically modified seeds.

REEL Cotton

The REEL (Responsible Environment Enhanced Livelihoods) cotton is an agricultural program that provides the farmers with three-year training on sustainable practices for cotton crop farming. The project was created in 2010, run by CottonConnect, which works together with leading brands and retailers. The REEL Cotton Program involved more than 20,000 farmers from countries like India, Pakistan, China, and Peru. The result from the training is increased cotton yields and income for the farmers, reducing at the same time the hazardous impact on the human health and environment (Responsible Environment Enhanced Livelihoods, 2016).

The Framers, producing cotton under the requirements of REEL Cotton are encouraged to reduce the number and volume of pesticides applied and to record their use. The cotton, produced under the REEL label, is not treated with pesticides Class Ia and Class Ib or other pesticides, which are prohibited by international conventions (Responsible Environment Enhanced Livelihoods, 2016).

REEL Cotton Program supports the organic cotton growth that produces cotton fibers of good quality. The trained farmers are made acquainted with several aspects of organic farming and good practices for organic cotton growth. REEL Cotton is an implementation partner for the Better Cotton Initiative for farmers in China and India, which are trained and supported to produce Better Cotton for multiple brands.

e^3 Cotton

e^3 Cotton is a sustainable cotton crop of Bayer CropScience, which offer to the market two types of cotton seeds: Certified FiberMax® and Authentic Stoneville®. The farmers, joining the e^3 program, are obliged to use Bayer branded cotton seeds, which count close to 40% of the cotton seeds market share in the United States (E3 – Sustainable Grown Cotton, 2018). Though Bayer is a globally oriented company, the e^3 cotton program is currently available for US farmers only, due to the content claims process and fibers traceability. Farmers are not specially trained, but their performance is self-evaluated through an online tool, called the Fieldprint Calculator, and assessed by third-party audits.

The Fieldprint Calculator does not include information about the pesticides used. Bayer CropScience declares that the cotton growers are encouraged to use integrated pest management, however (E3 – Sustainable Grown Cotton, 2018).

e^3 Cotton is not an organic one: Bayer CropScience does not sell non-treated seeds. As for the others, both types of cotton seeds are available: conventional and genetically modified. It has to be mentioned that the policy of Bayer CropScience is zero-tolerant to child labor (E3 – Sustainable Grown Cotton, 2018).

CONCLUSION: FROM ORGANIC TO SUSTAINABLE OR "BETTER" COTTON – WHERE IS THE SOLUTION?

Many apparel and textile selling companies have switched to offering both conventional and organic cotton, supporting the organic cotton textiles and the organic cotton growth by special labeling. Part of the marketing strategies of these companies was to especially mention the countenance of organic agriculture, which preserves the environment and human health.

However, the average consumers rejected to buy organic cotton items, because of their higher price. In the 2015-2016 season, the price for conventional cotton was 0.61 USD per pound vs. 2.2 USD per pound for the organic cotton (Kessenides, 2016). The result was that the apparel and other brands started to support the Better Cotton Initiative. Though it was not clearly defined, the shift was from organic to sustainable cotton.

However, it is clear that only the growth of organic cotton does not involve pesticides. That means that all discussed in this chapter problems, related with directed or non-directed exposure of humans to pesticides, will not appear. Is this real possibility for the world to produce cotton only via organic agriculture? It seems not.

Sustainable cotton is advertised as the best possible alternative of organic cotton. Antoshak (2013) defined it as "practical cotton": a crop that can be produced without a break while preserving the environment. It can be done via proven agricultural practices, better technology and ecological "cotton chain" that involves textile producers and brands, as well as retailers. It also means that the fields available today for cotton crop production will be available also tomorrow.

Over the past years, Ikea, Zara, Nike, Levi-Strauss, Marks & Spencers, Adidas, and H&M, among others, have been involved in the Better Cotton Initiative (BCI), which aims to produce and use sustainable cotton at acceptable prices. Sustainable cotton does not necessarily mean organic cotton, even though organic cotton is not excluded from BCI. The main driving force in BCI is to preserve the low price of cotton and cotton products while taking the necessary steps to reduce the pressure on the environmental issues: by using fewer pesticides, especially the most dangerous for human health and the environment, by reducing the use of water, and preserving the soil. IKEA, which consumes 1% of the global cotton production, introduced the use of Better Cotton in 2009 (Tan, 2017). In 2015 70% of all the cotton products of the brand were Better Cotton.

Better Cotton Initiative banns the pesticides Class Ia and Ib, but allows the use of other pesticides, like the glyphosate, for example. BCI is also neutral concerning the Bt cotton, which also requires the application of pesticides. The customers must be informed and to make their choice which initiatives to support buying the respective cotton textiles and cotton clothes.

REFERENCES

Action, P. (2007). *The Deadly Chemicals in Cotton. Environmental Justice Foundation in collaboration with Pesticide Action*. London, UK: Development House.

Alavanja, M. C., Dosemeci, M., Samanic, C., Lubin, J., Lynch, C. F., Knott, C., ... Blair, A. (2004). Pesticides and lung cancer risk in the agricultural health study cohort. *American Journal of Epidemiology*, *160*(9), 876–885. doi:10.1093/aje/kwh290 PMID:15496540

Alavanja, M. C., Samanic, C., Dosemeci, M., Lubin, J., Tarone, R., Lynch, C. F., ... Blair, A. (2003). Use of agricultural pesticides and prostate cancer risk in the Agricultural Health Study cohort. *American Journal of Epidemiology*, *157*(9), 800–814. doi:10.1093/aje/kwg040 PMID:12727674

Ali, T., Ismail, M., Asad, F., Ashraf, A., Waheed, U., & Khan, Q. M. (2018). Pesticide genotoxicity in cotton picking women in Pakistan evaluated using comet assay. *Drug and Chemical Toxicology*, *41*(2), 213–220. doi:10.1080/01480545.2017.1343342 PMID:28721745

Angelova, R. A. (2018), Organic Cotton: Technological and Environmental Aspects. In *Proc. of XXIII Int. Scientific Conference FPEPM*, September 17 – 20 (pp. 351-356).

Antoshak, R. (2013). Sustainable Cotton, the e3 Program, and the Better Cotton Initiative. Retrieved from http://rantoshak.blogspot.com/2013/07/sustainable-cotton-e3-program-and.html

Athreya, B. (2006). *Submission to US Department of Labor in response to Federal Register notice FR Doc. E6-20561 published November 29, 2006*. In Request for Information on Efforts by Certain Countries to Eliminate the Worst Forms of Child Labor.

Baron, R. L. (1994). A carbamate insecticide: A case study of aldicarb. *Environmental Health Perspectives*, *102*(Suppl. 11), 23–27. doi:10.1289/ehp.94102s1123 PMID:7737038

Benbrook, C. M. (2016). Trends in glyphosate herbicide use in the United States and globally. *Environmental Sciences Europe*, *28*(1), 3. doi:10.118612302-016-0070-0 PMID:27752438

Bennett, R., Buthelezi, T. J., Ismael, Y., & Morse, S. (2003). Bt cotton, pesticides, labour and health: A case study of smallholder farmers in the Makhathini Flats, Republic of South Africa. *Outlook on Agriculture*, *32*(2), 123–128. doi:10.5367/000000003101294361

Better Cotton Principles and Criteria. (2018). Version 2.0, March 2018. Retrieved from https://bettercotton.org/about-better-cotton/better-cotton-standard-system/production-principles-and-criteria/

Blasi, D. A., & Drouillard, J. (2002). Composition and feeding value of cottonseed feed products for beef cattle. Kansas State University, Agricultural Experiment Station and Cooperative Extension Service.

Bouchard, M. F., Chevrier, J., Harley, K. G., Kogut, K., Vedar, M., Calderon, N., ... Eskenazi, B. (2011). Prenatal exposure to organophosphate pesticides and IQ in 7-year-old children. *Environmental Health Perspectives*, *119*(8), 1189–1195. doi:10.1289/ehp.1003185 PMID:21507776

Budavari, S. (1989). *An Encyclopedia of Chemicals, Drugs, and Biologicals. The Merck Index*. Rahway, NJ: Merck and Co. Inc.

Cameron, P. J. (2007). Factors influencing the development of integrated pest management (IPM) in selected vegetable crops: A review. *New Zealand Journal of Crop and Horticultural Science*, *35*(3), 365–384. doi:10.1080/01140670709510203

Chemicals Program of the United Nations Environment Programme. (2004). *Childhood pesticide poisoning: information for advocacy and action.* Retrieved from http://www.who.int/ceh/publications/pestpoisoning.pdf

Chen, X. H., Wang, F. L., Zhang, R., Ji, L. L., Yang, Z. L., Lin, H., & Zhao, B. (2016). Evidences of inhibited arbuscular mycorrhizal fungal development and colonization in multiple lines of Bt cotton. *Agriculture, Ecosystems & Environment*, *230*, 169–176. doi:10.1016/j.agee.2016.05.008

Clay, J. (2013). *World agriculture and the environment: a commodity-by-commodity guide to impacts and practices*. Washington, DC: Island Press.

Cohn, B. A., Wolff, M. S., Cirillo, P. M., & Sholtz, R. I. (2007). DDT and breast cancer in young women: New data on the significance of age at exposure. *Environmental Health Perspectives*, *115*(10), 1406–1414. doi:10.1289/ehp.10260 PMID:17938728

D'Haenens, J. P., McDonald, K. W., Langley, R. L., Higgins, S. A., Scott, R., Farquhar, P. N., & Meggs, W. J. (2013). Aldicarb: A case series of watermelon-borne carbamate toxicity. *Journal of Agromedicine*, *18*(2), 174–177. doi:10.1080/1059924X.2013.766141 PMID:23540307

Damalas, C. A., & Hashemi, S. M. (2010). Pesticide risk perception and use of personal protective equipment among young and old cotton growers in northern Greece. *Agrociencia*, *44*(3).

De Bleecker, J., Willems, J., Van Den Neucker, K., De Reuck, J., & Vogelaers, D. (1992). Prolonged toxicity with intermediate syndrome after combined parathion and methyl parathion poisoning. *Journal of Toxicology. Clinical Toxicology*, *30*(3), 333–345. doi:10.3109/15563659209021548 PMID:1512808

Dewan, A., Bhatnagar, V. K., Mathur, M. L., Chakma, T., Kashyap, R., Sadhu, H. G., ... Saiyed, H. N. (2004). Repeated episodes of endosulfan poisoning. *Journal of Toxicology. Clinical Toxicology*, *42*(4), 363–369. doi:10.1081/CLT-120039542 PMID:15461244

Dich, J., & Wiklund, K. (1998). Prostate cancer in pesticide applicators in Swedish agriculture. *The Prostate*, *34*(2), 100–112. doi:10.1002/(SICI)1097-0045(19980201)34:2<100::AID-PROS4>3.0.CO;2-O PMID:9465941

Dowling, K. C., Costella, R. G., & Lemley, A. T. (2018). Modeling the Movement of a Rapidly Degrading Solute, Methomyl, in Dynamic Soil-Water Systems. *Mechanisms Of Pesticide Movement Into Ground Water*, *101*.

E3 – Sustainable Grown Cotton. (2018). Retrieved from https://www.e3cotton.us/

European Food Safety Authority (EFSA). (2015). Conclusion on the peer review of the pesticide risk assessment of the active substance glyphosate. *EFSA Journal*, *13*(11), 4302.

Extension Toxicology Network. (2003). Exotoxnet—A Pesticide Information Project. U.S. Department of Agriculture, Extension Service, and the National Agricultural Pesticide Impact Assessment Program.

Eyer, F., Meischner, V., Kiderlen, D., Thiermann, H., Worek, F., Haberkorn, M., ... Eyer, P. (2003). Human parathion poisoning. *Toxicological Reviews*, *22*(3), 143–163. doi:10.2165/00139709-200322030-00003 PMID:15181664

Garry, V. F. (2004). Pesticides and children. *Toxicology and Applied Pharmacology*, *198*(2), 152–163. doi:10.1016/j.taap.2003.11.027 PMID:15236951

Gbaruko, B. C., Ogwo, E. I., Igwe, J. C., & Yu, H. (2009). Organophosphate induced chronic neurotoxicity: Health, environmental and risk exposure issues in developing nations of the world. *African Journal of Biotechnology*, *8*(20).

Glin, L. J., Kuiseau, J., Thiam, A., Vodouhé, D. S., Dinham, B., & Ferrigno, S. (2006). *Living with Poison: Problems of Endosulfan in West Africa cotton growing systems*. London: PAN UK.

Gruere, A., & Plastina, A. (2010). Some Alternatives to Conventional Cotton: Organic Cotton, Fairtrade Cotton, Cotton Made In Africa and Better Cotton Initiative. *Cotton*, (May-June), 5-9.

Infante-Rivard, C., & Weichenthal, S. (2007). Pesticides and childhood cancer: An update of Zahm and Ward's 1998 review. *Journal of Toxicology and Environmental Health. Part B*, *10*(1-2), 81–99.

International Agency for Research on Cancer. (2015). Some organophosphate insecticides and herbicides: Diazinon, Glyphosate, Malathion, parathion, and Tetrachlorvinphos. *IARC Monographs on the Evaluation of Carcinogenic Risks to Humans*, 112.

Jabbar, A., Masud, S. Z., Parveen, Z., & Ali, M. (1993). Pesticide residues in cropland soils and shallow groundwater in Punjab Pakistan. *Bulletin of Environmental Contamination and Toxicology*, *51*(2), 268–273. doi:10.1007/BF00198891 PMID:8353391

Jin, S., Bluemling, B., & Mol, A. P. (2015). Information, trust and pesticide overuse: Interactions between retailers and cotton farmers in China. *NJAS Wageningen Journal of Life Sciences*, *72*, 23–32. doi:10.1016/j.njas.2014.10.003

Joint Meeting on Pesticide Residues. (2004). *Report of the Joint Meeting of the FAO Panel of Experts on Pesticide Residues in Food and the Environment and the WHO Core Assessment Group on Pesticide Residues*. Retrieved from http://www.fao.org/home/en/

Kessenides, D. (2016, October 20). Forget Organic, Retailers Increasingly Are Turning to Sustainable Cotton. *Bloomberg*. Retrieved from https://www.bloomberg.com/news/articles/2016-10-20/forget-organic-retailers-increasingly-are-turning-to-sustainable-cotton

Kumar, R., Kranthi, S., Nitharwal, M., Jat, S. L., & Monga, D. (2012). Influence of pesticides and application methods on pest and predatory arthropods associated with cotton. *Phytoparasitica*, *40*(5), 417–424. doi:10.100712600-012-0241-5

Landrigan, P. J., & Belpoggi, F. (2018). The need for independent research on the health effects of glyphosate-based herbicides. *Environmental Health*, *17*(1), 51. doi:10.118612940-018-0392-z PMID:29843729

Lari, S. Z., Khan, N. A., Gandhi, K. N., Meshram, T. S., & Thacker, N. P. (2014). Comparison of pesticide residues in surface water and ground water of agriculture intensive areas. *Journal of Environmental Health Science & Engineering*, *12*(1), 11. doi:10.1186/2052-336X-12-11 PMID:24398360

Leeman, W. R., Van Den Berg, K. J., & Houben, G. F. (2007). Transfer of chemicals from feed to animal products: The use of transfer factors in risk assessment. *Food Additives and Contaminants*, *24*(1), 1–13. doi:10.1080/02652030600815512 PMID:17164211

Lehmann, G. M., LaKind, J. S., Davis, M. H., Hines, E. P., Marchitti, S. A., Alcala, C., & Lorber, M. (2018). Environmental chemicals in breast milk and formula: Exposure and risk assessment implications. *Environmental Health Perspectives*, *126*(9), 096001. doi:10.1289/EHP1953 PMID:30187772

MacDonald, S. A., & Vollrath, T. L. (2005). *The forces shaping world cotton consumption after the multifiber arrangement*. Washington, DC: US Department of Agriculture.

Mancini, F., Van Bruggen, A. H., Jiggins, J. L., Ambatipudi, A. C., & Murphy, H. (2005). Acute pesticide poisoning among female and male cotton growers in India. *International Journal of Occupational and Environmental Health*, *11*(3), 221–232. doi:10.1179/oeh.2005.11.3.221 PMID:16130962

Musa, S., Gichuki, J. W., Raburu, P. O., & Mul, C. (2011). Organochlorine and organophosphorus pesticide residues in water and sediment from Yala/Nzoia River within Lake Victoria basin, Kenya. *Journal of Ecology and the Natural Environment*, *3*(12), 392–399.

Nanda, S., Kumar, M., Kumar, A., Behal, S., & Nanda, S. (2016). Malwa region, The focal point of cancer cases in Punjab: A Review study. *International Journal of Current Research in Multidisciplinary*, *1*(3), 41–45.

Niehoff, N. M., Nichols, H. B., White, A. J., Parks, C. G., D'aloisio, A. A., & Sandler, D. P. (2016). Childhood and adolescent pesticide exposure and breast cancer risk. *Epidemiology (Cambridge, Mass.)*, *27*(3), 326–333. doi:10.1097/EDE.0000000000000451 PMID:26808595

Ntow, W. J. (2005). Pesticide residues in Volta Lake, Ghana. *Lakes and Reservoirs: Research and Management*, *10*(4), 243–248. doi:10.1111/j.1440-1770.2005.00278.x

Pastor Ciscato, C. H., Gebara, A. B., & de Souza Spinosa, H. (2002). Pesticide residues in cow milk consumed in Sao Paulo City (Brazil). *Journal of Environmental Science and Health. Part. B, Pesticides, Food Contaminants, and Agricultural Wastes*, *37*(4), 323–330. doi:10.1081/PFC-120004473 PMID:12081024

Pay, E. (2009). *The market for organic and fair-trade cotton fibre and cotton fibre products*. Rome, Italy: Food and Agriculture Organization of the United Nations.

Pazou, E. Y. A., Lalèyè, P., Boko, M., Van Gestel, M. A., Ahissou, H., Akpona, S., ... Van Straalen, N. M. (2006). Contamination of fish by organochlorine pesticide residues in the Ouémé River catchment in the Republic of Bénin. *Environment International*, *32*(5), 594–599. doi:10.1016/j.envint.2006.01.007 PMID:16494946

Pesatori, A. C., Sontag, J. M., Lubin, J. H., Consonni, D., & Blair, A. (1994). Cohort mortality and nested case-control study of lung cancer among structural pest control workers in Florida (United States). *Cancer Causes & Control*, *5*(4), 310–318. doi:10.1007/BF01804981 PMID:8080942

Pesticide Action Network UK. (2000). *Methyl parathion*. Pesticide News No 36. Retrieved from http://www.pan-uk.org/pestnews/actives/methylpa.htm

Reports of the Joint Meeting of the FAO Panel of Experts on Pesticide Residues in Food and the WHO Core Assessment Group. (2003). Retrieved from http://www.fao.org/ag/AGP/AGPP/Pesticid

Responsible Environment Enhanced Livelihoods. (2016). REEL COTTON Code of Conduct, Version 1.0. Retrieved from http://cottonconnect.org/wp-content/uploads/reel-code-1.0.pdf

Rother, H. A. (2000). Influences of pesticide risk perception on the health of rural South African women and children. *African Newsletter on Occupational Health and Safety*, *10*(2), 11.

Rubin, C., Esteban, E., Kieszak, S., Hill, R. H. Jr, Dunlop, B., Yacovac, R., ... Pearce, K. (2002). Assessment of human exposure and human health effects after indoor application of methyl parathion in Lorain County, Ohio, 1995-1996. *Environmental Health Perspectives*, *110*(Supplement 6), 1047–1051. doi:10.1289/ehp.02110s61047 PMID:12634138

Rüchardt, A. F. (2017). *Cotton Made in Africa, Annual Report*. Hamburg, Germany: Aid by Trade Foundation.

Samsonov, Y. N., & Pokrovskii, L. M. (2001). Sensitized photodecomposition of high disperse pesticide chemicals exposed to sunlight and irradiation from halogen or mercury lamp. *Atmospheric Environment*, *35*(12), 2133–2141. doi:10.1016/S1352-2310(00)00494-5

Santhakumar, M., & Balaji, M. (2000). Acute toxicity of an organophosphorus insecticide monocrotophos and its effects on behaviour of an air-breathing fish, Anabas testudineus (Bloch). *Journal of Environmental Biology*, *21*(2), 121–123.

Statista. (2018a). Global Cotton Production 1990-217. Retrieved from https://www.statista.com/statistics/259392/cotton-production-worldwide-since-1990/

Statista. (2018b). Global Cotton Price Since 1990. Retrieved from https://www.statista.com/statistics/259431/global-cotton-price-since-1990/

Statista. (2018c). Global Cotton Production 2017/2018, by country. Retrieved from https://www.statista.com/statistics/263055/cotton-production-worldwide-by-top-countries/

Statista. (2018d). Top Cotton Exporting Countries 2017/2018. Retrieved from https://www.statista.com/statistics/191895/leading-cotton-exporting-countries/

Statista. (2018e). Top Cotton Importing Countries 2017/2018. Retrieved from https://www.statista.com/statistics/191896/leading-cotton-importing-countries/

Statista. (2018f). Vegetable Oils: Global Consumption by oil type 2013/14 to 2017/2018. Retrieved from https://www.statista.com/statistics/263937/vegetable-oils-global-consumption

Striepe, B. (2011). Cotton: The dirty truth about "The Fabric of our Lives." *Crafting a Green World*. Retrieved from http://craftingagreenworld.com/2011/10/11/the-dirty-side-of-cotton/

Sustainable Cotton Project. (2018). Media Kit. Retrieved from https://www.keepandshare.com/doc/6827338/media-kit-pdf-7-1-meg?da=y

TanD. (2017). Cotton. Retrieved from https://greenstitched.com/tag/cotton/

Tariq, M. I., Afzal, S., & Hussain, I. (2004). Pesticides in shallow groundwater of bahawalnagar, Muzafargarh, DG Khan and Rajan Pur districts of Punjab, Pakistan. *Environment International*, *30*(4), 471–479. doi:10.1016/j.envint.2003.09.008 PMID:15031006

Tariq, M. I., Afzal, S., & Hussain, I. (2006). Degradation and persistence of cotton pesticides in sandy loam soils from Punjab, Pakistan. *Environmental Research*, *100*(2), 184–196. doi:10.1016/j.envres.2005.05.002 PMID:16009361

Textile Exchange. (2017). *Preferred Fiber & Materials Market Report*. Retrieved from https://textileexchange.org/downloads/2017-preferred-fiber-materials-market-report/

Thurman, E. M., Zimmerman, L. R., Scribner, E. A., & Coupe, R. H. (1998). Occurrence of cotton pesticides in surface water of the Mississippi embayment. *U.S. Geological Survey Fact Sheet*, *4*, 22–98.

Townsend, T. (1997, May). World Cotton Outlook. International Cotton Advisory Committee (ICAC). In *Proceedings of the 73 rd Annual Convention of the American Crop Shippers Association* (pp. 22-24).

US Department of Agriculture, National Agricultural Statistics Service. (2004). *Agricultural Chemical Usage, 2003 Field Crops Summary 2004*. Collingdale, PA: Diane Publishing Co.

van Duijn, H., & Maas, M. (2017). Organic Cotton's Threshold Moment. *Organic Cotton Accelerator*. Retrieved from http://www.organiccottonaccelerator.org/wp-content/uploads/dlm_uploads/2017/03/OCA-Organic-Cottons-Threshold-Moment-2017.pdf

Waliszewski, S. M., Pardio, V. T., Waliszewski, K. N., Chantiri, J. N., Aguirre, A. A., Infanzon, R. M., & Rivera, J. (1997). Organochlorine pesticide residues in cow's milk and butter in Mexico. *The Science of the Total Environment*, *208*(1-2), 127–132. doi:10.1016/S0048-9697(97)00270-2 PMID:9496657

Webster, L. R., McKenzie, G. H., & Moriarty, H. T. (2002). Organophosphate-based pesticides and genetic damage implicated in bladder cancer. *Cancer Genetics and Cytogenetics*, *133*(2), 112–117. doi:10.1016/S0165-4608(01)00576-3 PMID:11943336

Yadav, I. C., Devi, N. L., Syed, J. H., Cheng, Z., Li, J., Zhang, G., & Jones, K. C. (2015). Current status of persistent organic pesticides residues in air, water, and soil, and their possible effect on neighboring countries: A comprehensive review of India. *The Science of the Total Environment*, *511*, 123–137. doi:10.1016/j.scitotenv.2014.12.041 PMID:25540847

Yarsan, E., Tanyuksel, M., Celik, S., & Aydin, A. (1999). Effects of aldicarb and malathion on lipid peroxidation. *Bulletin of Environmental Contamination and Toxicology*, *63*(5), 575–581. doi:10.1007001289901019 PMID:10541675

Zahm, S. H., & Ward, M. H. (1998). Pesticides and childhood cancer. *Environmental Health Perspectives*, *106*(Supplement 3), 893. PMID:9646054

Zapata, A. M., Santamaría, M. R., Alvarez, M. I., Salazar, S. V., & Müller, U. (1996). Organochlorine pesticide residues in cow's milk, Nicaragua. *Boletin de la Oficina Sanitaria Panamericana. Pan American Sanitary Bureau, 120*(6), 483–490.

Zia, M. S., Khan, M. J., Qasim, M., & Rehman, A. (2009). Pesticide residue in the food chain and human body inside Pakistan. *Journal of the Chemical Society of Pakistan, 31*, 284–291.

KEY TERMS AND DEFINITIONS

BCI Cotton: The cotton is produced as a part of the Better Cotton Initiative (BCI). It is not necessarily organic cotton. BCI requires the use of minimum personal protective equipment for people, working with pesticides. It is "technology neutral" to Bt cotton.

Cleaner Cotton™: This is cotton produced within the Sustainable Cotton Project (SCP), which supports US farmers. It does not involve organic cotton and Bt cotton production.

CmiA Cotton: This is the acronym for "Cotton Made in Africa." It is not necessarily organic cotton. The child labor is strictly prohibited.

Conventional (Non-Organic) Cotton: The most produced cotton crop in the world, which require the application of pesticides.

e³ Cotton: This is sustainable cotton of Bayer CropScience. e³ is not an organic cotton. The child labor is strictly prohibited.

Fair Trade Cotton: Cotton, certified by a fair-trade organization: means that the cotton producers receive a fair price for their cotton yield. It is not necessarily organic cotton.

Genetically Modified Cotton: Known also as Bt Cotton, which is one of the two types of genetically modified cotton crops. It produces toxins, which kills some of the insects. Still requires the application of pesticides.

Organic Cotton: A cotton crop, which is produced via organic methods and does not involve application of pesticides.

REEL Cotton: The REEL (responsible environment enhanced livelihoods) cotton is an agricultural program run by CottonConnect. It is not necessarily organic cotton.

Chapter 11
A Panel Asymmetric Causality Between Health and Climate Change:
Empirical Evidence From EU Regions

Reyhan Cafri
Iskenderun Technical University, Turkey

Pınar Kaya Samut
Atılım University, Turkey

ABSTRACT

As climate change threatens human life and health by causing severe storms, floods, temperature fluctuations and droughts, it is predicted that in the coming decades, most of the global population will be impacted and the lives of millions will be at risk. In this context, the article investigates the existence of a symmetric and asymmetric causality between climate change and health between 1990 and 2015 for European countries, including EU, EFTA member and EU candidate states. In the first stage of the analysis, health scores are estimated by cluster and discriminant analyses; in the second stage, the relationships among these scores and climate variables are examined. The country-specific findings are obtained for the health effects of climate change variables according to factors such as geographical structure and seasonal characteristics. According to the results, while the health effects of changes in temperature and greenhouse emissions differ from country to country, the reduction in precipitation for nearly half of the countries is found to have a negative effect on health.

INTRODUCTION

The adverse effects of the increasing world population and, consequently, increased human activity, in the environment have together caused global climate change, which has great ramifications for present and future generations. According to National Aeronautics and Space Administration (NASA) (2014), climate change is defined as the change in the normal temperature in a given period of time, or in the

DOI: 10.4018/978-1-5225-7635-8.ch011

amount of rain in a year. With the industrial revolution, increase in the greenhouse gases in the atmosphere and rising air pollution caused the world's average temperature to increase and rainfall patterns to change. Subsequently, an increasing trade volume through globalization continues to force countries to increase production, causing environmental pollution. As a result, this has become a factor included in all literature which addresses accelerating climate change (Idso & Idso, 2001; Vitousek, Mooney, Lubchenco, & Melillo, 1997; Zachos & Dickens, 2008). Due to damages as a result of global climate change, studies on the social and economic effects of this subject have started to draw attention. The fact that climate change threatens both present and future generations has raised a number of concerns. For this reason, this issue has been intensively discussed in national and international platforms. The concepts of growth and development, being previously among the main targets of economies, have been replaced by sustainable growth and development, and intensive studies have been initiated to improve the adaptation and resistance of a sustainable environment to climate change (Swart, Robinson, & Cohen, 2003; Soubbotina, 2004).

The concept of sustainability was introduced by the United Nations Environment and Development Commission's "Common Future" report published in 1987. According to this report, humanity has the capability of sustaining development by ensuring its daily needs, without jeopardizing the ability to respond to the future generations' needs (Brundtland, 1987). Besides this, sustainability is defined as ensuring the continuity of the diversity and productivity of biological systems according to the science of ecology. Climate change and disaster risk for sustainable improvement of life for future generations among sustainable development goals have been considered as one of the areas to be focused on mainly within the scope of strategic planning.

Climate change has environmental and socio-economic problems as well as direct and indirect effects on human life. These effects are caused by hot/cold air waves, air pollution, and allergens. On the other hand, the indirect effects of climate change, as a result of changes in the ecosystem, cause vectors to multiply or change in the habitat, resulting in infectious diseases such as malaria, tuberculosis, and AIDS. In addition, diseases such as dysentery, cholera, and typhoid are diseases that are indirectly caused by climate change. Besides, natural disasters such as rising water levels as a result of melting glaciers and hurricanes cause injuries and deaths. Moreover, these natural disasters can cause loss of production and hunger by deepening poverty due to economic loss. It is also stated that extreme weather affects people physically and weakens their psychological health (McMichael, 2013; Patz, Campbell-Lendrum, Holloway, & Foley, 2005; WHO, 2012).

While the impact of climate change on health is felt globally, different countries are experiencing these effects at different levels. According to the estimates of the World Health Organization, climate change is expected to negatively affect the lives and health of billions of people over the next decades. It is stated that climate change affects the most basic health needs such as clean air, safe water, sufficient food and adequate shelter. According to researches carried out by the World Health Organization, it is stated that exposure to air pollution causes heart and respiratory diseases, and also exposure to polluted air during pregnancy negatively affects infants' health (The European Economic Area (EAA), 2015). As a result of droughts caused by the increase in air temperatures and the decrease in rainfall, water, and food shortages are bound to occur. According to the studies on the effects of droughts, nutritional insufficiency, increased risk of infectious diseases, acute and chronic diseases that are increasing after inadequate and unclean water consumption are the main health problems caused by drought. Climate change is thought to affect food production especially in cereals. So, reducing the productivity of agriculture increases the risk of starvation and malnutrition, leading to infant and child deaths (McMichael & Haines, 1997).

In addition, drought caused by climate change is among the direct impacts that negatively affect health through food and water wars as a result of migration (Myers & Kent, 1995). Moreover, mosquitoes are susceptible to a series of vertebrate and invertebrate predators found in permanent water masses. Drought periods can eliminate predators from wetlands, resulting in safe havens for mosquitoes. It is claimed that mosquitoes can multiply and lead to infectious diseases (Landesman, Allan, Langerhans, Knight, & Chase, 2007). The long-term drought caused by extreme weather events is associated with mental problems and increases in people with mental disorders are among the estimates (Berry, Bowen, & Kjellstrom, 2010). Another point of view, excessive drought caused by fires may cause air pollutants and may cause respiratory distress (Epstein, 2001).

In the literature, generally, the studies about health are inclined to use life expectancy or mortality rates as indicators alongside carbon dioxide emission and average temperatures. Also, studies on the relationship between climate change and health are generally theoretically oriented or included only scenario analyses. In this study, different from these approaches, the effects of climate change on human health will be addressed in a comprehensive way by a variety of variables and detailed econometric analysis.

In this study, it is aimed to reveal the relationship between climate change and health for the period of 1990-2015 through symmetric and asymmetric causality analyses for the EU and EFTA states, all of which have a stronger and leading position in international efforts for climate change as a global problem, and the EU candidate countries. For this purpose, firstly the health indices of the countries will be established by Cluster and Discriminant analyses, and then the asymmetric causality between the obtained health scores and climate change variables will be examined. The rate of child mortality under the age of five, life expectancy, sanitation, and tuberculosis ratio will be used as health variables. Firstly, a dependent variable will be created by cluster analysis to form a health index consisting of these variables. For this, the European countries will be divided into two groups as healthy and healthier with the help of a Two-step Cluster analysis. By coding the countries as 1 and 2, for each year, the dependent variable of discriminant analysis will be obtained. By taking this dependent variable and four health variables as independent variables in the Discriminant Analysis, the health scores of the countries will be estimated for the period of 1990-2015.

At the second stage of the study, symmetric and asymmetric causality between the obtained health variable and the climate change variables will be analyzed by Hatemi-J Test. In the study, this causality relationship will be analyzed with six different variables that cause climate change, and the effects on human health will be examined one by one and in depth. One of the most important gases that cause climate change is carbon dioxide, which causes the greenhouse effect, resulting in temperature rises (Quadrelli & Peterson, 2007). Also, one of the air pollutants that adversely affect the environment and human health is nitrous oxide (N_2O), whose emission is also considered here. The environmental protection policies aimed at reforestation and increasing investments in renewable energy are known to mitigate the existing disadvantages. In this context, temperature averages and change, average precipitation, CO_2 emissions, N_2O emissions and renewable energy consumption will be taken into consideration for climate change. However, since the forest area in some countries has not changed or changed little for years, it can cause a near singular matrix problem, hence its exclusion from our analysis.

This study consists of six sections. The purpose and the importance of the study appear in the introduction. The literature on this subject is mentioned in section two. The next two sections introduce the data and method. Section five contains the findings, followed by the conclusions and political implications in section six.

LITERATURE REVIEW

In the early 1990s, studies on climate change and health were often discussed theoretically about the effects of climate change on potential health. One of these studies is the study on the health effects of ozone depletion. In this study, how the increases in ultraviolet radiation and climate change, which is exacerbated by human activities, triggers diseases such as skin cancer, respiratory disorders, infectious diseases, and allergy are explained (Longstreth, 1991). In another study, the effects of climate change on infectious diseases are discussed and it is emphasized that new and effective methods are needed for the control of vectors (Shope, 1991). In a study investigating the effects of climate change on malaria disease based on scenario analysis, it was concluded that the incidence of infection is susceptible to climate change in Africa regions where it is less endemic in Southeast Asia and South America (Martens, Niessen, Rotmans, Jetten, & McMichael, 1995). One of the basic studies on this subject is the study on the direct and indirect effects of climate change on health caused by greenhouse gases (McMichael & Haines, 1997). For the 45 major US cities, an analysis of the relationship between climate change and mortality rates, the study concluded that there was an increase in mortality rates for most cities. In addition, the study estimates a significant net increase in air-related mortality rates in the event of predicted warming by using models estimating climate change for 2020 and 2050 (Kalkstein & Greene, 1997).

In the greenhouse effect, the solar rays that heat the earth upon reflection are trapped by gases such as carbon dioxide, methane, and vapor. For this, such gases play a role in the warming of the earth by keeping the sun's heat within the atmosphere for a long time. Apart from such natural processes, the increase in greenhouse gases that occur as a result of human-induced activities exacerbates the effect. The largest share in the acceleration of this natural effect belongs to the energy sector with the use of fossil fuels. In addition to this, deforestation, industrial activity and uncontrolled urbanization increase the release of greenhouse gases in to the atmosphere (Idso & Idso, 2001). Eventually, this excess gas causes extreme weather events such as very high or low temperatures, torrential rain, floods, drought, and storms, all of which are clear signs of climate change.

Because climate change is an important risk factor in terms of human health, the issue has begun to attract attention in the literature. Climate change and health issues are often reported by international organizations such as World Health Organization (WHO) and the United Nations. In these reports, it is emphasized that the health effects of climate change will affect a majority of the world's population over the next decades and put the lives of millions of people at risk. Climate change affects human health directly and indirectly through a series of mechanisms.

While heat waves, physical hazards that occur as a result of the floods and storms, asthma, respiratory diseases and vectorial infectious diseases are among the direct effects, drought, agricultural malfunctions resulting in inadequate nutrition, conflicts over the depleting resources such as water, fisheries, fertile lands, and displacement of the population are among the indirect effects. It is emphasized that in long periods of drought, not only water shortage and food insufficiency but also as a result of increasing fire risks, immigration, lack of access to health services and increasing poverty are among the negative impacts on health. Besides, climate change will adversely affect normal human development by causing malnutrition and exposure to toxic contaminants in the prenatal period and childhood. It is noteworthy that water-borne diseases such as trachoma and scabies spread easily due to lack of hygiene during water-shortage periods, and that diarrhea in children under five also spikes as a result of water transportation from unsafe sources. (McMichael, Woodruff, & Hales, 2006; Portier et al., 2013; WHO, 2008; WHO, 2014)

It is suggested that climate change, which causes physical disturbances as well as extreme weather events, can cause chronic stress and mental disorders as a result of factors such as damage to property, loss of loved ones, and geographical shifts in populations. In addition, increased nighttime heat due to hot air waves and high humidity will cause bad sleep, triggering poor mental health. Moreover, mental disorders persist as psychoactive drugs become ineffective during heat waves (Portier et al., 2013; Berry, Waite, Dear, Capon, & Murray, 2018).

There are a limited number of empirical studies as well as reports and theoretical work by international organizations. Mostly, they examine the relation between temperature and mortality. It is emphasized that people in warmer cities are affected by cold weather, people in colder cities are influenced by hot weather, and that apart from the seasonal role of cold air, infections and hematological changes are more likely to occur among infants and the elderly.

In addition, it is stated that there is a "U" relationship between temperature and the mortality rate. Accordingly, when the temperature is at normal levels, the mortality rate is considered to be lower and stable, while this rate is higher when temperatures are above and below normal levels (McMichael et al., 2006). Supporting the "U" hypothesis, Rice (2003) emphasized that the presence of atmospheric carbon dioxide at 0.0037% (370 ppm) poses no threat to human health and has adverse effects at low or high concentrations. Sensitivity analysis in the study found that exposure to carbon dioxide above or below the normal rate poses a risk to particularly vulnerable people, and those who have hypertension, coronary artery disease and heart failure are endangered. Rooney et al. (1998) observed an increase of 8.9% in deaths due to temperature fluctuations and 38% in air pollution in their study of the effects of temperature fluctuations and air pollution on mortality in July and August 1995 in England and Wales. Extreme deaths were found in all age groups, but it was determined that the increase in mortality in women was related to cerebrovascular and respiratory infections.

In another study that tackles the relationship between temperature and mortality rates, these rates were estimated with regard to extreme temperatures in the summer of 1986-1987 in Madrid, especially in the age range of 65-74 and 74+ years by univariate and multivariate ARIMA models. The finding was that death rate increases by up to 28% for each degree above 36.5 °C, especially in 75+ women for circulatory failure reasons (Diaz et al., 2002).

Similarly, it is suggested that women are more likely to die as a result of natural disasters. Although such events impact all individuals, it was seen that on average in 141 countries women die more than men. This effect is stronger in countries where women have lower social, economic and political status, while it is almost equal in countries where women have a similar status to men (WHO, 2014).

Keatinge et al. (2000) examined the relationship between climate and mortality for people aged 65-74 years in Finland, Germany, the Netherlands, the United Kingdom, Italy, and Greece. The lowest temperature range in northern Finland is 14.3-17.3 °C, while in Athens it is 22.7-25.7 °C. It was also found that for all regions, deaths due to colds were higher than those due to temperature.

Healy (2002) also investigated the effect of extreme colds on mortality rates in the EU-14 region with Poisson regression, by associating it with housing, macroeconomic factors, lifestyle, socioeconomic status, and healthcare. The authors concluded that extreme cold increased mortality rates in Portugal, Spain, and Ireland. It has been suggested that these seasonal mortality rates can be reduced through the development of socio-economic factors such as the increase in health spending in public expenditures and the distribution of more equitable income.

In his study, Pope III et al. (2009) used life expectancy as well as the mortality rate as health variables and investigated the relation between air pollution and life expectancy in the 80s and 90s in the USA by regression analysis. As a result, a decrease in air pollution provided a 15% increase in life expectancy.

Pandey et al. (2005) investigated the effects of three air pollutants, suspended particulate matter (SPM), nitrogen dioxide (NO_2) and sulfur dioxide (SO_2) for Delhi on health risks of infants, children and adults and, as a result, they found that children are the most at risk due to air pollution and that nitrogen dioxide is the most effective air pollutant among the three.

The carbon dioxide released into the atmosphere is absorbed by the oceans and land. While the available studies are related to extreme weather events, Sirila et al. (2012) addressed water pollution in their work. The effects on human health are revealed by Monte-Carlo simulations. In addition, sensitivity analysis has revealed that a higher risk of carcinogen occurs as a result of adversely affecting the quality of drinking water. Patz (2002) argues that industrialized countries are using carbon capture and storage technologies to meet carbon reduction targets.

In this context, they compared the risk of death due to leakage in carbon dioxide storage areas and the risk of death in the absence of this technology. As a result, carbon dioxide storage sites have been found to have a lower risk of mortality than other natural or socially accepted risks, despite the risk of death from a possible leak. As a result of climate change, health is generally thought to be adversely affected in the literature. However, in some cases, it is suggested that climate change will have positive contributions to health. For example, in some places that are extremely cold, the air becomes more moderate and that's due to winter sickness decrease. Moreover, it is claimed that fewer pollens due to less production will lead to less asthma and allergens, and water-borne diseases will be reduced in places where heavy rainfall is reduced (McMichael et al., 2006).

DATA

In this study, for the purpose of analyzing the effects of climate change on health, four health and six climate variables were used. These variables are presented along with their definitions and measurement information in Table 1. The data was taken from the World Bank database (World Development Indicators) (The World Bank, 2014). The analysis was conducted between 1990 and 2015 for 35 European countries including 28 EU, 3 EFTA, and 4 EU candidate countries. While the sample includes all EU countries, Serbia and Montenegro from EU candidate countries and Liechtenstein from EFTA countries were excluded due to lack of data. The analyses cover 1990-2015 due to the availability of data, and the missing values for some countries going back 2 or 3 years were filled in by linear interpolation.

METHODOLOGY

Cluster and Discriminant Analyses

In the first stage of the study, health indices were generated with linear discriminant functions (DF) and dependent variables of DFs are defined by cluster analysis. Cluster analysis is a multivariate statistical technique that allows individuals to group by taking similarities into account and uses distance measures, correlation measures, or similarity measures of quality data to identify these similarities (Hair, Black,

Table 1. Model variables

	Definition	Measurement
Health indicators		
mortality	Mortality rate, under- 5	Per 1 000 live births
Life expect.	Life expectancy at birth	Total (years)
sanitation	Improved sanitation facilities	% of the population with access
tuberc	Incidence of tuberculosis	Per 100 000 people
Climate indicators		
CO_2	Carbon dioxide emissions	Metric tons per capita
temp.	Temperature averages	°C
tempdif	Temperature change	(Highest °C – lowest °C) during the year
prec	Average precipitation	In depth (mm per year)
N_2O	Nitrous oxide emissions	Thousand metric tons of CO_2 equivalent
renecon	Renewable energy consumption	% of total final energy consumption

Babin, & Anderson, 2010). It is expected that the homogeneity within the clusters formed in the cluster analysis and the heterogeneity between the clusters are high.

Cluster analysis is basically divided into two categories as hierarchical and non-hierarchical clustering. While in hierarchical clustering analysis the number of clusters occurs as the result of the analysis, in non-hierarchical clustering, it is determined from the beginning by researchers. Besides, in the hierarchical method, clustering is accomplished with the help of agglomerative or divisive method by using distance measures, whereas, in the case of hierarchical, grouping is performed by considering the within-cluster variance with K-means cluster method (Everitt, Landau, Leese, & Stahl, 2011).

In this study, a Two-stage cluster method which is a hybrid clustering technique formed by K-means and hierarchical methods is applied. In the first stage of the method, namely, pre-clustering step, observations are subdivided into smaller sub-clusters using a modified cluster features tree. In the second stage, called the clustering stage, each of these sub-clusters is defined as an initial cluster, and the clusters are combined until optimal clustering is achieved by agglomerative hierarchical clustering method (Bacher, Wenzig, & Vogler, 2004). The number of clusters can be determined by the researcher as well as by the model. In the Two-step cluster analysis, as the distance measure, log-likelihood or the Euclidean distance measure can be applied. Besides, The Schwarz's Bayesian information criterion (BIC) or the Akaike Information Criterion (AIC) is used to achieve optimal clusters. The relative contribution of the variables in the clusters is examined by the t-test for continuous variables and the chi-square ($\chi 2$) test for categorical variables (Rundle-Thiele, Kubacki, Tkaczynski, & Parkinson, 2015).

The European countries subjects to the present paper were separated into two clusters as healthy and less-healthy by Two-step cluster analysis and coded by 1 and 2 to form the dependent variable of the discriminant function. Discriminant analysis is a multivariate statistical method developed by R. A. Fisher in 1936. This powerful descriptive and classificatory technique multivariate statistical method is used to identify the factors that differentiate two or more pre-classified groups and to predict which group can be assigned upon observation from outside the group (Brown & Wicker, 2000). In discriminant analysis, a discriminant function composed of one dependent and one or more independent variable is estimated. The dependent variable should be measured on a categorical scale and the independent variables on a range or ratio scale. The discriminant function (DF) takes the following form (Hair et al., 2010):

$$Z_{ij} = a + W_1X_{1k} + W_2X_{2k} + \ldots + W_nX_{nk} \quad (1)$$

where

Z_{jk} = discriminant Z score of discriminant function j for object k
a = intercept
W_i = discriminant weight for independent variable i
X_{ik} = independent variable i for object k

While one DF is estimated for two categorical dependent variables, k-1 DFs are estimated for k grouped multiple discriminant analysis. The mathematical weights calculated for each discriminator variable are called 'discriminant coefficients' and indicate which variable is more discriminatory. The discriminant score for each function is calculated by multiplying each case's independent variable raw score and its coefficient. The average discriminant score of the cases belonging to a group represents the centroids of this group (Brown & Wicker, 2000).

Discriminant analysis has some assumptions such as multivariate normality, linearity, homogeneity of variance-covariance matrices, the absence of multicollinearity, and singularity (See for details: Tabachnick & Fidell, 2013). Multivariate normality of independent variables is testing by the Box's M test. The validity of the estimated DF is examined by Eigenvalue, Canonical Correlation and Wilk's Lambda values that give these ratios, and by Chi-Square Test which analyses the variability related to group differences. If the ratio of between-groups variability to within-group variability is high, this function is assumed as a successful and valid discriminant function (Sharma, 1996). In addition, classification accuracy is evaluated by hit rates and cross-validation. Hit ratio is calculated by dividing the number of correctly classified observations in each group by the total number of observations.

Panel Causality Tests

In the second stage of the study, the causal relationship between health and climate change is investigated using Two-step Cluster and Discriminant analyses - derived scores at the first stage. In order to apply causality analysis, it is necessary to determine the level of integration of the series (stationary levels) by unit root tests at first. However, second-generation unit root tests are used if there is cross-section dependency which means that a shock in one country affects other countries, and first-generation unit root tests are applied if such dependency does not exist. In this context, the cross- section dependency is tested by the CD test given in Equation 2, which is based on the sum of the correlation coefficients $\hat{p}_{ij}$ to determine which generation unit root tests should be applied.

$$CD = \sqrt{\frac{2T}{N(N-1)}} \left(\sum_{i=1}^{N-1} \sum_{J=i+1}^{N} \hat{p}_{ij} \right) \Rightarrow N(0,1) \quad (2)$$

According to the CD test, the H_0 hypothesis indicates that there is no relationship between cross sections, while the alternative hypothesis (H1) shows that there is a relationship (Pesaran, 2004).

The CADF test, a second-generation unit root test, which is applied to determine the level of integration or stationary levels of the variables and is valid under the cross- section dependency, is the extended version of the ADF regression calculated by considering the horizontal averages of first differences and the lag levels of each country. The regression model for CADF is:

$$\Delta y_{it} = a_i + b_i y_{i,t-1} + c_i \overline{y}_{t-1} + d_i \Delta \overline{y}_t + e_{it} \tag{3}$$

Here, the i index represents the cross-section (country), the index t is time and $\Delta y_{it} = y_{it} - y_{i,t-1}$.(Pesaran, 2007).

In the study, symmetric and asymmetric Hatemi-J Panel Causality Tests are applied in investigating the causality between the series. In the panel causality tests that give the general findings for all countries, the level values are included to the analysis when the variables are stationary (I(0)); the differences are included in the case of non-stationary (I(1)). On the other hand, heterogeneous panel causality test considers maximum stability levels.

The first causality test used in the literature is the Granger (1969) causality test. According to the definition of Granger causality, X is the Granger cause of Y, if the predictive values of Y obtained from the regression in which the past values of X are used as explanatory variables are more successful when compared to the case where the past values of X are not used (Granger, 1969). The series must be stable in Granger test. On the other hand, Toda-Yamamoto (1995) causality test generated after can be used without controlling the cointegration relationship both in the conditions of stable or non-stable. However, the important thing about this test is the lag numbers and the greatest degree of integration of the vector autoregressive model (VAR). However, Hacker and Hatemi-J (2006) has shown that the Toda-Yamamoto Test is not strong in small samples. For this reason, Hacker and Hatemi-J has developed a new method that includes the Bootstrap distribution in order to eliminate the weaknesses of the test. Yet, Toda-Yamamoto or Hacker and Hatemi-J (2006) tests accept the effects of positive and negative shock as identical. It was first proposed by Granger and Yoon (2002) that the effect of positive and negative shocks may be different and they examined the hidden co-integration relationship between the cumulative positive and negative components of the series. Inspired by this study, Hatemi-J (2012) investigated the causal relationship between negative and positive components of variables by developing Granger and Yoon's hidden co-integration analysis for causality analysis. In the light of this information, the causality between the negative and positive components of the variables representing climate indicators and health will be investigated by the Hatemi-J (2012) test.

For the Hatemi-J asymmetric causality analysis, the first step is to separate the variables into positive and negative components. To investigate the causal relationship between the two series as y_{1t} and y_{2t}, one can express $\varepsilon_{1i} = \varepsilon_{1i}^{+} + \varepsilon_{1i}^{-}$ and $\varepsilon_{2i} = \varepsilon_{2i}^{+} + \varepsilon_{2i}^{-}$.the components $\varepsilon_{1i}^{+} = \max\left(\varepsilon_{1i}, 0\right)$, $\varepsilon_{2i}^{+} = \max\left(\varepsilon_{2i}, 0\right)$, $\varepsilon_{1i}^{-} = \min\left(\varepsilon_{1i}, 0\right)$ and $\varepsilon_{2i}^{-} = \min\left(\varepsilon_{2i}, 0\right)$.are written as defined. Then, the negative and positive components are replaced instead of ε_{1t} and ε_{2t}:

$$y_{1t} = y_{1t-1} + \varepsilon_{1t} = y_{1,0} + \sum_{i=1}^{t} \varepsilon_{1i}^{+} + \sum_{i=1}^{t} \varepsilon_{1i}^{-}$$

$$y_{2t} = y_{2t-1} + \varepsilon_{2t} = y_{2,0} + \sum_{i=1}^{t} \varepsilon_{2i}^{+} + \sum_{i=1}^{t} \varepsilon_{2i}^{-} \tag{4}$$

Here, the positive and negative shocks of each variable are cumulatively expressed as $y_{1t}^{+} = \sum_{i=1}^{t} \varepsilon_{1i}^{+}$, $y_{1t}^{-} = \sum_{i=1}^{t} \varepsilon_{1i}^{-}$, $y_{2t}^{+} = \sum_{i=1}^{t} \varepsilon_{2i}^{+}$, and $y_{2t}^{-} = \sum_{i=1}^{t} \varepsilon_{2i}^{-}$. The causality relationship between the obtained positive and negative components is investigated by the Dumitrescu-Hurlin panel causality test (2012), which takes into account both heterogeneity and cross- section dependence and which can be used in the presence or absence of a cointegrated relationship. The basic hypothesis of the test is that there is no causality relation between the variables and the semi-asymptotic $\tilde{Z}_{N,T}^{HNC}$ statistic used in the case where the cross section size is larger than the time dimension is calculated as in Eq.5.

$$\tilde{Z}_{N,T}^{HNC} = \frac{\sqrt{N}\left[W_{N,T}^{HNC} - N^{-1}\sum_{i=1}^{N} E\left(W_{0,T}\right)\right]}{\sqrt{VarN^{-1}\sum_{i=1}^{N} Var\left(W_{0,T}\right)}} \tag{5}$$

Here, standardized $Z_{N,T}^{HNC}$ the statistic is obtained by $W_{N,T}^{HNC}$ panel statistic which is attained by taking the average of N units Wald $\left(W_{0,T}\right)$ statistics obtained from the Granger causality analysis calculated for each cross section unit.

Relevant statistics are calculated for the first, second and third lags, and it can be said to be causality when a statistically significant causality is attained for at least two lags (Dumitrescue & Hurlin, 2012).

The relationship between the statistically significant positive and negative components in the Dumitrescu-Hurlin panel causality analysis was analyzed by the Emirmahmutoğlu and Kose (EK) Panel Causality test which gives the causality results separately for each country. The EK panel causality test, which takes cross section dependency into account, can be used in the presence or absence of cointegration.

$$z_{i,t} = \mu_i + A_{i1} Z_{i,t-1} + \ldots + A_{ik} Z_{i,t-k_i} + \sum_{l=k_i+1}^{k_i + d\max_i} A_{il} Z_{i,t-1} + u_{i,t} \tag{6}$$

In the EK test statistic shown in Eq. 6, A_{ik} represents the parameter matrix, and $k_i + d\max_i$ (where k_i is the lag structure and $d\max_i$ is the maximal order of integration) indicates the maximum number of lags of the VAR model (Emirmahmutoglu & Kose, 2011).

EMPIRICAL RESULTS

This study investigates the asymmetric and symmetric causality between climate change and health. In the first stage of the study, the health indices of these countries are obtained by Two-Step Cluster and Discriminant analyses. In the second stage, the symmetric and asymmetric causality between these health scores and the climate change variables were analyzed. The results concerning these models appear in the following.

Obtaining Health Indices by Two-Step Cluster and Discriminant Analyses

At this stage, for 35 European countries, the health indexes for the years 1990-2015 are established. For this purpose, the rate of child mortality under the age of five, life expectancy, sanitation, and tuberculosis ratio were used as variables. Firstly, the countries were divided into two clusters as healthy and less healthy by Two-Step Cluster analysis, and by coding the countries as 1 and 2, the binary variables were attained for each year. These variables were taken as dependent variables in the Discriminant analysis, and then the health scores of each country for 1990-2015 were estimated.

In the Two-step Cluster method, the log-likelihood method is used as the distance measure and the BIC as the clustering criterion. Also, at the beginning of the process, the number of clusters was determined as 2. "Mortality" and "Tuberculosis" were taken after being converted to positive contributor variables, while "life expectancy" and "sanitation" were taken directly due to having a positive meaning by nature. The "mortality rate" values were transformed into the "survival rate" by subtracting from 1000 and the "incidence of tuberculosis" values were changed to "non-existence of tuberculosis incidents" by subtracting from 100 000. The generated variable was used as a dependent variable of the Discriminant Function (DF).

The DF established for health indicators is shown in Eq.7. The dependent variable of the function is a categorical variable obtained by the cluster analysis. On the other hand, the independent variables are the health variables measured on the ratio scale. These health variables were employed without any conversion because of the structure of the DF. By estimating the DF for each year, the health scores for 35 European countries for 1990-2015 were attained.

$$D = b_0 + b_1 X_1 + b_2 X_2 + b_3 X_3 + b_4 X_4 \tag{7}$$

$$\mathrm{D} = \begin{cases} 1, & healthy \\ 2, & less\,healthy \end{cases}$$

or

$$D = \begin{cases} 1, & less\, healthy \\ 2, & healthy \end{cases}$$

$X_1 : mortality; X_2 : life\ expect; X_3 : sanitiation; X_4 : tuberc.$

The validity of all estimated DFs was examined, with the result that they can all be used for prediction. Since the sample volume is larger than 30, it can be said that the sampling is normally distributed according to the Central Limit Theorem. To support this, the Box's M multiple normality test was performed and, although some functions have multiple normal distributions, some do not. For these, the individual normality of variables with Kolmogorov-Smirnov and Shapiro-Wilk tests was analyzed and the normality distributed finding was obtained in the majority.

The high ratio of between-groups variability to within-group variability indicates that DF is valid and has a high predictive power. To test the validity, Eigenvalue, Canonical Correlation, and Wilk's Lambda values were used, as well as Chi-Square test. The Wilk's λ values which give the ratio of the sum of squares within the group to the sum of the squares for all DFs are found close to 0. As a result of $\chi 2$ tests, the H_0 hypothesis was rejected. Thus, it is concluded that the discriminatory of the obtained functions is at a satisfactory level. In addition, the eigenvalues of the functions are sufficiently large and canonical correlation values are more than 0.70, supporting the validity of the DFs.

The predictive validity of DFs is tested with the accuracy of classification, and it is expected that the difference between the observed values and the estimated values is small. The degree of accordance of all estimated DFs ranged from 97.1% to 100%, which is the result of the consistency of the estimation results.

The health scores were estimated by the DFs of the European countries for 1990-2015, and these were used in the second stage to analyze the symmetric and asymmetric causal relationship between health and climate change. European countries were sorted according to their 25-year average score of health scores, and divided into two groups as healthy and less-healthy by general average (see the county groups in Table 2).

According to these results, the healthiest country is Switzerland, followed by Iceland and Sweden. The group of healthy countries consists of 17 EU countries and all the EFTA members. When the less-healthy countries group is concerned, it is seen that there are 11 EU countries with all of EU candidate and potential candidate countries. According to the 25-year average scores, the least healthy country is Latvia. When Latvia and Switzerland's 2015 health data are evaluated together, the difference between the health indicators of these countries are seen apparently. In 2015, Latvia and Switzerland have mortality rates of 7.9 and 4.1; life expectancy, 74.12 and 83.20; sanitation, 87.8 and 99.9, and tuberculous ratio, 41 and 7.3, respectively.

The Symmetric and Asymmetric Causality Between Health and Climate Change

After establishing the health index for the 1990-2015 for 35 countries, the causality between this index and the climate change indicators was tested. The cross-sectional dependency and the unit root test results from the preliminary tests to be performed before the transition to the causality analysis for symmetric variables, negative and positive components are given in Annex A, B, and C, respectively. As a result of the CD test, the presence of cross section dependency on all variables was determined. According to

Table 2. The healthy and less healthy countries

Healthy countries		Less Healthy countries	
Countries	**Scores**	**Countries**	**Scores**
Switzerland	1.23	Slovenia	-0.09
Iceland	1.14	Czech Republic	-0.42
Sweden	1.11	Bosnia and Herzegovina	-0.45
Italy	1.09	Albania	-0.48
Spain	1.03	Slovakia	-0.65
France	0.95	Croatia	-0.69
Norway	0.86	Macedonia. Rep. of	-0.74
Netherlands	0.78	Bulgaria	-0.83
Malta	0.77	Poland	-0.96
United Kingdom	0.71	Romania	-1.05
Belgium	0.65	Lithuania	-1.30
Austria	0.63	Hungary	-1.30
Cyprus	0.60	Estonia	-1.56
Greece	0.58	Turkey	-1.72
Germany	0.52	Latvia	-1.77
Luxembourg	0.43		
Finland	0.40		
Ireland	0.25		
Denmark	0.22		
Portugal	0.07		

the results of the unit root test, in the causality analysis of Dumitrescu-Hurlin, the difference of series is taken if the series is not stationary and the level of the series is taken if the series is stationary. Besides, in the EK heterogeneous causality analysis, the maximum integration ratios of the series have a great importance. Therefore, there is no need to take the difference of the series. Asymmetric relations are shown when variables are divided into positive and negative shocks; otherwise, it is referred symmetrical relations.

The symmetrical relationship is a causal relationship between two variables, but it does not show which component is affected by this component. Table 3 shows both symmetric and asymmetric causality results. Accordingly, it appears that there is a symmetric causality from carbon dioxide towards health. When we look at the asymmetric relationships, it is concluded that a positive shock from the amount of carbon dioxide is a cause for the positive shock to health. In addition, the presence of causality from a positive shock of carbon dioxide to a negative shock of health is detected. Here, the statistical significance of the Dumitrescu-Hurlin results $\left(\tilde{Z}_{N,T}^{HNC}\right)$ between the asymmetric shocks means that there is causality in at least one country.

There is causality from N_2O towards health, just like CO_2 towards health. It is seen that there are countries where the increase of N_2O affects health negatively, as well as countries which are effected positively.

Given the temperature increase, which is one of the most important indicators of climate change, the temperature averages, as well as temperature changes, are also included in the analyses as an important variable for the climate. In some countries, the increase in the difference between the hottest and the coldest of the year and the decline in some countries has been found to affect health negatively.

When the precipitation regimes are examined, it is found that positive shocks in some countries affect health positively, while in some countries negative shocks in the rainfall affect it negatively. Lastly, the health effects of the use of renewable energy sources consumption also differ from country to country. Positive shocks in the consumption of renewable energy sources in some countries are positively affecting health as expected. On the other hand, in some countries, negative shocks in the consumption of renewable energy sources are affecting health negatively, indicating that indirect use of other sources of energy has increased.

In Table 3, causality associations that are statistically significant do not show for which countries these relations are valid. If the results are statistically significant, then this relationship should be considered for at least one country; when it is meaningless, it shows that there is no causality relation for all countries.

Table 3. The result of symmetric and asymmetric panel causality test

Hypothesis	$\tilde{Z}^{HNC}_{N,T}$ (lag=1)	$\tilde{Z}^{HNC}_{N,T}$ (lag=2)	$\tilde{Z}^{HNC}_{N,T}$ (lag=3)
$H_0: \Delta CO_2 \neq> \text{Health}$	0.513	4.136***	2.799***
$H_0: \Delta CO_2^+ \neq> \text{Health}^+$	-2.002**	4.091***	1.788*
$H_0: \Delta CO_2^- \neq> \text{Health}^-$	0.197	-0.377	1.541
$H_0: \Delta CO_2^+ \neq> \text{Health}^-$	14.953***	9.039***	7.189***
$H_0: \Delta N_2O \neq> \text{Health}$	4.612***	6.929***	2.689***
$H_0: \Delta N_2O^+ \neq> \text{Health}^+$	-1.510	-2.159**	-1.988**
$H_0: \Delta N_2O^- \neq> \text{Health}^-$	2.501**	1.891*	0.497
$H_0: \Delta N_2O^+ \neq> \text{Health}^-$	9.793***	5.574***	3.616***
$H_0: \text{temp} \neq> \text{Health}$	2.627***	2.843***	0.899

continued on following page

Table 3. Continued

Hypothesis	$\tilde{Z}_{N,T}^{HNC}$ (lag=1)	$\tilde{Z}_{N,T}^{HNC}$ (lag=2)	$\tilde{Z}_{N,T}^{HNC}$ (lag=3)
$H_0 : \Delta temp^{+} \neq> Health^{+}$	3.873***	0.193	-1.879*
$H_0 : \Delta temp^{-} \neq> Health^{-}$	-1.222	-1.246	-1.731*
$H_0 : \Delta temp^{+} \neq> Health^{-}$	-1.597	-2.704***	-3.274***
$H_0 : tempdif \neq> Health$	-1.817*	-2.673***	-2.359**
$H_0 : \Delta tempdif^{+} \neq> Health^{+}$	-1.571	-1.877*	-1.572
$H_0 : \Delta tempdif^{-} \neq> Health^{-}$	-1.804*	-1.108	2.392**
$H_0 : \Delta tempdif^{+} \neq> Health^{-}$	19.991***	13.867***	9.234***
$H_0 : prec \neq> Health$	1.052	0.934	0.757
$H_0 : \Delta prec^{+} \neq> Health^{+}$	13.102***	11.942***	7.996***
$H_0 : \Delta prec^{-} \neq> Health^{-}$	4.797***	2.665***	5.073***
$H_0 : \Delta prec^{+} \neq> Health^{-}$	-0.688	0.022	2.616***
$H_0 : renecon \neq> Health$	7.123***	6.207***	6.054***
$H_0 : \Delta renecon^{+} \neq> Health^{+}$	8.542***	6.608***	5.483***
$H_0 : \Delta renecon^{-} \neq> Health^{-}$	21.041***	12.416***	8.353***
$H_0 : \Delta renecon^{+} \neq> Health^{-}$	-0.145	1.511	1.989*

Note: *, **, *** refer to a significance level of 10%, 5% and 1%, respectively.

Heterogeneous panel causality analysis was conducted to determine in which countries there exits statistically significant causality. Concerning this, the results are given in Table 4.

Countries in which a positive shock from CO_2 emissions, one of the important indicators suggested to cause climate change, have identified a causality towards a positive shock of health are Czech Republic, Lithuania, Malta, Romania, Turkey, Switzerland. In the literature, it is suggested that higher income people are healthier because they have better nutrition and better quality healthcare (Lorentzen et al., 2008; Pritchett & Summers, 1993). In this framework, it is considered that the increase in CO_2 emis-

Table 4. The countries according to the asymmetric causality results

Causality	Countries
$\Delta CO_2^+ \neq>$ Health$^+$	Czech Republic, Lithuania, Malta, Romania, Turkey, Switzerland
$\Delta CO_2^+ \neq>$ Health$^-$	Bulgaria, Croatia, Czech Republic, Germany, Romania, Slovakia
$\Delta N_2O^+ \neq>$ Health$^+$	Malta, Albania
$\Delta N_2O^- \neq>$ Health$^-$	Belgium, Croatia, Cyprus, Estonia, Ireland, Italy, Lithuania, Macedonia, Poland, Portugal, Spain, Albania, Norway
$\Delta N_2O^+ \neq>$ Health$^-$	Austria, Estonia, Albania
Δtemp$^+ \neq>$ Health$^+$	Belgium, Denmark, Finland, France, Germany, Hungary, Ireland, Italy, Luxembourg, Netherlands, Sweden, United Kingdom, Norway
Δtemp$^+ \neq>$ Health$^-$	Austria, Latvia, Lithuania
Δtempdif$^- \neq>$ Health$^-$	Finland, France, Luxembourg, Malta, Norway, Switzerland
Δtempdif$^+ \neq>$ Health$^-$	Austria, Croatia, Cyprus, Estonia, Hungary, Italy, Malta, Slovakia, Turkey
Δprec$^+ \neq>$ Health$^+$	Hungary, Ireland, Iceland, Norway
Δprec$^- \neq>$ Health$^-$	Croatia, Estonia, Finland, Greece, Hungary, Latvia, Lithuania, Macedonia, Malta, Poland, Portugal, Romania, Slovakia, Spain, Bosnia and Herzegovina, Albania
Δrenecon$^+ \neq>$ Health$^+$	Greece, Ireland, Macedonia, Netherlands, Slovenia
Δrenecon$^- \neq>$ Health$^-$	Bulgaria, Croatia, Cyprus, Denmark, Macedonia, Romania, Bosnia and Herzegovina

sions for these countries positively affects health by increasing income because of the increase in per capita income and the better health together with increasing income in parallel with the increase in growth and employment. Again from this point, the countries where the increase in nitrous oxide, measured as the equivalent of carbon emissions, has a positive effect on health through income-increasing effect are Malta and Albania.

Bulgaria, Croatia, Czech Republic, Germany, Romania, Slovakia are among the countries where the increase in CO_2 emissions affects the health negatively. In the meantime, Austria, Estonia, and Albania are the countries where the increase in nitrous oxide affects health negatively, the countries where the negative shocks on nitrous oxide negatively affect health are Belgium, Croatia, Estonia, Ireland, Italy, Lithuania, Macedonia, Poland, Portugal, Spain, Albania, Norway. For Estonia and Albania, it is seen that the increase or decrease of nitrous oxide affects health negatively. It is noted that both countries are in less healthy group countries as a result of cluster analysis. This indicates that the increase in N_2O may reduce winter sickness due to the increase in temperature, or that it may positively affect health as it is an income-enhancing factor. At the same time, it also affects health negatively in terms of causing air pollution. It shows that both effects are strong, both positive and negative.

When you look at the results related to temperature, countries where the increase in temperature affects health positively are Belgium, Denmark, Finland, France, Germany, Hungary, Ireland, Italy, Luxembourg, Netherlands, Sweden, United Kingdom, Norway. On the other hand, among the countries where the increase in temperature affects health negatively, there are countries like Austria, Latvia, and Lithuania.

Austria, Croatia, Cyprus, Estonia, Hungary, Italy, Malta, Slovakia and Turkey are the countries where the increase in temperature differences affects health negatively, while in Croatia, Estonia, Finland, Greece, Hungary, Latvia, Lithuania, Macedonia, Malta, Poland, Portugal, Romania, Slovakia, Spain, Bosnia and Herzegovina, and Albania the negative shocks in the precipitation, that is, the decrease, affects health negatively. It is noted that the increase or decrease in the difference between the coldest and the hottest, that is, temperature fluctuation, negatively affect Malta's health. In terms of precipitation regimes, while the increase in average precipitation in Hungary had a positive effect on health, it was found that the negative shocks in precipitation affected health adversely.

The countries where the increase in the consumption of renewable energy sources affects health positively are Greece, Ireland, Macedonia, Netherlands, and Slovenia. Besides, Bulgaria, Croatia, Cyprus, Denmark, Macedonia, Romania, Bosnia and Herzegovina are the countries where negative impacts on the consumption of renewable energy sources affect health adversely.

FUTURE RESEARCH DIRECTIONS

The rise in the temperature, the change in temperature differences and the variation of precipitation regimes usually come to mind when speaking of climate change. Generally, it is often argued that the factors behind these changes are the increase in carbon dioxide, methane, and nitrous oxide gases. However, according to the results obtained in the paper, in some countries, these gases contribute to health positively because they increase the income. In this study, the findings were obtained by taking countries as panels. Therefore, as the general average of countries is taken into account, concentrations of changes in temperature or precipitation changes or emissions increases are ignored in certain regions of the country. In the future studies, micro-based and country-specific research is recommended for remarkable results in the analyses. Factors that reflect climate change such as temperature, emissions, and precipitation regimes are phenomena that cannot be determined according to the sharp borders of the cities and states of the countries and, therefore, there is also the issue of spatiality in such a context. As a result, it is recommended to also incorporate the spatial effect into econometric analyses in future studies.

CONCLUSION

In this study, the effects of climate change on health were investigated for 35 European countries between 1990 and 2015. In the first stage, whether the countries are healthy or not are determined by using cluster analysis method. Later, the scores belonging to these variables were determined by discriminant analysis. Thus, health variables were created for each country. According to the results obtained, it is determined that the countries which are in the best condition of health are Switzerland, Iceland, and Sweden. It is noteworthy that there are 17 EU countries and all EFTA countries in the healthier country cluster. Eleven EU countries and all candidate countries are found to be in the less healthy country group.

Climate change was measured by greenhouse gas, temperatures, and the average precipitation. In addition, renewable energy consumption has also been taken into account on the assumption that the use of renewable energy sources, rather than fossil fuel use, could reduce greenhouse gas emissions and, thus, mitigate the adverse effects of climate change.

The causality between each variable representing climate change and the health variable was first obtained for all countries by the causality analysis. According to the results of asymmetric causality analysis, the increase in greenhouse gas emissions in some countries adversely affects health. In some countries, there were also results that indirectly affect health due to an increase in income or a reduction in winter sickness by moderating air. Similar to the effect of greenhouse gases, causalities from positive shocks of temperatures to positive and negative shocks of health vary depending on the country. Regarding the temperature changes, a causality from the negative or positive shocks of the difference between the coldest and the hottest during the year towards the negative shocks of health was obtained. This result supports the finding that cold or hot extreme weather events affect health in a negative way. Although there is no significant symmetric causality relationship between mean precipitation and health, there is a hidden causality relation. Positive shocks in precipitation have a positive effect on health in some regions, while it is concluded that in some regions it has a negative effect on health. Regarding renewable energy, it is seen that asymmetrically there is a positive contribution to health in any case. While positive shocks that occur from renewable energy consumption are determined as a causation towards the positive shocks of health, negative shocks that occur from renewable energy consumption are determined as a causation towards the negative shocks of health.

Among the findings of heterogeneous causality, it is found that carbon dioxide emission in Switzerland, which is the healthiest country, affects health positively and a decrease of the differences between the temperatures affects health negatively. Latvia, which is the least healthy country, found that the increase in temperatures and the decrease in precipitation negatively affected health.

As a result, the reflections of climate change on health differ from country to country. In this context, it is important to identify the biological sensitivities, socio-economic situation, cultural adequacy and structure, and population which is more vulnerable in order to minimize the negative impacts of climate change on health and to provides appropriate healthcare support.

It is known that transportation takes up an important share of human-induced greenhouse gas emissions. Reducing these emissions is expected to affect health in a positive way with a reduction in air pollution. Human health will be positively impacted in relation to air quality, with less dependence on personal vehicles, the use of public transport or cycling, or preferring to walk certain distances. Besides, it is thought that it will be effective in decreasing the mortality rate with fewer traffic accidents and increasing physical activity by walking, cycling and fighting obesity.

Renewable energy sources seem to have a great potential to mitigate the negative impacts of climate change on health. It would be appropriate for countries to invest in a variety of renewable energy sources, such as bioenergy, geothermal energy, direct solar energy, geothermal energy, and ocean or wind energy. However, since renewable energy sources have high costs in the first stage, fossil fuel consumption is preferred. On the other hand, the transition to sustainable energy sources is important in order to reduce the negative impact on the environment and human health. In this context, the development of technologies to reduce the costs of renewable energy sources should be encouraged.

REFERENCES

Bacher, J., Wenzig, K., & Vogler, M. (2004). SPSS twoStep cluster - a first evaluation. In *RC33 Sixth International Conference on Social Science Methodology: "Recent Developments and Applications in Social Research Methodology,"* Amsterdam, The Netherlands.

Berry, H. L., Bowen, K., & Kjellstrom, T. (2010). Climate change and mental health: A causal pathways framework. *International Journal of Public Health, 55*(2), 123–132. doi:10.100700038-009-0112-0 PMID:20033251

Berry, H. L., Waite, T. D., Dear, K. B., Capon, A. G., & Murray, V. (2018). The case for systems thinking about climate change and mental health. *Nature Climate Change, 8*(4), 282–290. doi:10.103841558-018-0102-4

Brown, M. T., & Wicker, L. R. (2000). Discriminant analysis. In H.E.A. Tinsley & S.D. Brown (Eds.), handbook of applied multivariate statistics and mathematical modeling (Ch. 8, pp. 209-235). London, UK: Academic Press.

Brundtland, G. H. (1987). *Our Common Future. World Commission on Environment and Development.* Oxford: Oxford University Press.

Díaz, J., Jordan, A., García, R., López, C., Alberdi, J., Hernández, E., & Otero, A. (2002). Heat waves in Madrid 1986–1997: Effects on the health of the elderly. *International Archives of Occupational and Environmental Health, 75*(3), 163–170. doi:10.100700420-001-0290-4 PMID:11954983

Dumitrescu, E. I., & Hurlin, C. (2012). Testing for Granger non-causality in heterogeneous panels. *Economic Modelling, 29*(4), 1450–1460. doi:10.1016/j.econmod.2012.02.014

EAA. (2015). Air Quality in Europe – *2015 Report.* Retrieved from https://www.eea.europa.eu/publications/air-quality-in-europe-2015

Emirmahmutoglu, F., & Kose, N. (2011). Testing for granger causality in heterogeneous mixed panels. *Economic Modelling, 28*(3), 870–876. doi:10.1016/j.econmod.2010.10.018

Epstein, P. R. (2001). Climate change and emerging infectious diseases. *Microbes and Infection, 3*(9), 747–754. doi:10.1016/S1286-4579(01)01429-0 PMID:11489423

Everitt, B. S., Landau, S., Leese, M., & Stahl, D. (2011). *Cluster analysis* (5th ed.). United Kingdom: John Wiley & Sons, Ltd. doi:10.1002/9780470977811

Fisher, R. A. (1936). The use of multiple measurements in taxonomic problems. *Annals of Human Genetics, 7*(2), 179–188.

Ghai, D., & Vivian, J. M. (2014). *Grassroots environmental action: people's participation in sustainable development.* Routledge.

Granger, C. W. J. (1969). Investigating causal relations by econometric models and cross spectral methods. *Econometrica, 37*(3), 424–438. doi:10.2307/1912791

Granger, C. W. J., & Yoon, G. (2002). *Hidden cointegration*. University of California.

Hacker, R. S., & Hatemi-J, A. (2006). Tests for causality between integrated variables using asymptotic and bootstrap distributions: Theory and application. *Applied Economics*, *38*(13), 1489–1500. doi:10.1080/00036840500405763

Hair, J. F., Black, W. C., Babin, B. J., & Anderson, R. E. (2010). *Multivariate data analysis: A global perspective*. New Jersey: Pearson.

Hatemi-J, A. (2012). Asymmetric causality tests with an application. *Empirical Economics*, *43*(1), 447–456. doi:10.100700181-011-0484-x

Healy, J. D. (2003). Excess winter mortality in Europe: A cross country analysis identifying key risk factors. *Journal of Epidemiology and Community Health*, *57*(10), 784–789. doi:10.1136/jech.57.10.784 PMID:14573581

Idso, S. B., & Idso, K. E. (2001). Effects of atmospheric CO_2 enrichment on plant constituents related to animal and human health. *Environmental and Experimental Botany*, *45*(2), 179–199. doi:10.1016/S0098-8472(00)00091-5 PMID:11275225

Kalkstein, L. S., & Greene, J. S. (1997). An evaluation of climate/mortality relationships in large US cities and the possible impacts of a climate change. *Environmental Health Perspectives*, *105*(1), 84–93. doi:10.1289/ehp.9710584 PMID:9074886

Keatinge, W. R., Donaldson, G. C., Cordioli, E., Martinelli, M., Kunst, A. E., Mackenbach, J. P., ... Vuori, I. (2000). Heat related mortality in warm and cold regions of Europe: Observational study. *BMJ (Clinical Research Ed.)*, *321*(7262), 670–673. doi:10.1136/bmj.321.7262.670 PMID:10987770

Landesman, W. J., Allan, B. F., Langerhans, R. B., Knight, T. M., & Chase, J. M. (2007). Inter-annual associations between precipitation and human incidence of West Nile virus in the United States. *Vector Borne and Zoonotic Diseases (Larchmont, N.Y.)*, *7*(3), 337–343. doi:10.1089/vbz.2006.0590 PMID:17867908

Longstreth, J. (1991). Anticipated public health consequences of global climate change. *Environmental Health Perspectives*, *96*, 139–144. doi:10.1289/ehp.9196139 PMID:1820256

Lorentzen, P., McMillan, J., & Wacziarg, R. (2008). Death and development. *Journal of Economic Growth*, *13*(2), 81–124. doi:10.100710887-008-9029-3

Martens, W. J., Niessen, L. W., Rotmans, J., Jetten, T. H., & McMichael, A. J. (1995). Potential impact of global climate change on malaria risk. *Environmental Health Perspectives*, *103*(5), 458–464. doi:10.1289/ehp.95103458 PMID:7656875

McMichael, A. J. (2013). Globalization, climate change, and human health. *The New England Journal of Medicine*, *368*(14), 1335–1343. doi:10.1056/NEJMra1109341 PMID:23550671

McMichael, A. J., & Haines, A. (1997). Global climate change: The potential effects on health. *BMJ: British Medical Journal*, *315*(7111), 805–809. doi:10.1136/bmj.315.7111.805 PMID:9345177

McMichael, A. J., Woodruff, R. E., & Hales, S. (2006). Climate change and human health: Present and future risks. *Lancet*, *367*(9513), 859–869. doi:10.1016/S0140-6736(06)68079-3 PMID:16530580

Myers, N., & Kent, J. (1995). *Environmental exodus: an emergent crisis in the global arena*. New York: Climate Institute.

NASA. (2014). What is climate change? Retrieved from https://www.nasa.gov/audience/forstudents/k-4/stories/nasa-knows/what-is-climate-change-k4.html

Pandey, J. S., Kumar, R., & Devotta, S. (2005). Health risks of NO2, SPM and SO_2 in Delhi (India). *Atmospheric Environment*, *39*(36), 6868–6874. doi:10.1016/j.atmosenv.2005.08.004

Patz, J. A. (2002). A human disease indicator for the effects of recent global climate change. *Proceedings of the National Academy of Sciences of the United States of America*, *99*(20), 12506–12508. doi:10.1073/pnas.212467899 PMID:12271143

Patz, J. A., Campbell-Lendrum, D., Holloway, T., & Foley, J. A. (2005). Impact of regional climate change on human health. *Nature*, *438*(7066), 310–317. doi:10.1038/nature04188 PMID:16292302

Pesaran, H. M. (2007). A Simple Panel Unit Root Test in the Presence of Cross Section Dependence. *Journal of Applied Econometrics*, *22*(2), 265–312. doi:10.1002/jae.951

Pesaran, M. H. (2004). General Diagnostic Tests for Cross Section Dependence in Panels. *CESifo*. Retrieved from https://ssrn.com/abstract=572504

Pope, C. A. III, Ezzati, M., & Dockery, D. W. (2009). Fine-particulate air pollution and life expectancy in the United States. *The New England Journal of Medicine*, *360*(4), 376–386. doi:10.1056/NEJMsa0805646 PMID:19164188

Portier, C. J., Tart, K. T., Carter, S. R., Dilworth, C. H., Grambsch, A. E., Gohlke, J., ... Maslak, T. (2013). A human health perspective on climate change: A report outlining the research needs on the human health effects of climate change. *Journal of Current Issues in Globalization*, *6*(4), 621–710.

Pritchett, L., & Summers, L. H. (1993). *Wealthier is healthier* (Vol. 1150). World Bank Publications.

Quadrelli, R., & Peterson, S. (2007). The energy–climate challenge: Recent trends in CO_2 emissions from fuel combustion. *Energy Policy*, *35*(11), 5938–5952. doi:10.1016/j.enpol.2007.07.001

Rice, S. A. (2003). Health effects of acute and prolonged CO2 exposure in normal and sensitive populations. In *Second Annual Conference on Carbon Sequestration* (pp. 5-8).

Rooney, C., McMichael, A. J., Kovats, R. S., & Coleman, M. P. (1998). Excess mortality in England and Wales, and in Greater London, during the 1995 heatwave. *Journal of Epidemiology and Community Health*, *52*(8), 482–486. doi:10.1136/jech.52.8.482 PMID:9876358

Rundle-Thiele, S., Kubacki, K., Tkaczynski, A., & Parkinson, J. (2015). Using two-step cluster analysis to identify homogeneous physical activity groups. *Marketing Intelligence & Planning*, *33*(4), 522–537. doi:10.1108/MIP-03-2014-0050

Sharma, S. (1996). *Applied multivariate techniques*. USA: John Wiley & Sons.

Shope, R. (1991). Global climate change and infectious diseases. *Environmental Health Perspectives*, *96*, 171–174. doi:10.1289/ehp.9196171 PMID:1820262

Siirila, E. R., Navarre-Sitchler, A. K., Maxwell, R. M., & McCray, J. E. (2012). A quantitative methodology to assess the risks to human health from CO_2 leakage into groundwater. *Advances in Water Resources*, *36*, 146–164. doi:10.1016/j.advwatres.2010.11.005

Soubbotina, T. P. (2004). *Beyond Economic Growth: An Introduction to Sustainable Development* (2nd ed.). Washington, DC: World Bank. doi:10.1596/0-8213-5933-9

Swart, R., Robinson, J., & Cohen, S. (2003). Climate change and sustainable development: Expanding the options. *Climate Policy*, *3*, S19–S40. doi:10.1016/j.clipol.2003.10.010

Tabachnick, B. G., & Fidell, L. S. (2013). *Using multivariate statistics* (6th ed.). USA: Pearson Education.

Toda, H. Y., & Yamamoto, T. (1995). Statistical inference in vector autoregressions with possibly integrated processes. *Journal of Econometrics*, *66*(12), 225–250. doi:10.1016/0304-4076(94)01616-8

Vitousek, P. M., Mooney, H. A., Lubchenco, J., & Melillo, J. M. (1997). Human domination of Earth's ecosystems. *Science*, *277*(5325), 494–499. doi:10.1126cience.277.5325.494

World Health Organization (WHO). (2008). *Climate change and health*. Retrieved from http://www.who.int/iris/handle/10665/126809

World Health Organization (WHO). (2012). *Atlas of health and climate*. Retrieved from http://www.who.int/globalchange/publications/atlas/en/

World Health Organization (WHO). (2014). *Gender, climate change and health*. Retrieved from http://www.who.int/globalchange/publications/reports/gender_climate_change/en/

Zachos, J. C., Dickens, G. R., & Zeebe, R. E. (2008). An early cenozoic perspective on greenhouse warming and carbon-cycle dynamics. *Nature*, *451*(7176), 279–283. doi:10.1038/nature06588 PMID:18202643

ADDITIONAL READING

Allende, A., Marín, A., Buendía, B., Tomás-Barberán, F., & Gil, M. I. (2007). Impact of combined postharvest treatments (UV-C light, gaseous O_3, superatmospheric O_2 and high CO_2) on health promoting compounds and shelf-life of strawberries. *Postharvest Biology and Technology*, *46*(3), 201–211. doi:10.1016/j.postharvbio.2007.05.007

Demetriades, J., & Esplen, E. (2008). The gender dimensions of poverty and climate change adaptation. *IDS Bulletin*, *39*(4), 24–31. doi:10.1111/j.1759-5436.2008.tb00473.x

Fankhauser, S., & McDermott, T. K. (Eds.). (2016). *The Economics of Climate-Resilient Development*. Edward Elgar Publishing. doi:10.4337/9781785360312

Flynn, J., Slovic, P., & Mertz, C. K. (1994). Gender, race, and perception of environmental health risks. *Risk Analysis*, *14*(6), 1101–1108. doi:10.1111/j.1539-6924.1994.tb00082.x PMID:7846319

Fröhlich-Nowoisky, J., Kampf, C. J., Weber, B., Huffman, J. A., Pöhlker, C., Andreae, M. O., ... Su, H. (2016). Bioaerosols in the Earth system: Climate, health, and ecosystem interactions. *Atmospheric Research*, *182*, 346–376. doi:10.1016/j.atmosres.2016.07.018

Hallegatte, S., & Rozenberg, J. (2017). Climate change through a poverty lens. *Nature Climate Change*, *7*(4), 250–256. doi:10.1038/nclimate3253

Mearns, R., & Norton, A. (Eds.). (2009). *Social dimensions of climate change: equity and vulnerability in a warming world*. World Bank Publications.

Ruosteenoja, K., Carter, T. R., Jylhä, K., & Tuomenvirta, H. (2003). *Future climate in world regions: an intercomparison of model-based projections for the new IPCC emissions scenarios*. Helsinki: Finn. Environ. Inst.

Selvey, L. A. (2015). Climate change is harmful to our health: Taking action will have many benefits. *The Medical Journal of Australia*, *203*(10), 397–398. doi:10.5694/mja15.00655 PMID:26561899

KEY TERMS AND DEFINITIONS

Causality: To give statistically significant information on a time series values about the future values of another time series.

Cluster Analyses: A multivariate statistical analysis method that groups individuals or objects according to their common characteristics.

Cross-Section Dependence: The situation of a shock coming from a horizontal section that affects other horizontal sections as well.

Discriminant Analyses: A multivariate statistical method which is used to identify the factors that differentiate two or more pre-classified groups by estimating a function.

Ecosystem: Interactions between living things and the inanimate environment surrounding them.

Renewable Energy: The energy continuously obtainable from the sources in nature, such as the wind and the sun.

Sanitation: Measures taken to maintain hygiene and healthy environment.

Sustainable Development: Without harming natural resources, to ensure economic growth by protecting the environment and fight against poverty.

Unit Root Test: A test for determining whether the mean, variance and covariance of a time series are independent of time.

Vectors: The living creatures which reserve and carry organisms that cause the diseases without harming the carrier.

APPENDIX

Table 5. Annex A

Variable	CD_{LM} stat.	CADF (Level)	CADF (1. Difference)	Degree Of Integration
health	5.72 (0.000)	-3.243 (-2.16)	....	I(0)
CO_2	30.90 (0.000)	-2.639 (-2.65)	-5.312 (-2.65)	I(1)
N_2O	38.42 (0.000)	-1.967 (-2.65)	-4.831 (-2.65)	I(1)
temp	65.37 (0.000)	-4.260 (-2.65)	....	I(0)
tempdif	39.10 (0.000)	-4.808 (-2.16)	....	I(0)
prec	18.12 (0.000)	-4.297 (-2.16)	....	I(0)
renecon	66.67 (0.000)	-2.716 (-2.65)	....	I(0)

Note: Below the CD statistic are the probability values and below the CADF t-bar statistics are 5% critical values.

Table 6. Annex B

Variable	CD_{LM} stat.	CADF (Level)	CADF (1. Difference)	Degree Of Integration
$health^-$	115.67 (0.000)	-2.905 (0.002)	....	I(0)
CO_2^-	100.11 (0.000)	0.436 (0.669)	-11.621 (0.000)	I(1)
N_2O^-	109.62 (0.000)	0.629 (0.735)	-4.962 (0.000)	I(1)
$temp^-$	118.08 (0.000)	2.521 (0.994)	-8.890 (0.000)	I(1)
$tempdif^-$	118.70 (0.000)	0.678 (0.751)	-10.507 (0.000)	I(1)
$prec^-$	118.04 (0.000)	0.445 (0.672)	-6.083 (0.000)	I(1)
$renecon^-$	103.27 (0.000)	-1.850 (0.032)	....	I(0)

Note: Below the CD statistic are probability values and below the CADF standardized Ztbar statistics for negative components are the p-values.

Table 7. Annex C

Variable	CD_{LM} stat.	CADF (Level)	CADF (1. Difference)	Degree Of Integration
$health^+$	116.83 (0.000)	-2.712 (0.003)	....	I(0)
CO_2^+	104.13 (0.000)	1.899 (0.971)	-9.099 (0.000)	I(1)
N_2O^+	108.25 (0.000)	-0.858 (0.195)	-6.942 (0.000)	I(1)
$temp^+$	119.22 (0.000)	0.895 (0.815)	-8.301 (0.000)	I(1)
$tempdif^+$	117.84 (0.000)	-0.585 (0.279)	-10.065 (0.000)	I(1)
$prec^+$	109.98 (0.000)	-0.167 (0.434)	-5.181 (0.000)	I(1)
$renecon^+$	112.55 (0.000)	0.396 (0.654)	-9.001 (0.000)	I(1)

Note: Below the CD statistic are probability values and below the CADF standardized Ztbar statistics for positive components are the p-values.

Section 2

Social and Political Aspects of Environmental Health

Chapter 12
Agbiotech, Sustainability, and Food Security Connection to Public Health

Ike Valentine Iyioke
Michigan State University, USA

ABSTRACT

Supporters of agricultural biotechnology have maintained a high enthusiasm for its role in improving agricultural yields and enhancing sustainability, for instance, in Africa. However, critics are deeply skeptical. This chapter sketches some of the main arguments on both sides to provide a summary analysis. The discussion includes multiple climatic, socioeconomic, and public policy drivers that have collided with the ability of the average person to achieve food security. If food security is to be understood as a matter of human health, then its definitions and designs must recognize food's many roles in creating positive public health outcomes. Hence, the discussion expands to include an integrative model of food security linking sociocultural, public policy, and ecological aspects to public health. The chapter concludes that extensive work must be done to steer policy initiatives toward common sense sustainability paths to achieve food security and/or sovereignty.

INTRODUCTION

Food—how it is produced, stored, processed, distributed, and consumed—has posed challenges throughout human history. After air, water and food are next in importance for human existence. In a world split between resource-rich and resource-poor nations, it is difficult to ensure a sufficient, safe, and nutritious food supply. The polarity of impact only gets more pronounced when the focus shifts to considerations for income and wealth inequality and with social exclusion and disadvantages (Burns, 2004). While many rich nations experience their version of food (in)security (rather than food's availability), poor nations are inundated with a host of unmet targets from production to consumption. Either way, public health is compromised when food is not served right.

DOI: 10.4018/978-1-5225-7635-8.ch012

This chapter provides a brief description of the food security concept. This chapter discusses factors related to the switch from traditional to mechanized industrial methods, including agricultural biotechnology (or agbiotech). This analysis includes a review of the consequences attending these methods. An attempt is made to illustrate the main arguments between supporters and doubters of agbiotech. This is followed with an analysis of how both sides differ in their understanding and grounding of sustainability (i.e., risks and capabilities of biotechnology).

Because eating is an ethical act, this chapter also examines the ethical implication of food production and consumption. This includes multiple climatic and socioeconomic or public policy drivers that have collided with the ability of the average person to achieve food security. Definitions and designs for food security must recognize food's many roles in creating positive public health outcomes. The chapter concludes that a significant amount of work is needed to steer policy initiatives toward common sense sustainability paths in its aim for plentiful, accessible, and nutritious food across the globe.

BACKGROUND ON AGBIOTECH

Agricultural biotechnology is the ability to translate and apply genomic knowledge using technological and scientific techniques to accelerate breeding of complex plant, animal, and microorganism traits leading to finished products. Central to this process is the scientist's understanding of DNA, the main constituent of chromosomes of organisms, which are manipulated to increase agricultural productivity. "By identifying genes that may confer advantages on certain crops, biotechnology enhances breeders' ability to make improvements in crops and livestock (BRIEF #1, 2004)."

It is a marked departure from about 10,000 years ago since traditional farmers have improved wild plants and animals through the selection and breeding of desirable characteristics using basic methods. This practice led to the domestication of plants and animals commonly used in crop and livestock agriculture. But advancements in the twentieth century and beyond, brought forth sophisticated methods which enable breeders to select traits resulting in increased yield, disease and pest resistance, drought resistance and enhanced flavor ("What is Agricultural Biotechnology?," 2004).

Methods commonly used in agbiotech are:

- **Genetic Engineering:** Which transfers useful characteristics (such as resistance to a disease) into a plant, animal or microorganism by inserting genes (DNA) from another organism
- **Molecular Marking:** Which examines the DNA of an organism to precisely select plants or animals that possess a desirable gene, even in the absence of a visible trait.
- **Molecular Diagnostics:** Which detects genes or gene products that are very precise and specific to more accurately diagnose crop and livestock diseases.
- **Vaccination:** For protection against some infectious illnesses in for example, chickens and cattle.
- **Tissue Culturing:** The regeneration of plants in the laboratory from disease-free planting materials for crops such as citrus, pineapples, avocados, mangoes, bananas, coffee and papaya ("What is Agricultural Biotechnology?," 2004).

HOW DO YOU DECONSTRUCT THE 'FOOD SECURITY' CONCEPT?

The fusion of food and security as a concept presupposes the factorial vagaries (from production to consumption) associated with the nourishing substance that humans eat or drink to sustain life, provide energy, promote growth, and ensure good health. The term "security" evokes its antonym, "danger." Hence, food is conceptualized in terms of its susceptibility to being in "harm's way" because attempts must be made to ensure its safety and to handle it with care.[1] This attribute of fragility (delicacy/delicateness) seems to defy a simple definition for food security.

Maxwell and Smith (1992), Smith, Pointing, and Maxwell (1993), and Hoddinott's (1999) inventorying of more than 200 definitions and formulations (e.g., DEFRA, 2006) typify the difficulty with its delineation. Food security has proven to be a cornucopia of ideas that periodically melts into other forms as it is examined. The many attempts at finding an accurate conceptual meaning of food security has been due to its long evolutionary process. It is a metamorphosis that may be far from over as:

No single existing survey instrument will ever be able to collect all needed indicators at the desired periodicity, and no single institution has either the mandate or the ability to measure and monitor food security in its many dimensions on a global scale (Carletto & Banerjee, 2013, p. 31).

On both personal and collective levels, how can one tell when he/she is slipping into food insecurity? Is food security best considered by means of production (supply side), in terms of access (demand side), or both? Does enough food entail its availability? Does availability translate to access? Does access to food mean access to any type of food, including preferred or culturally acceptable foods and foods with nutritional value? Questions like these have bothered analysts. Similar to measuring health vital signs, these questions point to indicators by which food security is ascertained, quantified, and qualified as means of determining an operational definition.

Renzaho and Mellor (2010) traced this tortuous path to the 1948 Declaration of Human Rights by the United Nations General Assembly. Article 25 discusses the inalienable rights of every human, including the right to an adequate standard of living such as rights to food (United Nations, 1948). The provision was bolstered later by Article 11 of the International Covenant on Economic, Social, and Cultural Rights adopted by the General Assembly (United Nations, 1966).

However, the food security concept took on a more definitive form at the World Food Conference in 1974, resulting in the Universal Declaration on the Eradication of Hunger and Malnutrition. Hence, food security was made to mean the "availability at all times, of adequate world food supplies of basic foodstuffs to sustain a steady expansion of food consumption and to offset fluctuations in production and prices" (United Nations, 1974).

In the 1983 Food and Agriculture Organization Director General's Report, emphasis went beyond food availability to include physical and economic access to food to meet dietary needs (FAO, 1983). Citing Anderson (1990), Renzaho and Mellor (2010) highlighted the definition of food security by the United States Department of Agriculture as:

Access by all people at all times to enough food for an active, healthy life and includes at a minimum: (a) the ready availability of nutritionally adequate and safe foods, and (b) the assured ability to acquire acceptable foods in socially acceptable ways (e.g., without resorting to emergency food supplies, scavenging, stealing, and other coping strategies) (p. 1575).

Despite its frequent use, Renzaho and Mellor (2010) conclude that this definition misjudges the political and economic situations across the globe. While the nature of food insecurity tends to look alike in developing and developed countries, the environmental setting in which it occurs differs significantly. One of such similarities is the existence of droughts, but others like armed conflicts, inadequate agricultural policies, and poor governance combine to negatively impact household livelihood. "For many countries experiencing natural and man-made disasters, and whose population's livelihood relies on migration wages, kinship support, wild animal, and food hunting are part of their normal livelihood mechanism" (Renzaho & Mellor, 2010, p. 3).

In emerging economies of the Pacific region, however, the causes of food insecurity cover a wide gamut such as high population density, diminishing and high incidences of labor migration within islands and overseas, weakening soil fertility, right to own land, and natural disasters. (Renzaho & Mellor, 2010, p. 3)

Three broad shifts are reflective of the successive definitions as noted by Maxwell (1996). They ae shifts that continue to preoccupy policy makers, international organizations, and many governments: (1) global and national to household and individual; (2) food-first perspective to livelihood perspective; and (3) objective indicators to subjective perceptions.

Hovering over the categories is the aspiration to meet a satisfactory level of food security. Thus, the relevant question has been: When is food supply sufficient, acceptable, or suitable? A similar question was raised by Pinstrup-Andersen (2009, p. 5), "Is it enough to meet economic demand and if so, at what price; or is it enough to meet energy and nutrient requirements?" Answers have been varied, including, understanding food security as a "minimal level of food consumption" (Reutlinger & Knaap, 1980); as a "target level" (Siamwalla & Valdes, 1980); as "enough food for life" (Krackt, 1981); as "the basic food needed" (FAO, 1983); as "enough for active, healthy life" (World Bank, 1986); as "adequate to meet nutritional needs" (Barraclough & Utting, 1987); and, as supply "for all family members to live healthy" (Sahn, 1989). On a country-by country basis,

National food sovereignty was and still is used to measure the extent to which a country has the means to make available to its people the food needed or demanded, irrespective of whether the food is domestically produced or imported. A country that does not produce the food it needs, or its population is prepared to buy and does not have the hard currency to import what is missing, would not be food sovereign (Pinstrup-Anderson, 2009, p. 5)

A pre-eminent definition of 'food security' is the proposal at the World Food Summit that food security is attained when "all people, at all times, have physical and economic access to sufficient, safe, and nutritious food to meet the dietary needs and food preferences for an active and healthy life" (FAO, 1996).

Beyond this, suggestions have been proposed that anthropometric measures may target pertinent policies and programs. "If nutritional security is the goal of interest, estimates of access to food should be combined with estimates of access to clean water and good sanitation" (Pinstrup-Anderson, 2009, p. 5). Anthropometric measures account for factors and considerations shaping food production, access, and consumption. These include the subtle fact that the ability to acquire enough food is not necessarily the same as actual food acquisition. Also, other household needs including goods and services, often compete with food acquisition. "The extent to which individual food security results in good nutrition depends on a set of non-food factors such as … access to primary health care" (Pinstrup-Anderson, 2009, p. 6).

Nutritional adequacy, while necessary, is not enough condition for food security. Hence, an objective set of measurements would include qualitative aspects and quantitative measures along with individual preferences, consistency with local food habits, cultural acceptability, and human dignity. Whether at the level of individual, household, or country, these requirements are a function of age, state of health, size, workload, environment, and behavior (Maxwell, 1996). Certainty and stability attributes have been added to food assessment and action to deconstruct it into more complete dimensions (Coates, 2013).

Of all the assessment indices, food availability and/or accessibility presents a major challenge given the neo-Malthusian projection of the world's teeming population, estimated to reach 9 billion by 2050 (United Nations, 2015). Hence, the global demand for food is predicted to increase for decades to come. Expert forecasts project that competition for natural resources such as land, water, energy, and the wild life "will affect our ability to produce food, as will the urgent requirement to reduce the impact of the food system on the environment" (Godfray et al., 2010, p. 812).

In addition to efforts to provide food security for a quantum projection of the world's population, a demand for environmentally and socially sustainable food is desirable. This effort would have to be more thoughtful than those of the 18th and 19th century Industrial and Agricultural Revolutions, and the 20th-century Green Revolution; given that it is constrained as never before by ecological degradation and dwindling natural resources.

CAN AGBIOTECH ELIMINATE HUNGER?

Studies of the benefits of biotechnology for agriculture have rapidly proliferated. For example, biotechnology promises far greater benefits to agricultural sustainability for Africa – a continent routinely and derisively labeled as synonymous with hunger and disease. To rid Africa of such pejorative image, some authors, including Thomson (2008) and Machuka (2001) – whose views will receive focused review shortly – suggest that biotechnology holds the wand to eliminate Africa's hunger and create agricultural sustainability. Such views have been sustained even in more recent literature (for instance, Henessy, Gupta & Kowalski, 2014; Arthur & Yobo, 2014).

Thomson (2008) noted that Africa should take advantage of agbiotech breakthroughs. These include initiatives related to insect-resistant maize and cotton, virus-resistant crops, drought-tolerant crops, and improved varieties of local crops like bananas, cassava, sorghum, and sweet potatoes. Thomson (2008), in her argument that Africa has a unique set of agriculture traits, discussed the continent's "lack of a dominant farming system, predominance of rain-fed agriculture as opposed to irrigation, and prevalence of soils of poor fertility" (p. 905). In her view, this points to the cyclically deficiency of low agricultural productivity and the limited amount of organic material available to be returned to the soil after harvesting. Therefore, Africa urgently needs to "improve the nutrient status of agricultural lands, many of which are acidic, low in phosphorous and high in toxic aluminum" (Thomson, 2008, p. 905).

Thomson (2008) acknowledged that the world is awash with enough food to go around (barring endemic distribution challenges, wars, corruption, and lack of infrastructure). Nonetheless, Thomson (2008) still thinks that genetically modified (GM) crops, which provide increased yields, could hold the ace; while also recognizingd constraints to attaining this goal, including consumer concerns related to GM foods.

Though more strident, Machuka's (2001) posture is nearly identical to Thomson's as it ascribes setbacks to crop production in sub-Saharan Africa (SSA),[2] including, pests, diseases, weeds, environmental degradation, and soil nutrient depletion. He identifies also, inadequate use of synthetic and other forms of modern farming methodologies and food processing mechanisms, poor roads networks.

Due to the prime place farming occupies in generating income and sustenance for most of Africa's population, Machuka (2001) is unflinching that the ultimate answer is "biotechnology for Africa, now" (p. 17). His claim for agbiotech goes beyond substantial contributions toward increasing food production to "preserving declining resources such as forests, soil, water, and arable land" (Machuka, 2001, p. 17).

Interestingly, Machuka's approach urges that agbiotech should empower the local people by building on indigenous traditions, techniques, experience, and knowledge accumulated over the millennia. This will avert "cut and paste" approaches borne out of possible ulterior motives. Granted that they may provide short-term, quick-fix solutions to unique problems, they are not of any use to "small-scale farmers in Africa who have developed their own unique crops, cropping, and farming systems that cannot be changed without their full and careful involvement" (Machuka, 2001, p. 18)

Despite making a few valid points, many would view Thomson and Machuka's propositions as a run-of-the-mill selling pitch favoring agbiotech. Concerns revolve around their inability to factor in fundamental challenges that beset agricultural production in Africa. These include:

- The role of strangulating lending conditions by international monetary agencies (such as International Monetary Fund [IMF] and the World Bank)
- Absence of large-scale agricultural investments by many African governments
- Inconsistent and lackluster agricultural programs and policies
- Factional strife and political unrest often initiated by neocolonial and/or other foreign influences
- Effects of trade and agricultural protectionism by Western countries, particularly the U.S.
- Damaging effects of the agbiotech industry

Also, it is largely true that much of Africa relies predominantly on rain-fed agricultural practices as opposed to irrigation. Yet it is hardly convincing that the nutrient status of agricultural lands (in the 11.7 million square-mile land area and the adjacent islands) are fraught with acidity, low in phosphorous and high in toxic aluminum, and hence unproductive. On this score alone, Thomson (2008) claimed, Africa cannot afford synthetic nutrients. Curiously, both Thompson (2008) and Machuka (2001) acknowledged a surplus of food in the world if only distribution, political, and economic policy constraints got out of the way. Nevertheless, they are undeterred in their conviction that much of Africa's agricultural and sustainability challenges will evaporate with the full embrace of agbiotech.

It warrants noting that the country of South Africa was the first in the world to adopt GM technology. Before genetically modified organism (GMO) legislation was in place, the South African government issued a permit for the commercial release in 1997 of MON810 maize, which contains Monsanto's patented *Bt gene Cry1Ab* and embodies much of the controversy surrounding GMOs (AfricaFocus Bulletin, 2013). This led to Monsanto colonizing the production of staple food by large-scale commercial farmers through aggressive acquisitions in the South African seed industry and patent laws protecting Monsanto's GM technology. Also, the technology came with the promise to ease pest management, save on pesticides, and reduce loss of yield through pest damage. The promise decisively failed. Monsanto's MON89034 subsequent replacement for insect resistance, MON810, also failed. Similar disastrous outcomes have been documented across the Global South (AfricaFocus Bulletin, 2013).

There has been a long suspicion about the biotech industry's aggressive marketing of their product as a key contributor in the global fight against hunger. The 2002 famine in Southern Africa was widely viewed as an opportunity to force-feed agbiotech on the people of that region by "expanding the market access and control of transnational corporations and undermining local smallholder production" (Zerbe, 2004, p. 593).

The truth remains that this expensive technology is being deployed in lucrative commodity crops for the sake of profit. For instance, the four dominant GM crops on the market (soya, maize, cotton, and canola) are not primarily valued for their contribution to African and global food security (AfricaFocus Bulletin, 2013). It is no longer a secret that the development of new seed technology through genetic modification and other methods is presented as a key component for raising productivity of African agriculture. If truth must be told, it actually serves to lure African farmers into international value chains in which the profits from what should be common resources are concentrated in the hands of private multinational companies. (AfricaFocus Bulletin, 2012, p. 14)

It was probably with good intention that in 2007 the Bill and Melinda Gates and Rockefeller Foundations established the Alliance for a Green Revolution for Africa (AGRA). Curiously, that initiative has not only become formal U.S. foreign policy but integral to the G8 approach to the problem of food security across the African continent. AfricaFocus analysts feel dubious that AGRA's initiative has transformed into official American policy and engages large global corporations in food production on African soil with African resources. Food security refers to linking Africa's biodiverse, local foods to the global market. Yet global agricultural markets are controlled by very few corporations. It is not hard to see how such an agenda prioritizes feeding Wall Street while threatening African smallholder food producers and Africa's food sovereignty.

The preceding argument has made clear how the promise of biotechnology has failed to raise the fortunes of the world's hunger-stricken population and the smallholder farmers who struggle to feed them. Instead, it has been profiting from the insecurities of the world's hungry without solving their hunger. Agbiotech's slogan remains that it has the where-with-all to erase deepening world hunger and resolve food insecurity, particularly in the Global South. However, with the Global North's reluctance to fully embrace transgenic foods, agbiotech has swerved toward the Global South as a ready market "in much the same way as the tobacco industry shifted its market focus southward" (McMichael, 2004, p. 140).

Surely, agbiotech's promises to solve food insecurity remain largely unproven. Its methods have faced renewed challenge by the natural time of traditional processes of selection and evolution. McMichael (2004) sums up its true purpose:

- Control of technology and markets
- Reduction of global biodiversity to transgenic monocultures
- Rejection of diversity of knowledge embedded in the cultures of the world's peasant farmers

In fact, the patenting of living organisms is widely viewed by Africans as biopiracy because it gives sole ownership to the corporation that inserted one gene. It does not recognize the innovations of thousands who developed the cultivar. Benefit sharing does not occur.

PROMISE TO IMPROVE FOOD PRODUCTION OR GENE SNATCHING?

The emergence of AGRA, as well as its recent posture, has analysts scratching their heads. One manifestation of this worry is the unexpressed goal of the AGRA and U.S. agroindustry: to access African genetic wealth for gene technologies and animal or plant breeding for corporate profit. Apparently, AGRA advocates policies that access the genetic wealth of indigenous populations without recognition—neither for their knowledge nor for the genetic parent materials. Likewise, they neither have plans to share benefits with those who cultivated and bred the plants and animals over centuries (Oguamanam, 2012; AfricaFocus Bulletin, 2012).

AfricaFocus further notes AGRA's technological approach to food production which radically differs from the 1960s Green Revolution whereby hybrid seeds developed for increased yields during that era remained in the public domain, to be freely exchanged among all farmers. Acting like a cartel, AGRA-sponsored seeds are most often privatized by the corporate seed breeder (AfricaFocus Bulletin, 2012). Every year the farmer must return to buy expensive seeds and can neither replant the next generation nor save or exchange the seeds among themselves for further experimentation. Patenting of living organisms (in this case, seeds) is recognized by U.S. law and advanced through its bilateral trade agreements, even as the American government refuses to sign on to the International Treaty for Plant Genetic Resources for Food and Agriculture (IT-2004) that ensures farmers' rights to save, exchange, and breed any seeds. The treaty also disallows patents for 64 crops and fodders, an aggregate representing most crops providing human nutrition (AfricaFocus Bulletin, 2012).

There is more to be said about the world's most valuable plant genetic resources, the majority of which are found in the Global South, home of "land races." According to Thompson and Hannah (2008), land races are crop varieties that have been grown over several centuries by indigenous farmers by selecting valuable traits through an ingenious process. Scientific advances that involve extracting valuable traits from the seeds of land races have been successfully carried out by industrial plant breeders from the Global North. Hence, "biotechnology has brought this set of concerns to the forefront of public attention in conjunction with legal debates over the patentability of genes and genetic sequences and over the status of patents" (Thompson & Hannah, 2008, p. 243).

The fear that agricultural genetic diversity of crops is being lost at an alarming rate is not new. For instance, Esquinas-Alcázar (2005, p. 946) warned that "given the enormous interdependence of countries and generations on this genetic diversity, this loss raises critical socio-economic, ethical, and political questions." Citing numerous instances and fingering the U.S. and Europe as major culprits, Kelbessa (2012) exasperated over the common practice where foreign corporations, colluding with some local African intellectuals, freely obtain knowledge and resources from peasant farmers. They erect legal protection for this knowledge without acknowledging the indigenous farmers, local authorities, and community within which the knowledge originally developed. Not only do innovators of this knowledge not receive any economic compensation for their research, they are unaware that pilfering of their indigenous knowledge is widespread (Kelbessa, 2012)

It is only fair that indigenous people should be compensated for the fact that their lands hold some of the world's stock of natural biological resources even as scientists from western countries have helped to extract them via bioprospecting. According to Millum (2010, p. 25), "We must build a robust defense for this intuition if we are to put it into practice and enforce it." Anything short of that is "biopiracy." This point has been a lightning rod of sorts.

Some critics accept the basic utilitarian rationale for patents, but question whether patents in biotechnology are really beneficial. Others see the utilitarian view of patents simply as a subterfuge to allow the growth of capitalist social relations and corporate power. Still others stress the view that indigenous people who discover uses for plants and who develop germplasm through generations of trial and error have a prior claim that vitiates this utilitarian rationale. These arguments are linked with concerns about intellectual property rights in the domain of human medicine, where patenting of genes and gene processes are sometimes said to violate human dignity (Thompson & Hannah, 2008, p. 244).

Discoveries in transgenic science come in leaps and bounds. The landmark event that made the most waves may be the successful cloning[3] of Dolly the Sheep from an adult cell at a Scottish research institute in July 1996. Not surprisingly, those waves (despite the sheep's demise six years later) still reverberate. Claims include GM cows that are primed to produce milk comparable to human milk, GM chickens that will not transmit bird flu, and GM grains, fruits, grass, and vegetables that have long been around and many more that are destined to land on our dinner tables.

The frequent dose of these claims signpost scientific milestones that jolt the minds and naturally prompt curiosity. There is the promise of biotechnology that will enable humans to be smarter, improve memories, increase strength and agility, live longer, be more resistant to disease, and enjoy richer emotional lives. Despite (re)assurances on the benefits of biotechnology (and in some cases because of it), the fact is that transgenic science is a process by which scientists alter an organism's genome by transferring one or more genes from another species or breed. This is done to determine the function of the inserted gene. It is not surprising that some people have paused to ponder the unforeseen/unforeseeable consequences. In addition, individuals are considering unexplored options and possibilities. It is understandable if the feeling of wonder and questioning metamorphosizes into doubt and unwillingness to put wholesale trust on this type of science. After all, not all scientific discoveries are or have been beneficial.

AGBOITECH OR TRADITIONAL AGRICULTURAL METHODS?

A major opposition to agbiotech is the ethical dialogue approach with roots in Oromo ecotheology and represents the voiceless indigenous marginalized natives such as found in Africa. Its methods teach positive relationship between God, humanity, the natural environment and nonhuman creation. The argument of retaining the natural environment and promoting an ecological balance through well-established indigenous agrarian methods is in opposition to the characteristics of agbiotech. According to Kelbessa (2005), it is absurd that indigenous people must relinquish their identity in the quest for western development, democracy, and human rights. It is even more so because western or western-trained academics have failed to carefully study indigenous environmental knowledge. The result has been that most Africans now active in conservation do so with the Western methods of wildlife management. Thus, by promoting the European management systems, the growth of an African conservation ethic suffers (Kelbessa, 2005).

When these imports confront the African environment, they tend to relentlessly exert control over traditional African land ethics with unaccustomed practices by using natural resources as objects for exploitation and profit making.

A related threat to indigenous and local ways of life is the commercialization and privatization of knowledge. In this regard, large transnational corporations are gaining control over the production and distribution of knowledge and life as a whole.

Agricultural production through large-scale intensive farming has been the model response in the fight against hunger. However, its methods are suspect. Industrial agriculture is wasteful, highly polluting, monopolistic (concentrated in the hands of few corporations), and, in fact, a major threat to food security. Other crises it has spurned (i.e., genetic erosion, disease susceptibility, and environmental stresses) need urgent re-examination. To the contrary, "small farming continues to offer more productive, stable, biodiverse, and place-based culinary alternatives" (McMichael, 2004, p. 151).

Traditional farming methods akin to agroecology offer several advantages over the conventional agroindustrial approach. These methods provide ecological principles for the design and management of sustainable and resource-conserving agricultural systems. Altieri, Rosset, & Thrupp (1998), have summarized the advantages thus:

- Agroecology relies on indigenous farming knowledge and selected modern technologies to manage diversity, incorporate biological principles and resources into farming systems and intensify agricultural production.
- It offers the only practical way to restore agricultural lands that have been degraded by conventional agronomic practices.
- It provides for an environmentally sound and affordable way for smallholders to intensify production in marginal areas.
- It has the potential to reverse the anti-peasant bias of strategies that emphasize purchased inputs as opposed to the assets that small farmers already possess, such as their low opportunity costs of labor.

WHAT ETHICAL LINES TO DRAW?

The fact that concerns have been raised about the enduring need for mankind to have food for normal body functioning is a clear indication of its ethical obligation. Indeed, the relief of hunger is a major claim on mankind's ethical responsibilities. It should not sit well with mankind's conscience that there is more than enough food to go around but are yet unwilling to device a reliable architecture to make that possible. Policy makers within governments ought to develop strategies to promote the interests of the citizenry to whom it is accountable. According to Rush (2013, p. 37), "Ensuring national food security is clearly one such strategy. Failure to protect citizen's interests in such a fundamental way would profoundly undermine the moral legitimacy of government."

Not everyone is getting the food they need, when they need it, and how they need it. This immediately raises the ethical question: Why is food not being produced and provided appropriately? It is a presupposition that certain actions that would ensure equity and access to food have been poorly applied or ignored. It is an ethical concern that there is not a lack of food but an unwillingness to establish equitable distribution apparati due to inordinate drive for profits at the expense of the disadvantaged.

As noted, concerns over agbiotech are rife, such as the use of rDNA in manipulating plant and animal genomes and others that are general to other forms of technology. The many issues surrounding agricultural biotechnology and their embedded ethical implications come under five themes: (1) impact on human health (i.e., food safety); (2) impact on the environment; (3) impact on non-human animals; (4) impact on farming communities in the developed and developing world; and (5) shifting power relations (e.g., the rising importance of commercial interests and multinationals; Thompson & Hannah, 2008).

At first glance, the agbiotech system seems wonderful. However, its underbelly is loathful. Industrial farming no longer commands the revolutionary status it once did; its exploitative methods are unsustainable to producing safe and healthy food. As noted by the Union of Concerned Scientists (UCS), industrial agriculture regards the farm as a production line where "inputs" (i.e., seedlings, pesticides, feed, and fertilizer) result in "outputs" (i.e., corn, chickens, and cattle). Hence, the primary drive, irrespective of everything else, is to increase yield per acre or pound of meat and minimize production costs, usually by exploiting economic scale (UCS, 2001).

In hindsight, pioneers of the Industrial Age must be disappointed that no one foresaw the trail of havoc—a great source of concern to environmental ethicists—from industrial agriculture that is witnessed today. According to Horrigan, Lawrence, and Walker (2002), the ills of agbiotech make a long list. It contributes to:

Numerous forms of environmental degradation, including air and water pollution, soil depletion, diminishing biodiversity, and fish die-offs. Meat production contributes disproportionately to these problems, in part because feeding grain to livestock to produce meat—instead of feeding it directly to humans—involves a large energy loss, making animal agriculture more resource intensive than other forms of food production. The proliferation of factory-style animal agriculture creates environmental and public health concerns, including pollution from the high concentration of animal wastes and the extensive use of antibiotics, which may compromise their effectiveness in medical use. At the consumption end, animal fat is implicated in many of the chronic degenerative diseases that afflict industrial and newly industrializing societies, particularly cardiovascular disease and some cancers. The pesticides used heavily in industrial agriculture are associated with elevated cancer risks for workers and consumers and are coming under greater scrutiny for their links to endocrine disruption and reproductive dysfunction (p. 445).

It is argued that GMOs have demonstrable benefits and the potential to increase the cost-efficiency of crop production. In addition, GMOS can build wealth for farmers and seed companies. Therefore, it should not be ethically justifiable to deny the public these obvious benefits unless it could be proven that GMOs pose a hazard to human health. However, the fact that there is some chance of a hazardous outcome to the public (slight or severe), criticisms from proponents of individual rights are justified. For instance, there is the risk of allergic reaction associated with GMOs, something that is common with proteins (Thompson & Hannah, 2008). Moreover, the assertions that GMOs have demonstrable benefits of some sort, are spurious. They do not fully account for unforeseen (but probably foreseeable) future safety issues posed to humans and the environment. Similarly, it is hard to understand why some are comfortable with granting "potential benefits" of GMOs but reluctant when considering "potential harm" to the public. It is equally misleading to claim that GMOs are more valuable and cost-effective than traditional crop production. The opposite has been proven to be the case. The issue with agbiotech may be largely economic. It is also significantly ethical given that hapless small holder farmers would lose their livelihood in the ruthless fight for patent rights.

There is also the claim that the slim probability of serious health effects on 'a minute segment' of the public should not outweigh the overwhelming economic and technological benefits. In other words, the interest of a trifle percentage does not match the opportunity of achieving the classic consequentialist utilitarian goal that maximizes benefits for the majority. Such claims are a conscious effort to inaccurately label the public (represented by the smallholder farmer) as "the minority" while a handful of agbiotech businesses become "the many." Huge profits and immense political clout do not make the biotech companies representative of the interest of the public. It does not matter that corporations have become powerful institutions that inordinately drive much of the public policies. One is not persuaded that the agbiotech industry should be accorded fiduciary status. It is hubris to use the biotech industry to shape the destiny of the vulnerable class. To do so for economic gains is ethically repugnant, especially when it is done under the pretext of solving world hunger.

Also, even as it might seem harsh to prohibit GMOs without a beyond-any-shred-of-doubt evidence that they pose a hazard to human health, the reverse logic ought to be noted. Inability to provide evidence is not a lack of proof of evidence. Thus, the present argument hints at the precautionary principle. It is a disposition that considers the course of action to be taken when an activity raises threats of harm to human health or the environment, even if some cause and effect relationships are not fully established. Lessons ought to be drawn from the 1992 Rio Declaration prescription:

In order to protect the environment, the precautionary approach shall be widely applied by States according to their capabilities. Where there are threats of serious or irreversible damage, lack of full scientific certainty shall not be used as a reason for postponing cost-effective measures to prevent environmental degradation. (United Nations, 1992)

Philosophers have analyzed environmental ethics using several approaches. They are duties to posterity (our obligations to consider and lessen the negative impacts of our actions on future generations) and eco-centric ethical values (our obligations to care for nature for its own sake). A general consequence of this analysis is that they manifest themselves as impacts on human beings (Thompson & Hannah, 2008).

WHAT DOES FOOD SECURITY GOT TO DO WITH PUBLIC HEALTH?

In 1920, Charles Winslow, an influential figure in public health, described the goal of public health as preventing disease, prolonging life, and promoting health and efficient functioning. These are all key words that relate to the popular Food and Agricultural Organization's (FAO) (1996) definition of food security. Further, public health's target to reduce the impact of disease and improve health and quality of life hinge on three key concepts in the pursuit of food security: (1) prevention; (2) population; and (3) justice. Public health seeks to protect against exposure to harmful or unhealthy substances or experiences, provide basic healthy amenities (i.e., portable water and a nutritious food supply), and attend to the needs, desires, and attributes of the population as a unit (Bouldin, 2010). Likewise, the all-encompassing food security concept connotes that, "In order to have robust nutrition outcomes, food both in terms of quantity and nutritional value, is important. But, so are access to healthcare, optimal hygiene, and adequate childcare services (Fanzo, 2015, p. 17).

The causal framework for nutrition demonstrates the importance of such sectors as agriculture and food, health, education, environment, water, and sanitation (WHO-UNICEF, 2015). In sum, public health and food security are so entwined that it is impossible to discuss one in isolation of the other.

Obviously, food supply is indispensable to human life and human development is crucial to achieving food security. These two dependent variables continue to experience intractable tensions. The result is a seething food crisis that pervades even during plenty. The evidential consequence and the intergenerational links between food access and nutritional status at different stages of the life course are telling. As one in every three persons worldwide is saddled with some form of malnutrition, it has thus been called a scourge in the world (DFID, 2011). Sobering statistics by Fanzo (2015) described the daunting challenges that stand in the way to provide "plentiful, healthy and nutritious food for all in an environmentally sustainable and safe manner, while addressing the multiple burdens of undernutrition, overweight and obesity and micronutrient deficiencies" (p. 15). Rather than do the needful, the agbiotech industry exerts the power of technology for other purposes.

Nutrients are the essential ingredients the body absorbs and utilizes for nourishment, growth, health, and social well-being (Fanzo, 2014). Inadequate supply of nutrients can lead to a chain of events through the life cycle. For instance, poor nutrition *in utero* can extend into adolescent and adult life. It can also span generations. This can mean early deaths for mothers, infants, and young children. Even when they survive, potential exists for impaired or irreversible physical and social development in the young. Subsequently, the result is poor health in adulthood affecting both individual well-being and social and economic development of nations (Black et al., 2013; Hoddinot, Rosegrant, & Torero, 2012).

Research has unquestionably linked a swelter of impacts of erratic global climatic changes to food production. The climatic changes include more intense heatwaves, rising sea levels, blizzards with more snow storms, frequent forest fires, bizarre record rainfalls, and longer and/or shorter seasons. The conclusions of Porter et al. (2014, p. 502) is that "little is known about combined effects of climate change factors on food quality." This offers little comfort to anyone eager to see direct deleterious impacts from climate change on human health. However, that claim is probably misleading. Citing Ceccarelli et al., (2010, p. 627), the same report says that:

Climate change will have some adverse impacts on food quality through biotic and abiotic stresses. These changes may affect crop quality by altering carbon and nutrient uptake and biochemical processes that produce secondary compounds during grain development and maturation. This in turn could impact human and livestock health by altering nutritional intake and/or affect economic value by altering traits to processers or the consumers.

Figure 1. Poor nutrition and impacts throughout the life cycle

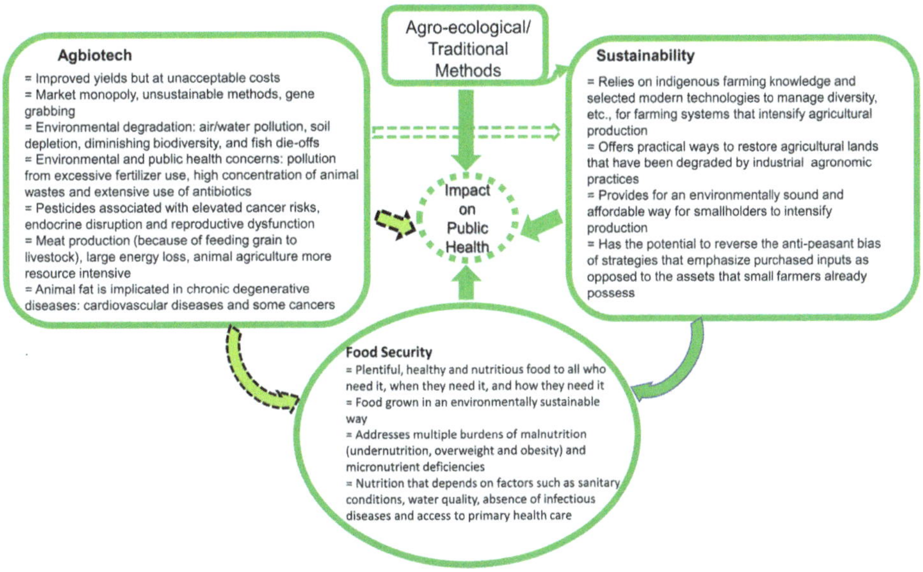

Climate change is primarily a problem of excessive carbon dioxide (CO_2) in the atmosphere. This carbon overload is caused mainly because humans burn massive amounts of fossil fuels like coal, oil, and gas or cut down and burn large swarths of forests which otherwise serve as a carbon sink (Union of Concerned Scientists, n.d.). In terms of agricultural production, it is hard to ignore the impacts of increased levels of CO_2. Porter et al. (2014) chronicled the effect of CO_2 on agricultural yields and human health. For example, cereals grown in elevated CO_2 show a decrease in protein (Ainsworth & McGrath, 2010; DaMatta, Grandis, Arenque, & Buckeridge, 2010; Erbs et al., 2010; Fernando et al., 2012; Högy et al., 2009; Pikki, Vorne, Ojanpera, & Pleijel, 2007). Meta-analysis of 228 experimental observations finds decreases between 10% and 14% in edible portions of wheat, rice, barley, and potato; there was a decrease of only 1.5% in soybeans, a nitrogen-fixing legume, when grown in elevated CO_2 (Taub, Miller, & Allen, 2008). Elevated CO_2 can lower the nutritional quality of flour produced from grain cereals and cassava (Erbs et al., 2010; Gleadow, Evans, McCaffery, & Cavagnaro, 2009; Högy et al., 2009). When coupled with increased crop and pathogen biomass, elevated CO_2 can result in increased severity of the *Fusarium pseudogramearum* pathogen, which leads to shriveled grains with low market value (Melloy et al., 2010). The only counter argument to this mountain of evidence is the claim by Duval et al. (2011) that elevated CO_2 can increase crop yield and overall yield of mineral.

CONCLUSION

This chapter was premised on the concentric link between public health, attainment of food security through sustainable means, and the promise of agbiotech. What has become apparent is the paradoxical reality accompanying each of the variables. Presently, agrobiotechnology research raises ethical, safety, and intellectual property rights issues. There is the question of whether we can provide plentiful, healthy, and nutritious food to all who need it, when they need it. Also, there is the lingering concern whether this can be done in an environmentally sustainable way while addressing the multiple burdens of malnutrition (i.e., undernutrition, overweight, and obesity) and micronutrient deficiencies. The drastic increase in grain yields in the past decades belies the growth in productivity and calories available per capita and pervasive malnutrition. “Though nutrition is critical to human health, it has yet to be systematically integrated into assessments of agricultural and food systems” (Remans, Wood, Saha, Anderman, & DeFries, 2014, p. 174). Likewise, the 2017 Global Hunger Index (GHI) shows that 52 out of 119 countries have levels of hunger that are serious, alarming, or extremely alarming. Despite a 27% decline since 2000, one in nine people (or 815 million worldwide) go to bed hungry each night (www.globalhungerindex.org/).

The approach of agbiotech must be revisited if its promise to wipe out hunger has failed and if its real passions are market monopoly, unsustainable methods, and gene grabbing. The combined effect of neo-colonial market influence by the Global North and the total control of crop-development agro-multinationals may be a threat to the diverse system of traditional farmers who would be forced into ‘bioserfdom.’

The colossal failure of many of the newly developed or hybridized crop and plant species in the Global South is dispiriting. The report of the International Assessment of Agricultural Knowledge, Science and Technology for Development (IAASTD) approved by 57 governments in Johannesburg presents a disturbing account of the failure of industrial farming. It calls for a fundamental change in farming to better address soaring food prices, hunger, social inequities, and environmental disasters (AfricaFocus Bulletin, 2009). The report notes that small-scale farmers and agro-ecological methods provide a way to

Figure 2. Agbiotech, sustainability, and food security impacts on public health

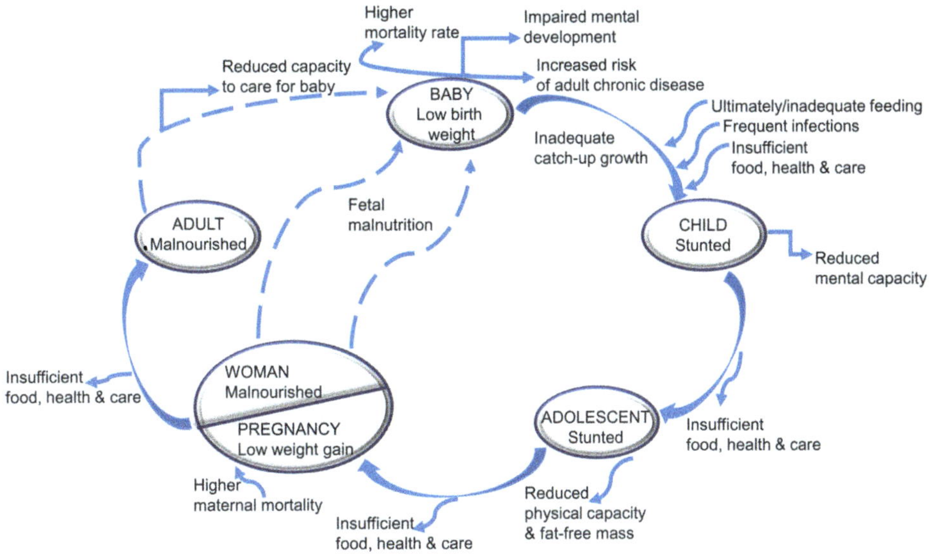

avert the current food crisis while meeting the needs of both local and international communities. More equitable trade arrangements and increased sharing of knowledge to support agroecologically-based approaches in both small farm and large-scale sectors are urgently required.

Food security cannot focus on meeting life's barest minimum. Instead, it should aim to pursue a good life. Hinderances to this goal still exist due to unsustainable agricultural practices, gauging market prices, climate change, land degradation, etc., vis-a-vis global demand (due to population increases and diet changes). Access to desired food is likely to increase substantially in the future, including a host of negative impacts on public health.

REFERENCES

AfricaFocus Bulletin. (2009, January 22). Africa: Agricultural knowledge.

AfricaFocus Bulletin. (2012). Africa: The hidden issue of "gene grabbing."

AfricaFocus Bulletin. (2013). Africa: Monopolizing maize.

Ainsworth, E., & McGrath, J. (2010). Direct effects of rising atmospheric carbon dioxide and ozone on crop yields. In D. Lobell & M. Burke (Eds.), *Climate change and food security: Adapting agriculture to a warmer world* (pp. 109–130). New York, NY: Springer.

Altieri, M. A., Rosset, P., & Thrupp, L. A. (1998). *The potential of agroecology to combat hunger in the developing world. A 2020 Vision for Food, Agriculture, and the Environment, 2020 Brief 55*. Washington, DC: International Food Policy Research Institute.

Arthur, G., & Yobo, K. (2014). Genetically Modified Crops in Africa. In M. Ahuja & K. Ramawat (Eds.), *Biotechnology and Biodiversity* (pp. 17–37). New York, NY: Springer.

Ayala, A., & Meier, B. (2017). A human rights approach to the health implications of food and nutrition insecurity. *Public Health Reviews*, *38*(10), 1–22. doi:10.118640985-017-0056-5 PMID:29450082

Barraclough, S., & Utting, P. (1987). *Food security trends and prospects in Latin America, Working paper no. 99.* Helen Kellogg Institute for International Studies, University of Notre Dame, USA.

Black, R., Victora, C., Walker, S., Bhutta, Z., Christian, P., de Onis, M., ... Uauay, R. (2013). Maternal and child undernutrition and overweight in low-income and middle-income countries. *Lancet*, *382*(9890), 427–451. doi:10.1016/S0140-6736(13)60937-X PMID:23746772

Bouldin, E. (2010). History and development of public health. In E. Andresen & E. Bouldin (Eds.), *Public health foundations: Concepts and practices* (pp. 3–24). San Francisco, CA: John Wiley & Sons, Inc.

Burns, C. (2004). *A review of the literature describing the link between poverty, food insecurity and obesity with specific reference to Australia. Centre for Physical Activity and Nutrition Research School of Exercise and Nutrition Sciences, Deakin University Melbourne.* Australia: VicHealth.

Carletto, C., & Banerjee, A. (2013). Towards better measurement of household food security: Harmonizing indicators and the role of household surveys. *Global Food Security*, *2*(1), 30–40. doi:10.1016/j.gfs.2012.11.006

Ceccarelli, S., Grando, S., Maatougui, M., Michael, M., Slash, M., Haghparast, R., ... Nachit, M. (2010). Plant breeding and climate changes. *The Journal of Agricultural Science*, *148*(06), 627–637. doi:10.1017/S0021859610000651

Coates, J. (2013). Build it back better: Deconstructing food security for improved measurement and action. *Global Food Security*, *2*(3), 188–194. doi:10.1016/j.gfs.2013.05.002

DaMatta, F., Grandis, A., Arenque, B., & Buckeridge, M. (2010). Impacts of climate changes on crop physiology and food quality. *Food Research International*, *43*(7), 1814–1823. doi:10.1016/j.foodres.2009.11.001

DEFRA. (2006). Food security and the UK: An evidence and analysis paper. Department for Environment, Food and Rural Affairs, Food Chain Analysis Group, London, UK.

Department for International Development (DFID). (2011, September). *Scaling up nutrition: The UK's position paper on undernutrition.* London, UK: DFID. Retrieved from https://assets.publishing.service.gov.uk/government/uploads/system/uploads/attachment_data/file/67466/scal-up-nutr-uk-pos-undernutr.pdf

Duval, B. D., Dijkstra, P., Natali, S. M., Megonigal, J. P., Ketterer, M. E., Drake, B. G., ... Hungate, B. A. (2011). Plant-soil distribution of potentially toxic elements in response to elevated atmospheric CO_2. *Environmental Science & Technology*, *45*(7), 2570–2574. doi:10.1021/es102250u PMID:21405117

Erbs, M., Manderscheid, R., Jansen, G., Seddig, S., Pacholski, A., & Weigela, H. (2010). Effects of free-air CO_2 enrichment and nitrogen supply on grain quality parameters and elemental composition of wheat and barley grown in a crop rotation. *Agriculture, Ecosystems & Environment*, *136*(1-2), 59–68. doi:10.1016/j.agee.2009.11.009

Esquinas-Alcázar, J. (2005). Protecting crop genetic diversity for food security: Political, ethical and technical challenges. *Nature Reviews. Genetics*, *6*(12), 946–953. doi:10.1038/nrg1729 PMID:16341075

Fanzo, J. (2014). Strengthening the engagement of food and health systems to improve nutrition security: Synthesis and overview of approaches to address nutrition. *Global Food Security*, *3*(3-4), 183–192. doi:10.1016/j.gfs.2014.09.001

Fanzo, J. (2015). Ethical issues for human nutrition in the context of global food security and sustainable development. *Global Food Security*, *7*, 15–23. doi:10.1016/j.gfs.2015.11.001

Fernando, Panozzo, J., Tausz, M., Norton, R., Fitzgerald, G., & Seneweera, S. (2012). Rising atmospheric CO_2 concentration affects mineral content and protein concentration of wheat grain. *Food Chemistry*, *133*(4), 1307–1311. doi:10.1016/j.foodchem.2012.01.105

Food and Agricultural Organization (FAO). (1983). *World food security: A reappraisal of the concepts and approaches* [Director General's Report]. Rome, Italy: FAO.

Food and Agricultural Organization (FAO). (1996). *Rome declaration on world food security*. Rome, Italy: World Food Summit.

Gleadow, R., Evans, J. R., McCaffery, S., & Cavagnaro, T. R. (2009). Growth and nutritive value of cassava are reduced when grown in elevated CO_2. *Plant Biology*, *11*(1), 76–82.

Godfray, H. C. J., Crute, I. R., Lawrence, D., Pretty, J. N., Thomas, S. M., Beddington, J. R., ... Toulmin, C. (2010). Food security: The challenge of feeding 9 billion people. *Science*, *327*(5967), 812–818. doi:10.1126cience.1185383 PMID:20110467

Henessy, W., Gupta, A., & Kowalski, S. (2014). Practice driving policy: Agbiotech transfer as capacity building. In S. Smith, P. Philips, & D. Castle (Eds.), *Handbook on agriculture, biotechnology and development* (pp. 314–342). Cheltenham, UK: Edward Elgar Publishing Limited. doi:10.4337/9780857938350.00028

Hoddinot, J., Rosegrant, M., & Torero, M. (2012). *Investments to reduce hunger and undernutrition. Copenhagen Consensus 2012 Challenge Paper, Hunger and Malnutrition*. Washington, DC: International Food Policy Research Institute.

Hoddinott, J. (1999). *Operationalizing household food security in developing projects: An introduction Technical Guide no. 1*. Washington, DC: International Food Policy Research Institute.

Högy, P., Wieser, H., Köhler, P., Schwadorf, K., Breuer, J., Franzaring, J., ... Fangmeier, A. (2009). Effects of elevated CO_2 on grain yield and quality of wheat: Results from a 3-year free-air CO_2 enrichment experiment. *Plant Biology*, (Suppl. 1), 1160–1169. PMID:19778369

Horn, F., & Breeze, R. (n.d.). Agriculture and food security. Agricultural Research Service, United States Department of Agriculture, Washington, DC.

Horrigan, L., Lawrence, R. S., & Walker, P. (2002). How sustainable agriculture can address the environmental and human health harms of industrial agriculture. *Environmental Health Perspectives*, *110*(5), 445–456. doi:10.1289/ehp.02110445 PMID:12003747

Kelbessa, W. (2005). *The utility of ethical dialogue for marginalized voices in Africa*. Retrieved from http://pubs.iied.org/pdfs/13508IIED.pdf?

Kelbessa, W. (2012). Environmental injustice in Africa. In H. McDonald (Ed.), *Pragmatism and Environmentalism 9* (Vol. 1, pp. 99–132). New York, NY: Rodopi.

Krackt, U. (1981). Food security for people in the 1980s. *Paper prepared for discussion at the North-South Food Roundtable Meeting*, Washington DC.

Machuka, J. (2001). Agricultural biotechnology for Africa. African scientists and farmers must feed their own people. *Plant Physiology*, *126*(1), 16–19. doi:10.1104/pp.126.1.16 PMID:11351064

Maxwell, S. (1996). Food security: A post-modern perspective. *Food Policy*, *21*(2), 155–170. doi:10.1016/0306-9192(95)00074-7

Maxwell, S., & Smith, M. (1992). Part 1: Household food security: A conceptual review. In S. Maxwell & T.R. Frankenberger (Eds.), Household food security: Concepts, indicators, measurements: A technical review (pp. 4-72). United Nations Children's Fund, New York, NY.

McMichael, P. (2004). Biotechnology and food security: Profiting on insecurity. In L. Beneria & S. Bisnath (Eds.), *Global tensions: Challenges and opportunities in the world economy* (pp. 137–154). New York, NY: Routledge.

Melloy, P., Hollaway, G., Norton, J. L., Norton, R., Aitken, E., & Chakraborty, S. (2010). Production and fitness of *Fusarium pseudogramearum inoculum* at elevated carbon dioxide in FACE. *Global Change Biology*, *16*(12), 3363–3373. doi:10.1111/j.1365-2486.2010.02178.x

Millum, J. (2010). How should the benefits of bioprospecting be shared? *The Hastings Center Report*, *40*(1), 24–33. doi:10.1353/hcr.0.0227 PMID:20169653

Oguamanam, C. (2013). Intellectual Property, Ag-biotech and the Right to Adequate Food: A Critical African Perspective.

Pikki, K., Vorne, V., Ojanpera, K., & Pleijel, H. (2017). Impact of elevated O_3 and CO_2 exposure on potato tuber micronutrients. *Agriculture, Ecosystems & Environment*, *118*(1-4), 55–64. doi:10.1016/j.agee.2006.04.012

Pinstrup-Anderson, P. (2009). Food security: Definition and measurement. *Food Security*, *1*(1), 5–7. doi:10.100712571-008-0002-y

Porter, J. R., Liyong, X., Challinor, A. J., Cochrane, K., Howden, S. M., Iqbal, M. M., … Ziska, L. (2014). Food security and food production systems. In C. Field et al. (Eds.), Climate change 2014: Impacts, adaptation, and vulnerability, Part A: Global and Sectoral Aspects (pp. 485-533). New York, NY: Cambridge University Press.

Remans, R., Wood, S., Saha, N., Anderman, T., & DeFries, R. (2014). Measuring nutritional diversity of national food supplies. *Global Food Security*, *3*(3-4), 174–182. doi:10.1016/j.gfs.2014.07.001

Renzaho, A., & Mellor, D. (2010). Food security measurement in cultural pluralism: Missing the point or conceptual misunderstanding? *Nutrition (Burbank, Los Angeles County, Calif.)*, *26*(1), 1–9. doi:10.1016/j.nut.2009.05.001 PMID:19804955

Reutlinger, S., & Knapp, K. (1980). *Food security in deficit countries.* World Bank.

Ruel, M., Garrett, J., Yosef, S., & Olivier, M. (2017). Urbanization, food security and nutrition. In Se. de Pee et al. (Eds.), *Nutrition and Health.* New York, NY: Springer. doi:10.1007/978-3-319-43739-2

Rush, E. (2013). Ethics of food security. In Q. Farmar-Bowers, V. Higgins, & J. Millar (Eds.), *Food security in Australia* (pp. 35–48). Boston, MA: Springer. doi:10.1007/978-1-4614-4484-8_3

Sahn, D. (1989). A conceptual framework for examining the seasonal aspects of household food security. In D. Sahn (Ed.), *Seasonal variability in third world agriculture: The consequences for food security* (pp. 67–77). Baltimore, MD: John Hopkins University Press.

Siamwalla, A., & Valdes, A. (1980). Food security in developing countries. *Food Policy*, *5*(4), 258–272. doi:10.1016/0306-9192(80)90055-X

Smith, M., Pointing, J., & Maxwell, S. (1993). *Household food security, concepts and definitions: An annotated bibliography. Development Bibliography No. 8.* Brighton, UK: Institute of Development Studies, University of Sussex.

Taub, D., Miller, B., & Allen, H. (2008). Effect of elevated CO_2 on the protein concentration of food crops: A meta-analysis. *Global Change Biology*, *14*(3), 565–575. doi:10.1111/j.1365-2486.2007.01511.x

The World Bank. (1986). Poverty and hunger: Issues and options for food security in developing countries. World Bank Policy Study.

Thompson, P., & Hannah, W. (2008). Food and agricultural biotechnology: A summary and analysis of ethical concerns. In U. Stahl, U. Donalies, & E. Nevoigt (Eds.), *Advances in biochemical engineering/biotechnology* (pp. 229–264). Berlin, Germany: Springer.

Thomson, J. (2008). The role of biotechnology for agricultural sustainability in Africa. *Philosophical Transactions of the Royal Society*, *363*(1492), 905–913. doi:10.1098/rstb.2007.2191 PMID:17761472

Union of Concerned Scientists (UCS). *Why does CO_2 get most of the attention when there are so many other heat-trapping gases?* UCS.

United Nations. (1966). *The international covenant on economic, social and cultural rights.* Adopted by the General Assembly of the United Nations on December 16, 1966.

United Nations. (1974). *Report of the World Food Conference.* New York, NY: United Nations.

United Nations. (1975). *Report of the World Food Conference.* Rome: UN.

United Nations. (1992). *Sales No. E.73.II.A.14 and corrigendum.* Rio de Janeiro, Brazil: United Nations.

United Nations. (2015). *World population projected to reach 9.7 billion by 2050.* Department of Economic and Social Affairs, UN.

United Nations. (1948). *Universal declaration of human rights.* Adopted by the General Assembly of the United Nations on December 10, 1948. Retrieved from http://www.un.org/en/universal-declaration-human-rights/index.html

What is Agricultural Biotechnology? (2004). U.S. Agency for International Development, Agricultural Biotechnology Support Project II, and the Program for Biosafety Systems.

WHO-UNICEF-USAID. (2015). *Improving nutrition outcomes with better water, sanitation and hygiene: practical solutions for policies and programs.* Retrieved from https://www.unicef.org/media/files/IntegratingWASHandNut_WHO_UNICEF_USAID_Nov2015.pdf

Zerbe, N. (2004). Feeding the famine? American food aid and the GMO debate in Southern Africa. *Food Policy, 29*(6), 593–608. doi:10.1016/j.foodpol.2004.09.002

ADDITIONAL READING

Cohen, M., & Garrett, J. (2010). The food price crisis and urban food (in)security. *Environment and Urbanization, 22*(2), 467–482. doi:10.1177/0956247810380375

Fenning, T. M., & Gershenzon, J. (2003). European agbiotech crisis? *Nature Biotechnology, 21*(4), 1–2. doi:10.1038/nbt0403-360 PMID:12665816

Institute for Responsible Technology. (n.d.). Retrieved from https://responsibletechnology.org/gmo-education/

Loring, P., & Gerlach, S. (2009). Food, culture, and human health in Alaska: An integrative health approach to food security. *Environmental Science & Policy, 12*(4), 466–478. doi:10.1016/j.envsci.2008.10.006

Meyer, H. (2011). Systemic risks of genetically modified crops: The need for new approaches to risk assessment. *Environmental Sciences Europe, 7*(23), 1–11.

Morgan, K. (2009). Feeding the city: The challenge of urban food planning. *International Planning Studies, 14*(4), 341–348. doi:10.1080/13563471003642852

Ricroch, A. e., Bergé, J. & Kuntz, M. (2010). *Is the Suspension of MON810 Maize Cultivation by Some European Countries Scientifically Justified?* ISB News Report.

KEY TERMS AND DEFINITIONS

Agbiotech: A collection of scientific techniques to improve plants, animals, and microorganisms.

Agroecology: Agroecology is the study of the methods of ecological processes applied to agricultural production systems. These methods provide ecological principles applied for the design and management of sustainable and resource-conserving agricultural systems.

Food Security: When all people have physical and economic access to sufficient, safe, and nutritious food to meet the dietary needs and food preferences for an active and healthy life.

Food Sovereignty: Is a term coined by members of Via Campesina in 1996 and refers to the right of everyone to healthy and culturally appropriate food produced through ecologically sound and sustainable methods, and their right to define their own food and agriculture systems.

GMO: A GMO (genetically modified organism) is the result of a laboratory process where genes from the DNA of one species are extracted and artificially forced into the genes of an unrelated plant or animal to achieve an improved product. This process also may be called either genetic engineering (GE) or genetic modification (GM). GMOs are also known as "transgenic" organisms.

Public Health: The science of preventing disease, prolonging life, and promoting health and efficient functioning.

Sustainability: The pursuit of global environmental viability via avoidance of the depletion of natural resources to maintain an ecological balance.

ENDNOTES

1 Other approaches have been considered in discussing agriculture and food security. Horn and Breeze (n.d.) called attention to the growing threat on the American agriculture and food supply system, as well as its vulnerability to bioterrorism and biological warfare. They cover three major areas: (1) agriculture, the science and art of farming; (2) biological warfare, the use of disease-spreading microorganisms, toxins, and pests against enemy armed forces or civilians; and (3) terrorism, the use of terror or violence to intimidate, subjugate, and demoralize, especially as a political weapon or policy. On their part, Ayala and Meier (2017) used international human rights law as a critical role in guiding governments that are struggling to protect the health of their populations, particularly among the most susceptible groups, in responding to food and nutrition insecurity. Still, others have examined trends, unique characteristics, challenges, and distinctive factors and conditions that shape urban poverty, food insecurity, and malnutrition with a view to designing programs and policies to improve the lives of urban dwellers (Ruel, Garrett, Yosef, & Olivier, 2017).

2 Many authors are either unaware or nonchalant (or both) about the debasing connotation of dividing Africa between north and south of the Sahara. With the intent to project what they see as the backward "Black Africa" they expose their ignorance of the historical antecedents of the continent. The SSA reference is a fictional neo-colonial ploy promoting superficial divisions and comparisons. It gives the impression that, due to their proximity to Europe, all countries north of the Sahara are self-sufficient and have nothing in common with the rest of Africa. That is far from the truth.

3 This is not to confuse the meaning of cloning with that of gene modification in biotechnology. Although they are not the same, the two fall under transgenic science.

Chapter 13
Pharmaceuticals in Environment:
Global Concerns and Regulations

Alka Bali
Panjab University, India

ABSTRACT

Pharmaceuticals and personal care products (PPCPs) constitute an integral part of modern healthcare systems which enter the environment through various routes. Because of their inherent biological activity, their presence in soil and the aquatic environment poses several eco-toxicological problems. Antibiotic contamination of soil and water bodies is leading to the development of microbial resistance to antibiotics and this has been recognized by several global bodies like WHO and EPA. Effective steps need to be taken in this regard including increased awareness, reduced pharmaceutical discharges in environment, green and sustainable pharmaceutical practice by pharmaceutical industry and healthcare professionals and improved remediation/bioremediation methods. This chapter outlines the various anticipated routes of exposure of pharmaceuticals to the environment along with their detrimental effects, fate and degradation in aquatic and terrestrial environments. The chapter also dwells upon the role of various regulatory bodies and plausible measures that may be adopted to alleviate the problem.

INTRODUCTION

Pharmaceuticals and personal care products (PPCPs) are the broad group of compounds designed for cure and treatment of various diseases in human and veterinary healthcare setup. These have been an integral part of modern healthcare system and are primarily intended to improve health and the quality of life in the general population. The US FDA has approved over one lakh compounds making up thousands of prescriptions, as well as over the counter (OTC) marketed drug products. Further, there are a large number of drug molecules not approved by the FDA which are in therapeutic use in other countries. Majority of pharmaceuticals are drugs or pharmaceutical excipients and are synthetic/ semi-synthetic molecules belonging to various therapeutic categories such as antibiotics, anti-inflammatory drugs, an-

DOI: 10.4018/978-1-5225-7635-8.ch013

tidepressants, antihypertensives, hormonal drugs, etc. Several compounds have their origins in natural sources including plants, animals, marine products, bacteria or fungi. Pharmaceuticals are utilized for their various therapeutic applications and subsequently, these are excreted from the body along with their metabolites (i.e., breakdown products) as part of normal biochemical elimination processes and enter the environment through various routes. Pharmaceuticals also enter the environment as discharges from the pharmaceutical industry effluents or unused medical products. Veterinary pharmacy is another source of pharmaceuticals entering the environment. Fig. 1 gives a concise representation of the various routes through which pharmaceuticals gain entry into the soil and aquatic environment. In recent years, there has been an increased awareness about this issue (Steger-Hartmann, & Schweinfurth, 2006)

Several of these PPCPs are known to be incompletely removed by wastewater treatment process systems and finally enter rivers, streams, lakes or landfills. Possible harmful contribution of pharmaceuticals towards environmental populations remained a non-existent topic for a long time till early 90s when studies conducted in this area provided an insight that production of pharmaceuticals resulted in the generation of 50-100 times of pharmaceutical and solvent waste (Sheldon, 2007). Various studies suggested that measures are needed to be taken by the pharmaceutical industry to reduce environmental pollution and to introduce greener approaches towards generation. Pharmaceutical pollution is a dynamic entity because life expectancy has been progressively increasing over the years, so the consumption of pharmaceuticals, especially by the elderly population, will also proportionately increase resulting in an increase in pharmaceutical pollution of the environment. Hence, dynamics of the problem needs to be considered for true assessment of the problem. Research in this area has considerably evolved over this decade, beginning with detection and analysis of these micro-pollutants to evaluation of toxicity aspects of pharmaceuticals and presently, risk assessment and risk management issues are being targeted. This book chapter highlights the environmental risks associated with the regular use of pharmaceuticals, their ubiquitous contamination of environment and the role of regulatory agencies in preventing health hazards associated with their environmental exposure. A brief overview of the current status and risks involved are discussed along with the methods and approaches to ameliorate the situation. For greater details, the reader is advised to consult the more specific texts and reviews (e.g., Kummerer, 2009a, 2009b).

Figure 1. Sources of pharmaceuticals in the environment

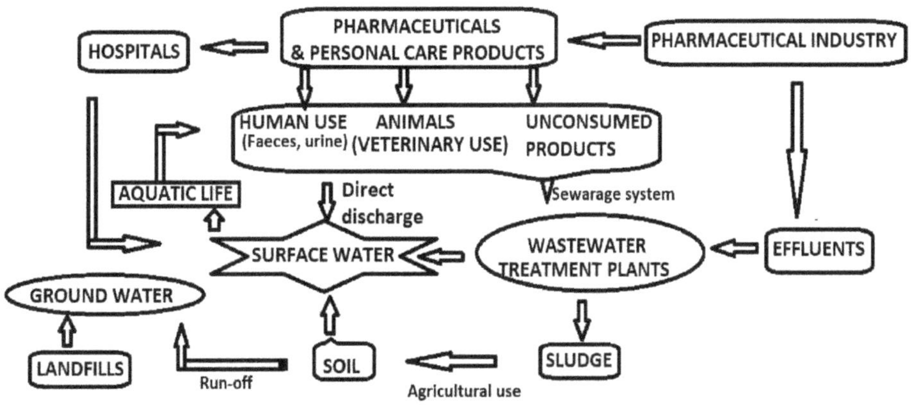

PHARMACEUTICALS IN ENVIRONMENT: GRAVITY OF THE PROBLEM

The presence of APIs (active pharmaceutical ingredients) in the environment is a topic of current interest and is increasingly being highlighted in scientific literature worldwide (Christensen, 1998; Halling-Sørensen et al., 1998; Liebig, Moltmann, & Knacker, 2006). With advances in analytical technology, even trace levels of pharmaceuticals in the environment come within detectable limits. This has not only increased public awareness but also raised concerns about the potential long-term impact of PPCPs on human health and the aquatic environment. Several API (active pharmaceutical ingredient) residues are being detected in drinking water, surface waters (such as rivers and lakes), ground waters, sediments and soils. Several studies and review articles have been published in recent years relating to acute toxicities of different pharmaceutical substances. Toxic effects involve inhibition of enzymes like cyclooxygenase, behavioural changes, reproductive changes, etc. among others.

The persistence of PPCPs pharmaceuticals in the environment (PiE) could pose a greater environmental threat than agricultural pesticides as pharmaceuticals are primarily designed and intended to affect physiological processes in human beings or animals in veterinary pharmacy (Kolpin et al., 2002; Loffler, Rombke, Meller, & Ternes, 2005). The situation cannot be stated as alarming from published studies, including ones from the World Health Organisation (WHO) that concluded that pharmaceuticals in drinking water are less likely to affect human health at the levels detected (WHO's 2012 Technical Report on Pharmaceuticals in Drinking Water). According to this report, the concentrations of pharmaceuticals in treated drinking water are generally well below 50 ng/L (50 parts per trillion). Yet, chronic (long-term) exposure of non-target organisms to pharmaceuticals is an emerging cause of concern which has been accepted by the UN Environment Assembly in its recent 'The Frontiers Report' launched in 2017. This concern is not at all misplaced considering the fact that pharmaceutical substances are inherently, bioactive molecules and their effects on various organisms could be substantial.

Endocrine Disrupting Compounds

Endocrine disrupting agents are the chemicals that interfere with the endocrine systems in humans and animals resulting in various hormonal changes with resultant immunological and neurological effects. A wide range of toxic and carcinogenic chemicals are known to cause endocrine disruption, including dioxins, polychlorinated biphenyls, DDT and other pesticides, and plasticizers such as bisphenol A. However, several pharmaceuticals also happen to be unfortunate inclusions in this list. Some drugs are hormones or hormonal mimics that can affect several aquatic species, e.g., some are capable of feminizing or masculinizing fish (Ternes, 2014). For example, estrogenic drugs 17α-, 17β-ethinyloestradiol and estrone (Fig. 2) are known to be significant contributors towards feminization of male fish in effluent-dominated rivers due to their estrogenic properties (Snyder, Villeneuve, Snyder, & Giesy, 2001, Snyder & Benotti, 2010). The apparent widespread feminization of male fish in rivers has invited significant attention from regulators in Europe, the United Kingdom, the United States, and Japan as reliable laboratory data has confirmed that steroidal estrogens are capable of initiating these estrogenic effects in wild fish at concentrations present in effluents and in the aquatic environment (Gross-Sorokin, Roast, & Brighty, 2006). Based on this study, the Environment Agency of England and Wales had concluded that available evidence for endocrine disruption in fish warrants development of a risk management strategy for monitoring estrogenically active effluents being released in aquatic environment.

Figure 2. Steroidal compounds and oxytocics as endocrine disruptors

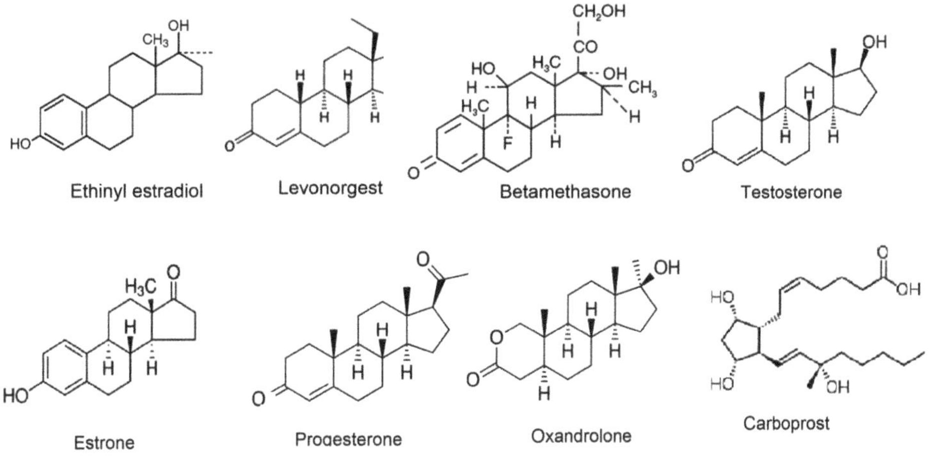

Nearly 90% of the estrogen load in environment comes from animal manure from concentrated animal-feeding operations and it is normally not treated unless it is to be discharged into water bodies. Another study has concluded that feminization of wild fish in U.K. rivers is linked to both steroidal estrogens and xenoestrogens and other contaminants with antiandrogenic properties (Jobling, Burn, Thorpe, Williams, & Tyler, 2009). Recent papers have highlighted the role of a group of fungicides, the azoles (e.g., ketoconazole) (Matthiessen & Weltje, 2015) and commonly used antidiabetic drug metformin (Bienkowski, 2018) in causing masculinization of fish. Studies show that azole drugs bring about masculinization or defeminization in fish possibly by inhibition of the Cytochrome P450 enzyme aromatase (CYP19) (Matthiessen, & Weltje, 2015).

Endocrine disrupting compounds (EDCs) are arousing global concern as an emerging pollutant class because of subsequent exposure of human beings and other animals who are dependent upon these aquatic animals for food (Ismail, Wee, & Aris, 2017). Although there is no complete list of endocrine disruptors available, several steroidal drugs like estrogens, testosterone, progesterone, androgens, contraceptives, and oxytocics are listed in the NIOSH (National Institute for Occupational Safety and Health) Hazardous Drug Alert. Kumar & Xagoraraki (2010) have developed a comprehensive ranking system (termed as EOC Rank system) for prioritizing the monitoring of a total of 100 pharmaceuticals and personal care products and endocrine-disrupting chemicals (together called as Emerging organic contaminants or EOCs) in the stream/source waters and finished drinking water in the U.S.

Antibiotic Contamination of Soil and Water Resources

A major area of concern is excessive level of the reported antibiotic contamination of soil and water bodies leading to development of microbial resistance to antibiotics (Fig. 3). Their recalcitrant nature results in significant exposure of the microorganisms to these drugs. Existing strains of microbes undergo mutations in presence of these antibiotic drug residues present resulting in generation of newer antibiotic-resistant strains. A recent study done on water resources in Hyderabad, South India, a major production area for the global bulk drug market, has concluded that the environmental specimens collected from 28 different sampling sites were contaminated with antimicrobials. Corresponding microbiological

Figure 3. Various types of antimicrobial (antibiotics, sulphonamides) pharmaceutical wastes in soils and water bodies

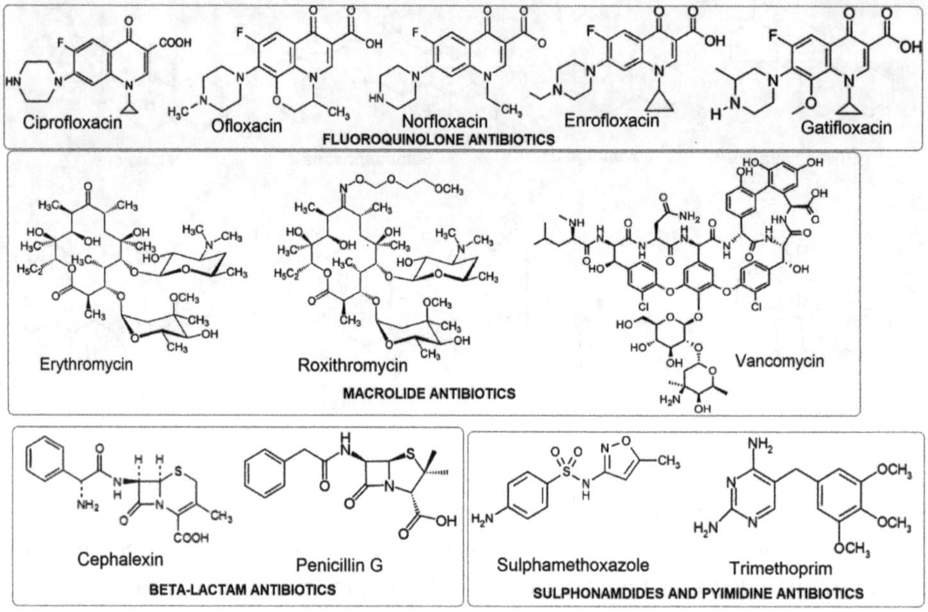

analyses also correspondingly revealed an extensive presence of extended-spectrum beta-lactamase and carbapenemase-producing strains of Enterobacteriaceae and non-fermenters in more than 95% of the samples (Lübbert et al., 2017). These strains have been termed as the modern day 'superbugs.' These resistant superbugs are a cause of grave concern as they have multiplied manifold in huge numbers worldwide, creating a situation of health emergency. There are several of other reports where bacteria resistant to antibiotics have been found in the aquatic environment (Kummer, 2009b; Watkinson, Murby, & Costanzo, 2007). The presence of vancomycin and ampicillin-resistant strains of *Enterococcus faecium* have been reported from wastewaters in England (Caplin, Hanlon, & Taylor, 2008). It is still not clear whether the role of antimicrobials in the development of resistant strains of bacteria and in transfer of resistance is significant at concentrations found for antimicrobials in the environment. However, all these studies do suggest a definitive correlation between the two. Hou et al (2015) have studied the distribution of sulfonamides, selected antibiotics (tetracyclines, quinolones, and macrolides) and antiparasitics (nitrofurans) in livestock manure and amended soils of China. Maximum prevalence levels were found for tetracyclines followed fluoroquinolones, sulphonamides nitrofurans and macrolides in this order. Amended soils showed higher concentrations of tetracyclines (TCs) compared to sulphonamides (SAs) or other veterinary antibiotics because TCs are strongly adsorbed onto the soil organic matter through cation exchange.

Fluoroquinolone antibiotics are one of the most frequently prescribed medicines as therapeutic agents in human and animal health care. This drug class has also become one of the major contaminants in the waste water bodies, and these drugs are not completely removed during the commonly employed treatment processes (Riaz et al., 2018). Their presence in the irrigation water, bio-solids and livestock manure has been reported to adversely affect the soil micro-environment as these tend to interact with soil in several ways with resultant impact on the soil flora and fauna. Fluoroquinolones (FQs) bind strongly to the topsoil, reducing the threat of surface water and groundwater contamination. But their strong binding to soil and sediments further delays their biodegradation and this can explain the observed recalcitrant nature of FQs (Sukul & Spileller, 2007).

The worsening problem of antibiotic resistance has been taken very seriously by the World Health Organization (WHO) which has launched new guidelines on use of antimicrobials. This class of drugs has particularly serious implications with respect to environmental contamination due to their inherent resistance to undergo biodegradation, the reason being that these have actually been developed as antimicrobials (Larsson, 2014). 'The Frontiers Report' released by the United Nations Environment Assembly (2017) has particularly raised concern at the role of the environment in the emergence and spread of resistance to antimicrobials.

Cytotoxic Substances in Environment

Chemotherapeutics used as antineoplastic or cytostatic agents are cytotoxic drugs used to disrupt the proliferation of tumour cells and these are known to contaminate the ecosystems (Fig. 4). These drugs can introduce cytotoxic and/or mutagenic lesions to the DNA and RNA of organisms thus, disrupting their cells. Compared to other classes of drugs like NSAIDs (non-steroidal anti-inflammatory drugs), antibiotics and lipid regulators, these are prescribed in much smaller doses. As a result, these are generally present in the environment at levels below the current levels of analytical detection (LOD value in sub-nanograms/mL) set by the guideline of the European Medicines Agency (EMA). A particular class of these agents, termed as the alkylating agents, are recognized to contribute significantly to environmental pollution. For example, the alkylating anticancer agent cyclophosphamide has been shown to cause modification of the life history parameters and proteome profile of *Daphnia magna* clones (Grzesiuk et al., 2018). Kovacs et al. (2015) have demonstrated histopathological changes in the liver and kidney of *Danio rerio* (zebrafish) as a result of chronic two-generation exposure to the cytotoxic drug 5-fluorouracil (5-FU) at environmentally relevant concentrations (10 ng/L). This exposure impaired their DNA integrity and induced massive whole-transcriptome changes. However, in a later study (Kovacs et al., 2016) low acute and sub-chronic toxicity was reported for four cytostatic drugs 5-fluorouracil, cisplatin, etoposide and imatinib mesylate on zebrafish. A comparative *in vitro* toxicological study conducted with the cytotoxic drugs, 5-FU, cisplatin and etoposide towards zebrafish liver (ZFL) cells, human peripheral blood lymphocytes and human hepatoma (HepG2) cells by Gajski et al. (2016) has demonstrated higher toxicity of these agents on ZFL cells thus, raising concerns about their impact on aquatic organisms. Kümmerer, Haiß, Schuster, Hein, & Ebert, (2016) have investigated the possibility of an underestimation of potential risks related to the presence of anticancer drugs with respect to the trigger value stated in EMA and FDA guidelines. They have identified a total of 102 environmentally relevant antineoplastic agents. Pharmaceuticals in environment typically exist at low concentrations as complex mixtures, hence, a so-called 'cocktail effect' is postulated to be of eco-toxicological significance (Gajski et al., 2016). Several studies have been conducted investigating synergistic effects of mixtures of various cytotoxic drugs (Kundi et al., 2016; Eleršek et al., 2016).

Figure 4. Cytotoxic agents present as wastes in soils and water bodies

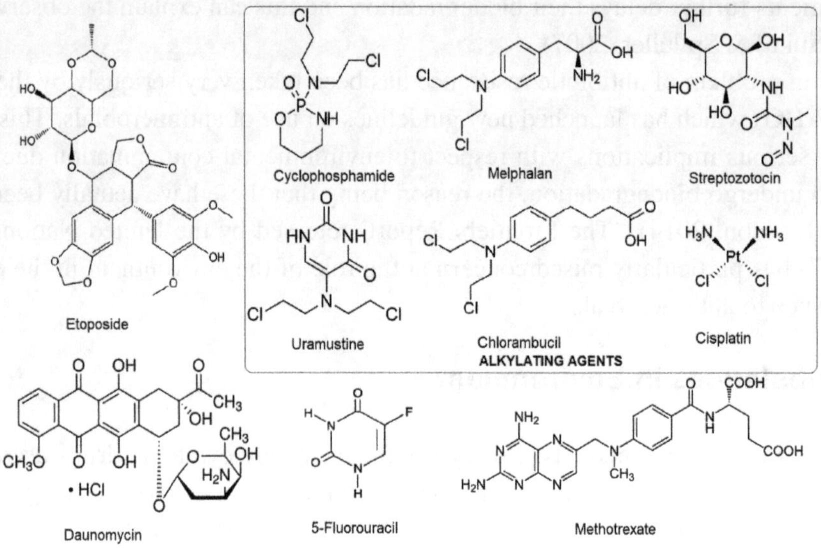

NSAIDs in Environment

Non-steroidal anti-inflammatory drugs (NSAIDs) (Fig. 5) are the most frequently prescribed drugs with high rates of disposal into municipal wastes and landfills. Their presence results in variable levels of alteration of biochemical and microbial activity of soils which disturbs the soil functioning (Cycoń,

Figure 5. Pharmaceutical wastes belonging to different drug classes

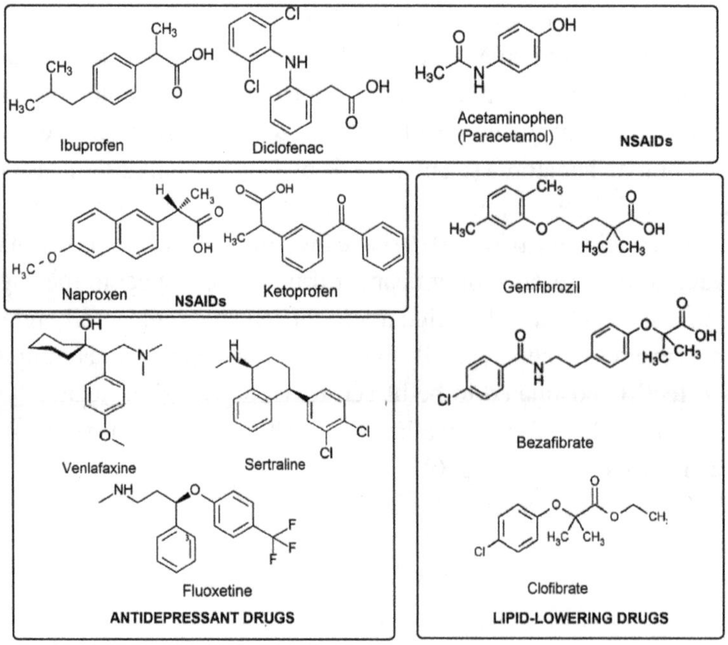

Borymski, Żołnierczyk, & Piotrowska-Seget, 2016). Five most frequently prescribed NSAIDs ibuprofen, diclofenac, naproxen, ketoprofen and indomethacin have been quantified in river resources of Czech Republic (Marsik et al., 2017). Ibuprofen was the most abundant anti-inflammatory analgesic in surface waters attributed to its high consumption and poor elimination profile by the conventional water treatment processes. This was followed by naproxen, diclofenac and ketoprofen and indomethacin in decreasing order of concentrations.

Paracetamol (acetaminophen), a widely used antipyretic, analgesic and antiinflammatory drug and its structural analogs easily accumulate in aquatic environment and have been detected in surface waters, wastewater, and drinking water worldwide (Wu, Zhang, & Chen, 2012). Excessive use of an unlicensed veterinary product containing the anti-inflammatory drug diclofenac has been linked to the decline of the vulture population on the Indian sub-continent. Worldwide, nearly 61% of the vulture species are endangered with extinction, with most significant declines in regions of Asia and Africa previously rich in vulture population (Ogada, Keesing, & Virani, 2012). In Asia, the population of Gyps vultures has slid down by more than 95% due to diclofenac poisoning. The drug was banned by regional governments in 2006, but its veterinary use has continued illegally resulting in exposure of vultures to high levels of diclofenac when they directly feed on cattle carcasses. For diclofenac, the effective concentration for chronic fish toxicity is in the range of wastewater concentrations. Another factor which has been largely ignored is the ecotoxicology of transformation products of drugs. For example, studies relating to toxicological assessment of naproxen and its photo-degradation products in aquatic organisms have shown that photo-transformation products of the drug had higher toxicities than the parent drug, although genotoxicity was not detected (Isidori et al., 2005).

Antidepressant Drugs

Aquatic animals especially fish exposed to antidepressant drugs (Fig. 5) present in water have altered neurotransmitter concentrations and behaviour (Australian water association, 2018). The antidepressant drug oxazepam causes alteration in the behaviour and feeding rate of wild fish *Perca fluviatilis* (Heynen, Fick, Jonsson, Klaminder, & Brodin, 2016) at environmentally relevant concentrations. Similarly, chronic exposure to the selective serotonin reuptake inhibitor (SSRI), fluoxetine (Prozac) has been linked to developmental delays in *Rana pipiens* larvae (Foster, Burton, Basu, & Werner, 2010). Fluoxetine (Prozac) and its active metabolite norfluoxetine are the most frequently detected antidepressants in the brains of wild-caught fish as they bio-accumulate in brain areas (Schultz et al., 2010). Fluoxetine has also raised concerns over potential neuroendocrine disruption in teleost fish (Mennigen, Stroud, Zamora, Moon, & Trudeau, 2011). Other frequently detected antidepressant drugs are sertraline, and its transformation product norsertraline (Schultz et al., 2010). A behavioural study with four commonly prescribed antidepressants, fluoxetine, sertraline, venlafaxine, and bupropion (alone and in mixtures) showed that exposure to venlafaxine and bupropion and mixtures of the four drugs slowed down predator avoidance behaviours in larval fathead minnows (*Pimephales promelas*) (Painter et al., 2010).

Fibrates (Lipid Lowering Drugs)

Lipid regulating drugs (fibrates) (Fig. 5), employed to control hypercholesterolemia, have demonstrated varying degrees of toxicity to various aquatic species. Lipid regulating drug gemfibrozil and diclofenac have demonstrated acute and chronic toxicity to three freshwater species (*Daphnia magna, Pseudokirch-*

neriella subcapitata, Lemna minor) and altered biomarker expression in zebra mussel (*Dreissena polymorpha*). These results suggest toxicity of the two drugs to aquatic species at environmentally relevant concentrations (Quinn, Schmidt, O'Rourke, & Hernan, 2011). Toxicity of the two drugs to the marine mussel (*Mytilus spp.*) has also been reported by Schmidt, O'Rourke, Hernan, & Quinn (2011). Bezafibrate, another lipid-lowering drug has been reported as potential endocrine disruptor in male zebrafish (*Danio rerio*) (Velasco-Santamaría, Korsgaard, Madsen, & Bjerregaard, 2011). Clofibrate is another widely prevalent lipid lowering drug in the aquatic environment which can alter lipid metabolism in male fathead minnows (*Pimephales promelas*) (Weston, Caminada, Galicia, & Fent, 2009).

Several other classes of pharmaceuticals have demonstrated varying levels of ecotoxicity in aquatic and soil environments. Aquatic monitoring of pharmaceuticals in countries like European Union, the USA and China has highlighted the gravity of the problem. A recent study by the German Federal Environment Agency (UBA) has confirmed the presence of as many as 156 pharmaceuticals in Germany in surface water, groundwater and drinking water.

Antihypertensives in Environment

Antihypertensives (Fig. 6) are one of the most commonly used class of drugs today and this is a cause of considerable environmental concern. Several ecotoxicological studies have been directed towards risk assessment of antihypertensives like atenolol, propranolol, metoprolol and verapamil. More than 45 reports are available relating to their immediate and long-term toxicity in environment (Godoy, Kummrow, & Pamplin, 2015a). Beta blockers like propranolol, atenolol and metoprolol have been most frequently detected in the aquatic environment posing hazards to non-target organisms of both fresh and marine water species. Their ecotoxicity evaluation has been recently carried out on varied organisms, such as marine bacteria (*Vibrio fischeri*), green algae (*Scenedesmus vacuolatus*), soil/sediment bacteria (*Arthrobacter globiformis*) and duckweed (*Lemna minor*). Based on toxicological data from the green

Figure 6. Antihypertensive drugs as pharmaceutical wastes

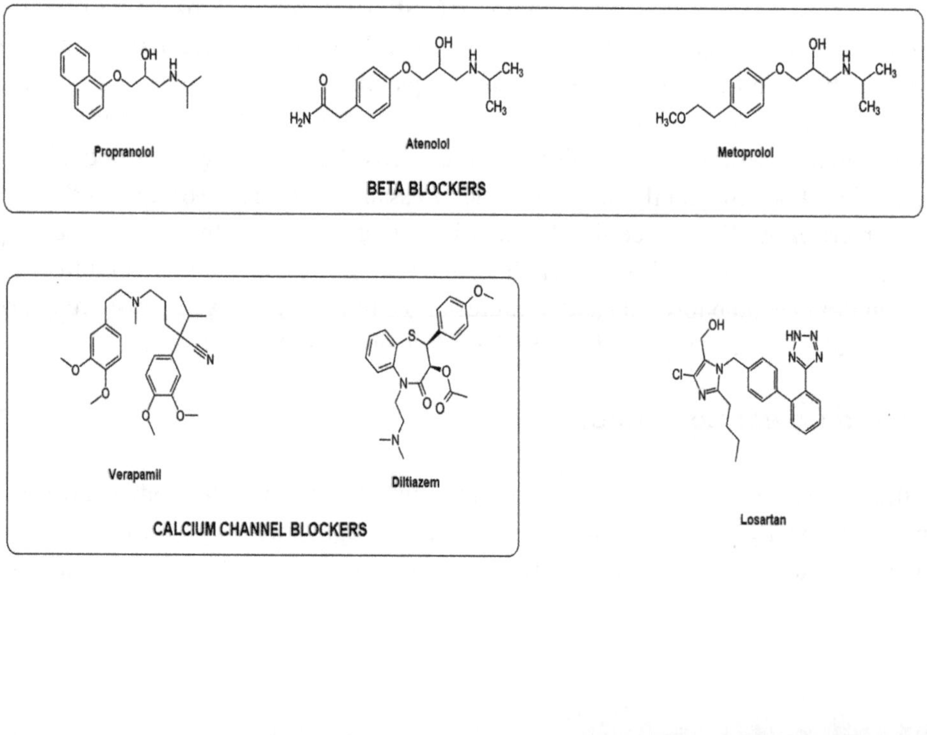

algae test, propranolol and metoprolol have been found to be harmful to aquatic organisms (Maszkowska et al., 2014). The concern is escalated by the fact that these are amongst the drugs achieving highest maximum concentrations in surface waters. A recent report investigates the toxic effects of propranolol (and a NSAID, paracetamol) in the neotropical fish species *Phalloceros harpagos* after their acute and chronic exposure (Pereira et al., 2018). In a recent review report, amount of amlodipine and verapamil (belonging to another class of antihypertensives, i.e., calcium channel blockers) in effluents and freshwater systems has been reported to exceed the therapeutic hazard values (THV) 28% of the time (Saari, Scott, & Brooks, 2107). Losartan is an antihypertensive drug under the most recent class of angiotensin II receptor antagonists. Ecotoxicological evaluation of this drug to *Lemna minor* has shown that losartan poses risk to most aquatic matrices (Godoy, Kummrow, & Pamplin, 2015b)

Inhalation Anesthetics

Halogenated general anesthetics (Fig. 7) such as halothane, enflurane, isoflurane, desflurane, sevoflurane and nitrous oxide (N_2O) are routinely employed during surgery. The emission of these volatile anaesthetics into the environment and its contribution towards ozone depletion in the stratosphere and greenhouse effect has been globally recognized (Langbein et al., 1999; Ryan & Nielsen, 2010). Although these gases are present in the atmosphere at a combined concentration of about 100,000 times lower than carbon dioxide (CO_2), these contribute to a global warming effect of approximately 10% to 15%. This is indicated by their global warming potential (GWP) of 1750. Their vapors are eliminated by exhalation without being metabolized inside the body and hence, these are discharged as waste directly into the atmosphere. The anesthetic use of nitrous oxide alone, a well-known greenhouse gas, contributes almost 3.0% of the total emissions in the United States (Ishizawa, 2011).

Figure 7. Inhalation anaesthetics as pharmaceutical wastes

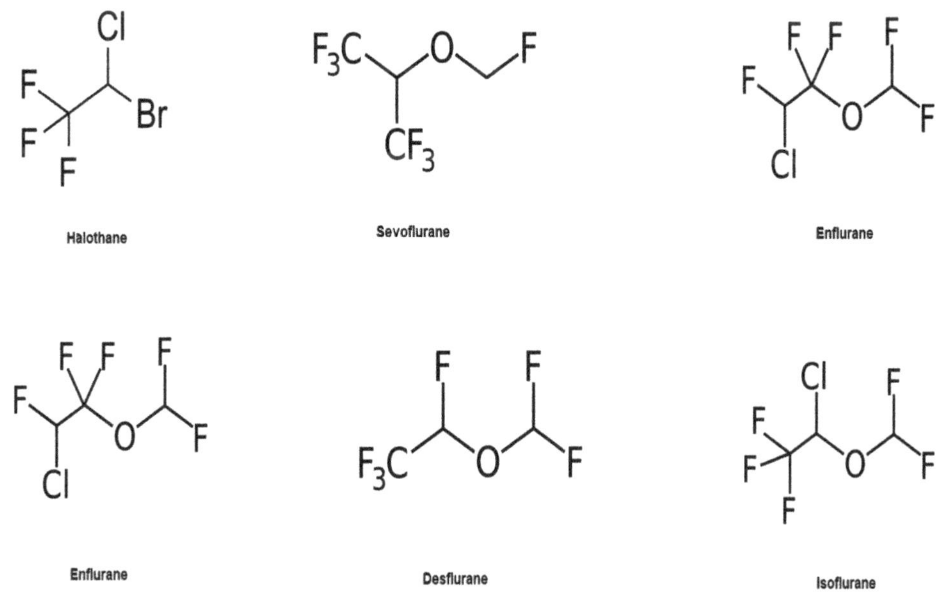

REPORTED STUDIES ON FATE TRANSPORT AND DEGRADATION OF PHARMACEUTICALS

A particular concern regarding the environmental impact of pharmaceuticals and personal care products is that many of these compounds are inherently designed to be lipophilic in order to be able to pass through biological membranes. This imparts them characteristics to be biologically persistent to retain their therapeutic efficacy. Studies have provided evidence of occurrence of more than 160 different APIs (active pharmaceutical ingredients) in the aquatic environment. Concentrations of pharmaceuticals in surface water and effluent from sewage treatment plants (STPs) have been shown to range from ng/L to µg/L. As a consequence, there has been a growing interest not only regarding the presence of pharmaceuticals in the environment but also regarding their fate in various environments. The topic has been reviewed recently (Li, 2014). Dissipation of pharmaceuticals in the aquatic environment is controlled by different processes including aerobic and anaerobic bio-degradation, abiotic transformation such as photo-degradation, hydrolysis and sediment sorption. Most important processes for removal of pharmaceuticals from the dissolved phase are aerobic and anaerobic bio-degradation. As drug compounds are often resistant to hydrolysis, this reaction can be considered as negligible for most human drugs. Direct and indirect photolysis is principal route of abiotic transformation of pharmaceuticals in surface waters.

There are primarily three fates for drugs: first, mineralization to form carbon dioxide and water (Halling- Sørensen et al., 1998), e.g. aspirin (Richardson and Bowron, 1985). Second case is that of lipophilic substances which are not readily degradable and get partly retained in the sludge. Latter is usually dispersed in fields where it may affect the micro-environment. Thirdly, parent lipophilic drug can metabolize to a more hydrophilic form. These metabolites are also persistent and pass on through waste water treatment plants to enter rivers and various water bodies.

Pharmaceuticals are utilized for their numerous pharmacological effects. Once taken inside the body, these undergo various metabolism reactions to be bio-transformed into different chemical substances called as their metabolites (Fig. 8).

Figure 8. Metabolic biotransformation reactions of pharmaceuticals (diclofenac and ibuprofen) inside the body

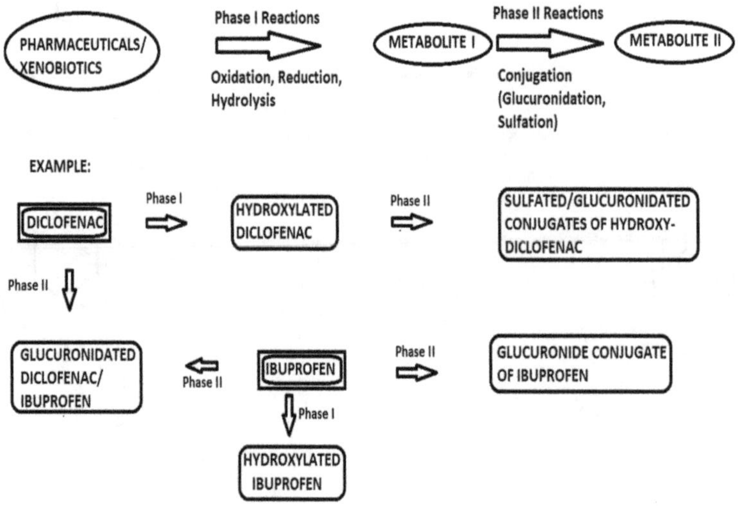

The environmental fate of ten selected pharmaceuticals and pharmaceutical metabolites has been reported by Loffler et al (2005) in water and sediment systems. Amongst these, four ^{14}C-labeled drugs (paracetamol, iopromide, ibuprofen, and diazepam) have been analyzed by radio-TLC analysis whereas, six non-labeled drugs (clofibrate, oxazepam, carbamazepine, 2-hydroxyibuprofen, 10,11-dihydro-10,11-dihydroxycarbamazepine and ivermectin) have been analyzed by LC-tandem mass spectrometry. The NSAID drugs ibuprofen, 2-hydroxyibuprofen, and paracetamol displayed a low persistence with DT_{50} ((time required for 50% dissipation of the initial concentration) values of NMT 20 days (water/sediment system). A moderate persistence was found for drugs ivermectin and oxazepam (DT_{50} 15 and 54 days, respectively). Iopromide, also exhibited a moderate persistence and was converted into at least four transformation products. The drugs diazepam, carbamazepine, 10,11-dihydro-10,11-dihydroxy carbamazepine, and clofibrate, exhibited high persistence (DT_{90} values of > 365 d) in the water/sediment system. An elevated level of sorption onto the sediment was observed for ivermectin, diazepam, oxazepam, and carbamazepine. Another study has been conducted on soil sorption, photo-degradation, and chemical transformation of NSAID drugs naproxen and ibuprofen (Vulava, Cory, Murphey, & Ulmer, 2016). Naproxen is degraded by photochemical oxidation to the extent of more than 90% (Felis, Marciocha, Surmacz-Gorska, & Miksch, 2007). Analgesic drugs, ibuprofen and diclofenac are also effectively removed from aquatic environment by photo-degradation (Felis & Miksch, 2009).

A study with natural steroidal estrogens, estrone, 17β-estradiol, estriol and 17α-estradiol, has shown that conventional wastewater treatment methods (through sorption by sludge and subsequent biodegradation) efficiently remove 17β-estradiol (85-99%), but estrone removal is poor (25-80%). In sewage treatment plants (STPs), elimination rates of various estrogenic hormonal drugs varies from 0% to 90% depending on the type of treatment process and various other parameters including hydraulic and sludge retention times (Combalbert & Hernandez-Raquet, 2010). Fate, transport and biodegradation approaches for natural estrogenic hormones in environment and engineered systems has been investigated by Khanal et al (2006). Further, Silva, Otero, & Esteves (2012) have reviewed various conventional and advanced processes (including physical, biological and advanced oxidation processes) for elimination of natural estrogens- estrone, 17β-estradiol and estriol along with a synthetic estrogen, 17α-ethinylestradiol from aquatic ecosystems. Photo-degradation has been found to be a major degradation route for pharmaceuticals and other chemicals in environment along with other factors such as oxygen, nitrate ions, nitrite ions, etc. Studies with a widely prevalent drug in wastewaters and landfills diclofenac have shown that the drug is photodegradable (Zhang et al., 2011) and more than 90% of the drug is eliminated photolytically from waters in presence of natural sunlight (Poiger, Buser, & Muller, 2009). In this study, the drug first degraded to 8-chlorocarbazole-1-acetic acid, which photo-degraded at an even faster rate than the parent drug itself. Another photo-degradation product, carbazole-1-acetic acid was formed only in the presence of an H-source (e.g., methanol). In the absence of an H-source/air, the product formed was hydroxycarbazole-1-acetic acid. Fate of diclofenac in municipal wastewater plant has been reviewed (Vieno & Sillanpää, 2014). Similarly, salicylic acid has also been found to be photodegraded in aquatic environment by pseudo-first-order reaction kinetics (Gangwang, G. Liu, H. Liu, Zhang, & Wang, 2012). These studies showed that the photo-degradation rate decreased with increasing initial oxygen concentration and increased with increasing oxygen levels. Further, nitrate ions (NO_3^-) and nitrite ions (NO_2^-) also increased the photo-degradation rates. Fluoroquinolone (FQ) antibiotics used in human and veterinary medicine are excreted as parent compound, as conjugates (Phase II metabolism), or as oxidation, dealkylation, hydroxylation, or decarboxylation products of the parent drugs (Phase I metabolic reactions). A significant amount of FQs and their metabolites enter the soil as a part of urine, feces or manure. Although these are not removed completely by various removal processes, wastewater treatment is an efficient method for their elimination (79%-87%) before these enter various water bodies. FQs are also amenable to photodegradative reactions in aqueous medium including oxidation, dealkylation, and cleavage of the piperazine ring system (Sukul & Spiteller, 2007).

Nitrate-induced photo-degradation of atenolol in aqueous solution has been investigated by Ji, Zeng, Ferronato, Chovelon, & Yang (2012) and they have concluded that photo-degradation is very effective mechanism for reduction of atenolol toxicity in natural waters. The photolytic degradation of the drug follows pseudo-first-order kinetics and is affected by various ionic concentrations including nitrate, bicarbonate and hydroxyl ions.

Recently, the presence of abused psychoactive drugs including cocaine, cannabinoids, opiates, etc. have been reported in surface and wastewaters (Boleda, Galceran, & Ventura, 2007; Castiglioni, Zuccato, Chiabrando, Fanelli, & Bagnati, 2008). Nałecz-Jawecki (2007) has evaluated *in vitro* biotransformation of the antidepressant drug fluoxetine by High Performance Liquid Chromatography (HPLC), mass spectrometry (MS) and eco-toxicological tests. A recent study has been reported on eco-toxicological assessment of 43 pharmaceuticals representing diverse classes of drugs, including antibiotics, anti-depressants, anti-inflammatory drugs, sex hormones, lipid regulators and β-blockers with respect to their possible impact on the Mediterranean aquatic environment (Desbiolles, Malleret, Tiliacos, Wong-Wah-Chung, & Laffont-Schwob, 2018). Snyder and Benotti (2010) have reviewed pharmaceuticals endocrine disrupting compounds in drinking water and highlighted various issues associated with their fate and transport. Natural processes like seasonal flow, climate change, prolonged drought, etc. can drastically alter environmental concentrations of these compounds. Studies with abiotic degradation pathways of the NSAID ibuprofen in the presence of a major mineral component of soil (kaolinite clay) (Rubasinghege et al., 2017) have shown that the rate and extent of ibuprofen degradation is greatly dependent upon the presence of clay particles and solar radiation. Adsorption over clay surface by interaction with surface silanols was the predominant mechanism in absence of light whereas, in presence of solar radiations, the drug degraded to various degradation products, the most abundant being 4-acetylbenzoic acid. The latter showed higher toxicity towards algae compared to the parent drug but overall mixture of all degradation products had lower toxicity than ibuprofen.

In a study, the performances of the conventional activated sludge (CAS) treatment and two pilot-scale membrane bioreactors (MBRs) have been assessed in eliminating 31 pharmaceutical substances. The most ubiquitous contaminants in the sewage water were found to be NSAIDs- ibuprofen & acetaminophen, antibiotic- ofloxacin, β-blocker- atenolol, hypoglycaemic drug- glibenclamide, lipid regulator- bezafibrate, and a diuretic- hydrochlorothiazide. Other drugs included ketoprofen, diclofenac, and azithromycin. The anti-epileptic drug carbamazepine and the diuretic hydrochlorothiazide were unaffected by any of the three treatments and other drugs were also not incompletely removed by any of the processes (Radjenović, Petrović, & Barceló, 2009).

Although physical/chemical degradation of various drugs and chemicals plays a major role in their degradation and removal from the environment, degradation of these xenobiotics by biological mechanisms is being widely pursued in various eco-friendly bioremediation approaches. These approaches are based on utilization of various biological processes in microorganisms, plants and enzymes (bacterial bioremediation, mycoremediation, phytoremediation, etc.). These approaches have been recently reviewed (Bali, 2017). For example, paracetamol wastewater is mainly treated by chemical oxidation processes, but its biodegradation is being considered as a low-cost, environment friendly option (Wu, Zhang, & Chen, 2012). Microbial biodegradation of various steroidal estrogens is also known to play a vital role in determining their fate and transport in built and natural environments. Estrogens can be degraded through abiotic degradation and by growth-linked as well as non-growth-linked reactions in the presence of selective microorganisms (Yu, Deeb, & Chu, 2013).

REGULATORY CONTEXT

In the recent years, there has been an increased awareness about the presence of pharmaceuticals and PPCPs in surface water and potable water resources. Several reports on measurements done on surface water or waste water for presence of various PPCPs are available in literature. In the regulatory context, it has become imperative to carry out an environmental risk assessment (ERA) for new PPCPs (Liebig et al., 2006). ERA involves the evaluation of the exposure assessment based on reliably predicted or measured environmental concentrations (PECs or MECs) of chemicals.

In US, there are several regulatory bodies which oversee the management aspects of pharmaceutical wastes. These include the US Environmental Protection Authority (EPA), Drug Enforcement Administration (DEA), Occupational Safety and Health Administration (OSHA), State Environmental Protection Agencies and Local Publicly Owned Treatment Works (POTW). Chemical wastes are categorized as hazardous or non-hazardous wastes. Hazardous wastes are further divided into two main categories:

1. **Listed Wastes:** These are the commercial chemical products recognized as acutely hazardous. These are further subcategorized into F, K, P and U lists.
2. **Characteristic Wastes:** These have to be regulated as they exhibit some hazardous properties, e.g., ignitable, reactive, corrosive and toxic characteristics.

Several pharmaceuticals figure in two of the four lists, i.e., P and U lists.

P-listed pharmaceuticals are the drugs categorized as acutely hazardous (LD_{50} value of 50 mg/kg or lesser) under Resource Conservation and Recovery Act (RCRA) of the United States. There are eight pharmaceuticals currently included in the P-list (Table 1. Epinephrine (adrenergic agent) and nitroglycerin (antianginal drug) are the most common P-listed drugs in use. The USEPA and many state environmental protection agencies (but not all) have provided exclusions for these two drugs. The empty containers and transdermal patches discarded for P-listed drugs are also treated as hazardous wastes.

Twenty-one drugs are included in the U-list of pharmaceutical wastes (termed as U-Listed Pharmaceuticals) (Table 2).

More than 100 chemotherapy agents (used for treatment of cancer) are currently in market. Amongst these, one is P-listed and eight are U-listed pharmaceuticals (Table 2. However, bulk quantities of 'all'

Table 1. P-Listed pharmaceutical wastes

Pharmaceutical	Waste Code	Pharmaceutical	Waste Code
Arsenic trioxide	P012	Phentermine	P046
Epinephrine	P042	Physostigmine	P204
Nicotine	P075	Physostigmine salicylate	P188
Nirtroglycerine	P081	Warfarin<0.3%	P001

Table 2. U-Listed pharmaceutical wastes

Pharmaceutical	Waste Code	Pharmaceutical	Waste Code
Chloral Hydrate	U034	Paraldehyde	U182
Chlorambucil	U034	Phenol	U188
Cyclophosphamide	U034	Reserpine	U200
Daunomycin	U034	Resorcinol	U201
Dichlorodifluoromethane	U034	Saccharin	U202
Diethylstilbestrol	U034	Selenium sulfide	U205
Hexachlorophene	U034	Streptozotocin	U206
Lindane	U129	Trichloromonofluromethane	U121
Melphalan	U150	Uracil Mustard	U237
Mercury	U151	Warfarin<0.3%	U248
Mitomycin C	U010		

these agents have to be managed as hazardous wastes. Several pharmaceutical companies and hospitals have been discarding "bulk" P- or U- listed chemotherapy agents as trace chemotherapy waste as there are no particular RCRA regulations for trace chemotherapy waste. This is one area in which enforcement strategy needs to be implemented.

The US EPA has released a 'ten-step blueprint for healthcare facilities in the United States'. The original version was published on 15th April 2006 which has been revised and published in 2008 (EPA, 2008). All of the above described information relating to categorization and treatment of various types of pharmaceutical wastes has been included in this document.

Recognizing this environmental impact of pharmaceuticals, several countries have developed formal environmental risk assessment (ERA) guidelines for pharmaceuticals. For example, these legal guidelines are a part of the registration dossier for pharmaceutical products in Europe and the United States. It is not easy to directly and exclusively relate an environmental effect to the release of one particular pharmaceutical contained in a product. Thus, European legislation includes a prospective ERA for registra-

Table 3. P- and U-Listed Chemotherapy Agents

Chemotherapy Agent	Waste Code
Arsenic trioxide	**P012**
Chlorambucil	**U035**
Cyclophosphamide	**U058**
Daunomycin	**U059**
Diethylstilbestrol	**U089**
Melphalan	**U150**
Mitomycin C	**U010**
Streptozotocin	**U206**
Uracil Mustard (Uramustine)	**U237**

tion of human and veterinary products and for all new marketing applications for human and veterinary medicinal products. In this regard, studies are formally conducted to evaluate the environmental fate of the APIs and assess their potential toxicity to various environmental species. The information garnered from these studies is compiled in ERA expert reports submitted in support of US/EU drug filings.

The European Medicines Agency (EMEA) has laid down guidelines outlining the process of the environmental risk assessment for human drugs. These guidelines encompass a two-tiered assessment program: first is a modelling step for the scenario of an environmental exposure and a subsequently, the second step relates to the environmental fate and effects testing.

The World Health Organization (WHO) has taken serious cognizance of the worsening problem of antibiotic resistance and it has launched new guidelines on use of medically important antimicrobials in food-producing animals (WHO guidelines on use of medically important antimicrobials in food-producing animals, 2007). WHO has recommended that farmers and the food industry should stop the routine use of antibiotics for prevention of diseases or for promotion of growth in healthy animals. The intention is to reduce their use in animals so that their effectiveness may be preserved for human medicine by reducing the chances of development of resistance. 'The Frontiers Report' launched by the United Nations Environment Assembly at UN Environment headquarters in Nairobi (Dec. 5, 2017) has included antimicrobial resistance amongst the six emerging areas of concern. Most importantly, it has particularly highlighted the role of the environment in the emergence/spread of resistance to antimicrobials and development of ferocious superbugs. The UN Environment chief Erik Solheim has stated that "We could be spurring the development of ferocious superbugs through ignorance and carelessness."

All these regulations have resulted in several drug manufacturing units designing and operating their manufacturing processes and facilities and formulating policies to minimize discharges of pharmaceuticals into the wastewater and to ensure disposal of returned or waste pharmaceutical products in an environment friendly manner (Pfizer, 2018; GlaxoSmithKline, 2016). Several industrial houses are setting up pre-treatment plants for wastewater treatment using additional technologies to ensure that APIs posing health risks are eliminated prior to discharge, e.g., methods like incineration may be followed rather than disposing them off in landfills. Unfortunately, situation in developing countries in the Asian subcontinent is quite different. Here, specific guidelines are either non-existent or regulations are not enforced stringently and the effluents from pharmaceutical companies contribute to various forms of environmental pollution. Unfortunately, the regulatory agencies in developed countries also do not consider environmental norms of the companies from which they are procuring the drugs for manufacturing drug products. As an example, the Good Manufacturing Practices (GMPs) norms to be fulfilled by drugs manufacturing companies to sell their products in the UK do not include environmental practices as one of the criteria to be inspected by regulatory agency for medicines and medical devices in the UK.

Hospitals and other healthcare facilities can play a crucial role in alleviating this problem through effective management of drug inventory. Two case studies have been reported (EPA, 2008) where two hospitals implemented proper management programs to reduce the quantity of outdated medicines and resultant pharmaceutical waste. An inventory reduction project was undertaken at Falls Memorial Hospital at Minnesota which resulted in significant reduction of pharmaceutical waste but also reduced the hospital expenses. This included preparation of therapeutic substitution lists and reduction of number of stocked medicines belonging to the same therapeutic class in the formulary. Using these substitution lists, the patient on a particular drug could be switched to another drug of the same class which was included in the formulary. In the second case at Hennepin County Medical Center (HCMC), Minneapolis, Minnesota, reverse distribution system was introduced in the hospital as a part of waste reduction project to ensure that maximum drugs were used before their expiration period. This resulted in over $80,000 in cost savings and reduction of 378 lbs. of pharmaceutical waste.

WHAT NEEDS TO BE DONE?

Although, awareness of the problem is there, limited steps have been taken to recognize pharmaceutical contaminants in water sources and to device measures to reduce them (Deziel, 2014; Kummerer, 2010). This is probably due to the fact that the problem does not apparently look like a major issue in present context. However, this can also be attributed to limited data available on contamination and the problem may actually be more deep-seated than it could be envisaged.

During the course of drug development programs of human pharmaceuticals, considerable amount of data relating to the pharmacological, pharmacokinetic and toxicological parameters is generated. This information can be used to develop substance-specific test programs for evaluation of potential environmental risk additionally taking into account their patient usage patterns and pharmacodynamic parameters. Laenge, Steger-Hartmann, & Schweinfurth (2006) have suggested that the environmental risk evaluation process included as a part of drug approval process should be a focused assessment strategy based on the existing therapeutic requirements in light of the current knowledge. Research needs to be directed towards newer methods of decomposition of drugs in wastes. For example, Bojanowska-Czajka et al (2015) have studied the radiolytic decomposition of the three widely used drugs diclofenac, ibuprofen and carbamazepine (antiepileptic) as a function of absorbed dose of gamma radiations. The possibility of decomposition of all the drugs has been investigated in river water samples as well as hospital waste. Another degradation method for the antibiotic ciprofloxacin and sulfonamide antibiotic sulfamethoxazole has been assessed by ferrous-activated persulfate with possible implications in remediation of groundwater laden with antibiotics (Ji, Ferronato, Salvador, Yang, & Chovelon, 2014). Degradation of antibiotics in the river water matrix was found to be comparable to Milli-Q water, implying that the method is suitable for depleting the antibiotics under environmentally relevant conditions.

Photocatalytic degradation of another persistent pharmaceutical from wastewaters carbamazepine has been reported using titanium dioxide (TiO_2) and zinc oxide (ZnO) nanoparticles prepared in the presence of water-soluble whey powder as stabilizer (Mohapatra et al., 2014). Another method based on advanced oxidation treatment of wastewater and wastewater sludge also resulted in complete removal of carbamazepine (Mohapatra, Brar, Tyagi, Picard, & Surampalli, 2014). Recently, degradation and mineralization of amoxicillin, a beta-lactam antibiotic included in the WHO list of essential medicines has been studies by UVC-activated persulfate-based photo-degradation in various aqueous media (Kattel, Kaur, Trapido, & Dulova, 2018). The treatment was found to degrade the drug completely.

Eco-pharmacovigilance (EPV) is a pragmatic approach which can be employed to assess and minimize the potential risks presented by pharmaceutical residues in environment. It is an emerging area of research being proposed as a new means of risk assessment and scientific understanding of the problem in which an individual drug or a specific group/class of pharmaceuticals is targeted on a prioritized basis. It is a feasible, economical and customized approach to reduce the environmental concentrations and risks of pharmaceuticals. Being a developing branch of science, its encompassments and methodologies are yet to be decided. Although, it is impractical to implement this for all pharmaceuticals, still it can be carried out for a selected group or class of drugs which have extensive use in medicine, e.g., NSAIDs (Holm et al., 2013; He, Wang, Liu, & Hu, 2017; Wang, He, Yan, & Hu, 2017). An example may be cited of a recent literature report on targeted eco-pharmacovigilance for ketoprofen which has given certain recommendations based on available ecotoxicity data on the drug. These include close monitoring of the drug in natural environment, reduction of drug residues in environment through source control, encouraging urine source separation and treatment and controlled use of ketoprofen in veterinary settings (Wang, Zhao, Zhang, & He, 2018).

FUTURE RESEARCH DIRECTIONS

Future research in this area should target various aspects with one common goal of reducing pharmaceutical contaminants in the environment. This should begin with reduction of pharmaceutical discharges into land and water through proper use and disposal guidelines. Reduction of environmental exposure resulting from improper drug disposal at the level of patient warrants increased awareness. There needs to be a heightened level of communication and cooperation between patients, physicians, retailers and pharmaceutical companies to ensure that unused or expired products are returned by retailers (and others in the supply chain) to the manufacturer. Physicians and pharmacists need to sensitize and educate the patients about proper use of medicines and return of unused medicines to the pharmacy. Secondly, database on risks posed by different drug classes needs to be expanded. Combinations of several management strategies are required to palliate the risks presented by pharmaceuticals. These include pharmaceutical-return programs, sophisticated effluent treatment strategies in consultation with various stakeholders and laying emphasis on development of "green" pharmaceuticals. Comprehensive eco-toxicological studies are available for very few substances due to which the knowledge regarding the fate, transportation of a vast section of pharmaceuticals is virtually non-existent. There is practically no data for risk assessment of metabolites or other transformation products of most of the drugs in use. The main obscurity with respect to drug pollutants is what fractions of drug residues occurring in environment are coming from discarded unused drugs (Ruhoy & Daughtonm, 2007). Hence, work needs to be directed towards enhancing this knowledge base so that the obtained information can be utilized in development of green pharmacy. Limits and/or thresholds for APIs in different environmental areas and in drinking water have to be laid down. Plausible environmental risks posed by the launch of a new pharmaceutical product must be assessed *via* tracking its usage and exposure aspects.

Third and the most important research is the development of more effective remediation measures for removal of drug contaminants from land and aquatic environment. More efficient sewage treatment methods should be devised considering the pharmaceutical contaminants in a particular geographical area. Effective bioremediation measures need to be developed to overcome the various drawbacks of chemical and physical treatments.

Drug producers are expected to follow Good Manufacturing Practices (GMP) guidelines, but unfortunately, these guidelines do not cover the environmental aspects. Hence, it is the need of the hour that various pharmaceutical companies not only follow the Good Manufacturing Practices (GMP) norms but also adopt green and sustainable pharmacy practices. They must consider long-term environmental aspects in the design and launch of new APIs so that more environmentally benign pharmaceuticals reach the market. Last but not the least, in order to educate the physicians as well as pharmacists about environmental aspects of drugs, this information could be included in the syllabi of the undergraduate and post graduate pharmacy and medicine programs.

CONCLUSION

Pharmaceutical contamination of terrestrial and water resources is an emerging global problem. The available database on the toxicity aspects of pharmaceuticals at levels encountered in the environment is abysmally low, especially in the developing countries. Pharmaceuticals are gaining access to our water bodies and soils through a variety of routes and we are not even having adequate knowledge about the gravity of the problem. There has been an increased sensitization and awareness about the problem as evidenced from an escalation of literature reports in recent years. However, lot still needs to be done to assess the level of contaminations of various classes of pharmaceuticals. Pharmaceutical industry, hospitals along with every member of the healthcare chain need to join hands together to practice green pharmacy with an aim to reduce deleterious environmental impacts. Eco-pharmacovigilance measures are needed to assess and circumvent these problems which may not appear to be urgent but will definitely escalate in long-term if not adequately addressed at growing stage itself.

REFERENCES

Australian Water Association. (2018). *Antidepressant drugs in water affect fish behaviour.* Retrieved from http://www.awa.asn.au/AWA_MBRR/Publications/Latest_News/Antidepressant_drugs_in_water_affect_fish_behaviour.aspx

Bali, A. (2017). Bioremediation of Pharmaceutical Wastes. In J. N. Bhakta (Ed.), *Handbook of Research on Inventive Bioremediation Techniques* (pp. 364–393). Hershey, PA: IGI Global. doi:10.4018/978-1-5225-2325-3.ch016

Bienkowski, B. (2018). Diabetes Drug Makes Male Minnows More Female. *Scientific American*. Retrieved from https://www.scientificamerican.com/article/diabetes-drug-makes-male-minnows-more-female/

Bojanowska-Czajka, A., Kciuk, G., Gumiela, M., Borowiecka, S., Nałęcz-Jawecki, G., Koc, A., ... Trojanowicz, M. (2015). Analytical, toxicological and kinetic investigation of decomposition of the drug diclofenac in waters and wastes using gamma radiation. *Environmental Science and Pollution Research International*, *22*(24), 20255–20270. doi:10.100711356-015-5236-6 PMID:26308920

Boleda, M. R., Galceran, M. T., & Ventura, F. J. (2007). Trace determination of cannabinoids and opiates in wastewater and surface waters by ultra-performance liquid chromatography-tandem mass spectrometry. *Journal of Chromatography. A*, *1175*(1), 38–48. doi:10.1016/j.chroma.2007.10.029 PMID:17980892

Caplin, J. L., Hanlon, G. W., & Taylor, H. D. (2008). Presence of vancomycin and ampicillin-resistant *Enterococcus faecium* of epidemic clonal complex-17 in wastewaters from the south coast of England. *Environmental Microbiology*, *10*(4), 885–892. doi:10.1111/j.1462-2920.2007.01507.x PMID:18093157

Castiglioni, S., Zuccato, E., Chiabrando, C., Fanelli, R., & Bagnati, R. (2008). Mass spectrometric analysis of illicit drugs in wastewater and surface water. *Mass Spectrometry Reviews*, *27*(4), 378–384. doi:10.1002/mas.20168 PMID:18421768

Christensen, F. M. (1998). Pharmaceuticals in the environment--a human risk? *Regulatory Toxicology and Pharmacology*, *28*(3), 212–222. doi:10.1006/rtph.1998.1253 PMID:10049792

Combalbert, S., & Hernandez-Raquet, G. (2010). Occurrence, fate, and biodegradation of estrogens in sewage and manure. *Applied Microbiology and Technology*, *86*(6), 1671–1692. doi:10.100700253-010-2547-x PMID:20354692

Cycoń, M., Borymski, S., Żołnierczyk, B., & Piotrowska-Seget, Z. (2016). Variable effects of non-steroidal anti-inflammatory drugs (NSAIDs) on selected biochemical processes mediated by soil microorganisms. *Frontiers in Microbiology*, *7*, 1969. doi:10.3389/fmicb.2016.01969 PMID:28018307

Daughton, C. G. (2003). Cradle-to-cradle stewardship of drugs for minimizing their environmental disposition while promoting human health. I. Rationale for and avenues toward a green pharmacy. *Environmental Health Perspectives*, *111*(5), 757–774. doi:10.1289/ehp.5947 PMID:12727606

Desbiolles, F., Malleret, L., Tiliacos, C., Wong-Wah-Chung, P., & Laffont-Schwob, I. (2018). Occurrence and eco-toxicological assessment of pharmaceuticals: Is there a risk for the Mediterranean aquatic environment? *The Science of theTotal Environment, 639*, 1334-1348.

Deziel, N. (2014). Pharmaceuticals in wastewater treatment plant effluent waters," *Scholarly Horizons: University of Minnesota, Morris Undergraduate Journal, 1*(2).

Eleršek, T., Milavec, S., Korošec, M., Brezovšek, P., Negreira, N., Zonja, B., ... Filipič, M. (2016). Toxicity of the mixture of selected antineoplastic drugs against aquatic primary producers and their behaviour under the applied exposure conditions. *Environmental Science and Pollution Research International*, *23*(15), 14780–14790. doi:10.100711356-015-6005-2 PMID:26755176

Environmental Protection Agency. Managing Pharmaceutical Waste: A 10-Step Blueprint for Healthcare Facilities in the United States, *U.S. Environmental Protection Agency*. Retrieved from http://www.hercenter.org/hazmat/tenstepblueprint.pdf

Federal Environment Agency. (2013). *Pharmaceuticals in the Environment – A first Compilation of German Monitoring Data*. Retrieved from www.umweltbundesamt.de/sites/default/files/medien/377/dokumente/compilation-pharmaceuticalsintheenvironment_uba.pdf

Felis, E., Marciocha, D., Surmacz-Gorska, J., & Miksch, K. (2007). Photochemical degradation of naproxen in the aquatic environment. *Water Science and Technology*, *55*(12), 281–286. doi:10.2166/wst.2007.417 PMID:17674860

Felis, E., & Miksch, K. (2007). Removal of analgesic drugs from the aquatic environment using photochemical methods. *Water Science and Technology*, *60*(9), 2253–2259. doi:10.2166/wst.2009.668 PMID:19901456

Foster, H. R., Burton, G. A., Basu, N., & Werner, E. E. (2010). Chronic exposure to fluoxetine (Prozac) causes developmental delays in Rana pipiens larvae. *Environmental Toxicology and Chemistry*, *29*(12), 2845–2850. doi:10.1002/etc.345 PMID:20836066

Gangwang, G., Liu, G., Liu, H., Zhang, N., & Wang, Y. (2012). Photodegradation of salicylic acid in aquatic environment: effect of different forms of nitrogen. *The Science of the Total Environment, 435-436*, 573-577.

Gajski, G., Gerić, M., Žegura, B., Novak, M., Nunić, J., Bajrektarević, D., ... & Filipič, M. (2016). Genotoxic potential of selected cytostatic drugs in zebrafish liver cell line, human hepatoma HepG2 cells and human lymphocytes. *Environmental Science and Pollution Research International*, *23*(15), 14739–14750. doi:10.100711356-015-4592-6 PMID:25943512

GlaxoSmithKline. (2016). *GSK Public policy positions: Pharmaceuticals in the environment.* US: GlaxoSmithKline Communications and Government Affairs.

Godoy, A. A., Kummrow, F., & Pamplin, P. A. (2015a). Occurrence, ecotoxicological effects and risk assessment of antihypertensive pharmaceutical residues in the aquatic environment--A review. *Chemosphere, 138*, 281–291. doi:10.1016/j.chemosphere.2015.06.024 PMID:26091869

Godoy, A. A., Kummrow, F., & Pamplin, P. A. (2015b). Ecotoxicological evaluation of propranolol hydrochloride and losartan potassium to Lemna minor L. (1753) individually and in binary mixtures. *Ecotoxicology (London, England)*, *24*(5), 1112–1123. doi:10.100710646-015-1455-3 PMID:25847105

Gross-Sorokin, M. Y., Roast, S. D., & Brighty, G. C. (2006). Assessment of feminization of male fish in English rivers by the environment agency of England and Wales. *Environmental Health Perspectives*, *114*(Supplement 1), 147–151. doi:10.1289/ehp.8068 PMID:16818261

Grzesiuk, M., Mielecki, D., Pilżys, T., Garbicz, D., Marcinkowski, M., & Grzesiuk, E. (2018). How cyclophosphamide at environmentally relevant concentration influences Daphnia magna life history and its proteome. *PLoS One*, *13*(4), e0195366. doi:10.1371/journal.pone.0195366 PMID:29621334

Halling-Sørensen, B., Nors Nielsen, S., Lanzky, P. F., Ingerslev, F., Holten Lützhøft, H. C., & Jørgensen, S. E. (1998). Occurrence, fate and effects of pharmaceutical substances in the environment--a review. *Chemosphere*, *36*(2), 357–393. doi:10.1016/S0045-6535(97)00354-8 PMID:9569937

He, B. S., Wang, J., Liu, J., & Hu, X. M. (2017). Eco-pharmacovigilance of non-steroidal anti-inflammatory drugs: Necessity and opportunities. *Chemosphere*, *181*, 178–189. doi:10.1016/j.chemosphere.2017.04.084 PMID:28437743

Heynen, M., Fick, J., Jonsson, M., Klaminder, J., & Brodin, T. (2016). Effect of bioconcentration and trophic transfer on realized exposure to oxazepam in 2 predators, the dragonfly larvae (*Aeshna grandis*) and the Eurasian perch (*Perca fluviatilis*). *Environmental Toxicology and Chemistry*, *35*(4), 930–937. doi:10.1002/etc.3368 PMID:26762222

Holm, G., Snape, J. R., Murray-Smith, R., Talbot, J., Taylor, D., & Sörme, P. (2013). Implementing ecopharmacovigilance in practice: Challenges and potential opportunities. *Drug Safety*, *36*(7), 533–546. doi:10.100740264-013-0049-3 PMID:23620169

Hou, J., Wan, W., Mao, D., Wang, C., Mu, Q., Qin, S., & Luo, Y. (2015). Occurrence and distribution of sulfonamides, tetracyclines, quinolones, macrolides, and nitrofurans in livestock manure and amended soils of Northern China. *Environmental Science and Pollution Research International*, *22*(6), 4545–4554. doi:10.100711356-014-3632-y PMID:25318415

Ishizawa, Y. (2011). Special article: General anesthetic gases and the global environment. *Anesthesia and Analgesia*, *112*(1), 213–217. doi:10.1213/ANE.0b013e3181fe02c2 PMID:21048097

Isidori, M., Lavorgna, M., Nardelli, A., Parrella, A., Previtera, L., & Rubino, M. (2005). Ecotoxicity of naproxen and its phototransformation products. *The Science of the Total Environment*, *348*(1), 93–101. doi:10.1016/j.scitotenv.2004.12.068 PMID:16162316

Ismail, N. A. H., Wee, S. Y., & Aris, A. Z. (2017). Multi-class of endocrine disrupting compounds in aquaculture ecosystems and health impacts in exposed biota. *Chemosphere*, *188*, 375–388. doi:10.1016/j.chemosphere.2017.08.150 PMID:28892772

Ji, Y., Ferronato, C., Salvador, A., Yang, X, & Chovelon, J. M. (2014). Degradation of ciprofloxacin and sulfamethoxazole by ferrous-activated persulfate: implications for remediation of groundwater contaminated by antibiotics. *The Science of the Total Environment, 472,* 800-808.

Ji, Y., Zeng, C., Ferronato, C., Chovelon, J. M., & Yang, X. (2012). Nitrate-induced photodegradation of atenolol in aqueous solution: Kinetics, toxicity and degradation pathways. *Chemosphere*, *88*(5), 644–649. doi:10.1016/j.chemosphere.2012.03.050 PMID:22497785

Jobling, S., Burn, R. W., Thorpe, K., Williams, R., & Tyler, C. (2009). Statistical modeling suggests that antiandrogens in effluents from wastewater treatment works contribute to widespread sexual disruption in fish living in English rivers. *Environmental Health Perspectives*, *117*(5), 797–802. doi:10.1289/ehp.0800197 PMID:19479024

Kattel, E., Kaur, B., Trapido, M., & Dulova, N. (2018). Persulfate-based photodegradation of a beta-lactam antibiotic amoxicillin in various water matrices. *Environmental Technology*, 1–28. doi:10.1080/09593330.2018.1493149 PMID:29932810

Khanal, S. K., Xie, B., Thompson, M. L., Sung, S., Ong, S. K., & Van Leeuwent, J. (2006). Fate, transport, and biodegradation of natural estrogens in the environment and engineered systems. *Environmental Science & Technology*, *40*(21), 6537–6546. doi:10.1021/es0607739 PMID:17144275

Kolpin, D. W., Furlong, E. T., Meyer, M. T., Thurman, E. M., Zaugg, S. D., Barber, L. B., & Buxton, H. T. (2002). Pharmaceuticals, Hormones, and Other Organic Wastewater Contaminants in U.S. Streams, 1999–2000: A National Reconnaissance. *Environmental Science & Technology*, *36*(6), 1202–1211. doi:10.1021/es011055j PMID:11944670

Kovacs, R., Bakos, K., Urbnyi, B., Kovesi, J., Gazsi, G., Csepeli, A., ... Horvath, A. (2016). Acute and sub-chronic toxicity of four cytostatic drugs in zebrafish. *Environmental Science and Pollution Research International*, *23*(15), 14718–14729. doi:10.100711356-015-5036-z PMID:26201655

Kovacs, R., Csenki, Z., Bakos, K., Urbanyi, B., Horvath, A., Garaj-Vrhovac, V., ... Filipic, M. (2015). Assessment of toxicity and genotoxicity of low doses of 5-fluorouracil in zebrafish (*Danio rerio*) two-generation study. *Water Research, 77*, 201–212. doi:10.1016/j.watres.2015.03.025 PMID:25889180

Kumar, A., Xagoraraki, I. (2010). Pharmaceuticals, personal care products and endocrine-disrupting chemicals in U.S. surface and finished drinking waters: a proposed ranking system. *The Science of the Total Environment, 408*(28), 5972-5989.

Kummerer, K. (2009a). The presence of pharmaceuticals in the environment due to human use—Present knowledge and future challenges. *Journal of Environmental Management, 90*(8), 2354–2366. doi:10.1016/j.jenvman.2009.01.023 PMID:19261375

Kummerer, K. (2009b). Antibiotics in the environment—a review—part II. *Chemosphere, 75*(4), 435–441. doi:10.1016/j.chemosphere.2008.12.006 PMID:19178931

Kummerer, K. (2010). Pharmaceuticals in the environment. *Annual Review of Environment and Resources, 35*(1), 57–75. doi:10.1146/annurev-environ-052809-161223

Kümmerer, K., Haiß, A., Schuster, A., Hein, A., & Ebert, I. (2016). Antineoplastic compounds in the environment—Substances of special concern. *Environmental Science and Pollution Research International, 23*(15), 14791–14804. doi:10.100711356-014-3902-8 PMID:25475615

Kundi, M., Parrella, A., Lavorgna, M., Criscuolo, E., Russo, C., & Isidori, M. (2016). Prediction and assessment of ecogenotoxicity of antineoplastic drugs in binary mixtures. *Environmental Science and Pollution Research International, 23*(15), 14771–14779. doi:10.100711356-015-4884-x PMID:26139396

Laenge, R., Steger-Hartmann, T., & Schweinfurth, H. (2006). The environmental risk assessment of human pharmaceuticals in the overall EU regulatory affairs process. *Regulatory Toxicology and Pharmacology, 45*(3), 223–228. doi:10.1016/j.yrtph.2006.04.001 PMID:16716476

Langbein, T., Sonntag, H., Trapp, D., Hoffmann, A., Malms, W., Röth, E. P., ... Zellner, R. (1999). Volatile anaesthetics and the atmosphere: Atmospheric lifetimes and atmospheric effects of halothane, enflurane, isoflurane, desflurane and sevoflurane. *British Journal of Anaesthesia, 82*(1), 66–73. doi:10.1093/bja/82.1.66 PMID:10325839

Larsson, D. G. J. (2014). Antibiotics in the environment. *Upsala Journal of Medical Sciences, 119*(2), 108–112. doi:10.3109/03009734.2014.896438 PMID:24646081

Li, W. C. (2014). Occurrence, sources, and fate of pharmaceuticals in aquatic environment and soil. *Environmental Pollution, 187*, 193–201. doi:10.1016/j.envpol.2014.01.015 PMID:24521932

Liebig, M., Moltmann, J. F., & Knacker, T. (2006). Evaluation of measured and predicted environmental concentrations of selected human pharmaceuticals and personal care products. *Environmental Science and Pollution Research International, 13*(2), 110–119. doi:10.1065/espr2005.08.276 PMID:16612900

Löffler, D., Römbke, J., Meller, M., & Ternes, T. A. (2005). Environmental fate of pharmaceuticals in water/sediment systems. *Environmental Science & Technology, 39*(14), 5209–5218. doi:10.1021/es0484146 PMID:16082949

Lübbert, C., Baars, C., Dayakar, A., Lippmann, N., Rodloff, A. C., Kinzig, M., & Sörgel, F. (2017). Environmental pollution with antimicrobial agents from bulk drug manufacturing industries in Hyderabad, South India, is associated with dissemination of extended-spectrum beta-lactamase and carbapenemase-producing pathogens. *Infection*, *45*(4), 479–491. doi:10.100715010-017-1007-2 PMID:28444620

Maszkowska, J., Stolte, S., Kumirska, J., Łukaszewicz, P., Mioduszewska, K., Puckowski, A., ... Białk-Bielińska, A. (2014). Beta-blockers in the environment: Part II. Ecotoxicity study. *The Science of the Total Environment*, *15*(493), 1122–1126. doi:10.1016/j.scitotenv.2014.06.039 PMID:24975494

Matthiessen, P., & Weltje, L. (2015). A review of the effects of azole compounds in fish and their possible involvement in masculinization of wild fish populations. *Critical Reviews in Toxicology*, *45*(5), 453–467. doi:10.3109/10408444.2015.1018409 PMID:25899164

Mennigen, J. A., Stroud, P., Zamora, J. M., Moon, T. W., & Trudeau, V. L. (2011). Pharmaceuticals as neuroendocrine disruptors: Lessons learned from fish on Prozac. *Journal of Toxicology and Environmental Health. Part B, Critical Reviews*, *14*(5-7), 387–412. doi:10.1080/10937404.2011.578559 PMID:21790318

Mohapatra, D. P., Brar, S. K., Daghrir, R., Tyagi, R. D., Picard, P., Surampalli, R. Y., & Drogui, P. (2014). Photocatalytic degradation of carbamazepine in wastewater by using a new class of whey-stabilized nanocrystalline TiO_2 and ZnO. *The Science of the Total Environment*, *485-486*, 263–269. doi:10.1016/j.scitotenv.2014.03.089 PMID:24727044

Mohapatra, D. P., Brar, S. K., Tyagi, R. D., Picard, P., & Surampalli, R. Y. (2014). Analysis and advanced oxidation treatment of a persistent pharmaceutical compound in wastewater and wastewater sludge-carbamazepine. *The Science of the Total Environment*, *470-471*, 58–75. doi:10.1016/j.scitotenv.2013.09.034 PMID:24140682

Nałecz-Jawecki, G. (2007). Evaluation of the in vitro biotransformation of fluoxetine with HPLC, mass spectrometry and eco-toxicological tests. *Chemosphere*, *70*(1), 29–35. doi:10.1016/j.chemosphere.2007.07.035 PMID:17764718

Oaks, J. L., Gilbert, M., Virani, M. Z., Watson, R. T., Meteyer, C. U., Rideout, B. A., ... Khan, A. A. (2004). Diclofenac residues as the cause of vulture population decline in Pakistan. *Nature*, *427*(6975), 630–633. doi:10.1038/nature02317 PMID:14745453

Ogada, D. L., Keesing, F., & Virani, M. Z. (2012). Dropping dead: Causes and consequences of vulture population declines worldwide. *Annals of the New York Academy of Sciences*, *1249*(1), 57–71. doi:10.1111/j.1749-6632.2011.06293.x PMID:22175274

Painter, M. M., Buerkley, M. A., Julius, M. L., Vajda, A. M., Norris, D. O., Barber, L. B., ... Schoenfuss, H. L. (2009). Antidepressants at environmentally relevant concentrations affect predator avoidance behavior of larval fathead minnows (*Pimephales promelas*). *Environmental Toxicology and Chemistry*, *28*(12), 2677–2684. doi:10.1897/08-556.1 PMID:19405782

Pereira, B. V. R., Matus, G. N., Costa, M. J., Santos, A. C. A. D., Silva-Zacarin, E. C. M., do Carmo, J. B., & Nunes, B. (2018). Assessment of biochemical alterations in the neotropical fish species *Phalloceros harpagos* after acute and chronic exposure to the drugs paracetamol and propranolol. *Environmental Science and Pollution Research International*, *25*(15), 14899–14910. doi:10.100711356-018-1699-6 PMID:29546518

Pfizer. (2018). *Pharmaceuticals in the environment (PIE).* US: Pfizer Inc.

Poiger, T., Buser, H., & Müller, M. D. (2001). Photodegradation of the pharmaceutical drug diclofenac in a lake: Pathway, field measurements, and mathematical modelling. *Environmental Toxicology and Chemistry*, *20*(2), 256–263. doi:10.1002/etc.5620200205 PMID:11351424

Quinn, B., Schmidt, W., O'Rourke, K., & Hernan, R. (2011). Effects of the pharmaceuticals gemfibrozil and diclofenac on biomarker expression in the zebra mussel (*Dreissena polymorpha*) and their comparison with standardised toxicity tests. *Chemosphere*, *84*(5), 657–663. doi:10.1016/j.chemosphere.2011.03.033 PMID:21489596

Radjenović, J., Petrović, M., & Barceló, D. (2009). Fate and distribution of pharmaceuticals in wastewater and sewage sludge of the conventional activated sludge (CAS) and advanced membrane bioreactor (MBR) treatment. *Water Research*, *43*(3), 831–841. doi:10.1016/j.watres.2008.11.043 PMID:19091371

Riaz, L., Mahmood, T., Khalid, A., Rashid, A., Ahmed Siddique, M. B., Kamal, A., & Coyne, M. S. (2018). Fluoroquinolones (FQs) in the environment: A review on their abundance, sorption and toxicity in soil. *Chemosphere*, *191*, 704–720. doi:10.1016/j.chemosphere.2017.10.092 PMID:29078193

Rubasinghege, G., Gurung, R., Rijal, H., Maldonado-Torres, S., Chan, A., Acharya, S., ... Piyasena, M. (2017). Abiotic degradation and environmental toxicity of ibuprofen: Roles of mineral particles and solar radiation. *Water Research*, *131*, 22–32. doi:10.1016/j.watres.2017.12.016 PMID:29258002

Ruhoy, I. S. & Daughtonm C. G. (2007). Types and quantities of leftover drugs entering the environment *via* disposal to sewage—revealed by coroner records. *The Science of the Total Environment, 388*, 137–148.

Ryan, S. M., & Nielsen, C. J. (2010). Global warming potential of inhaled anesthetics: Application to clinical use. *Anesthesia and Analgesia*, *111*(1), 92–98. doi:10.1213/ANE.0b013e3181e058d7 PMID:20519425

Saari, G. N., Scott, W. C., & Brooks, B. W. (2017). Global scanning assessment of calcium channel blockers in the environment: Review and analysis of occurrence, ecotoxicology and hazards in aquatic systems. *Chemosphere*, *189*, 466–478. doi:10.1016/j.chemosphere.2017.09.058 PMID:28957764

Schmidt, W., O'Rourke, K., Hernan, R., & Quinn, B. (2011). Effects of the pharmaceuticals gemfibrozil and diclofenac on the marine mussel (*Mytilus* spp.) and their comparison with standardized toxicity tests. *Marine Pollution Bulletin*, *62*(7), 1389–1395. doi:10.1016/j.marpolbul.2011.04.043 PMID:21652050

Schultz, M. M., Furlong, E. T., Kolpin, D. W., Werner, S. L., Schoenfuss, H. L., Barber, L. B., ... Vajda, A. M. (2010). Antidepressant pharmaceuticals in two U.S. effluent-impacted streams--Occurrence and fate in water and sediment, and selective uptake in fish neural tissue. *Environmental Science & Technology*, *44*(6), 1918–1925. doi:10.1021/es9022706 PMID:20121081

Sheldon, R. A. (2007). The E factor: Fifteen years on. *Green Chemistry*, *9*(12), 1273–1283. doi:10.1039/b713736m

Silva, C. P., Otero, M., & Esteves, V. (2012). Processes for the elimination of estrogenic steroid hormones from water: A review. *Environmental Pollution*, *165*, 38–58. doi:10.1016/j.envpol.2012.02.002 PMID:22402263

Snyder, S. A., & Benotti, M. J. (2010). Endocrine disruptors and pharmaceuticals: Implications for water sustainability. *Water Science and Technology*, *61*(1), 145–154. doi:10.2166/wst.2010.791 PMID:20057100

Snyder, S. A., Villeneuve, D. L., Snyder, E. M., & Giesy, J. P. (2001). Identification and quantification of estrogen receptor agonists in wastewater effluents. *Environmental Science & Technology*, *35*(18), 3620–3625. doi:10.1021/es001254n PMID:11783637

Sukul, P., & Spiteller, M. (2007). Fluoroquinolone antibiotics in the environment. *Reviews of Environmental Contamination and Toxicology*, *191*, 131–162. doi:10.1007/978-0-387-69163-3_5 PMID:17708074

Velasco-Santamaría, Y. M., Korsgaard, B., Madsen, S. S., & Bjerregaard, P. (2011). Bezafibrate, a lipid-lowering pharmaceutical, as a potential endocrine disruptor in male zebrafish (Danio rerio). *Aquatic Toxicology (Amsterdam, Netherlands)*, *105*(1-2), 107–118. doi:10.1016/j.aquatox.2011.05.018 PMID:21703979

Vieno, N., & Sillanpää, M. (2014). Fate of diclofenac in municipal wastewater treatment plant - a review. *Environment International*, *69*, 28–39. doi:10.1016/j.envint.2014.03.021 PMID:24791707

Vulava, V. M., Cory, W. C., Murphey, V. L., & Ulmer, C. Z. (2016). Sorption, photodegradation, and chemical transformation of naproxen and ibuprofen in soils and water. *The Science of the Total Environment*, *565*, 1063–1070. doi:10.1016/j.scitotenv.2016.05.132 PMID:27262983

Wang, J., He, B., Yan, D., Hu, X. (2017). Implementing ecopharmacovigilance (EPV) from a pharmacy perspective: A focus on non-steroidal anti-inflammatory drugs. *The Science of the Total Environment, 15,* 603-604, 772-784.

Wang, J., Zhao, S. Q., Zhang, M. Y., & He, B. S. (2018). Targeted eco-pharmacovigilance for ketoprofen in the environment: Need, strategy and challenge. *Chemosphere*, *194*, 450–462. doi:10.1016/j.chemosphere.2017.12.020 PMID:29227893

Watkinson, A. J., Murby, E. J., & Costanzo, S. D. (2007). Removal of antibiotics in conventional and advanced wastewater treatment: Implications for environmental discharge and wastewater recycling. *Water Research*, *41*(18), 4164–4176. doi:10.1016/j.watres.2007.04.005 PMID:17524445

Weston, A., Caminada, D., Galicia, H., & Fent, K. (2009). Effects of lipid-lowering pharmaceuticals bezafibrate and clofibric acid on lipid metabolism in fathead minnow (*Pimephales promelas*). *Environmental Toxicology and Chemistry*, *28*(12), 2648–2655. doi:10.1897/09-087.1 PMID:19522550

Wu, S., Zhang, L., & Chen, J. (2012). Paracetamol in the environment and its degradation by microorganisms. *Applied Microbiology and Technology*, *96*(4), 875–884. doi:10.100700253-012-4414-4 PMID:23053075

Yu, C. P., Deeb, R. A., & Chu, K. H. (2013). Microbial degradation of steroidal estrogens. *Chemosphere*, *91*(9), 1225–1235. doi:10.1016/j.chemosphere.2013.01.112 PMID:23517889

Zhang, N., Liu, G., Liu, H., Wang, Y., He, Z., & Wang, G. (2011). Diclofenac photodegradation under simulated sunlight: Effect of different forms of nitrogen and kinetics. *Journal of Hazardous Materials*, *192*(1), 411–418. PMID:21664047

KEY TERMS AND DEFINITIONS

API: Active pharmaceutical ingredients.

Chemotherapy Agents: Technically, the term refers to therapeutic chemical treatment originally used as anti-infective term (for mercury and arsenic which were used before antibiotics were discovered) but most commonly, it is used for drugs or drug combinations used for treatment of cancer.

Endocrine Disruptors: Are the chemicals that interfere with the functioning of various endocrine glands (e.g., thyroid, adrenal, and reproductive glands) and their hormones at extremely low concentrations, such as parts per billion (or even parts per trillion). These potent chemicals mimic/block a hormone, or in some other way enhance or disrupt normal hormone activity.

EOCs: Emerging organic contaminants including pharmaceuticals, personal care products, 'lifestyle' compounds, etc.

Global Warming Potential: GWP is a measure of how much heat a greenhouse chemical or gas traps within the atmosphere up to a specific time horizon (commonly, 20, 1000 or 500 years), with respect to carbon dioxide. The GWP value of carbon dioxide is taken as unity.

Hypercholesterolemia: Elevated cholesterol levels in the body.

LD_{50} Value: Oral lethal dose of a compound, i.e., the amount of compound which is lethal in 50% of the population. Lower the LD_{50} value more lethal is the compound.

NSAIDs: Non-steroidal anti-inflammatory drugs, one of the most frequently prescribed drug classes in inflammatory disorders and pain management.

PPCPs: Pharmaceuticals and personal care products.

Superbugs: Antibiotic-resistant strains formed by mutation of wild or normal strains as a result of excessive exposure to antibiotics.

Chapter 14
The Waste-Energy-Health Nexus:
The Social (In)Justice Dimension

Denis Andreas Sarigiannis
Aristotle University of Thessaloniki, Greece

Alberto C. Gotti
Eucentre Foundation, Italy

Spyros P. Karakitsios
Aristotle University of Thessaloniki, Greece

ABSTRACT

The main issues that pertain to the health burden from waste management and energy resource use are laid out highlighting the aspects that determine actual exposure and the socio-economic conditions that underlie them. Case studies covering biomass burning, acute and chronic exposure to urban and industrial waste are described. They refer to different areas in Europe and socio-economic strata focusing on susceptible population groups, which may be affected by enhanced exposure to environmental toxicants stemming from municipal and industrial waste management and domestic heating or cooking using biomass. These features make socio-economic status and the consequent social (in)justice a key determinant of overall exposure early in life. The latter results in a high probability of onset or exacerbation of adverse health outcomes both in the medium term and later in life. Additional factors that affect the health impacts of environmental exposures comprise choice of diet, education level of parents, access to green or blue space and housing condition.

INTRODUCTION

In recent years, it has been extensively recognized that sociodemographic inequalities formulate significant differences in exposure patterns, which are also reflected in health adversities (Gouveia, 2016). These inequalities, also described as environmental injustice, are observed at different levels of social organization, including differences among countries, within countries, within the urban envelope or even within communities. These differences describe both socioeconomic and demographic inequalities.

DOI: 10.4018/978-1-5225-7635-8.ch014

Very characteristic examples on how sociodemographic inequalities among countries are related to environmental exposure, are provided by harmonized biomonitoring studies, i.e. biomonitoring studies, where samples have been taken at the same period of time, related to specific age groups and the samples have been analysed under similar SOPs. Analysis of the socioeconomic aspects of exposure based on human biomonitoring (HBM) data provides useful insights on the effect that socioeconomic disparities have on exposure to chemicals at the country level. As shown in Figure 1, DDT levels in human samples (for the years 2001-2002 when data were available for most of the countries) were negatively correlated to average gross domestic product (GDP) per capita for the same period.

In Balkan countries, this might be related to the fact that DDT was the main biocide used to "eradicate" malaria worldwide, beginning in 1955. Small quantities of DDT were sprayed inside dwellings, and the malarial parasite vectors were either killed or repelled by the chemical. The program was thus successful in essentially wiping out malaria. Reduced hygiene conditions in countries with lower income, had favored the development of malaria but DDT was proven to be an effective countermeasure. However, due to its persistence and bioaccumulation potential, DDT levels continue to be higher in these countries compared to the rest of the European Region. High levels of DDT in countries of the former Soviet Union (FSU) reflect the fact that from 1950 to 1970 more than 20,000 tonnes of DDT were used annually. Most DDT was applied in southern regions of the FSU where agricultural activity was the more pronounced, such as Moldova and Ukraine followed by the Northern Caucasus region of Russia and the Central Asian republics. Figure 1 shows that even in 2001-2002, DDT concentrations found in human milk in countries such as Russia and Ukraine were quite high compared to other countries in Europe. DDT levels in the Czech Republic are high as well. Even though the country stopped production of DDT, HCH and other pesticides listed in the Stockholm Convention, significant contamination has been found in soil around sites where tonnes of obsolete pesticides, especially DDT and HCB, were buried (Beránek, 2005). This could lead to enhanced levels of human exposure through a horde of possible pathways and consequently could explain the relatively higher values of DDT in breast milk in the Czech population.

Similarly, comparison of exposure to DEHP with average GDP per capita (for year 2012, when human biomonitoring (HBM) data were also collected) shows that exposure to the restricted phthalates is negatively correlated to affluence (see Figure 2). This is an interesting conclusion which has to be investigated more in detail, in terms of sources to DEHP exposure and socioeconomic determinants, whether these are related to building materials emissions (e.g. vinyl flooring) or exposure due to object-to-mouth behavior involving toys with high content in DEHP. In Western Europe, DEHP represented in 2008 only 18% of the overall consumption of plasticizers. In comparison, DEHP represents 50% of the total use of plasticizers in the world. A putative explanatory hypothesis is that in countries with lower GDP cheaper imported plastic materials are preferred compared to the ones produced in the European Union. Thus, policies for consumer protection might not be adequate for public health protection if related only to products manufactured in the EU.

On the contrary, blood levels of PCDDs/PCDFs are positively correlated to gross domestic product per capita (Figure 3). More than ninety percent (90–98%) of typical human uptake of PCDDs/PCDFs comes from diet and especially from food of animal origin: meat, dairy products, or fish predominate, depending on the country (Liem et al., 2000). These statistics exclude of course potential occupational exposure sources (Malisch and Kotz, 2014). In different studies uptake from ambient sources (ingestion of soil and water, inhalation of air or dust) and miscellaneous non-dietary sources (transfer from paper; cigarette smoking) was estimated to be only in the range of up to 10% of the total average adult exposure (Liem et al., 2000). These higher exposure levels in countries with higher GDP per capita might be at-

Figure 1. Socioeconomic dimension of exposure to DDT. Exposure is higher in countries with lower GDP per capita

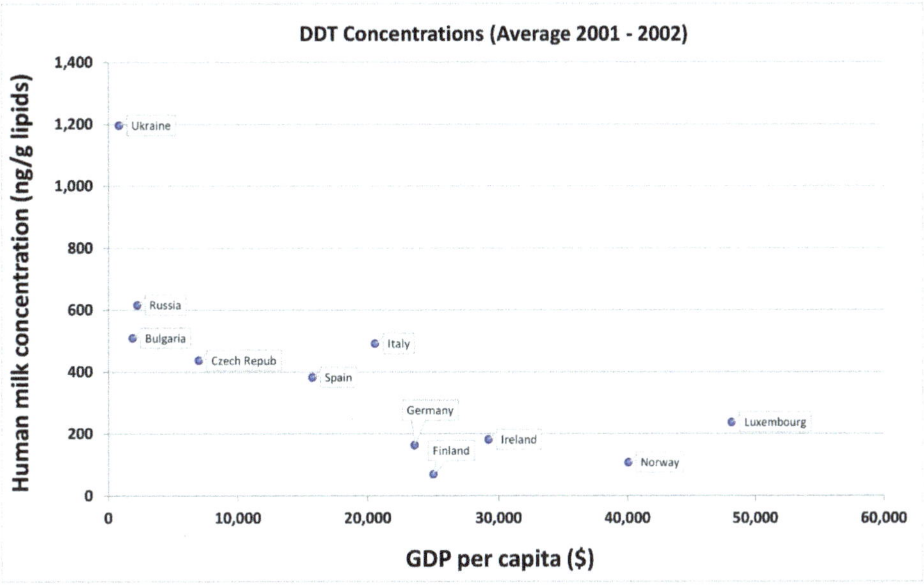

Figure 2. Socioeconomic dimension of exposure to phthalates: exposure to DEHP (in terms of total DEHP metabolites in urine) is higher in countries with lower GDP per capita
(World-Bank, 2013)

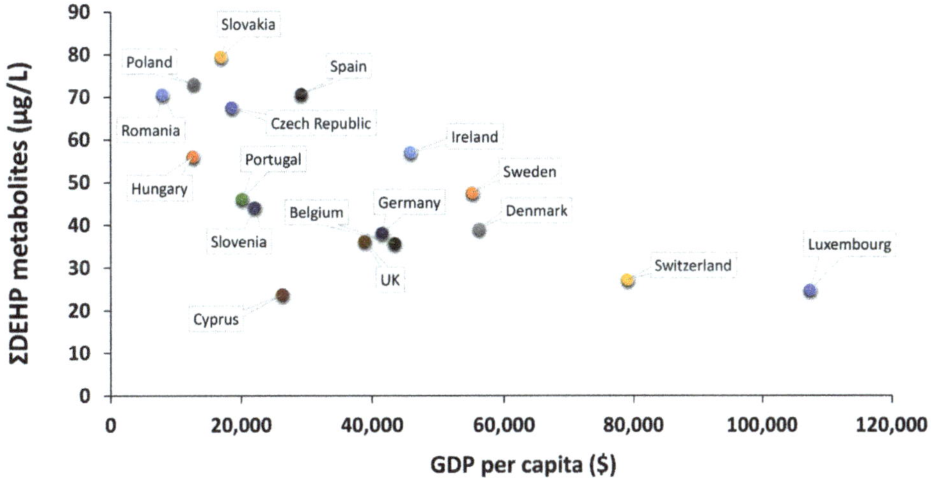

tributed to higher consumption of beef meat, dairy products and fish, where these compounds tend to accumulate more.

Inter-country differences in biomonitoring levels can also be associated to specific dietary patterns and consumer products use. In countries with intensive agriculture, pesticides levels are expected to be higher. Exposure to metals and PBT compounds is higher in coastal population, due to bioaccumulation and bio-magnification through the food web and the relatively higher consumption of seafood. On the

Figure 3. Socioeconomic dimension of exposure to PCDDs/PCDFs. Exposure is higher in countries with higher GDP per capita

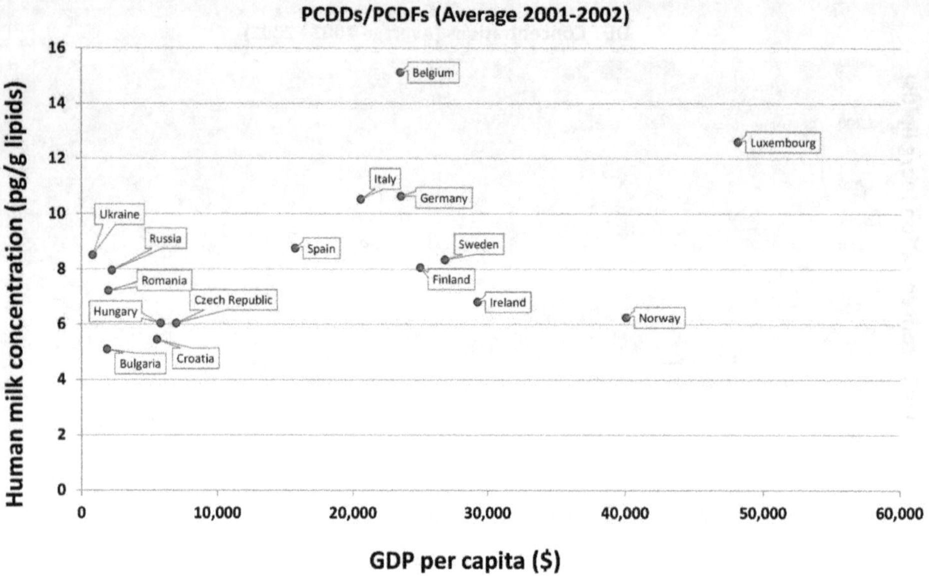

contrary, inter-country variability is limited for compounds that are not widespread in the environment and which are mostly found in consumer products. This was clearly illustrated in the latest results of DEMOCOPHES (Schindler et al., 2014) regarding bisphenol-A. Mean urinary levels of bisphenol-A were similar (ranging between 1.4 and 2.1 μg/L) in four countries with completely different socioeconomic and climatic conditions (Luxembourg, Slovenia, Spain and Sweden).

Differences within the urban canopy are usually referred as socio-spatial Inequalities; in large urban areas, inequalities show strong geographical patterns, characterized by well-defined hotspots (Shrestha et al., 2016). It has also to be noted that specific hotspots are associated with heightened vulnerability among population who belong to racial or ethnic minorities or are of low socio-economic status (SES), such as immigrants or Romani populations (Krista et al., 2009). These socially disadvantaged populations are usually resided in the urban areas close to industrial or other contamination sources, thus, subjected to higher exposure levels, especially in the case of an accidental release. This problem is not only related to Romani population, but it has been generally accepted that racial and socioeconomic disparities are detrimental for the residential proximity to industrial (Mohai et al., 2009) and waste management (Martuzzi et al., 2010) activities.

Finally, violent changes in the overall socioeconomic status in the country level, could result in significant environmental degradation. A typical example is the irrational use of biomass burning for space heating in Greece, that resulted in significantly increased PM levels in the ambient and in indoor air. Although the use of biomass for space heating was introduced in 2011 as a CO_2-neutral means to foster global warming mitigation, a series of austerity measures combined with the excessive rise in the taxation of light heating diesel, resulted in irrational use of biomass for residential heating in the winter of 2012-2013. This was followed by a significant increase of ambient and indoor air levels and, consequently of population exposure to PM10 and PM2.5 (Sarigiannis et al., 2014).

Given all the above, it is of particular interest to demonstrate how environmental injustice related to waste and energy sectors is translated into additional health burdens and to try to identify the different sociodemographic components that form exposure and adversities in health status. These pertain to:

- Use of biomass for domestic heating in urban centres in Europe
- Accidental fires in waste recycling plants - socio-economic minorities living nearby the waste management facility, enhancing thus the respective health risk from accidental operation.
- HERACLES waste study assessing long-term exposure of the population living nearby large sanitary landfills to endocrine disrupting chemicals such as plasticisers released from plastic and micro plastic waste.
- Exposure to industrial waste and its effects on the neurodevelopment of children living in proximity with industrial zones.

CASE STUDIES

Use of Biomass for Domestic Heating in Urban Centres in Europe

Indoor biomass burning for residential heating is a major source of indoor and outdoor air quality degradation. One of the major components of biomass burning is emitted PM. The association of biomass burning PM with potential health effects, as well as their toxicity potency in comparison to other PM combustion sources have been investigated through a controlled study of human exposure to wood smoke, epidemiological studies (observational or interventional), as well as with toxicological tests - a very comprehensive review on both perspectives was carried out by Naeher et al. (2007).

Over the last couple of years, the use of biomass as heating source was allowed in Greece as a CO_2-neutral means of space heating in the large metropolitan areas of Athens and Thessaloniki affecting more than half of the country's population. At the same time the use of light heating diesel was heavily taxed apparently to combat illegal trafficking of heating diesel. In the same period Greece faces a financial crisis with significant repercussions on the average household income. That combination of parameters resulted in increased use of biomass for residential heating in year 2012, followed by a significant increase of ambient air, indoor air and exposure to PM10 and PM2.5. In this study, we aim to quantify the health and socioeconomic effects related to that shift from light heating diesel to biomass burning, as well as to evaluate alternative scenarios of residential heating energy share.

Methodology

Study Design

To better identify the contribution of biomass burning to elevated PM and PAHs exposure and the respective impact on public health, a seven-month long monitoring and modeling study was designed including:

- Measurements of ambient air particles of aerodynamic diameter of 2.5 and 10 μm in two sampling locations, representative for the urban background levels and a traffic site as well.

- Measurements of indoor PM in 30 houses, including periods when an open fireplace was used or not for space heating. Details on the residential location characteristics are presented in Table 1.
- Chemical analysis of levoglucosan (a well-established tracer of biomass burning) and PAHs in the particle phase.
- Development of an indoor air pollution dispersion model that takes into account the interaction of outdoor penetration and the contribution of indoor sources.
- Assessment of personal exposure and actual population intake of PMx and PAHs in both the particle and gaseous phases, accounting for individual activity patterns and the related effect of activity intensity in inhalation rate and pollutants intake.
- Deposition of particles across the human respiratory tract, aiming at estimating the actual number of particles and toxic burden people are exposed to.
- Application of well-established exposure-response functions for mortality and morbidity (cardiovascular and respiratory hospital admissions) based on PMx exposure and development of a mechanistic methodology for estimating exposure to PAHs and the attributable lung cancer risk.
- Translation of potential health impact into monetary costs.

Our 7-month study included a wide variety of meteorological conditions. To better understand the differences between the cold period of the year (during which space heating was used) and the warm period of the year, the measurement dataset was divided as follows:

1. From October 5 to November 10 (2012) and from March 10 to April 15 (2013) the period was considered as warm. PM levels measured in this period were considered as representative for the rest of the warm period, based on the evaluation of older PM time series in Thessaloniki.
2. From November 10 (2012) to March 9 (2013) the period was considered as cold; the low ambient air temperatures induced the use of space heating in dwellings.

Scenario Analysis: Socioeconomic Components of Energy Share

The results of the 2012-2013 measurements were compared to the ones made in 2011-2012 to understand better the effect that different policy measures regulating the market price of heating fuel in tandem with the incumbent economic crisis in Greece and other countries in the European South may have on non-occupational exposure of the urban population to particulate matter and the associated health and monetary impact. Own-price elasticity of light heating oil was taken as el_{oil} = -0.39 (IOBE, 2013). A field survey encompassing ca. 300 households across the greater area of Thessaloniki implemented using the on-line SurveyMonkey tool provided consumer behavior information that was used to generate the cross-fuel elasticity table below.

The scenarios are based on reasonable assumptions and existing trends related to the energy market share of different fuels and heating systems (e.g. the market share of natural gas use for space heating had been increasing over the last years but it is currently stabilized to around 40%). However the interplay of multiple factors such as financial pressures or incentives might result in unexpected figures (as occurred with the increased biomass use), favoring one technological solution for space heating over another. Through analysis of specific scenarios, we highlighted the attributable differences in public health burden, should specific space heating practices be adopted. The different policy scenarios examined (and the corresponding average urban background concentrations) are presented in Table 4.

Table 1. Cross-price elasticities of alternative space heating energy carriers

	Light heating oil	Natural gas	Biomass	Electricity
Light heating oil	----	n/a	-0.97	-0.24
Natural gas	n/a	----	n/a	n/a
Biomass	-1.03	n/a	----	0.25
Electricity	-4.1	n/a	3.98	----

n/a: sufficient data non available to support the estimation of elasticity

Differences in the urban background concentration, which in turn were reflected in population exposure to PM for the intervention scenarios examined herein, were estimated based on a data assimilation algorithm coupling: (a) a regulatory atmospheric dispersion model (CALPUFF) (Scire, 2000b; Scire, 2000a) following a Langrangian Gaussian formulation applied on area sources that was supported by a refined and up-to-date emissions inventory at high spatial resolution; (b) the OSPM model (Berkowicz et al., 2008) for capturing traffic-related emissions taking into account street canyons; and (c) spatially distributed measurements of PMx concentrations using ground monitors across the Thessaloniki metropolitan area. The computed annual average concentrations at the receptor points for the OSPM and the CALPUFF models together with the observations from air pollution monitoring stations across the greater area of Thessaloniki are used as input to a spatial interpolation model employing ordinary kriging. The relative weight of the pollution estimates from atmospheric models and ground monitors are optimized to reduce the residual error based on an advanced Kalman filter formulation.

The following figure shows the resulting PM2.5 map of the metropolitan area of Thessaloniki in 2011. In order to simplify the estimation of the effect that different space heating fuels and technological options have on the atmospheric burden with particulate matter in Thessaloniki an empirical model was built, correlating the 2011-2013 ambient air concentration data, the distribution of fuel/technology used for these years and the respective PM emission factors. The latter are equal to 0.36, 2.16 and 160 mg PM2.5/MJ for natural gas (boilers), oil (boilers) and biomass burning (open and closed fireplaces, wood stoves, pellet and wood log boilers) as derived from both an extensive literature review and experimental work regarding boiler emission efficiencies for different types of fuel (Nussbaumer et al., 2008). The emission factor for biomass burning systems is a weighted average of the emission factors of each of the biomass combustion technologies considered weighed by the respective relative market shares (see table 5). The latter were derived through the field survey described above.

Table 2. Fuel/technology use distribution and corresponding urban background concentrations

Scenario	Oil	Natural gas	Biomass burning	Electricity	PM2.5 ($\mu g/m^3$)
2011-2012	44.0%	40.0%	5.6%	10.4%	41.2 (measured)
2012-2013	22.3%	40.0%	26.7%	15.7%	62.6 (measured)
Scenario 1	38.5%	41.5%	10.0%	10.0%	36.3
Scenario 2	43.5%	41.5%	5.0%	10.0%	28.4
Scenario 3	23.5%	62.5%	4.0%	10.0%	26.5
Scenario 4	20.0%	70.0%	0.0%	10.0%	20.0

Figure 4. PM2.5 concentration map in the greater area of Thessaloniki (2011)

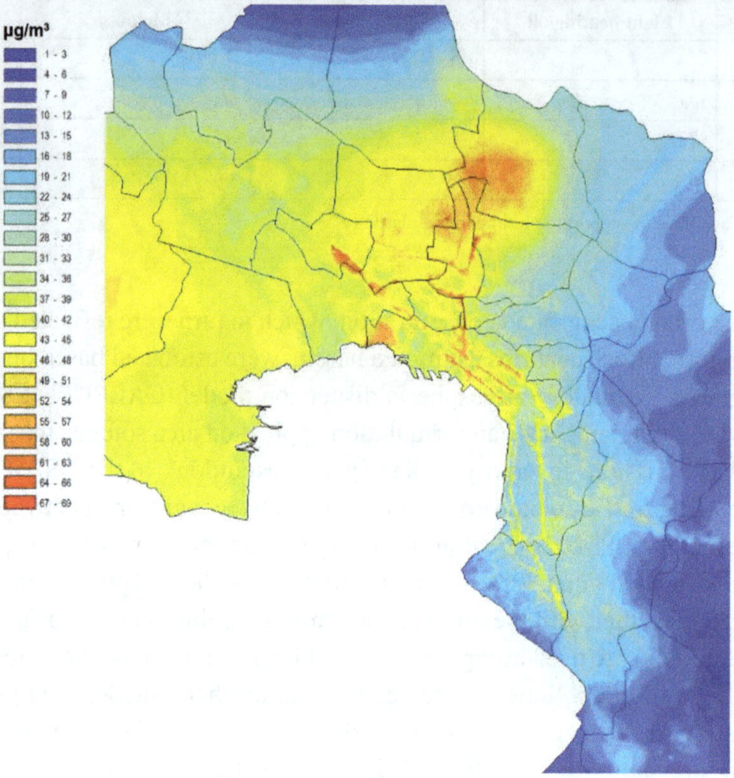

The following regression model for the interpolation of projected ambient air PM concentrations during the cold period of a given year was derived based on the emission factors and the comparison of the concentration data between 2011/2012 and 2012/2013 cold and warm period data:

$$C_{cold} = C_{warm} + a \cdot f_{oil} \cdot E_{oil} + b \cdot f_{ng} \cdot E_{ng} + c \cdot f_{bio} \cdot E_{bio}$$

where C_{warm} is the urban background concentration in the warm period of the same year, f_{oil}, f_{ng} and f_{bio} are the residential heating technological energy share for light heating oil, natural gas and biomass respec-

Table 3. Emission factors and relative market shares of biomass combustion technologies

Biomass burning technologies	Relative market share (%)	Average emission factor (mg PM2.5/MJ)
Open fireplace	30	160
Closed fireplace	10	41
Pellet boiler	10	21.6
Wood stove	40	240
Wood log boiler	10	96

tively and a, b, c are the regression coefficients (respectively equal to 0.95. 0.97 and 2) that fit best the results for the average winter urban background levels in the Thessaloniki area. Additional parameters that might affect the model were statistically insignificant, since the meteorological conditions between the two years did not differ substantially and long-range particulate pollution transport did not show significant variation for the duration of the study. During the cold period of 2011/2012 daily mean temperature, wind speed and precipitation were 12.1 °C, 3.7 km/h and 0.8 mm, while the respective values for 2012/2013 were 12.8 °C, 4.3 km/h and 1.3 mm. The number of heating degree days was higher during the 2011-2012 winter (1528 deg-days) compared to the 2012-2013 winter (1329 deg-days) (IOBE, 2013).

Results: Health Impact and Monetary Valuation

The estimated health impact and the corresponding monetary valuation for the selected mortality and morbidity indicators are illustrated in Figures 2 to 8. Overall, the number of excess deaths (Figure 2) attributed to PM exposure in the metropolitan area of Thessaloniki (with a population of more than 1m inhabitants) for 2011 are 1369, while the respective number for 2012 is 1287. What is significantly different between these two years is the distribution between the warm and the cold season. Despite the fact that the duration of the cold period is practically half the one of the warm period, in 2012 the impacts are higher in the cold period (728 out of 1288 annual deaths), in contrast to 526 cases out of 1369 (annually) in 2011. Thus, the air pollution burden associated with particulate matter during the cold season of 2012-2013 resulted in an estimate of more than 200 excess premature deaths attributable to airborne PM exposure than in the corresponding period in 2011-2012. Excess mortality during the cold period of the year corresponds to 3540 years of life lost (Figure 3) taking into account the population age distribution.

Similar figures are derived for morbidity indices: new cases of chronic bronchitis (Figures 5 and 6) dominate adverse health outcomes, followed by respiratory hospital admissions (Figure 7) and cardiovascular hospital admissions (Figure 8). In the remaining scenarios, impacts are gradually decreasing, reflecting the improvement of ambient and indoor air quality resulting from the reduction of biomass and the increase of natural gas use for space heating.

Monetary costs related to annual mortality are in the range of billion euro no matter whether we apply the the value of statistical life (VSL) or the value of a life year (VOLY) methodology. Following the

Figure 5. All cause mortality and related monetary cost

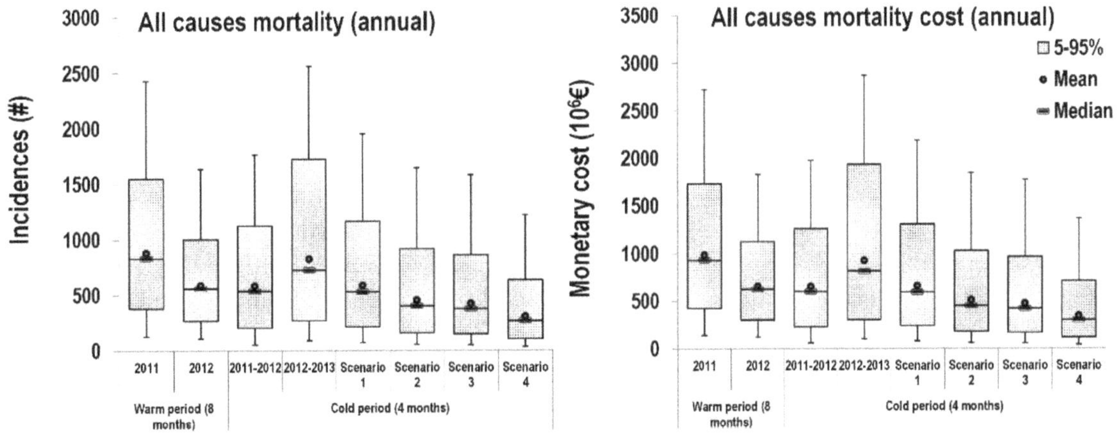

Figure 6. All cause mortality (expressed in YLL) and related cost of life years lost

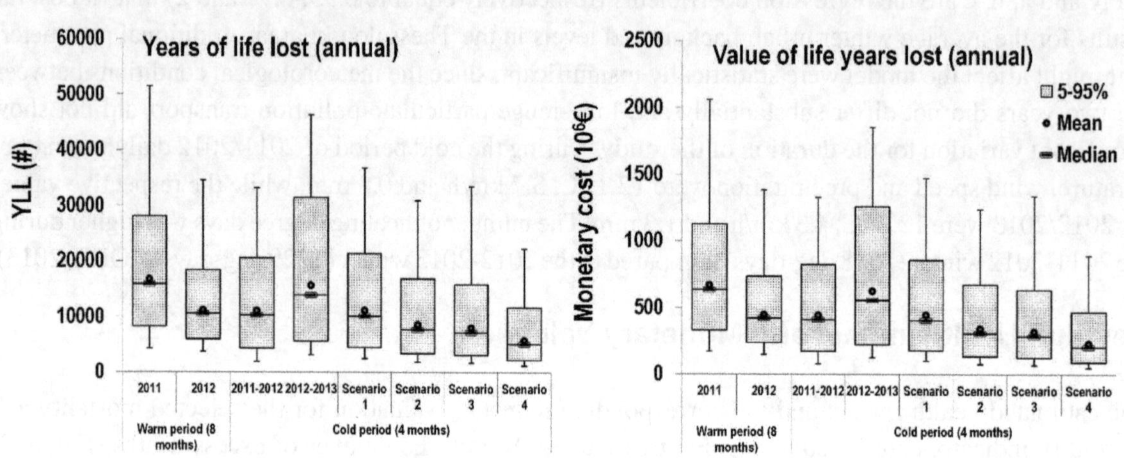

Figure 7. Infant mortality and related monetary cost

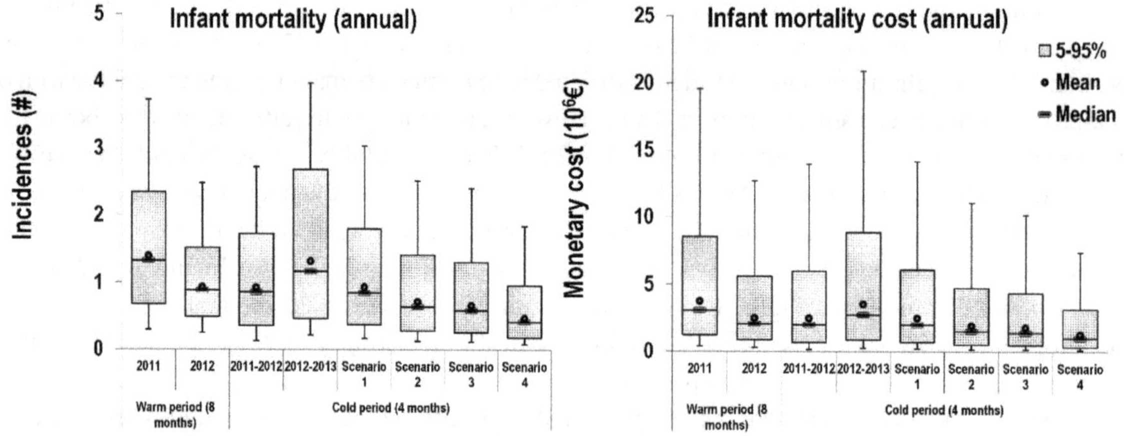

Figure 8. Chronic bronchitis (adults) new cases and related monetary cost

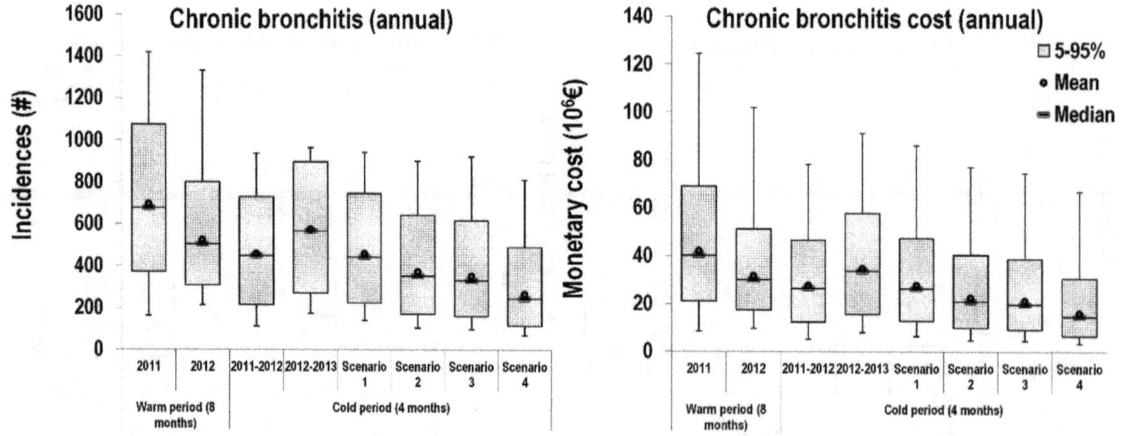

VOLY method, the estimated costs are about 30% lower, mainly reflecting the different costing structure of life expectancy lost according to the age pyramid of the population studied. Morbidity cost related to chronic bronchitis (especially for children) is, generally, one order of magnitude lower (hundreds of millions). Morbidity costs related to cardiovascular and respiratory morbidity (the most directly immediate effects of increased PM pollution) are in the range of million euros.

Scenario analysis showed that large benefits could be expected from potential policy interventions bearing changes in the composition of the fuel mix used for residential heating. These benefits are attributable to the differences in particulate emissions between biomass combustion and the competing fuels and space heating systems. The most effective way to achieving this result would seem to be a relaxation of the high taxation imposed in the last three years on heating oil in Greece.

Figure 9. Chronic bronchitis (children) new cases and related monetary cost

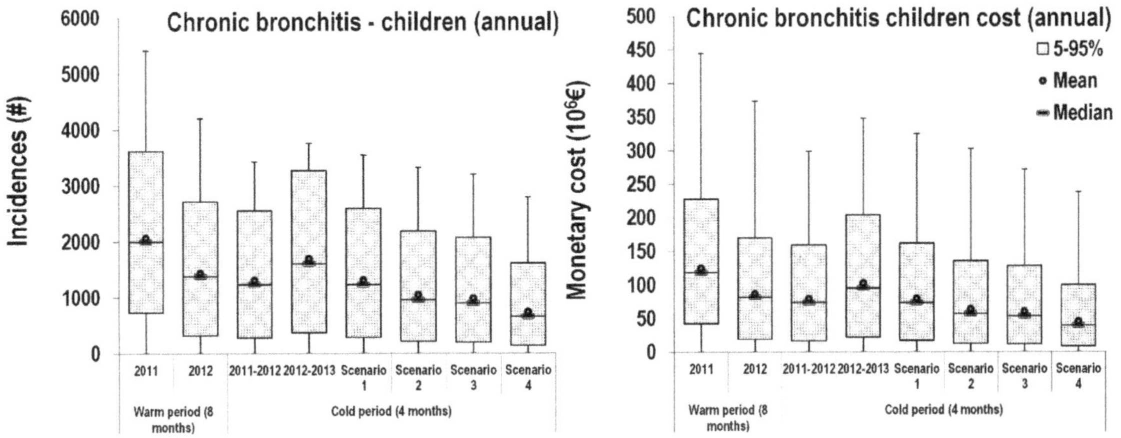

Figure 10. Respiratory hospital admissions and related monetary cost

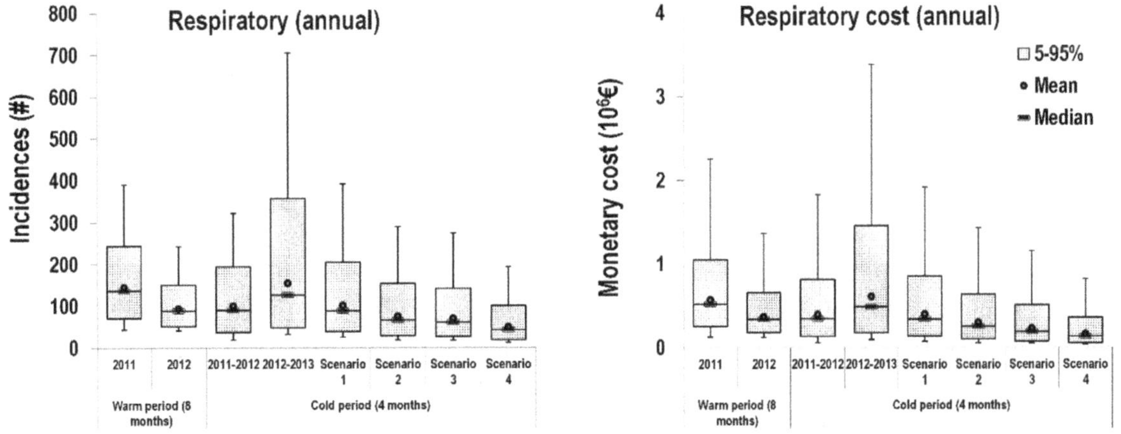

Figure 11. Cardiovascular hospital admissions and related monetary cost

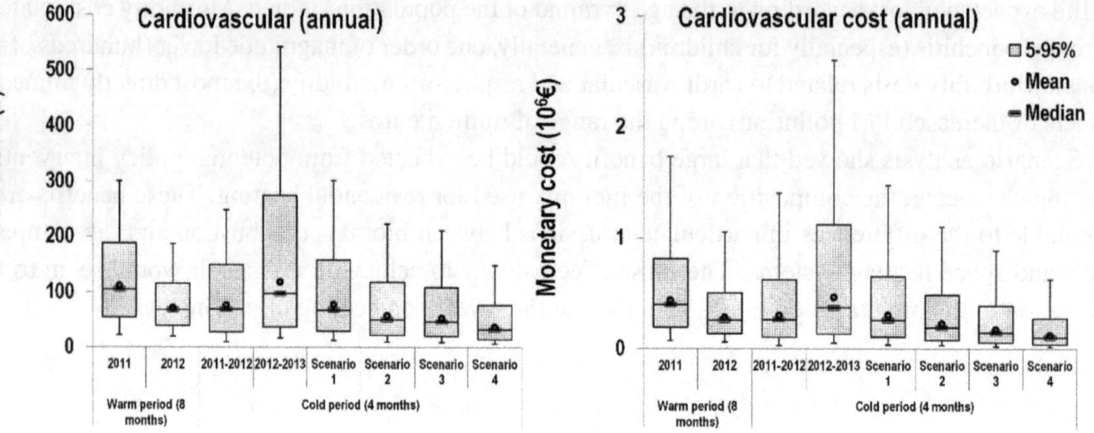

DISCUSSION

In this study the health impact and the associated monetary cost of non-occupational exposure to PM in the ambient and indoor air were assessed, focusing on the effect of the increased use of biomass as domestic heating source. Current methodological schemes for assessing impacts of biomass combustion rely on the association of indoor biomass burning with several adverse health outcomes. These studies are subject to major uncertainties related to the actual additional burden of exposure related to infiltration of outdoor air in the indoor air (Noonan and Balmes, 2010). Our methodology reduces these uncertainties by addressing the differences related to the variability of temporal emissions and the corresponding outdoor and indoor concentrations. In this way, the impact on the urban population is taken into account, distinguishing between households that use biomass for indoor space heating and the ones that do not do so. The contribution of biomass combustion indoors is very important since uncontrolled biomass burning results in significant degradation of the overall urban air quality with dire consequences on indoor air quality from ambient air penetration indoors. Moreover, biomass combustion sources emit particles directly into the indoor air burdening it even further. Quantifying the outdoor:indoor air interactions as in the present study is key for estimating correctly the overall health burden to the urban population. According to the WHO (2007), PM that originates from biomass burning is at least as harmful for public health as PM coming from different combustion sources (Naeher et al., 2007). This allows aggregate exposure to PM from different sources (traffic, other combustion and biomass burning) and environmental interactions (such as the outdoor-to-indoor air penetration) to be tackled within a unified modeling framework, providing thus an aggregate input for the estimation of the total health impact on the local population. Our team has shown recently that lung cancer risk from PAHs adsorbed onto PM emitted from biomass combustion is higher than the corresponding risk from PM in car exhaust (Sarigiannis et al., 2015). In this study, however, we shall adopt the WHO assumption and consider similar concentration-response functions to hold for PM emitted from all combustion sources.

Our results on health impacts concord with the ones derived by other recent studies. A direct comparison to a conceptually similar study carried out in Austria (Haluza et al., 2012), indicates that the expected health impact attributed to PM is higher in the city of Thessaloniki. This can be explained by the overall higher levels of PM, the incorporation of actual exposure and inhalation rate based on type and intensity of activity of the exposed population and of the indoor: outdoor interaction in our methodology. Moreover, we have used PM2.5 instead of PM10 as exposure metric, considering that this is more relevant for explaining the adverse health effects of biomass burning.

Compared to the intervention study of Johnston et al. (2013), we underestimate cardiac effects. This could be due to the relative paucity of mechanistic information characterizing epidemiological studies and the respective CRFs. Wood smoke particles are generally smaller than 1 μm, with a size distribution that peaks between 0.15 and 0.4 μm (Hays et al., 2002). As with other combustion mixtures, such as diesel and tobacco smoke, fresh wood smoke contains a large number of ultrafine particles (UFPs) with aerodynamic diameter smaller than 100 μm. UFPs condense rapidly as they cool and age. Considering that biomass-originated PM is characterized by very low aerodynamic diameter, PM2.5 is rather a proxy than the actual exposure metric. When ultrafine PM is emitted to the atmosphere it undergoes several transformations (hydroscopic growth, condensation etc.), which result in very fast particle growth and the formation of PM of larger aerodynamic diameter (Sarigiannis et al., 2002; Sarigiannis et al., 2004). Cardiovascular disease attributed to exposure to particulate matter is related primarily to translocation of ultrafine particles from the respiratory tract through the alveoli via systemic circulation. Thus, cardiovascular problems and health effects not attributed to lung or systemic inflammation seem to be associated primarily with exposure to UFPs rather than larger particles (Brook, 2008). Overall, the quantification of exposure to airborne PM and the assessment of the associated health impact would benefit greatly from the incorporation of mechanistic elements such as human respiratory tract deposition and oxidative stress potential in the determination of the CRFs used for health impact assessment.

Socioeconomic status affects the use of energy resources and the activity patterns related to specific exposure scenarios of variable intensity. Several studies have shown that variations in socioeconomic status may have significant impact on human exposure to pollutants. For example, children of lower socioeconomic status families are more vulnerable to asthma (Neidell, 2004; Pediatrics, 2000), while increased mortality due to exposure to PM10 concentrations has been associated with lower income (Forastiere et al., 2007). In addition, health status is also affected by behavioral factors, such as nutrition, smoking, alcohol consumption and physical activity (Arcus-Arth Broadwin & Lam, 2001; Newman, 2002); therefore, socioeconomically disadvantaged populations experience more often chronic diseases (e.g. COPD or hypertension) during their life (Lee et al., 1995). Families of higher socioeconomic status may also invest in their health and they may be more likely to seek preventive health care (Leaderer et al., 1999). Since 2009 significant reductions were observed in GDP and available income coupled to increased unemployment in Greek cities (IMF, 2012). All three are key determinants of population well-being. In the period 2012-2013 the dire economic situation of Greek households was burdened further by a heavy tax on light heating diesel, which resulted in a market price increase of ca. 50% in 2012-2013 compared to 2011-2012. The compounded effect of reduced available income and the dramatically increased retail price of heating oil and – to a lesser extent – of natural gas, led many households to much cheaper fuels such as woody biomass. This, in turn, resulted in the estimated increase of overall mortality attributed to PM in the cold season of 2012-2013 compared to the one in 2011-2012.

According to the WHO, indoor smoke is ranked as the second most important environmental health risk factor, after poor water/sanitation/hygiene. Among all major policy-relevant risk factors, indoor air pollution from solid fuel is tenth globally, and fourth in less developed countries (Naeher et al., 2007). Degradation of outdoor and indoor air quality amplifies the differences between high and low-income countries. In Greece, the main culprits for the health burden attributed to exposure to airborne particles has shifted recently from traffic to biomass use for heating; this observation is consistent and can be explained by the financial figures described in Figure 9.

The latter indicate the significant repercussions of the incumbent financial crisis on the average household income, which when combined with the simultaneous increase in the price of light heating diesel due to extra-heavy taxation led a large number of Greek households to energy poverty. The associated health effects are reckoned to be disproportionally high compared to the short-term potential financial gains from increased taxation and similar austerity measures. In practice, according to the Foundation for Economic and Industrial Research (IOBE, 2013), there were no actual financial benefits from the increased taxation of light diesel for space heating. On the contrary, the revenues from excise tax and VAT imposed on heating oil from the over-taxation were 187 million euro less than the previous year in Greece. This was due to the lower amount of heating oil taxed (2,629,931 kt in 2011-2012 compared to 1,335,083 kt in 2012-2013). Austerity measures resulted in a dramatic change in consumer behavior, with a consequent consumer shift to alternative fuels for space heating (such as illicit or unregulated biomass burning). This change resulted in both reduced tax revenues to the state and urban air quality deterioration, which would result in an increase of 40% in health burden costs between the winters of 2012-2013 and 2011-2012.

Figure 12. Financial figures and estimated mortality for the years 2011 and 2012

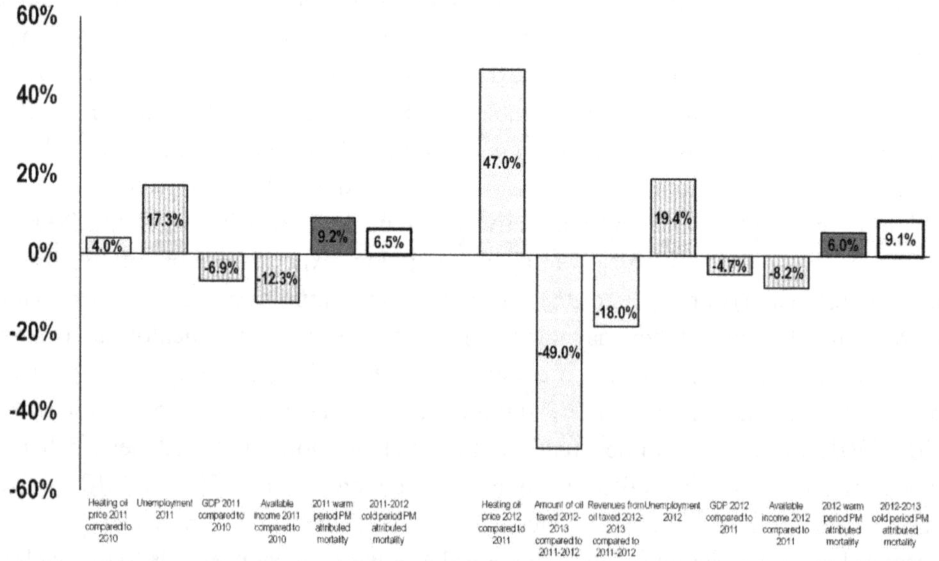

Accidental Fires in Waste Recycling Plants: Socio-Economic Minorities Living Nearby the Waste Management Facility, Enhancing Thus the Respective Health Risk From Accidental Operation

Introduction

Waste recycling is one of the main cornerstones of the EU waste management strategy (Farmer et al., 2015). It offers many advantages contributing to the circular economy and the sustainable and efficient use of natural and man-made resources. However, waste recycling facilities may be associated to adverse health outcomes in the aftermath of industrial accidents involving the inadvertent generation of toxic chemicals and their release into the environment. In addition, concerns have been raised with regard to the potential toxic content of recycled material.

Among the major concerns related to accidents in plastic recycling plants are the emissions of dioxins and furans (PCDDs/PCDFs). These compounds are characterized by high carcinogenic potency (Cole et al., 2003). Because PCDDs/PCDFs appears to be acting like a potent and persistent hormone agonist, it appears reasonable to incorporate mechanistic information on receptor-mediated events in risk assessments for TCDD. This information may be obtained from steroid receptor action and from molecular data on the Ah receptor (Lucier et al., 1993). This receptor-based toxicity, results in sex-dependent sensitivities, as a result of a set of sex-specific PCDD/PCDF-responsive genes. However, the estimation of the additional probability of cancer due to the additional exposure burden is quite difficult (Dong et al., 2016). A major obstacle is that an elevated short-term external exposure associated to the accidental event, has to be translated into long term risk estimates. Considering the significant persistence and bioaccumulation of PCDDs/PCDFs in the human body, assessing the actual internal dosimetry of this complex mixture is of particular importance. The biokinetics of TCDD are relatively well understood in adult humans (Kerger et al., 2006; Michalek and Tripathi, 1999; Milbrath et al., 2009). However, the impact of pregnancy and lactation on the elimination of TCDD and other dioxins is not clear (Emond et al., 2016). Additional insights regarding the biological perturbations induced by PCDDs/PCDFs exposure are provided by transcriptomics and metabolomics analysis, where altered levels of endogenous steroid metabolites and modified urinary bile acids profiles were identified as a result of acute exposure to PCDDs/PCDFs (Jeanneret et al., 2014). Taken together, these findings are compatible with an increased expression of cytochrome P450s, persistent hepatotoxicity, bile acid homeostasis dysregulation and oxidative stress. In *in vivo* studies (mice), serum metabolomics identified azelaic acid monoesters as significantly increased metabolites after TCDD treatment, due to downregulation of hepatic carboxylesterase 3 (CES3, also known as triglyceride hydrolase) expression in an arylhydrocarbon receptor (AhR)-dependent manner (Matsubara et al., 2012). The decreased CES3 expression was accomplished by TCDD-stimulated TGFβ-SMAD3 and IL6-STAT3 signaling, but not by direct AhR signaling, indicating that PCDDs/PCDFs affect additional pathways beyond the ones regulated by AhR. With regard to AhR deregulation, PCDDs/PCDFs exposure elicited metabolite and gene expression changes *in vivo* subjects (mice) associated with lipid metabolism and transport, choline metabolism, bile acid metabolism, glycolysis, and glycerophospholipid metabolism (Forgacs et al., 2012). From transcriptome analysis of mitogen-induced lymphocytes cultured with 10 nM TCDD, all AhR-dependent genes were induced by 1.2- to

13-fold and plasma TCDD was associated with decreased 7-ethoxyresorufin O-deethylase activity, as well as strong positive correlation between AhR and CYP1A1/ CYP1B1 expression (Landi et al., 2003).

Accidental fires in the plastic industry comprise one of the major events resulting in contamination of various environmental media to PCDDs/PCDFs of the surrounding area; air samples collected in the 5th day of such an event were found to contain over 1000 pg/m^3 TEQ (toxic equivalent quantity) of dioxin, exceeding background levels by 2,500–25,000 fold (Fernando et al., 2014). Based on the above, the current study aimed at calculating the health burden (in terms of cancer risk) of the Romani population living in the Aspropyrgos area (part of the greater Athens metropolitan area in Greece) due to increased exposure to dioxins and furans (PCDDs/PCDFs), emitted by an accidental fire in a plastics recycling plant in June 2015. The fire resulted in significant particle and gaseous emissions of several compounds related to plastic industry. In addition, release of dioxins and furans was a major concern, due to their persistence in environmental and biological matrices, as well as to their carcinogenic potency. In order to face the methodological problem mentioned above, a comprehensive methodology involving both measured data and complex internal exposure modelling was employed.

Methodology

Overall Study Design

In order to estimate the risk related to the PCDDs/PCDFs emitted during the fire, it was critical to estimate the long-term internal burden of exposure associated to this event. PCDDs/PCDFs are bioaccumulative and persistent with a half-life time of almost 7.5 years in humans. Hence, it is critical to translate the actual uptake during the accidental event (that lasted for a few days) into a long term (lasting for many years) internal exposure burden. The only scientifically sound way to translate these external doses into internal exposure to the target tissues was through the use of physiology based biokinetic (PBBK) models. To be able to perform this type of calculation, it was critical to be able to identify (a) the background exposure levels to PCDDs/PCDFs and (b) the additional burden of exposure due to this accidental event. Towards this aim, the following data were needed:

- Data on ambient air levels of PCDDs/PCDFs during the accidental event were obtained by various measurements of particulate matter (PM) and analysis of PCDDs/PCDFs in both the particle and gaseous phase.
- Human biomonitoring (HBM) data for estimating the background exposure to the exposed population. In practice, the HBM data of the local population collected from a previous study (before the accident) where used to estimate the equivalent background exposure that results in the corresponding HBM data; the additional exposure of the measured PCDDs/PCDFs was added to these background levels for a duration of 6 days.
- Metabolomics analysis data derived from blood samples of n=50 individuals, used for identifying perturbed metabolic pathways. Advanced bioinformatics algorithms were used to identify potential biomarkers and demonstrate how useful the selected metabolomics results are.

Applied Methodology

Integrated Exposure Assessment and Internal Exposure Modelling

Realistic exposure assessment is data-intensive, requiring detailed information at every step of the source-to-dose pathway. Aiming at associating external exposure estimates from short-term short-term ambient air contamination with long-term internal dose, the computational platform INTEGRA (Sarigiannis et al., 2015a) was used. INTEGRA brings together all available information within a coherent methodological framework for assessing the source-to-dose continuum for the entire life cycle of substances covering an extensive chemical space. The major component of INTEGRA is a computational platform that integrates environmental fate, exposure and internal dose dynamically in time. The platform is largely validated using human biomonitoring data from Europe and the USA and comprises the following components:

1. A multimedia model to account for multi-scale interactions affecting the environmental transport and fate of chemicals. The model takes into account interactions across various scales (e.g. continental, regional and local) and mass exchange among various phases and media (e.g. soil, air water and sediment).
2. Indoor micro-environmental modelling and detailed personal exposure assessment, including all potential exposure pathways and routes of exposure. It has to be noted that PCDDs/PCDFs are highly lipophilic compounds and they adsorb strongly on particles. As a result, for properly estimating exposure to PCDDs/PCDFs estimation of actual uptake of particles across the human respiratory tract is necessary. HRT particle deposition modeling was applied for the determination of PM deposition fraction (DF) to the three parts of the pulmonary system in order to estimate the uptake of PCDDs/PCDFs. Major mechanisms of PM deposition across HRT include diffusion, sedimentation and impaction. Secondary mechanisms involve interception and electrostatic deposition. Different HRT regions involve different deposition mechanisms, with regard to different PM size as follows:
    - **Naso-Pharyngeal Region (or upper respiratory tract – URT):** Impaction, sedimentation, electrostatic (particles > 1 μm)
    - **Tracheo-Bronchial (TB) Region:** Impaction, sedimentation, diffusion (particles < 1 μm)
    - **Pulmonary (P) Region:** Sedimentation, diffusion (particles < 0.1 μm)

Several parameters affect HRT deposition, including PM properties (concentration and size distribution), air flow parameters (lung capacity and breathing frequency) and HRT physiology (structure and morphology). All of these parameters have been taken into account in the approach applied herein.

HRT deposition was carried out using the Multiple Path Particle Deposition (MPPD) v. 2.1 model (de Winter-Sorkina and Cassee, 2002), which is incorporated in INTEGRA. Age-specific lung geometries representing 10 distinct ages from 3 months old to 21 years old are also provided. An idealized symmetric single-path model as well as a 5-lobe symmetric multiple-path model are available for use with each age setting (Mortensen, 1983; Mortensen, 1988; Mortensen et al., 1983). Software input includes morphological parameters of pulmonary system – functional residual volume (FRC), tidal volume (TV), upper respiratory tract (URT) volume, as well as breathing frequency (BF) for each age group

3. A generic PBBK model that incorporates life stage changes and physiological and metabolic efficiency change over an individual's lifetime (from conception till 80 years of age). The model is able to cover perinatal exposure including exposure routes such as lactation, being practically a mother-fetus interaction model. Advanced QSAR models are used to estimate physicochemical and biochemical parameters of the model in order to expand its applicability domain to a large chemical space (Sarigiannis et al., 2015b). The fundamentals of PBPK modelling are to identify the principal organs or tissues involved in the disposition of the chemical of interest and to correlate the chemical absorption, distribution, metabolism, and excretion within and among these organs and tissues in an integrated and biologically plausible manner. Within the boundary of the identified compartment (e.g., an organ or tissue or a group of organs or tissues), whatever inflows must be accounted for via whatever outflows or whatever is transformed into something else. This mass balance is expressed as a mathematical equation with appropriate parameters carrying biological significance. A generic equation, for any tissue or organ, is:

$$V_i \frac{dC_{ij}}{dt} = Q_i(CA_j - CV_{ij}) - Metab_{ij} - E\lim_{ij} + Absorp_{ij} - \Pr Binding_{ij}$$

where V_i represents the volume of tissue group i, Q_i is the blood flow rate to tissue group i, CA_j is the concentration of chemical j in arterial blood, and C_{ij} and CV_{ij} are the concentrations of chemical j in tissue group i and in the effluent venous blood from tissue i, respectively. $Metab_{ij}$ is the rate of metabolism for chemical j in tissue group i; liver, being the principal organ for metabolism would have significant metabolism and, with some exception, usually $Metab_{ij}$ is equal to zero in other tissue groups. $Elim_{ij}$ represents the rate of elimination from tissue group i (e.g., biliary excretion from the liver), $Absorp_{ij}$ represents uptake of the chemical from dosing (e.g., oral dosing), and $PrBinding_{ij}$ represents protein binding of the chemical in the tissue. All these terms are zero unless there is definitive knowledge that the particular organ and tissue of interest has such processes. A series of similar mass balance differential equations representing all of the interlinked compartments are formulated to express a mathematical representation, or model, of the biological system. This model can then be used for computer simulation to predict the time course behavior of any given parameter in the model. In the current study, the model was properly parameterized for PCDDs/PCDFs. The biokinetics of TCDD are relatively well understood in adult humans (Kerger et al., 2006; Michalek and Tripathi, 1999; Milbrath et al., 2009) and several key parameters (tissue partition coeficients and clearance rates) were used from literature. The key aspects characterizing TCDD biokinetics are very high lipophilicity (adipose:tissue blood patrition coefficient is equal to 220) and very slow elimination rate, resulting in a half-life elimination rate of 7.5 years, explaining its long persistance and bioaccumulation potential. Another important issue that needed to be addressed was the transfer of PCDDs/PCDFs through the placenta during pregnancy and maternal milk during lactation. The model describes mother fetus interactions by modelling the intra-placental properties that govern the transfer of xenobiotics and their metabolites from the mother to the fetus as it grows. The anthropometric parameters of the models are time dependent, so as to provide a lifetime internal dose assessment, as well as to describe the continuously changing physiology of the mother and the developing fetus. The model includes diffusive flow from the uterus to the placenta and back during pregnancy (Beaudouin et al., 2010). Excretion via lactation is described as an output from the mammary tissue compartment through a partitioning process between mammary tissue and milk, and milk withdrawal by suckling, as described for PCBs in rats (Lee et al., 2007) and further adopted for humans (Verner et al., 2008).

4. Inverse modelling for exposure reconstruction and human biomonitoring (HBM) data assimilation. This module allows the translation of HBM data into external exposure estimates i.e. the exposure that corresponds to the observed biomonitoring data (Sarigiannis et al., 2016). Depending on the detail of the ancillary information available, valid estimates about the contribution of the various pathways and routes can be made as well.

Human Biosamples, Metabolomics and Pathway Analysis

In a selected number of 50 individuals living in the area, blood sample was obtained for metabolomics analysis. 300 μl blood serum was transferred to 1.5 ml small Eppendorf tubes. At the same time, 50μl of each sample was placed in a falcon-type container for the preparation of the Quality Control QC sample and stored at -80 °C. A three-fold amount of ice-cold solvent, in this case 900 μl of methanol, was added to precipitate the sample proteins in the form of a white precipitate. These aliquots were centrifuged for 20 minutes in a standard centrifuge at 10,000 rpm. After completion of centrifugation, 950 μl of the supernatant was taken and placed in 1.50 ml small Eppendorf tubes and stored at -80 °C. When moving forward with the analysis, the samples were centrifuged for 5 minutes at 10,000rpm, because residue was observed at the bottom. 500 μl,were taken, using a special speed-vac device, evaporated and dried with N_2. The same procedure was followed for QC samples. In the next step, the samples were resuspended in 100μl of water. And then centrifuged for 20 minutes in a standard centrifuge at 10,000 rpm. 95 μl of the supernatant were taken and placed in special vials suitable for the Orbitrap autosampler. The samples at this stage were ready for analysis and placed in the cooled autosampler (4 °C) and analysed in a Thermo Scientific™ Orbitrap LC/MS-MS. After the analysis of positive and negative ionization, the m/z spectrums were processed with MZmine (Katajamaa et al., 2006). Baseline correction was carried out as there is usually an imbalance between spectra due to the introduction of a different noise value, followed by peak detection, chromatogram deconvolution (Alonso et al., 2015) and peak alignment using the random sample consensus algorithm (Zhao and Yu, 2017). Finally, metabolite identification was carried out using the MetaboSearch tool, where the metabolites identification based on m/z values was carried out on four bases simultaneously, including the Human MetabolomeDataBase (HMDB), the Madison Metabolomics Consortium Database (MMCD), the Metlin database and the LipidMaps database (Zhou et al., 2012). The next step after metabolite identification was the build-up of mechanistic hypotheses, i.e. setting the combination of identified metabolites within a plausible biological context. The specific work on metabolic pathway analysis was carried out using the Agilent Mass Profiler Professional (MPP). This is a powerful tool designed to accept input data, results obtained by sample analysis by LC/MS-MS, and provide high quality information about the observed relationships between samples or sample groups. It is noteworthy that in this study metabolic pathways were analyzed separately for each sample, i.e. at the end of the analysis 50 lists of metabolic pathways were generated based on the results obtained from the analysis of samples with LC/MS-MS.

Cancer Risk Potency

Mixtures of PCDDs/PCDFs are complex environmental mixtures of 210 interrelated chemicals composed of different dioxins and furans. For PCDD/PCDF mixtures, the reference chemical is 2,3,7,8 – tetrachlorodibenzo-p-dioxin (2,3,7,8–TCDD) because it is the most toxic and best-studied of the 210 PCDDs/PCDFs. The toxicity equivalence factor (TEF) methodology was developed by the U.S. Environmental Protection Agency to evaluate the toxicity and assess the risks of a mixture of structurally related chemicals with a common mechanism of action. A TEF is an estimate of the relative toxicity of a chemical compared to a reference chemical. Toxic Equivalents, or TEQs, are used to report the toxicity-weighted masses of mixtures of PCDDs/PCDFs. The TEQ method of PCDDs/PCDFs reporting is more meaningful than simply reporting the total number of grams of a mixture of variously toxic compounds because the TEQ method offers toxicity information about the mixture. Within the TEQ method, each PCDDs/PCDFs compound is assigned a Toxic Equivalency Factor, or TEF. This factor denotes the toxicity of a given dioxin compound relative to the toxicity of 2,3,7,8-TCDD, which is assigned the value of one. Other dioxin compounds are given equal or lower numbers, with each number roughly proportional to its toxicity relative to that of 2,3,7,8-TCDD. Developed by the World Health Organization, TEFs are used extensively by scientists and governments around the world (Van den Berg et al., 1998), finally expressing the so-called TEQ WHO (toxicity equivalent concentration in accordance with the methodology of the World Health Organization), that uses units of grams-TEQ. The EPA uses TEQ WHO to report emissions of PCDDs/PCDFs from known sources to the open environment in its Inventory of Sources of Dioxin in the United States and similar practices have been adopted worldwide, including all the data presented in this study. To obtain the number of grams-TEQ of a dioxin mixture, one simply multiplies the mass of each compound in the mixture by its TEF and sums them up.

EPA has classified 2,3,7,8-TCDD as a Group B2, meaning a probable human carcinogen (USEPA, 1985). With regard to 2,3,7,8-TCDD, EPA has calculated an inhalation cancer slope factor of $1.5 \cdot 10^5$ $(mg/kg/d)^{-1}$ and an inhalation unit risk estimate of 3.3×10^{-5} $(pg/m^3)^{-1}$ for 2,3,7,8-TCDD. A similar slope factor of $1.5 \cdot 10^5$ $(mg/kg/d)^{-1}$ has been proposed for orally administered 2,3,7,8-TCDD, which correspond to an oral unit risk factor of 4.5 $(\mu g/L)^{-1}$.

Results

Ambient Air Concentrations of PCDDs/PCDFs

Analysis of ambient air samples (both particle and gaseous phase) showed that the levels of PCDDs/PCDFs in the surrounding area were 1.8 pg/m3 TEQ WHO (toxicity equivalent concentration in accordance with the methodology of the World Health Organization). These levels are significantly higher than the ones reported in previous studies, where the atmospheric background concentration of a typical industrial site in the wider area of Athens was found to be equal to 0.1 pg/m^3 TEQ WHO, but in the same order of magnitude to the levels of landfill fires (Figure 13).

Figure 13. Levels of PCDDs/PCDFs (TEQ) at various Athens sub-areas, as well as during accidental fire events

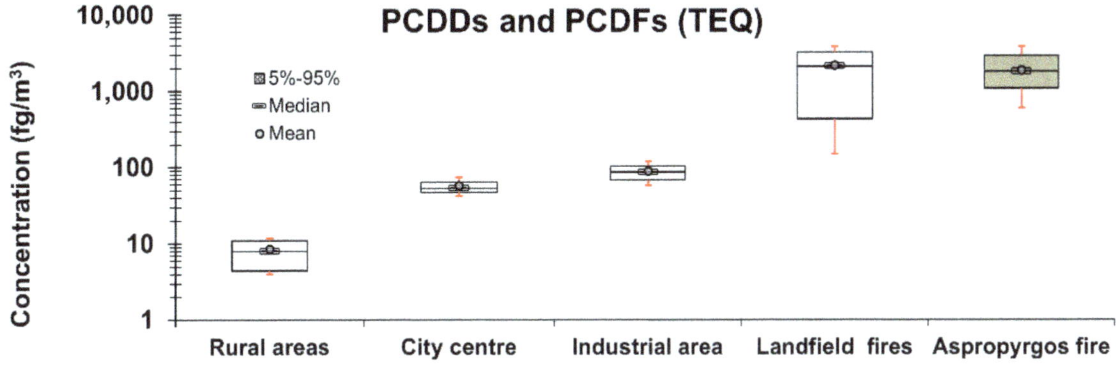

Internal Dose of PCDDs/PCDFs

To calculate the additional burden of exposure for the living population due to the accidental event, it was critical to estimate the actual background exposure to dioxins/furans. For this purpose, the data of a biomonitoring study held in Athens in 2006 (Costopoulou et al., 2006) were used, according to which the average PCDDs/PCDFs TEQ concentration in blood serum was equal to 7.3 pg/g lipids. Exposure reconstruction using biomonitoring data provided a comprehensive overview of the actual daily uptake from all potential pathways (e.g. ambient air and food) and routes (inhalation and oral). According to the biokinetic model, this blood concentration level corresponds to an equivalent daily intake of PCDDs/PCDFs of about 0.002 pg_TEQ/kg_bw/d. By using these uptake levels, the respective time course of the concentration of PCDDs/PCDFs in the blood for a period of 30 years is described with the blue solid line of Figure 2. As shown in Figure 14, exposure to the accidental fire fumes results in a significant increase of dioxin levels in the blood, up to 18 pg/g lipids (red thick line). Due to the PCDDs/PCDFs

Figure 14. Internal exposure to dioxins/furans under (a) usual conditions (continuous line) and (b) under accidental release (dotted line)

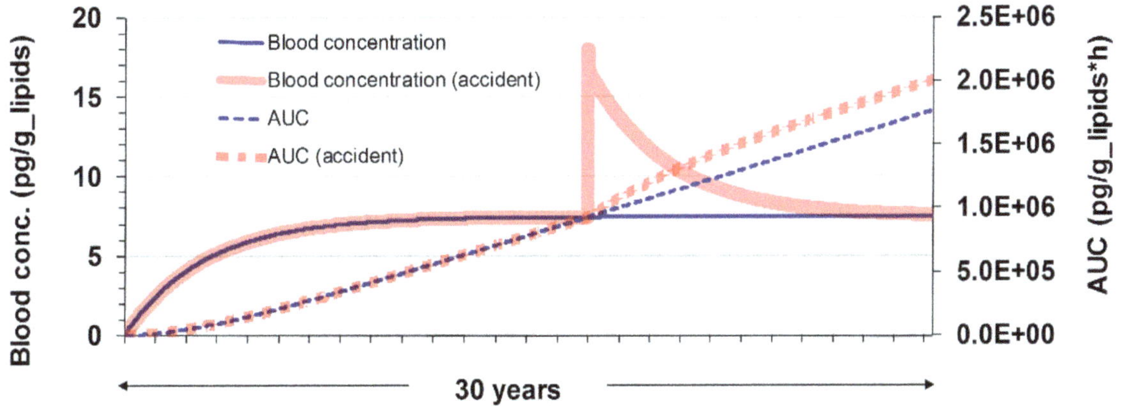

Figure 15. Estimated cancer risk for the exposed population before and after the accidental fire

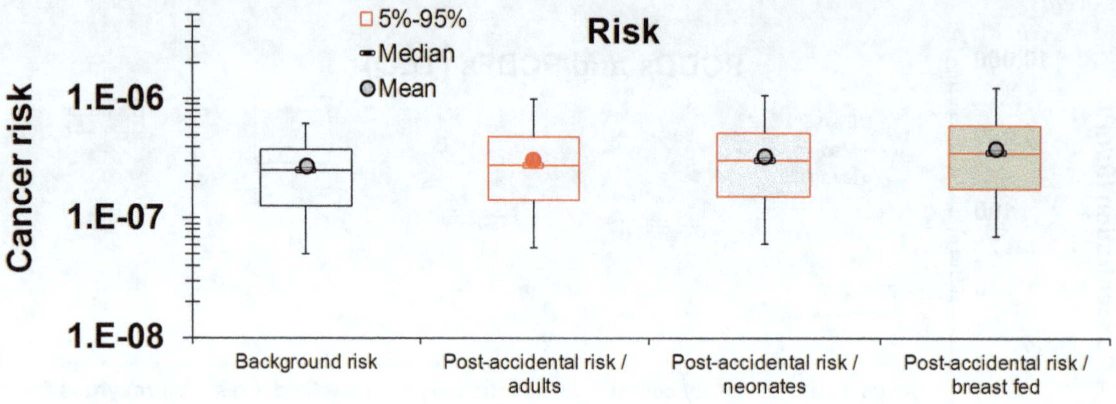

persistence, the concentrations in the blood will remain higher than the ones of the background for several years. The elevated exposure levels in adult mothers, are very important for the developing fetus. In the case of pregnant women exposure, the constantly elevated blood levels in the mother, result in similar levels of PCDDs/PCDFs in fetal blood. Considering that the fetus has a higher percentage of adipose tissue than adults, and thus a relatively higher capacity of lipophilic compound bioaccumulation, this additional burden of PCDDs/PCDFs at that early life stage, results in continuously higher internal exposure (AUC is almost 20% higher) during the entire lifespan. Similarly, the breast milk of exposed mothers is expected to have a concentration of PCDDs/PCDFs of almost 10 pg/g lipids, resulting in a significant exposure burden during the breast-feeding period, which in turn results in an increase of the entire lifespan AUC of almost 30%.

Estimation of Cancer Risk

This additional internal exposure burden which is also illustrated as the difference of the area under the curve (AUC) between the blue and the red dotted lines, will result in an increased risk of cancer associated with exposure to PCDDs/PCDFs. The obtained AUC was translated into a new equivalent chronic uptake dose, equal to 0.00226 pg_TEQ/kg_bw/d. Uptake estimates were translated into cancer risk estimates, using the slope factor proposed by the US Environmental Protection Agency (1985, 1997).

Accounting for variability in exposure estimates, fat and blood lipids content, distributions of exposure estimates were derived. Based on the background level of exposure to PCDDs/PCDFs of the general population the risk of chronic exposure was estimated (mean value) equal to $2.57 \cdot 10^{-7}$. For the population exposed over 6 days to the PCDDs/PCDFs fumes emitted from the recycling plant fire the respective risk (mean value) was up to $2.91 \cdot 10^{-7}$, indicating an increase of 13% in the 30-year cancer risk. It has to be noted that even the upper bounds of the post-accidental risk estimates are below 10^{-6} (Figure 15).

The respective risk is expected to be higher for neonates, whose mothers were exposed to the fumes of the accidental fire during pregnancy. The higher levels of PCDDs/PCDFs in the blood during pregnancy will result in continuously higher levels during their entire life span, resulting in an increase of the estimated lifetime risk of almost 20%. The estimated lifetime risk is expected to be even higher for neonates that are also breast fed; breast feeding is considered a major source of lifetime exposure to dioxins and the increased levels of exposure to PCDDs/PCDFs are considered to contribute to up to 32%.

Biosample and Metabolic Pathway Analysis

It has also to be noted that both the elevated internal exposure to PCDDs/PCDFs, and the activation of molecular pathways related to cancer have been verified by biomonitoring of the population leaving nearby the plastic recycling plant. For this purpose, human blood was sampled from 50 individuals, including both adults and children. Untargeted metabolomics analysis indicated that increased levels of unsaturated vs saturated fatty acids were identified compared to controls (population non-exposed to the fumes). This finding could indicate perturbation of cholesterol homeostasis; the latter, is highly related to AhR deregulation. The aryl hydrocarbon receptor does not only act as a transcription factor binding the dioxin responsive element (DRE) and activating metabolizing enzymes such as CYP1A1 and CYP1B1. AhR is also involved in the regulation of other pathways in a DRE-independent manner. As an example, AhR regulates cholesterol biosynthesis by interacting with the sterol element-binding protein 2 (SREPB2) transcription factor. Furthermore, cross-talks between AhR and some nuclear receptors such as the estrogen receptor (ER) and the androgen receptor (AR) are well described (Beischlag et al., 2008). AR itself influences cholesterol homeostasis by interacting with the liver X receptor (LXR), which can regulate sulfotransferases and thereby androgens activity (Jeanneret et al., 2014). Exposure to dioxins eventually leads to alterations in several metabolic pathways, including hepatic lipogenesis, perturbed TCA cycle, disrupted carbohydrate and amino acid metabolism as well as inhibition of de novo fatty acid biosynthesis. The results of this analysis, indicated the activation of pathways associated to cancer, thus verifying the hypothesis of increased cancer risk due to exposure to dioxins and furans. Additional identified pathways related to cancer included the sphingosine, the sphingosine-1-phosphate metabolism pathways, the Endothelin 1 receptor (ET-1R) pathway and the P450-dependent formation of polyunsaturated fatty acid epoxides. Sphingolipid metabolites, ceramide, sphingosine, and sphingosine 1-phosphate, have emerged as a new class of lipid biomodulators of various cell functions. These functions include adhesion, cellular growth and differentiation, apoptosis and surface antigens. As a result, altered sphingolipid metabolism contributes to cancer progression (Ryland et al., 2011). Endothelin 1 receptor (ET-1R) pathway is aberrantly expressed in human malignancies, potentially representing prognostic factors. Their activation by ligand stimulation initiate signaling cascades activating different downstream effectors, allowing precise control over multiple signaling pathways. The molecular events underlying these responses include the activation of transcriptional factors and coactivators, and downstream genes, acting as key players in tumor growth and progression (Rosanò and Bagnato, 2016). Finally, the perturbation of the cytochrome P450-dependent formation of polyunsaturated fatty acid epoxides, which is an important biochemical pathway creating mediators of inflammation and blood pressure regulation. Once formed these compounds can be incorporated into phospholipid membrane, and released by the action of phospholipase A2. The epoxides of arachidonic acid, i.e. the epoxyeicosatrieneoic acid or EETs, are putative endothelial derived hyperpolarization factors which increase the open state probability of Ca++ sensitive K+ channels, leading to vasodilation in arteriolar beds. The 11(12)-EET in particular appears to have potent functions in vasodilation, and are inhibitors of NFKb dependent inflammatory signalling, and PAI-1 activity. The 5(6)-EET appears unique, in that its metabolic transformation through cyclooxygenase activities produces potent vasoconstrictors. With the exception of the 5(6)-EET, these epoxy fatty acids are good substrates for the soluble epoxide hydrolase. Hydrolytic tranformation to vicinal diols eliminates vasoactive actions, however these vicinal diols have been reported to have other biological activites, including PPAR-alpha activation. Recent development of inhibitors of the soluble epoxide hydrolase are proving to have potent anti-inflammatory, anti-hypertensive, and anti-nociceptive properties (Panigrahy et al., 2010).

Discussion

The current study dealt with the assessment of long-term effects of exposure to PCDDs/PCDFs due to an accidental event occurred in a plastic recycling plant. Translating short term environmental contamination events into the equivalent long-term internal exposure and latent effect estimation represents a major scientific challenge. In order to addressing this issue, the comprehensive methodological framework INTEGRA was applied (Sarigiannis et al., 2014; Sarigiannis et al., 2016). Considering that the exposure burden due to the accidental event is not relevant to a long-term increase of external intake, by simply using a daily intake rate and a slope factor, would not allow us to properly account for the actual risk, resulting to significant underestimation, since the actual increase in the intake, would be accounted only for the 6 days of the fire. On the contrary, the use of internal dosimetry metrics, allowed us to track the AUC, which is a more realistic metric for associating exposure and effect. In addition, inter-individual variability of the population has been taken into account in terms of age, body fat, lipids in the blood and smoking status. As a result, due to the accidental event, an increase of the long-term cancer risk associated to PCDDs/PCDFs of 13% for the adult local population was estimated, while significantly elevated risk estimates were calculated for neonates (20% increased risk) who's their mothers were exposed during pregnancy and for breast fed infants (32% increased risk). The fact that the increase of the associated risk is in the range of 10^{-7}, indicates that the estimated risk is not negligible and is within the range of the background risk associated to PCDDs/PCDFs exposure from multiple sources. On the other hand, considering the continuous efforts for reducing the emissions of PCDDs/PCDFs in the environment and the continuously reducing levels globally identified in human matrices and especially analysis of human breast milk that is a non-invasive method, the additional burden of such type of accidental events will be more and more important. It has also to be taken into account that exposure to the specific event might be higher for part of the population (living closer to the center of the plume) and also that there are significant differences in the susceptibility of the population against carcinogenic agents. In this case the estimated risks could be higher (upper part of the risk estimates distribution), in the order of magnitude of 10^{-6}; the latter is considered as the acceptable risk for environmental factors. Moreover, the effect on the most vulnerable population (fetus and breast-feeding neonates) are expected to be significantly higher than the adults. This is the result of the major toxicokinetic characteristics of PCDDs/PCDFs; prenatal and postnatal exposure comprise a significant contributor of actual internal exposure to dioxins, providing the heritage of PCDDs/PCDFs initial burden of exposure. It is also important that metabolic pathway analysis revealed the perturbation of cancer-related pathways (AhR, sphingosine and sphingosine-1-phosphate metabolism, Endothelin 1 receptor and the P450-dependent formation of polyunsaturated fatty acid epoxides). It is interesting that these metabolic pathways indicate perturbations associated to cancer through different mechanisms of actions beyond the well-known AhR activation; changes of glycosphingolipids on the cellular membrane of cancer cells leads to significant changes of the antigenic properties, including the formation of tumor-associated carbohydrate antigens, and a loss of adhesion, as well as increased motility enhancing invasion and metastasis. On the other hand, ET-1R regulates cell proliferation, survival, motility, cytoskeletal changes, angiogenesis, metastasis as well as drug resistance, while cytochrome P450-derived metabolites of arachidonic acid, EETs and HETE may be involved in cancer in a few different ways: either in cell-autonomous tumor survival and growth or in modulating stromal processes, such as angiogenesis and inflammation that can support tumor progression (Panigrahy et al., 2010). Overall this is of particular important, demonstrating that under exposure to complex mixtures, such as the PCDDs/PCDFs mixture here in; it has been demonstrated that additional pathways might be activated, beyond the ones (AhR related pathways) related to the compound (TCDD) that is driving the mixture toxicity. This is a key finding that gives additional insights to already well-established concepts on mixture toxicology (Sarigiannis et al., 2009; Sarigiannis and Hansen, 2012), moving forward to intersecting pathways of toxicity, identified by metabolomics analysis. Metabolomics has the potential to inform and support the definition of adverse outcome pathways based on physiology-related data that incorporate particular key events. This includes the identification of previously undefined key events by measuring changes in endogenous metabolites involved in a wide variety of biochemical pathways, and associate these changes with exposure to specific combinations of exogenous compounds. In this study, starting from untargeted metabolomics, potential pathways of toxicity were hypothesized, based on changes of the metabolic profile of the individuals. Overall, this case provides additional evidence that the different elements of the connectivity paradigm can be functionally integrated among them to provide a coherent framework towards the development of adverse outcome pathways (Ankley et al., 2010; Gutsell and Russell, 2013). This has particular importance for the identification of human health risks associated to the various waste management options, pointing out that the identification of pre-clinical effect biomarkers through metabolomics analysis (Wishart et al., 2016) could effectively support the verification of potential risks. Finally, with regard to the study at hand, additional analysis has been foreseen, that includes analysis of both environmental and biological samples. The first ones will inform us about the fate of these persistent compounds and the potential exposure of the local population through additional exposure pathways. The second ones will provide us information whether the perturbations in metabolic pathways identified immediately after the accidental event are sustained. Towards this aim, further targeted metabolomics analysis will be carried out so as to provide quantitative detail on the dynamic metabolic fluxes and thus support mechanistically the persistence of the hypothesised pathways of toxicity.

Heracles Waste Study Assessing Long-Term Exposure of the Population Living Nearby Large Sanitary Landfills to Endocrine Disrupting Chemicals Such as Plasticisers Released From Plastic and Micro Plastic Waste

Introduction

The HERACLES Waste Study cohort in Greece, is a cohort study aiming at assessing the contribution of plasicizers associated to children neurodevelopment. The study has been established in 2012. Around 350 children aged 3 to 8 living in the proximity of a landfil between 0.5 and 12 km were enrolled.

Data Used in the Analysis

Exposure Factors

For the association, several exposure factors have been investigated, including:

- Exposure to plasticizers, including:
    - BPA
    - DEHP
    - BBzP
    - BiNP
- Additional proxies of exposure, such as
    - Distance from the contaminated sites

Exposure and Effect Modifiers

Additional factors considered as exposure and effects modifiers were included as well. These included:

- Sociodemographic parameters such as
    - Socioeconomic status
    - Mother education
    - Father education
    - Stress events
- Child anthropometric parameters and post-delivery factors
    - Child body mass index
    - Child gender
    - Breastfeeding
- Presence of micronutrients, minerals and vitamins
    - Se in the mother plasma during pregnancy, delivery and in cord blood
- Detailed dietary habits
    - Consumption of meat products (pork meat, beef, lamb, sausages)
    - Consumption of fish
    - Consumption of sea food
    - Consumption of poultry (eggs, chicken)
    - Consumption of dairy products (milk, yogurt)
    - Consumption of nuts
    - Consumption of fruits
    - Consumption of vegetables
    - Consumption of snacks (biscuits, chocolates)

Health Outcomes Investigated

The health outcomes considered in this study are relevant to the neurodevelopmental disorders in children estimated following the administration to the children or their parents and teachers the following four test batteries.

The Child Behavior Checklist (Achenbach and Rescorla, 2001), also called the Achenbach System of Empirically Based Assessment, is a report form to screen for emotional, behavioral, and social problems. The CBCL's questions are associated with problems on a syndrome scale in eight different categories: anxious/depressed, withdrawn/depressed, somatic complaints, social problems, thought problems, attention problems, rule-breaking behavior, and aggressive behavior. The CBCL also has a scale set to show scores associated with disorders from the Diagnostic and Statistical Manual of Mental Disorders (American Psychiatric Association., 2000): anxiety, oppositional defiant disorder, conduct problems, somatic problems, affective problems, and attention deficit disorder. Many studies have demonstrated a high rate of reliability between the scales of the CBCL and actual psychological diagnosis (Warnick et al., 2008).

The Cambridge Neuropsychological Test Automated Battery (CANTAB); it has been used to assess neurocognitive performance in modeling studies of Chronic Fatigue Syndrome (CFS) (Capuron et al., 2001; Robbins and Sahakian, 2002). CANTAB has modules for several neurocognitive functions and processes including psychomotor and motor speed, reasoning and planning abilities, memory and attention, and frontal, temporal and hippocampal dysfunctions. Thus, it allows assessment of neuro-cognitive dysfunctions associated with neurologic disorders and neuro-cognitive syndromes.

The Social Responsiveness Scale (SRS); it is often used to measure Autism Spectrum Disorders (ASD) severity. The Social Responsiveness Scale (SRS) is a parent and teacher-completed screening questionnaire measures social ability of children from 4 years to 18 years old. It is used primarily to measure Autism Spectrum Disorders (ASD) severity. Although SRS is frequently referred to as a measure of "social impairment," many SRS items describe other core features of ASD, including communication deficits and repetitive behaviors (Constantino et al., 2000), as well as symptoms not exclusively related to ASD diagnostic criteria (Grzadzinski et al., 2011).

The Wechsler Intelligence Scale for children – Fourth Edition (Wechsler, 2003); it is an individually administered measure of intelligence intended for children aged six years to 16 years and 11 months. WISC-IV yields measures of general intelligence as reflected in both verbal and nonverbal (performance) abilities and specific indices including verbal comprehension, perceptual reasoning, working memory and processing speed.

Results and Interpretation of EWAS Analysis

EWAS analysis results relevant to the Child Behavioral CheckList (CBCL) test battery results show that socio-cultural factors are strongly associated with children behavior. More specifically the mother school title and the age of the mothers at birth show both a robust statistical association (p-value<0.05 and in some cases p-value <0.01) with most of the CBCL indices considered. Looking at the volcano plots both parameters show a negative association with the CBCL scores indicating that lower educational level of the mothers as well as a lower age of the mother at the children birth may have negative impact on the children behavior.

The stress index was derived by merging the total number of stressful events detected by the mother and their average intensity is also playing an important role on the children behavior (p-value<0.05 and in some cases p-value < 0.01) showing a negative effect on both internalizing and externalizing problems indices such as anxiety and depression, withdrawal and depression and somatic complaints, aggressive and rule-breaking behavior. Of statistical significance is the association of the concentration of selenium in blood which appears to beneficially, especially with regard to Internalizing Problems and ADHD as measured by CBCL battery indices. These results confirm the antioxidant properties of selenium which is a well-known regulator of brain function (Dominiak et al., 2016). These positive properties that selenium possesses are attributed to its ability to be incorporated into selenoproteins as an amino acid. Several selenoproteins are expressed in the brain, in which some of them, e.g. glutathione peroxidases (GPxs), thioredoxin reductases or selenoprotein P, are strongly involved in antioxidant defense and in maintaining intercellular reducing conditions. Since increased oxidative stress has been implicated in neurological disorders higher levels of selenium in blood may be among the important factors protecting against those pathologies.

Breast feeding in the first months of children life is another parameter that shows a significant statistical association (p-value < 0.05) especially with the internalizing problems as measured by CBCL battery indices. Also, in this case, the association shows a negative sign indicating that breastfeeding and especially its duration during the first year of life results in a beneficial effect on anxiety/depression, withdrawal/depression and somatic complaints as reported by the CBCL indices.

CBCL indices as measured by teachers reveal slightly different patterns. Even though the socio-cultural factors such as mother school title still show robust associations with most of the Child Behavioral CheckList test battery outcomes, other variables appear to play an important role. Among them the distance of the residence address from the waste management site shows a strong association especially with the internalizing problems. The negative sign of the association corroborates the negative impact of living in areas close to the waste management site especially on anxiety/depression, withdrawal/depression and somatic complaints.

With regard to Attention Deficit Hyperactivity Disorder, breast feeding shows a strong association with Oppositional Defiant Disorder (ODD). Among the various food items considered, some of them show significant statistical association with CBCL indices. Consumption of pork (e.g. pork dishes, lard, bacon, salami) appears to be inversely associated (p-value <0.05) with the CBCL indices related to externalizing problems such as aggressive and rule-breaking behavior as well as with association with ODD or and with Conduct Problems. High consumption of chicken reveals a strong association with Attention Deficit Hyperactivity Disorder measured by the teachers. Consumption of cabbage and lentils appears to influence negatively Attention Deficit Hyperactivity Disorder, ODD and with Conduct Problems too. High consumption of coffee is associated with externalizing problems such as aggressive and rule-breaking behavior and with Attention Deficit Hyperactivity Disorder and Conduct Problems measured by the teachers. Fish consumption reveals opposite effects on the basis of the fish type: while higher consumption of sardines and/or salmon (also canned) appears to be statistically associated with ADHD, consumption of herring, mackerel and trout (also canned) indicates a beneficial effect on the CBCL indices related to Conduct Problems. Higher consumption of pine nuts and nuts as well as of white and wheat bread indicates a beneficial effect on externalizing problems such as aggressive and rule-breaking behavior. Finally, higher consumption of eggs and of beans are also associated to beneficial effects on internalizing problems (i.e. anxiety/depression, withdrawal/depression and somatic complaints) indices.

EWAS analysis results relevant to the Cambridge Neuropsychological Test Automated Battery (CANTAB) test battery results show that concentration of Manganese in the hair is associated (p-value <0.05) with the Spatial Working Memory (SWM) with a positive sign revealing that higher Manganese levels in the hair increase error generation. Socio-cultural factors show again significant statistic association with the outcomes of the CANTAB test battery. More in detail Mother School title appears to have a beneficial effect (p-value < 0.05) on the Stop Signal Task while Father School title on the spatial Working Memory Strategy index (p-value < 0.05). The stress index is also strongly associated (p-value <0.01) with the Spatial Working Memory (SWM) with a negative sign showing that higher stress levels decrease the error production.

EWAS analysis results relevant to the Social Responsiveness Scale (SRS) test battery show that also in this case socio-cultural factors are strongly associated with the Social Responsiveness Scale outcomes considered. Mother school title (p-value <0.000) and to a lower extent Father school title (p-value < 0.05) show both a robust statistical association the T scores of both the parents and teachers. Moreover, the associations have a negative direction demonstrating that lower educational level of the parents may have negative impact on the Autism Spectrum Disorder (ASD) impairments of children.

Distance of the residence address from the waste management site shows a good association (p-value <0.001) with the T scores of the teachers. The negative sign of the association confirms the potential negative impact of living in the areas close to the waste management site on ASD impairments of children. Breastfeeding in the first months of children life also shows a good statistical association (p-value <0.05) with T scores as reported by teachers. The association shows a negative sign indicating the positive effect of breastfeeding, and especially its duration during the first year of life, on ASD impairments of children.

Among the biomonitoring data selenium in blood appears to be inversely associated (p-value <0.05) with the T scores of the parents. The negative sign of the association supports the positive impact of selenium on the neurodevelopmental disorders. Among the different food items higher consumption of pork dishes (lard, bacon, sausage) (p < 0.01), coffee (p-value < 0.01), chicken (p < 0.05), breadsticks, crackers and rusks (p-value < 0.05) and lentils (p-value < 0.05) are associated with higher T scores of the SRS test battery indicating a potential negative effect on ASD impairments. On the contrary higher consumption of tomatoes (p-value < 0.001), white fish (e.g. codfish, rumble fish) (p-value < 0.01) and soft cheese (p-value < 0.05)) are related with lower T scores of the SRS test battery signifying a potential positive effect on ASD impairment of children.

EWAS analysis results relevant to the WISC-IV test results show that the variable distance of the residence address from the waste management site is a key factor associated with almost all the indices of the WISC IV test. More specifically this variable shows a robust statistical association (p-value <0.001) with the IQ, Verbal Comprehension index, Perceptual Reasoning index, Working Memory index. Analysis of the results show a positive association with the WISC IV scores indicating that living far from the waste management site has a positive impact on the children cognitive functions. Some interesting conclusions can be drawn from the analysis of food consumption patterns. Tomatoes consumption appears to be statistically (p-value <0.05) associated to IQ, Verbal Comprehension index and Working Memory index while cereal consumption reveals a strong association (p-value < 0.01) with the Perceptual Reasoning index. Both these food items show a positive sign meaning that their consumption has potential positive effects on the cognitive functions of the children. Epidemiological evidence suggests that consumption of lycopene, natural antioxidant presents in tomatoes, is able to reduce the risk of chronic diseases such as cancer, cardiovascular diseases as well as psychiatric syndromes (Story et al., 2010). In another study (Li and Zhang, 2007) reported that low serum levels of lycopene have been associated with increased

Figure 16. Association of intelligence quotient (from the WISC-IV test battery) with the environmental, dietary and exposure factors

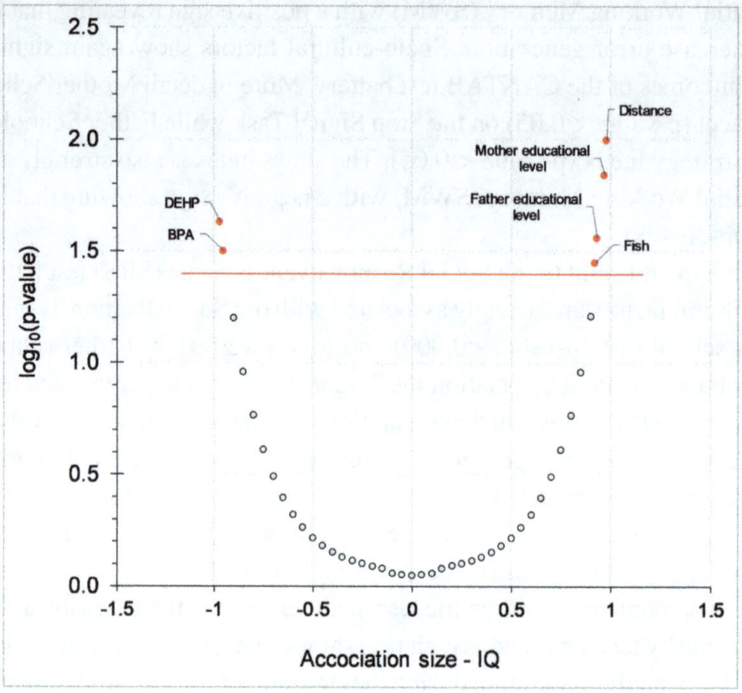

risk of psychiatric disorders. One review of 22 studies examining the association of breakfast cereal consumption and academic performance in children and adolescents concluded that breakfast consumption may improve cognitive function related to memory, test grades, and school attendance (Rampersaud et al., 2005). Among the plasticizers examined in the study, BPA and DEHP are statistically associated with lower IQ. This is probably related to perturbation of mitochondrial respiration, which in turn affects growth of neurons at critical developmental stages. On the other hand, sociodemographic factors such as mother and father educational level, hold a key role in children IQ. Similarly to the CBCL test battery, consumption of fish shows a dual behavior depending on the type of fish considered: higher consumption of white fish appears to have positive effects on the IQ and Verbal Comprehension index (p-value <0.001) while higher consumption of white fish reveals a negative effect (p-value <0.01) on Perceptual Reasoning index and Working Memory index.

Exposure to Industrial Waste and Its Effects on the Neurodevelopment of Children Living in Proximity With Industrial Zones

Introduction

Health impact assessment in industrially contaminated sites is a complex process that entails consideration of various technical, environmental, societal and health-related aspects coupled to the associated uncertainties. The key questions in this regard can be summarized as follows:

1. What type of compounds do we have to deal with? Typically, emissions vary significantly as a function of the industrially contaminated site activity type. Their intensity varies with the duration of activities, the environmental restoration measures applied and the amount of processed materials.
2. How are these compounds distributed in the environment? Of particular interest in this regard are the environmental compartments in which chemicals are released and the physicochemical properties of the released compounds.
3. What are the exposure levels to these compounds for on-site workers and the local population? Addressing this point requires assessing the contribution of multiple pathways and routes of exposure to the overall exposure burden, as well as reckoning the relative contribution of the industrially contaminated site sources to the exposure background in the vicinity.
4. How does exposure to industrially contaminated sites relate to adverse health outcomes? Answering the above requires integrated consideration of both epidemiological and toxicological evidence relating exposure to effects. This, however, would need to be sustained by the elucidation of the biological mechanisms underlying the exposure-to-effect continuum, i.e. the relevant adverse outcome pathway(s) linking the molecular biology of human disease onset and/or exacerbation and environmental co-exposure to the traditionally complex mixture of toxicants found in industrially contaminated sites.

The exposome (Wild, 2005) represents the totality of exposures from conception onwards, including the exogenous and endogenous exposures and modifiable risk factors that predispose to and predict disease. Unravelling it will help us understand the intricate web of relationships between environmental exposures, lifestyle, genetics and disease (Sarigiannis, 2015a). Such a process implies that environmental exposures and genetic variance are reliably measured and linked through mechanistic analysis of toxicity pathways. To understand the interaction between environmental exposure and disease, we need to capture the biological perturbations initiated by chronic exposure to environmental stressors and identify the ones that overcome the homeostasis barrier inducing alterations of the cell/tissue environment and cascade down to disease phenotypes.

Based on all the above and accounting for the methodological difficulties for a comprehensive assessment of the impact that waste sites may have on public health, the current study describes how the exposome can improve our understanding in the complex relationships between exposure to an ICS and the related health effects. The ultimate objective is to enable cost-effective prevention strategies that curb hazardous exposures with precision at the individual (or susceptible subgroup) level and only limited uncertainty at the community level. In this work we present a novel approach to health risk and impact assessment of industrially contaminated sites that explores the connectivity among the different information layers pertinent to environmental characterisation on the one hand and the different scales of biological organisation in human beings (from gene regulatory networks to cell/tissue function allostasis to organism physiological perturbations). We give examples of the application of the exposome connectivity paradigm in two case studies: the contamination of the water table in the Asopos river basin with Cr(VI) in the industrial zone outside of Athens, in the Attica region of Greece; and the contamination of the soil with toxic metals outside of Taranto in the Puglia region of Italy.

Methodology

Overall Methodological Concept of Exposome

Exposome science aims at elucidating the mechanistic processes that describe the source-to-dose continuum. Towards this aim, several methodological tools are employed related to environmental and human biomonitoring. Starting from environmental exposure, various sensors including in situ systems for regulatory monitoring of environmental media, personal, wearable and remote sensors are combined to determine the external exposome, feeding fusion algorithms for integrating functionally these datasets and filling adequately data gaps in space and time.

External exposures are translated into internal dose both at systemic level and at target tissues using physiology-based biokinetic models that consider the different routes of exposure and the chemical and biochemical interactions among the pollutant mixture components. Biological perturbations at different are captured with multiple –omics (including genomics, transcriptomics, proteomics and metabolomics) and post-omics technologies including epigenomics.

Identification of the perturbations results in the identification of putative pathways of toxicity, that are verified by targeted multi-omics and functional assays. Advanced bioinformatics tools such as support vector machines and clustering algorithms and systems biology models allow us to identify the functional links among the data derived from high throughput testing platforms and disease phenotypes providing thus phenotypic anchoring of the mechanistic hypotheses made earlier. Finally, translation of individual into community effects is carried out using advanced statistic tools that allow the understanding of the complex web of interconnection among the investigated parameters, such as the environment-wide association studies (EWAS) concept. In this context, the correlated environmental factors are not considered confounders; rather they are dealt with as co-variates, which are in "linkage disequilibrium" (LD) with each other. LD is a statistical construct that allows the identification of causal loci in genomic trait analysis. Borrowing the "linkage disequilibrium" from genomics research in EWAS allows us to discern the

Figure 17. Assessing health impacts of ICS using the exposome paradigm

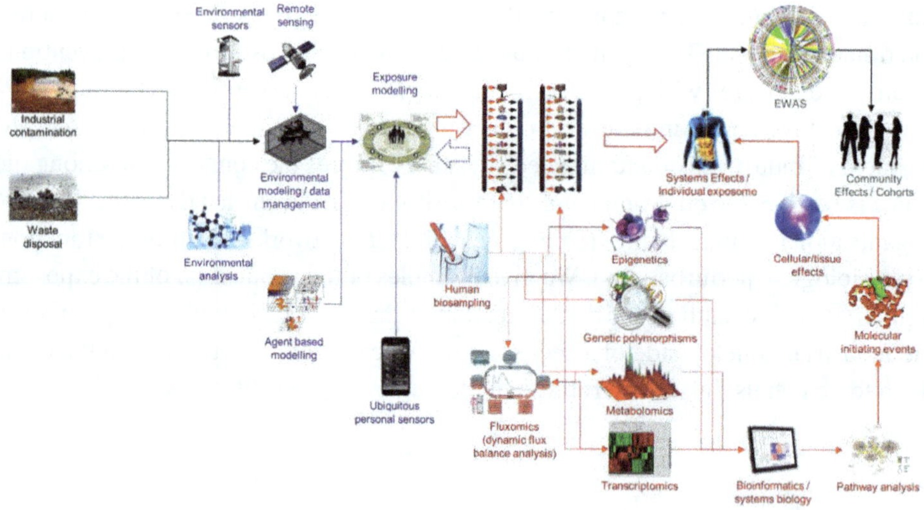

causal determinants that define the relationship between exposures to contaminants in ICS and adverse health outcomes. Our approach to implementing EWAS is a population-based data analysis approach that correlates multiple environmental factors to disease. The EWAS approach has been introduced by Patel et al. (2010) and it is based on the Genome-Wide Association Study (GWAS) paradigm. In EWAS, the place of the genome is replaced by the environment, i.e. the metrics of all the environmental exposures related to the population in the area. Specific metrics can be the amount of a chemical substance found in human matrices, a self-reported historical exposure and common well–being characteristics such as family and social economic status (SES). and the contamination of the soil with toxic metals outside of Taranto in the Puglia region of Italy. We integrated data from measurements of toxic metal contamination in soil samples, human biomonitoring in blood or urine of volunteers, questionnaires on dietary patterns and other behavioral traits that may affect exposure.

Assessment of Long-Term Exposure Effects on Child Neurodevelopment

The area of study (Taranto, Italy) is characterized by the presence of the largest steel transformation and production plant of Europe with a capacity to produce 10 million tons of steel annually, which corresponds to 40% of Italian steel production. The analysis focused on the exposure of more than 300 children aged between 6 and 12 years to heavy metals through biomonitoring samples that were collected and analysed. To assess potential neuropsychological and behavioral deficits in the study subjects four different test batteries were administered to children, their parents and teachers as appropriate. For the association, several exposure factors have been investigated, including:

- Exposure to heavy metals, such as Cd, Hg and As in urine, Pb in blood, Mn and Hg in hair
- Additional proxies of exposure, such as distance from the contaminated sites, concentration of heavy metals in the soil of the child address
- Additional factors considered as exposure and effects modifiers such as:
  - Sociodemographic parameters (socioeconomic status, mother education, father education, stress events)
  - Child anthropometric parameters and post-delivery factors (child body mass index, child gender, breastfeeding, presence of micronutrients, minerals and vitamins, Se in the mother plasma during pregnancy, delivery and in cord blood)
  - Detailed dietary habits, such as consumption of meat products (pork meat, beef, lamb, sausages), fish, sea food, poultry (eggs, chicken), dairy products (milk, yogurt), nuts, fruits, vegetables and snacks (biscuits, chocolates)
- Analysis of metabolomics profile from urinary samples and pathway analysis, for identifying the pathways that are perturbed and associated with the respective neurodevelopmental progress.
- Neurodevelopmental progress in children was estimated with the Wechsler Intelligence Scale for children – Fourth Edition (Wechsler, 2003), which is an individually administered measure of intelligence intended for children. WISC-IV yields measure of general intelligence as reflected in both verbal and nonverbal (performance) abilities and specific indices including verbal comprehension, perceptual reasoning, working memory and processing speed.

Results: Exposure to Metals and Neurodevelopmental Disorders in Taranto

The levels of heavy metals biomonitored and measured in the soil (for selected compounds) in the study area are illustrated in Figure 18.

Food consumption patterns influence neurodevelopmental indicators as well. Tomato consumption appears to be statistically (p-value < 0.05) associated with IQ (Figure 19), Verbal Comprehension index and Working Memory index while cereal consumption reveals a strong association (p-value < 0.01) with the Perceptual Reasoning index. Both food items are positively associated with cognition indices meaning that their consumption has potential positive effects on the cognitive functions of the children. Epidemiological evidence suggests that consumption of lycopene, a natural antioxidant present in to-

Figure 18. Levels of heavy metals in soil (aggregated levels in living areas, spot measurements in industrial site)

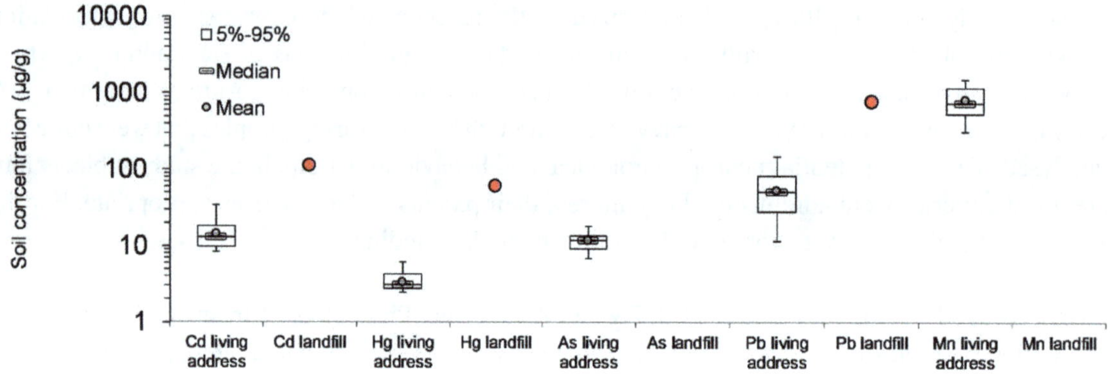

Figure 19. Association of IQ (from the WISC-IV test battery) with environmental, dietary and exposure factors

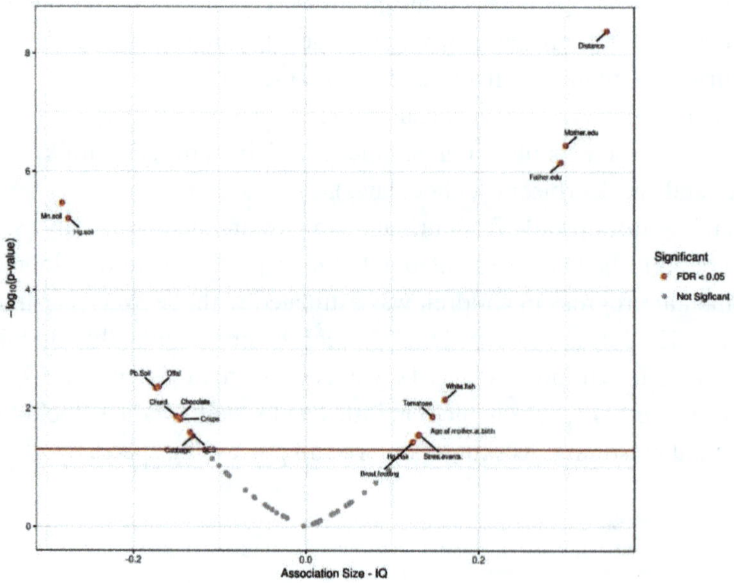

matoes, is able to reduce the risk of chronic diseases such as cancer, cardiovascular diseases as well as psychiatric syndromes. Consumption of fish showed a hybrid behavior depending on the type of fish and the neurodevelopmental indicator considered: higher consumption of white fish appears to have positive effects on the IQ and Verbal Comprehension index (p-value < 0.001) while higher consumption of white fish reveals a negative effect (p-value < 0.01) on Perceptual Reasoning index and Working Memory index. Among the sociodemographic parameters, it has been illustrated that the parental educational level is positively associated with IQ; in fact it is the second most significant parameter. Based on the metabolomics analysis and the subsequent bioinformatics analysis, several metabolic pathways were identified. Among the various pathways identified, the following ones have been associated to lower scores of neurological development: lactose degradation III, trehalose degradation II trehalase, sucrose degradation V for mammalians, UDP N acetyl D galactosamine biosynthesis II, glycogen degradation III, glycogen degradation II, GDP glucose biosynthesis, Glycolysis Gluconeogenesis, Hs AMP activated Protein Kinase .AMPK. Signaling WP1403 86073, Hs Cori Cycle WP1946 79691, mevalonate pathway I, cholesterol superpathway, geranylgeranyldiphosphate biosynthesis I via mevalonate.

The mevalonate cascade is a key metabolic pathway that regulates a variety of cellular functions and is thereby involved in the pathophysiology of many brain diseases, including neurodevelopmental and neurodegenerative disorders (Jiao et al., 2016). The mevalonate pathway was correlated with both the cholesterol and geranylgeranyldiphosphate biosynthesis pathways, resulting in central nervous system deregulation. For example, the key biochemical finding for mevalonate kinase deficiency is the accumulation of urinary mevalonic acid / mevalonolactone (Kanungo et al., 2013). Moreover 7-dehydrolesterol, the last compound before cholesterol biosynthesis, is involved in vitamin D_3 biosynthesis. Disactivation of the pathway blocks D_3 biosynthesis, a mechanism which has been associated with neurodevelopmental disorders. According to Kocovska et al. (Kocovska et al., 2012), vitamin D deficiency may be an environmental trigger for autism spectrum disorder (ASD) in individuals genetically predisposed for the broad phenotype of autism. Several pieces of indirect evidence exist that autophagy may degrade the glycogen in neurons, in a way similar to many other tissues. For example, defects in lysosomal enzyme acid alpha-glucosidase have been associated to glycogen accumulation in many tissues, including neurons (Sidman et al., 2008); the concentration of glycogen in neurons provokes neurodegenaration. Trehalose acts as a potent stabilizer of proteins able to preserve protein structural integrity and reduces aggregation of pathologically misfolded proteins (Emanuele, 2014). Trehalose is an mTOR-independent inducer of autophagy and, together with TSC, form a complex which is the key regulator of protein synthesis. Thus, they control cell growth (Zhou and Parada, 2012). Recent data suggest that the TSC1/2 complex influences also neural polarity.

DISCUSSION

From the various case studies described above, the socioeconomic components of exposure related to waste and energy activities were highlighted.

Regarding the use of biomass for energy, the case-study presented herein, dealt with the health and economic impact of the increased biomass use in Greece taking the example of Thessaloniki, the second largest city in the country and a major economic, industrial and commercial hub in Southeastern Europe. Results showed an increase of about 200 excess premature deaths (out of a population of almost 900,000 inhabitants) or 3400 YLL from all causes during the 2012-2013 winter compared to the 2011-2012 winter, that correspond to an additional health burden to an average cost ranging between 200 - 250 million euro (up to 1.2 billion). Considering the high overall cost, the heavy taxation of light heating diesel in Greece should be reconsidered. Thus, the effect of biomass displacement was evaluated by alternative scenario analysis, which clearly showed the benefits of policy interventions that would discourage the use of biomass as fuel source for domestic heating. Fiscal policies at the national level should take into account environmental health externalities and indeed consider how the increased public health burden would influence mid- and long-term financial turnovers. It has also to be noted, that health burden is not equally distributed within the urban canopy. From the latest PM measurements, it was identified that PM10 levels were inversely correlated with SES.

This is explained by the fact that people of lower SES are more susceptible to energy poverty, thus, more prone in less environment friendly options for space heating. At the same time, actual exposure to PM is even higher to the ones illustrated by ambient air spatial distribution figures; biomass burning appliances result in indoor PM emissions (also of PM of lower aerodynamic diameter), which in turn results in significantly higher PM exposure and uptake levels.

Based on the results of the study and taking into account the importance of public health and the related socioeconomic cost, specific interventions are recommended, such as:

- Reduction of the price of light heating diesel through relaxation of the related excise tax
- Financial incentives for light heating diesel replacement by natural gas or electricity
- Enhancement of the support given to residential energy conservation schemes and simplification of the relevant regulatory framework to ease the access of larger numbers of households to such programs.

Regarding the Romani population and the increased risks of dioxins/furans related cancer, it has to be considered that although waste recycling is considered one of the most environment friendly and sustainable waste management options, accidental events might result in significant contamination of the surrounding area, affecting adversely the population leaving nearby. The study herein, applied a comprehensive methodological framework for addressing one of the major problems related to acci-

Figure 20. Spatial distribution of PM10 levels in Thessaloniki, in relation to SES status

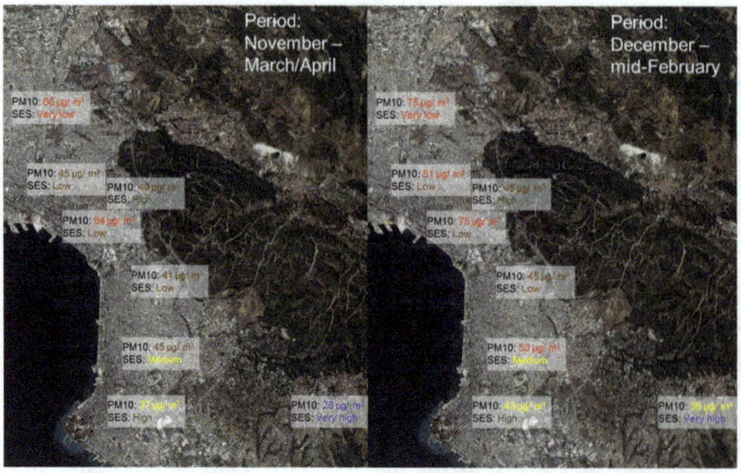

dental events and the release of biocumulative, persistent and toxic compounds, which is the translation of a short-term exposure event into a long-term exposure estimate. Towards this aim, the INTEGRA computational platform (Sarigiannis et al., 2015a) allowed the assimilation of different types of environmental and HBM data in order to estimate the chronic internal exposure to PCDDs/PCDFs. The TEQ concept for the mixture of PCDDs/PCDFs was employed to compute the associating risks using as a TEF reference compound 2,3,7,8-TCDD, which has a well-established slope factor. Based on the above, an average increase of 13% of cancer risk attributed to PCDDs/PCDFs was estimated for the exposed population. A key finding of the study was that neonates and breast-fed infants face even higher lifetime risks. These risks were quantified (20% and 32% respectively). The perturbation of pathways related to PCDDs/PCDFs mediated cancer, were also verified by metabolomics and metabolic pathway analysis. However, once more it has to be highlighted that the overall study concerns a minority that represents a very distinct socially disadvantaged population group, which is subjected to toxicants exposure in the case of accidental events.

With regard to the risks associated with proximity to industrially and waste contaminated sites, exposome science (Sarigiannis, 2015a; Sarigiannis, 2015b) can overhaul the current environmental health impact assessment paradigm, allowing us to effectively address the complexity related to the interplay of genetic, epigenetic, environmental, dietary and sociodemographic parameters. This requires coupling high dimensional biology and system science aiming at integration using big data analytics and bioinformatics. Towards this aim, the connectivity approach to the exposome elucidates toxicity pathways and assigns causal associations between environmental stressors and health. The application of the above methodology in typical industrially and waste contaminated sites, allowed us to conclude that proximity to industrial activities and exposure to heavy metals commonly found in industrial activities, combined with sociodemographic and dietary parameters, result in metabolic pathways perturbation that are mechanistically associated with lower neurodevelopmental scores in children and increased cancer risk for all age groups. Our analyses further demonstrate the protective role of specific dietary components that reduce oxidative stress at the cellular level. Elucidation of the interaction between environmental contamination and dietary elements highlights the importance of exposome-wide associations when addressing the linkage between environmental contamination and public health. Thus, understanding the complex interplay of the multitude of factors associated with environment and health, the contribution of sociodemographic factors either directly (e.g. educational level) or indirectly (quality of diet) is successfully attributed. From the analysis it was identified that the most influential parameters are the socio-economic-cultural conditions of the family. The positive effect of these factors on the neurodevelopmental cognitive functions is associated to the better quality of life, translated as nutrition of higher quality, lower exposure to environmental contamination and better educational activities and opportunities. Similarly, parent school title has been associated to cognitive development. Among the investigated parameters, specific dietary components seem to have either a positive or a negative influence, however, due to the lack of food residue data the associations are many times inconclusive. However, it is clearly demonstrated that foods with antioxidants (e.g. tomatoes) or foods rich omega 3 fatty acids (nuts, almonds, eggs) have a clearly beneficial effect on cognitive functions. Beyond the effect of these factors, exposure related parameters seem to be important in specific tests. Distance from the industrially and waste contaminated sites affects the outcomes of many indices of the four batteries test analyzed impacting negatively the population living in the areas closer to the industrially and waste contaminated sites, confirms the hypothesis that these are major pollution source for the population living in the area, eventually with additional pollutants than the ones described in the biomonitoring data. What it really is worth to be further investigated is the identification of synergies among heavy metals and plasticisers in children neurodevelopment. The preliminary findings of metabolic pathway analysis from cohort samples, revealed that alterations in urine metabolites associated with exposure to plasticisers are related to the TCA cycle, suggesting impaired mitochondrial respiration; the latter is central to energy metabolism and cellular signaling and plays fundamental roles several cellular processes. Inhibition of mitochondrial oxidative phosphorylation could also cause a defective mitochondrial energy production during the process of fetus formation and development that are reflected in early life motor development. The latter is enhanced by the oxidative stress induced by heavy metals (Sarigiannis and Salifoglou, 2016). This defective mitochondrial energy production during the process of fetus formation and development is reflected in early life motor development.

CONCLUSION

In terms of public health protection, it is obvious from all the above, that environmental injustice associated with waste and energy sectors, contributes to higher risks for the socially disadvantaged through multiple pathways:

- Higher exposure levels to contaminants emitted from the related activities: several factors contribute to higher exposure levels, related both to less environment friendly and to consumer behavior aspects. In this sense, the use of biomass for space heating is related to the degradation of both the air quality in the vicinity, as well as the residential indoor air quality, that result in higher exposure levels to PM and to the adsorbed toxic compounds (such as PAHs).

Similarly, poor consumer choices have been associated with elevated exposure to plasticisers. The purchasing of low-cost toys, food contact materials and building materials from non-EU origin, thus not fulfilling REACH restrictions on the use of the more toxic plasticisers such as DEHP, results in higher exposure levels, that are also reflected in children neurodevelopment. Other consumer choices of lower quality are associated to food; socially disadvantaged usually consume lower amounts of healthy foods such as fish (rich in omega-3 acids), and at the same time lower quality food products (higher amount of pesticides, preservatives and food additives).

- Proximity to industrially contaminated and waste management sites: Usually, socially disadvantaged populations live closer to sources of contamination related to industrial/energy production and waste management activities, as the result of the lower land prices closer to these areas. On the other hand, it has been evident that proximity to these types of contaminated sites is the most significant variable associated (inversely) with the children IQ. This indicates that multiple environmental contaminants (either heavy metals, or organic compounds) act cumulative (and eventually synergistically) towards deficient neurodevelopment. Cases like the Romani population located in Aspropyrgos, Greece, living within the close vicinity of waste management sites (recycling plant, among other industrial activities allocated in the area), serve as the best examples to highlight this problem.

- Lower educational level: Lower educational level is reflected in environmental exposure and health continuum in multiple aspects. A major component of educational level is highly associated with the perception of importance of healthy diet and lifestyle choices; as an example, it has been found in many studies that parental education level has been associated to higher levels of children exposure to second-hand tobacco smoke. Also, differences in parental education level are also reflected in terms of creative time and activities in the interaction with the children, which in turn is another significant determinant of child neurodevelopment.
- Lower quality of health services: Socially disadvantaged have limited access to quality health services and are less prone to regular medical exams, which in turn results in later diagnosis of potential adverse health outcomes and worst prognosis.

REFERENCES

Achenbach, T. M., & Rescorla, L. A. (2001). *Manual for the ASEBA school-age forms & profiles: an integrated system of mult-informant assessment*. Burlington: University of Vermont, Research Center for Children, Youth & Families.

Adler, N. E., & Newman, K. (Ed.). (2002). Socioeconomic Disparities In Health: Pathways And Policies.

Alonso, A., Marsal, S., & Julia, A. (2015). Analytical methods in untargeted metabolomics: State of the art in 2015. *Frontiers in Bioengineering and Biotechnology*, *3*, 23. doi:10.3389/fbioe.2015.00023 PMID:25798438

American Psychiatric Association. (2000). *Diagnostic and statistical manual of mental disorders*. Washington: American Psychiatric Association.

Ankley, G. T., Bennett, R. S., Erickson, R. J., Hoff, D. J., Hornung, M. W., Johnson, R. D., ... Villeneuve, D. L. (2010). Adverse outcome pathways: A conceptual framework to support ecotoxicology research and risk assessment. *Environmental Toxicology and Chemistry*, *29*(3), 730–741. doi:10.1002/etc.34 PMID:20821501

Arcus-Arth Broadwin, R. & Lam, R. (2001). Impacts of Socioeconomic Factors on Residential Indoor Air Quality and Human Health. *Environmental Toxicology and Human Health, 2*.

Beaudouin, R., Micallef, S., & Brochot, C. (2010). A stochastic whole-body physiologically based pharmacokinetic model to assess the impact of inter-individual variability on tissue dosimetry over the human lifespan. *Regulatory Toxicology and Pharmacology*, *57*(1), 103–116. doi:10.1016/j.yrtph.2010.01.005 PMID:20122977

Beischlag, T. V., Morales, J. L., Hollingshead, B. D., & Perdew, G. H. (2008). The Aryl Hydrocarbon Receptor Complex and the Control of Gene Expression. *Critical Reviews in Eukaryotic Gene Expression*, *18*(3), 207–250. doi:10.1615/CritRevEukarGeneExpr.v18.i3.20 PMID:18540824

Beránek, M. (2005). POPs Pesticides in the Czech Republic. The International POPs Elimination Project Czech Republic.

Berkowicz, R., Ketzel, M., Jensen, S. S., Hvidberg, M., & Raaschou-Nielsen, O. (2008). Evaluation and application of OSPM for traffic pollution assessment for a large number of street locations. *Environmental Modelling & Software*, *23*(3), 296–303. doi:10.1016/j.envsoft.2007.04.007

Brook, R. D. (2008). Cardiovascular effects of air pollution. *Clinical Science*, *115*(6), 175–187. doi:10.1042/CS20070444 PMID:18691154

Capuron, L., Ravaud, A., & Dantzer, R. (2001). Timing and specificity of the cognitive changes induced by interleukin-2 and interferon-alpha treatments in cancer patients. *Psychosomatic Medicine*, *63*(3), 376–386. doi:10.1097/00006842-200105000-00007 PMID:11382265

Cole, P., Trichopoulos, D., Pastides, H., Starr, T., & Mandel, J. S. (2003). Dioxin and cancer: A critical review. *Regulatory Toxicology and Pharmacology*, *38*(3), 378–388. doi:10.1016/j.yrtph.2003.08.002 PMID:14623487

Constantino, J. N., Przybeck, T., Friesen, D., & Todd, R. D. (2000). Reciprocal social behavior in children with and without pervasive developmental disorders. *Journal of Developmental and Behavioral Pediatrics*, *21*(1), 2–11. doi:10.1097/00004703-200002000-00002 PMID:10706343

Costopoulou, D., Vassiliadou, I., Papadopoulos, A., Makropoulos, V., & Leondiadis, L. (2006). Levels of dioxins, furans and PCBs in human serum and milk of people living in Greece. *Chemosphere*, *65*(9), 1462–1469. doi:10.1016/j.chemosphere.2006.04.034 PMID:16765419

de Winter-Sorkina, R., & Cassee, F. R. (2002). *From concentration to dose: factors influencing airborne particulate matter deposition in humans and rats*. Bilthoven: RIVM National Institute for Public Health and the Environment.

Dominiak, A., Wilkaniec, A., Wroczynski, P., & Adamczyk, A. (2016). Selenium in the Therapy of Neurological Diseases. Where is it Going? *Current Neuropharmacology*, *14*, 282–299. doi:10.2174/1570159X14666151223100011 PMID:26549649

Dong, Z., Yuan, G., & Hu, J. (2016). Uncertainty analysis in 2,3,7,8-tetrachlorodibenzo-p-dioxin (TCDD) cancer dose-response for three occupational cohorts. *Environment International*, *88*, 53–59. doi:10.1016/j.envint.2015.12.010 PMID:26708281

Emanuele, E. (2014). Can trehalose prevent neurodegeneration? Insights from experimental studies. *Current Drug Targets*, *15*(5), 551–557. doi:10.2174/1389450115666140225104705 PMID:24568549

Emond, C., DeVito, M., Warner, M., Eskenazi, B., Mocarelli, P., & Birnbaum, L. S. (2016). An assessment of dioxin exposure across gestation and lactation using a PBPK model and new data from Seveso. *Environment International*, *92-93*, 23–32. doi:10.1016/j.envint.2016.03.015 PMID:27045706

Farmer, T. D., Shaw, P. J., & Williams, I. D. (2015). Destined for indecision? A critical analysis of waste management practices in England from 1996 to 2013. *Waste Management (New York, N.Y.)*, *39*, 266–276. doi:10.1016/j.wasman.2015.02.023 PMID:25771762

Fernando, S., Jobst, K. J., Taguchi, V. Y., Helm, P. A., Reiner, E. J., & McCarry, B. E. (2014). Identification of the halogenated compounds resulting from the 1997 Plastimet Inc. fire in Hamilton, Ontario, using comprehensive two-dimensional gas chromatography and (ultra)high resolution mass spectrometry. *Environmental Science & Technology*, *48*(18), 10656–10663. doi:10.1021/es503428j PMID:25133985

Forastiere, F., Stafoggia, M., Tasco, C., Picciotto, S., Agabiti, N., Cesaroni, G., & Perucci, C. A. (2007). Socioeconomic status, particulate air pollution, and daily mortality: Differential exposure or differential susceptibility. *American Journal of Industrial Medicine*, *50*(3), 208–216. doi:10.1002/ajim.20368 PMID:16847936

Forgacs, A. L., Kent, M. N., Makley, M. K., Mets, B., DelRaso, N., Jahns, G. L., ... Reo, N. V. (2012). Comparative metabolomic and genomic analyses of TCDD-elicited metabolic disruption in mouse and rat liver. *Toxicological Sciences*, *125*(1), 41–55. doi:10.1093/toxsci/kfr262 PMID:21964420

Gouveia, N. (2016). Addressing Environmental Health Inequalities. *International Journal of Environmental Research and Public Health*, *13*(9), 858. doi:10.3390/ijerph13090858 PMID:27618906

Grzadzinski, R., Di Martino, A., Brady, E., Mairena, M. A., O'Neale, M., Petkova, E., ... Castellanos, F. X. (2011). Examining autistic traits in children with ADHD: Does the autism spectrum extend to ADHD? *Journal of Autism and Developmental Disorders*, *41*(9), 1178–1191. doi:10.100710803-010-1135-3 PMID:21108041

Gutsell, S., & Russell, P. (2013). The role of chemistry in developing understanding of adverse outcome pathways and their application in risk assessment. *Toxicology Research*, *2*(5), 299–307. doi:10.1039/c3tx50024a

Haluza, D., Kaiser, A., Moshammer, H., Flandorfer, C., Kundi, M., & Neuberger, M. (2012). Estimated health impact of a shift from light fuel to residential wood-burning in Upper Austria. *Journal of Exposure Science & Environmental Epidemiology*, *22*(4), 339–343. doi:10.1038/jes.2012.27 PMID:22569207

Hays, M. D., Geron, C. D., Linna, K. J., Smith, N. D., & Schauer, J. J. (2002). Speciation of gas-phase and fine particle emissions from burning of foliar fuels. *Environmental Science & Technology*, *36*(11), 2281–2295. doi:10.1021/es0111683 PMID:12075778

IMF. (2012). *World Economic outlook*. Washington, DC, U.S.A.: World Economic and Financial Surveys.

IOBE, Equating the Excise Duty Rates on Heating and Diesel Oil. Foundation for economic and industrial research, 2013.

Jeanneret, F., Boccard, J., Badoud, F., Sorg, O., Tonoli, D., Pelclova, D., ... Rudaz, S. (2014a). Human urinary biomarkers of dioxin exposure: Analysis by metabolomics and biologically driven data dimensionality reduction. *Toxicology Letters*, *230*(2), 234–243. doi:10.1016/j.toxlet.2013.10.031 PMID:24201000

Jiao, X., Ashtari, N., Balaei, M. R., Chen, Q. M., Badbezanchi, I., Shojaei, S., ... Marzban, H. (2016). Mevalonate Cascade and Neurodevelopmental and Neurodegenerative Diseases: Future Targets for Therapeutic Application. *Current Molecular Pharmacology*. PMID:26758948

Johnston, F. H., Hanigan, I. C., Henderson, S. B., & Morgan, G. G. (2013). Evaluation of interventions to reduce air pollution from biomass smoke on mortality in Launceston, Australia: Retrospective analysis of daily mortality, 1994-2007. *BMJ (Clinical Research Ed.)*, 346. PMID:23299843

Kanungo, S., Soares, N., He, M., & Steiner, R. D. (2013). Sterol metabolism disorders and neurodevelopment-an update. *Developmental Disabilities Research Reviews*, *17*(3), 197–210. doi:10.1002/ddrr.1114 PMID:23798009

Katajamaa, M., Miettinen, J., & Orešič, M. (2006). MZmine: Toolbox for processing and visualization of mass spectrometry based molecular profile data. *Bioinformatics (Oxford, England)*, *22*(5), 634–636. doi:10.1093/bioinformatics/btk039 PMID:16403790

Kerger, B. D., Leung, H.-W., Scott, P., Paustenbach, D. J., Needham, L. L., Patterson, D. G. Jr, ... Mocarelli, P. (2006). Age- and Concentration-Dependent Elimination Half-Life of 2,3,7,8-Tetrachlorodibenzo-p-dioxin in Seveso Children. *Environmental Health Perspectives*, *114*(10), 1596–1602. doi:10.1289/ehp.8884 PMID:17035149

Kocovska, E., Fernell, E., Billstedt, E., Minnis, H., & Gillberg, C. (2012). Vitamin D and autism: Clinical review. *Research in Developmental Disabilities*, *33*(5), 1541–1550. doi:10.1016/j.ridd.2012.02.015 PMID:22522213

Krista, H., Tamara, S., & Richard, F. (2009). Environmental justice and Roma communities in Central and Eastern Europe. *Environmental Policy and Governance*, *19*(4), 251–268. doi:10.1002/eet.511

Landi, M. T., Bertazzi, P. A., Baccarelli, A., Consonni, D., Masten, S., Lucier, G., ... Grassman, J. (2003). TCDD-mediated alterations in the AhR-dependent pathway in Seveso, Italy, 20 years after the accident. *Carcinogenesis*, *24*(4), 673–680. doi:10.1093/carcin/bgg002 PMID:12727795

Leaderer, B. P., Naeher, L., Jankun, T., Balenger, K., Holford, T. R., Toth, C., ... Koutrakis, P. (1999). Indoor, outdoor, and regional summer and winter concentrations of PM10, PM2.5, SO42-, H+, NH4+, NO3-, NH3, and nitrous acid in homes with and without kerosene space heaters. *Environmental Health Perspectives*, *107*, 223–231. PMID:10064553

Lee, K., Yanagisawa, Y., Spengler, J. D., & Billick, I. H. (1995). Classification of house characteristics based on indoor nitrogen dioxide concentrations. *Environment International*, *21*(3), 277–282. doi:10.1016/0160-4120(95)00025-G

Lee, S. K., Ou, Y. C., Andersen, M. E., & Yang, R. S. H. (2007). A physiologically based pharmacokinetic model for lactational transfer of PCB 153 with or without PCB 126 in mice. *Archives of Toxicology*, *81*(2), 101–111. doi:10.100700204-006-0130-0 PMID:16858609

Li, Y., & Zhang, J. (2007). Serum concentrations of antioxidant vitamins and carotenoids are low in individuals with a history of attempted suicide. *Nutritional Neuroscience*, *10*(1-2), 51–58. doi:10.1080/10284150701250747 PMID:17539483

Liem, A. K. D., Fürst, P., & Rappe, C. (2000). Exposure of populations to dioxins and related compounds. *Food Additives and Contaminants*, *17*(4), 241–259. doi:10.1080/026520300283324 PMID:10912239

Lucier, G. W., Portier, C. J., & Gallo, M. A. (1993). Receptor mechanisms and dose-response models for the effects of dioxins. *Environmental Health Perspectives*, *101*(1), 36–44. doi:10.1289/ehp.9310136 PMID:8390353

Malisch, R., & Kotz, A. (2014). Dioxins and PCBs in feed and food - Review from European perspective. *The Science of the Total Environment*, *491-492*, 2–10. doi:10.1016/j.scitotenv.2014.03.022 PMID:24804623

Martuzzi, M., Mitis, F., & Forastiere, F. (2010). Inequalities, inequities, environmental justice in waste management and health. *European Journal of Public Health*, *20*(1), 21–26. doi:10.1093/eurpub/ckp216 PMID:20061348

Matsubara, T., Tanaka, N., Krausz, K. W., Manna, S. K., Kang, D. W., Anderson, E. R., ... Gonzalez, F.J. (2012). Metabolomics identifies an inflammatory cascade involved in dioxin- and diet-induced steatohepatitis. *Cell Metabolism*, *16*(5), 634–644. doi:10.1016/j.cmet.2012.10.006 PMID:23140643

Michalek, J. E., & Tripathi, R. C. (1999). Pharmacokinetics of TCDD in veterans of Operation Ranch Hand: 15-year follow-up. *Journal of Toxicology and Environmental Health. Part A.*, *57*(6), 369–378. doi:10.1080/009841099157584 PMID:10478820

Milbrath, M. O., Wenger, Y., Chang, C. W., Emond, C., Garabrant, D., Gillespie, B. W., & Jolliet, O. (2009). Apparent half-lives of dioxins, furans, and polychlorinated biphenyls as a function of age, body fat, smoking status, and breast-feeding. *Environmental Health Perspectives*, *117*(3), 417–425. doi:10.1289/ehp.11781 PMID:19337517

Mohai, P., Lantz, P. M., Morenoff, J., House, J. S., & Mero, R. P. (2009). Racial and Socioeconomic Disparities in Residential Proximity to Polluting Industrial Facilities: Evidence From the Americans' Changing Lives Study. *American Journal of Public Health*, *99*(S3), S649–S656. doi:10.2105/AJPH.2007.131383 PMID:19890171

Mortensen, J. D. (1983). A Study of Age Specific Human Respiratory Morphometry: Final Report. University of Utah Research Institute.

Mortensen, J. D. (1988). *Age related morphometric analysis of human lung casts. Extrapolation of Dosimetric Relationships for Inhaled Particles and Gases*. San Diego, CA: Academic Press.

Mortensen, J. D., Young, J. D., Stout, L., Stout, A., Bagley, B., & Schaap, R. N. (1983). A numerical identification system for airways in the lung. *The Anatomical Record*, *206*(1), 103–114. doi:10.1002/ar.1092060112 PMID:6881547

Naeher, L. P., Brauer, M., Lipsett, M., Zelikoff, J. T., Simpson, C. D., Koenig, J. Q., & Smith, K. R. (2007). Woodsmoke health effects: A review. *Inhalation Toxicology*, *19*(1), 67–106. doi:10.1080/08958370600985875 PMID:17127644

Neidell, M. J. (2004). Air pollution, health, and socio-economic status: The effect of outdoor air quality on childhood asthma. *Journal of Health Economics*, *23*(6), 1209–1236. doi:10.1016/j.jhealeco.2004.05.002 PMID:15556243

Noonan, C. W., & Balmes, J. R. (2010). Biomass smoke exposures: Health outcomes measures and study design. *Inhalation Toxicology*, *22*(2), 108–112. doi:10.3109/08958370903008888 PMID:20044883

Nussbaumer, T., Czasch, C., Klippel, N., Johansson, L., & Tullin, T. (2008). Particulate Emissions from Biomass Combustion in IEA Countries. International Energy Agency (IEA) Bioenergy, Zürich, Switzerland.

Oracle. (2011). Oracle Crystal Ball Fusion Edition, version 11.0.

Panigrahy, D., Kaipainen, A., Greene, E. R., & Huang, S. (2010). Cytochrome P450-derived eicosanoids: The neglected pathway in cancer. *Cancer and Metastasis Reviews*, *29*(4), 723–735. doi:10.100710555-010-9264-x PMID:20941528

Pediatrics, A. A. o. (2000). Guide to Your Child's Allegies and Asthma. New York: V. Books.

Rampersaud, G. C., Pereira, M. A., Girard, B. L., Adams, J., & Metzl, J. D. (2005). Breakfast habits, nutritional status, body weight, and academic performance in children and adolescents. *Journal of the American Dietetic Association*, *105*(5), 743–760. doi:10.1016/j.jada.2005.02.007 PMID:15883552

Robbins, T. W., & Sahakian, B. J. (2002). *Computer Methods of Assessment of Cognitive Function. In Principles and Practice of Geriatric Psychiatry* (pp. 147–151). John Wiley & Sons, Ltd. doi:10.1002/0470846410.ch28

Rosanò, L., & Bagnato, A. (2016). β-arrestin1 at the cross-road of endothelin-1 signaling in cancer. *Journal of Experimental & Clinical Cancer Research: CR.*, *35*(1), 121. doi:10.118613046-016-0401-4 PMID:27473335

Ryland, L. K., Fox, T. E., Liu, X., Loughran, T. P., & Kester, M. (2011). Dysregulation of sphingolipid metabolism in cancer. *Cancer Biology & Therapy*, *11*(2), 138–149. doi:10.4161/cbt.11.2.14624 PMID:21209555

Sarigiannis, D. (2015a). Exposome science for public health protection and innovation. *Toxicology Letters*, *238*(2), S12–S13. doi:10.1016/j.toxlet.2015.08.154

Sarigiannis, D. (2015b). Unravelling the Exposome through integrated exposure biology. *Toxicology Letters*, *238*(2), S229–S230. doi:10.1016/j.toxlet.2015.08.680

Sarigiannis, D., Gotti, A., Karakitsios, S., Kontoroupis, P., & Nikolaki, S. (2012). Intera Platform: A Tool for Mechanistic Risk Assessment of Indoor Air Pollutants. *Epidemiology (Cambridge, Mass.)*, 23.

Sarigiannis, D., Karakitsios, S., Gotti, A., Handakas, E., & Papadaki, K. (2015a). INTEGRA: Advancing risk assessment using internal dosimetry metrics. *Toxicology Letters*, *238*(2), S110–S111. doi:10.1016/j.toxlet.2015.08.359

Sarigiannis, D., Karakitsios, S., Gotti, A., Loizou, G., Cherrie, J., Smolders, R., . . . Sleeuwenhoek, A. (2014). Integra: From global scale contamination to tissue dose. In *Proceedings - 7th International Congress on Environmental Modelling and Software: Bold Visions for Environmental Modeling, iEMSs 2014* (Vol. 2, pp. 1001-1008). Academic Press.

Sarigiannis, D., Marafante, E., Gotti, A., & Reale, G. C. (2009). Reflections on new directions for risk assessment of environmental chemical mixtures. *International Journal of Risk Assessment and Management*, *13*(3/4), 216–241. doi:10.1504/IJRAM.2009.030697

Sarigiannis, D., Papadaki, K., Kontoroupis, P., & Karakitsios, S. (2015b). Advanced QSAR models for use in toxicokinetic modelling. *Toxicology Letters*, *238*(2), S166–S167. doi:10.1016/j.toxlet.2015.08.568

Sarigiannis, D. A., Hansen, U. (2012). Considering the cumulative risk of mixtures of chemicals - A challenge for policy makers. *Environmental Health: A Global Access Science Source.*

Sarigiannis, D. A., Karakitsios, S. P., Handakas, E., Simou, K., Solomou, E., & Gotti, A. (2016). Integrated exposure and risk characterization of bisphenol-A in Europe. *Food and Chemical Toxicology*, *98*, 134–147. doi:10.1016/j.fct.2016.10.017 PMID:27769850

Sarigiannis, D. A., Karakitsios, S. P., Kermenidou, M., Nikolaki, S., Zikopoulos, D., Semelidis, S., ... Tzimou, R. (2014). Total exposure to airborne particulate matter in cities: The effect of biomass combustion. *The Science of the Total Environment*, *493*, 795–805. doi:10.1016/j.scitotenv.2014.06.055 PMID:25000575

Sarigiannis, D. A., Karakitsios, S. P., Zikopoulos, D., Nikolaki, S., & Kermenidou, M. (2015). Lung cancer risk from PAHs emitted from biomass combustion. *Environmental Research*, *137*, 147–156. doi:10.1016/j.envres.2014.12.009 PMID:25543545

Sarigiannis, D. A., & Salifoglou, A. (2016). Research directives toward deciphering adverse outcome pathways induced by environmental metallotoxins. *Current Opinion in Chemical Engineering*, *13*, 161–169. doi:10.1016/j.coche.2016.09.010

Sarigiannis, D. A., Soulakellis, N., Schäfer, K., Tombrou, M., Sifakis, N. I., Assimakopoulos, D., ... Saisana, M. (2002). ICAROS: An integrated computational environment for the assimilation of environmental data and models for urban and regional air quality. *Water Air and Soil Pollution Focus*, *2*(5/6), 641–654. doi:10.1023/A:1021357417913

Sarigiannis, D. A., Soulakellis, N. A., & Sifakis, N. I. (2004). Information Fusion for Computational Assessment of Air Quality and Health Effects. *Photogrammetric Engineering and Remote Sensing*, *70*(2), 235–245. doi:10.14358/PERS.70.2.235

Schindler, B. K., Esteban, M., Koch, H. M., Castano, A., Koslitz, S., Canas, A., ... Angerer, J. (2014). The European COPHES/DEMOCOPHES project: Towards transnational comparability and reliability of human biomonitoring results. *International Journal of Hygiene and Environmental Health*, *217*(6), 653–661. doi:10.1016/j.ijheh.2013.12.002 PMID:24405937

Scire, J., Robe, F. R., Fernau, M. E., & Yamartino, R. J. (2000b). *A user's Guide for the CALMET Meteorological Model (Version 5).* Concord: Earth Tech Inc.

Scire, J., Strimaitis, D. G., & Yamartino, R. J. (2000a). *A user's Guide for the CALPUFF Dispersion Model (Version 5).* Concord: Earth Tech Inc.

Shrestha, R., Flacke, J., Martinez, J., & van Maarseveen, M. (2016). Environmental Health Related Socio-Spatial Inequalities: Identifying "Hotspots" of Environmental Burdens and Social Vulnerability. *International Journal of Environmental Research and Public Health*, 13. PMID:27409625

Sidman, R. L., Taksir, T., Fidler, J., Zhao, M., Dodge, J. C., Passini, M. A., ... Shihabuddin, L. S. (2008). Temporal neuropathologic and behavioral phenotype of 6neo/6neo Pompe disease mice. *Journal of Neuropathology and Experimental Neurology*, *67*(8), 803–818. doi:10.1097/NEN.0b013e3181815994 PMID:18648322

Story, E. N., Kopec, R. E., Schwartz, S. J., & Harris, G. K. (2010). An update on the health effects of tomato lycopene. *Annual Review of Food Science and Technology*, *1*(1), 189–210. doi:10.1146/annurev.food.102308.124120 PMID:22129335

USEPA, U.S. Environmental Protection Agency. (1985). Health Assessment Document for Polychlorinated Dibenzo-p-Dioxin. Environmental Criteria and Assessment Office, Office of Health and Environmental Assessment, Office of Research and Development, Cincinnati, OH.

Van den Berg, M., Birnbaum, L., Bosveld, A. T., Brunstrom, B., Cook, P., Feeley, M., ... Zacharewski, T. (1998). Toxic equivalency factors (TEFs) for PCBs, PCDDs, PCDFs for humans and wildlife. *Environmental Health Perspectives*, *106*(12), 775–792. doi:10.1289/ehp.98106775 PMID:9831538

Verner, M. A., Charbonneau, M., Lopez-Carrillo, L., & Haddad, S. (2008). Physiologically based pharmacokinetic modeling of persistent organic pollutants for lifetime exposure assessment: A new tool in breast cancer epidemiologic studies. *Environmental Health Perspectives*, *116*(7), 886–892. doi:10.1289/ehp.10917 PMID:18629310

Warnick, E. M., Bracken, M. B., & Kasl, S. (2008). Screening Efficiency of the Child Behavior Checklist and Strengths and Difficulties Questionnaire: A Systematic Review. *Child and Adolescent Mental Health*, *13*(3), 140–147. doi:10.1111/j.1475-3588.2007.00461.x

Wechsler, D. (2003). *Wechsler Intelligence Scale for Children*. San Antonio, TX: Psychological Corporation.

WHO. (2007). Health relevance of particulate matter from various sources.

Wild, C. P. (2005). Complementing the genome with an "exposome": The outstanding challenge of environmental exposure measurement in molecular epidemiology. *Cancer Epidemiology, Biomarkers & Prevention*, *14*(8), 1847–1850. doi:10.1158/1055-9965.EPI-05-0456 PMID:16103423

Wishart, D., Mandal, R., Stanislaus, A., & Ramirez-Gaona, M. (2016). Cancer Metabolomics and the Human Metabolome Database. *Metabolites*, *6*(1), 10. doi:10.3390/metabo6010010 PMID:26950159

World-Bank. (2013). *World Development Indicators database* (Vol. 2014). World Bank.

Zhao, S., & Yu, G. (2017). A new image registration algorithm using SDTR. *Neurocomputing*, *234*, 174–184. doi:10.1016/j.neucom.2016.12.055

Zhou, B., Wang, J., & Ressom, H. W. (2012). MetaboSearch: Tool for Mass-Based Metabolite Identification Using Multiple Databases. *PLoS One*, *7*(6), e40096. doi:10.1371/journal.pone.0040096 PMID:22768229

Zhou, J., & Parada, L. F. (2012). PTEN signaling in autism spectrum disorders. *Current Opinion in Neurobiology*, *22*(5), 873–879. doi:10.1016/j.conb.2012.05.004 PMID:22664040

Chapter 15
Glyphosate Toxicology:
What We Can Learn From the Current Controversy

Sheldon Krimsky
Tufts University, USA

ABSTRACT

This chapter explores the glaring scientific differences in the human health assessment of the popular herbicide glyphosate between European and American institutions. The International Agency for Research on Cancer (IARC) classified glyphosate as a probable human carcinogen, while the U.S. Environmental Protection Agency (EPA) concluded that glyphosate is not likely to be carcinogenic to humans. Both IARC's and the EPA's carcinogenic risk assessment processes are discussed. This work reveals uncertainties in the sciences of toxicology and epidemiology, as well as assumptions made in their applications for evaluating glyphosate. These uncertainties, along with the political context of chemical risk assessment, are at the root of the divergent findings on the carcinogenic risks of glyphosate.

INTRODUCTION

By now it is widely understood that determining the safety of a chemical has become a heavily politicized activity. Notwithstanding the claims of regulatory bodies, that science-based evidence guides their health and environmental assessments of a chemical, we continue to see a significant divergence in the toxicological profiles among different sectors of the scientific community and between the agencies of different countries.

The battlegrounds over the safety of chemicals occur between non-profit groups and government regulatory agencies as well as between groups of scientists who position themselves on one side or the other on whether a chemical is safe enough or too dangerous to keep in commercial use.

What can explain the differences in the assessment of chemical safety? The published science behind any chemical assessment is available to all. The science of toxicology is not, at least overtly, embedded in an ideology. It is taught throughout the world utilizing principles and textbooks that are widely shared.

DOI: 10.4018/978-1-5225-7635-8.ch015

Since the Enlightenment empiricism has been the cornerstone of the physical and social sciences. We perform experiments and allow the data to determine whether a hypothesis has been confirmed or falsified. Sometimes it takes one elegant, well executed experiment to bring consensus to a community of scientists. That was the case when evidence from an eclipse confirmed Einstein's General Theory of Relativity that the path of light can be altered by a massive body.

In the science of chemical toxicology there are not *experimentum crucis* [crucial experiments] capable of bringing consensus to a problem. Every experimental result in toxicology can be dissected for the gaps in reaching a definitive conclusion that the chemical is hazardous. There are always more experiments to perform to reduce the uncertainties. Commercial interests exploit the uncertainties to derail any regulations by demanding more studies.

Of course, even if there were a consensus on how a substance affects the human body, there remains the normative question, "what is acceptable risk?" These decisions are made every time a new drug is introduced for approval by the U.S. Food and Drug Administration. (FDA). When there is a consensus on the drug's efficacy against a disease, there must be a decision on whether its benefits are worth the risks of the side effects that will accrue to some patients. And even when a drug is licensed by the regulatory body, individuals can decide for themselves whether the risk of side effects are worth the benefits claimed for the drug.

Industrial and agricultural chemicals once approved expose countless people who cannot easily protect themselves or opt out of being exposed to the chemical. As an example, the law regulating industrial chemicals in the United States, first passed in 1976 as the Toxic Substances Control Act (TSCA) had a forty-year run before it was amended in 2016. Within those forty years about 85,000 chemicals were introduced into consumer products, yet only five chemicals were highly regulated or banned (Krimsky, 2017). I will leave to the final section why it has been so difficult for regulatory agencies in the United States to fully evaluate, regulate and ban toxic chemicals.

In this chapter I shall focus on the agricultural herbicide glyphosate. After a brief discussion of its path to commercial use and its special role in genetically engineered crops, I shall examine the cancer hazard assessment carried out by the International Agency for Research on Cancer (IARC) and compare that with the similar assessment by the U.S. Environmental Protection Agency (EPA). While they had access to the same published science, their conclusions were vastly different. IARC found that glyphosate is a probable human carcinogen, while the EPA concluded that it was not a human carcinogen. I will be exploring the reasons for this divergence of views on glyphosate toxicology. Did they use different criteria for determining human carcinogenicity? Did they employ different models of carcinogenesis? Did they select the relevant studies differently? Were there political and economic forces affecting the decision? I shall also discuss the efforts by one of the leading manufacturers of glyphosate, Monsanto, through its product Roundup, to influence a finding that it was safe to use as labeled. My analysis is based largely on two documents, IARC's *Monograph on the Evaluation of Carcinogenic Risks to Humans* and EPA's *Revised Glyphosate Issue Paper* both released in 2017.

DISCOVERY OF GLYPHOSATE

In 1950 a Swiss chemist, Henri Martin, while working for a small pharmaceutical company, developed a new (phosphonomethyl) derivative of an amino acid glycine. Failing to find any pharmaceutical applications, it was left in storage and in the log books. After the company (Cilag) was sold, the research samples, including the glycine derivative, was passed on to a chemical company and eventually ended up at Monsanto. As reported by Dill et al (2010):

In its Inorganic Division, Monsanto was developing compounds as potential water-softening agents and over 100 related aminomethylphosphonic acid (AMPA) analogs were synthesized. When these compounds were tested as herbicides by Dr. Phil Hamm, two showed some herbicidal activity on perennial weeds.

When water has high concentrations of calcium, iron and magnesium it is said to be hard. Calcium and magnesium have two positive charges and iron has three. Since glyphosate is a negatively charged molecule, it can bond with the other molecules and pull them out of solution. In 1961 glyphosate was patented by the Stauffer Chemical Company as a descaling (metal binders) and chelating agent and was used to clean mineral deposits in pipes and boilers of residential and commercial hot water systems.

While Monsanto scientists were investigating glyphosate's potential water-softening properties, which were too weak to be commercially useful, they learned that it was a phytotoxicant and could kill weeds. A Monsanto chemist, John Franz, made analogs of AMPA to get a more potent herbicide. He synthesized the current form of glyphosate in 1970. It was first described by Franz and colleagues in the *Proceedings of the North Central Weed Science Society* (Baird et al., 1971). Monsanto gave the compound the trade name of Roundup. Franz received U.S. patent 3,799,758 on March 26, 1974 for glyphosate, which he assigned to Monsanto. The patent states:

In accordance with the invention it has been found that the growth of germinating seeds, emerging seedlings, maturing and established woody and herbaceous vegetation and aquatic plants can be controlled by exposing the emerging seedlings or above ground portions of maturing and established vegetation, or the aquatic plants to the action of an effective amount of glycines of the present invention...These compounds are effective as post-emergent phytotoxicants or herbicides... (John, 1974)

Glyphosate's herbicidal property is based on its inhibition of the enzyme EPSPS (present in plants, fungi and bacteria), which is necessary for the plants to synthesize amino acids, without which they cannot survive. Vertebrates, including humans, do not possess the same enzyme pathway. In the next development, Monsanto found that some bacteria survived in the presence of Roundup. Recombinant DNA technology had been in development for about a decade. Monsanto scientists worked on splicing the genes that made the bacteria tolerant to Roundup in plants. When that was achieved, a new class of genetically engineered herbicide-resistant crops was introduced into agriculture under the moniker "Roundup-ready seeds."

ROUNDUP'S COMMERCIAL APPLICATIONS

Monsanto received a license for Roundup on the basis of studies that classified it as a relatively safe herbicide. The fact that the chemical pathway (shikimate) that the herbicide disrupted in plants and bacteria does not exist in humans was a point in its favor. Through the 1970s and 1980s hundreds of products containing glyphosate were marketed in the United States for use in agriculture, forestry, home lawn care, and gardens. Today, an estimated 750 farm and garden products contain glyphosate (Landrigan and Belpoggi, 2018).

In 1985 an EPA panel classified glyphosate as a Class C chemical, which stipulates that there is suggestive evidence of carcinogenic potential, based on kidney adenomas in male mice. In 1991 the EPA downgraded its classification to Class E, which means "evidence of non-carcinogenic for humans."

Through an unexpected discovery in 1989 a Monsanto plant in Louisiana that manufactured Roundup released glyphosate residues into waste ponds. Monsanto' waste cleanup division discovered that the bacteria in the ponds developed a resistance to the herbicide. The genes that made the bacteria herbicide resistant became a subject of interest to the seed developers who sought a method of introducing them into soybeans.

After a set of agreements were reached among Monsanto, Agracetus, and Asgrow (later acquired by Monsanto), the method of transferring herbicide-resistant genes into soybeans proved successful and a major distributor of soybeans agreed to take on the genetically engineered seed. In 1992, Monsanto struck a deal with the giant seed company Pioneer to commercialize GMO soybeans and corn. By 1996 the first herbicide resistant seeds entered the U.S. market.

Monsanto heralded the herbicide-resistant crop technology as a breeding mechanism that would establish a new era of sustainable agriculture introducing high quality and safe herbicides (Kishore, G.M. et al., 1992). Charles Benbrook studied the use of herbicides before and after the introduction of herbicide-resistant seeds. He found that glyphosate applications rose globally nearly 15-fold since herbicide-resistant seeds were introduced into agriculture (Benbrook, 2016). Partly as a result of its expanded use, more attention was focused on the toxicology of glyphosate. This resulted in more laboratory studies and new agency reviews.

IARC'S ASSESSMENT OF GLYPHOSATE

The International Agency for Research on Cancer (IARC), an independent research arm of the World Health Organization (WHO), issued its evaluation on whether the herbicide glyphosate was a human carcinogen in 2015. Its report concluded: Glyphosate is probably carcinogenic to humans. That finding ignited a controversy among scientists and across national boundaries.

IARC was established as a world cancer agency in 1965 through a resolution of the World Health Assembly. It began its chemical monograph program in 1971. The stated aim of the program was to develop an instrument capable of evaluating the best evidence available at a given time on carcinogenic agents, in order to provide a sound scientific basis for cancer prevention (Saracci and Wild, 2015). The agency has strict procedures for developing a monograph on the carcinogenicity of a chemical that includes its choice of panelists, observers, conflicts of interest, and the choice of scientific studies.

For the monograph on glyphosate IARC established a Working Group of 18 scientists from nine countries including France, Chile, Italy, Australia, Canada, Finland, The Netherlands, New Zealand and the United States. Five categories of participants were invited to its meeting: the Working Group; additional specialists; representatives of national and international health agencies, such as the U.S. Centers for Disease Control; observers with relevant scientific credentials; and the IARC staff. It even had an observer from Monsanto.

Each participant including the IARC staff had to disclose any relevant financial interests covering four years related to the subject matter of the meeting. The declarations of interest are evaluated by IARC officials, who decide whether changes should be made in an individual's participation. The monograph panel reviews different types of studies that can reveal evidence for human carcinogenicity including:

cohort studies, case control studies, correlation or ecological (epidemiological) studies; intervention studies, and case reports.

IARC does not conduct studies, rather it reviews studies in the scientific literature. It will only accept data from studies in the public domain and available to independent scientific review. The panel will not accept studies from industry that has not gone through peer review and have been published. Evidence of human carcinogenicity is classified into one of five categories: carcinogen; probable carcinogen; possible carcinogen; not classifiable; and probably not a carcinogen. The IARC Working Group on glyphosate met on Lyon, France on March 3-10, 2015. Its carcinogenic assessment of glyphosate, along with several other pesticides, was published in a monograph in 2017 titled *Some Organic Phosphate Insecticides and Herbicides* (IARC, 2017).

The majority of IARC's report on glyphosate is devoted to the review and summary of relevant studies selected by the Working Group. The *Monograph* consisted of detailed charts with key characteristics of each study listed including organ sites, risk estimates and exposure categories. Their reviews include studies classified as case control, cohort, occupational, food residue, human excretion, and *in vitro* with human cells.

One of the main sources of evidence for IARC was a prospective cohort study conducted in IOWA and North Carolina called the Agricultural Health Study. The National Institutes of Health administered a survey to pesticide users (insecticides and herbicides), which questioned participants about crops grown, livestock raised, pesticide application methods, and protective equipment used. This type of survey is designed to acquire human exposure data, which are then correlated positively or negatively with disease outcomes. This population study is highly valued as the only published findings on people's exposure to glyphosate correlated with cancer for different sites. The total cohort assembled in 1997 comprised 75,000 adult study subjects. IARC cites seven reports from the Agricultural Health Study and several case control reports as central to its evaluation of the human carcinogenic potential of glyphosate.

At the beginning of its *Monograph,* IARC states that it uses the term "carcinogenic risk" to mean that an agent is capable of causing cancer and that the evaluation of such risks are made by international working groups of independent scientists and are qualitative in nature. While the Working Group found no correlation between exposure to glyphosate and prostate, breast, colorectal, skin, and pancreatic cancers, it did find an association between glyphosate and non-Hodgkin's lymphoma (NHL). The IARC monograph stated: Two large case-control studies of NHL [non-Hodgkin's lymphoma] from Canada and he USA, and two case-control studies from Sweden reported statistically significant increased risks of NHL in association with exposure to glyphosate (IARC, 2017). Even when adjusted for exposure to other pesticides, the risk of NHL persisted.

IARC referenced 269 scientific studies for its glyphosate monograph. It included both positive and negative findings in its assessment. The working group found limited evidence in humans for the carcinogenicity of glyphosate, and found sufficient evidence in animal studies to declare glyphosate a carcinogen. Based largely on the animal data and with limited human data, IARC reported that the weight of evidence convinced the Working Group that glyphosate was a probable human carcinogen.

"Weight of evidence" is generally not quantifiable. There are no scales to "weigh" the evidence. The "weighing of evidence" is a committee process that depends on the collective experience of panel members when they review the body of toxicology studies, the types and quality of studies, and the plausibility of cancer outcomes. Thus, the "weight of evidence" is the outcome of a consensus of panel members based on their collective experience. That is why it is critically important for panel members to be unbiased and non-conflicted by financial interests. Some panels may have a preference for human data and will not classify a chemical as a carcinogen unless the human epidemiological data, on its own, is convincing. Other toxicologists will use whatever human data is available and combine it with animal data.

There was no indication from its report that IARC departed from standard criteria or models of carcinogenicity or genotoxicity as it based its assessment on peer-reviewed and established toxicological assessments. Also, the *Monograph* provided no algorithm for "weighing the evidence" or for the integration of the diverse studies into a conclusion.

EPA'S ASSESSMENT OF GLYPHOSATE

The EPA has been engaged in the assessment of glyphosate at least as early as 1985, when it classified the chemical as a possible human carcinogen. In 1986 the EPA asked its FIFRA [Federal Insecticide, Fungicide, Rodenticide Act] Scientific Advisory Panel (SAP) to evaluate the carcinogenic potential of glyphosate. With the available evidence at the time the SAP listed glyphosate as a Group D chemical, which signifies that it is not classifiable as to its carcinogenicity. It recommended that the EPA undertake new studies. In 1991, when new rodent studies of glyphosate became available, the EPA's Carcinogenicity Peer Review Committee classified glyphosate as a Group E chemical (evidence of non-carcinogenicity in humans), thereby downgrading its risk. And in 2015, the EPA's Cancer Assessment Review Committee found that glyphosate is not likely to be carcinogenic to humans.

The EPA's Office of Pesticide Programs issued its revised assessment of glyphosate on December 12, 2017 in a 216-page document. After an introduction that discusses their systematic review of the literature, data collection and studies submitted to the agency, the report proceeds with an examination of the existing science on glyphosate and cancer sites. Since IARC only identified NHL as the only cancer site associated with glyphosate exposure, I shall focus on EPA's review of glyphosate and NHL and seek to understand why IARC and EPA differed on that association.

The EPA's lengthy study provided greater detail than that of IARC on how it evaluated individual studies, how it generated a literature review, and on the rating of studies as low, moderate or high quality. Like IARC, the EPA provided summary tables of individual studies. There are a few general comments that can be made about EPA's review of the science linking glyphosate and NHL. EPA considered the sample sizes used by IARC as too small. They also questioned the meta-analyses that combined data from different studies.

The EPA review committee looked at nine studies related to NHL published between 1990 and 2013, some that pooled data from other studies, a multi-center population-based study, a hospital-based case control study using questionnaire data, and meta-analyses. Some of EPA's evaluation of the quality of the data are as follows:

Many of the evaluated studies were limited by small sample sizes, which resulted in large confidence intervals and reduced the reliability of the results to demonstrate a true association (EPA, 2017).

Analyses were performed with 6 studies, which many would consider small for performing meta-analyses. Rarely will meta-analyses synthesize data from studies with identical study designs and methods (EPA, 2017).

The EPA report also was dubious about confounding factors in the studies that IARC used in its analysis. The report stated that: lack of adjustment for co-exposure to other pesticides in these analyses could partially explain the conflicting results between the cohort and the case-control studies (EPA, 2017). This is just a speculation. It is not at all generally expected that different study methods will yield identical results. You have to look at the trend lines. They also noted that the meta-analyses that were statistically significant were borderline. They argued that each study carries over "confounding issues inherent in each individual study" into the meta-analysis. Unless each study used in the meta-analysis are identical in method with no confounding factors, it will be subject to the criticism. However, rarely will meta-analyses claim there is such parity between studies, yet their results are widely accepted. Also cited was that publication bias may have played a role because positive results (adverse findings) are more likely to be published than results that show no effect.

The EPA review makes no reference to bias from studies by the pesticide and chemical industries. Those effects are well documented in the literature. The EPA also criticized the exposure data from individuals surveyed. It argued that investigators used proxy respondents for exposure assessment in the major agricultural study, which has the potential to increase recall bias.

The EPA report found deficiencies in each of the nine studies. For example, it stated: none of the studies in this evaluation of glyphosate exposure and risk of NHL accounted for other potential confounders, such as diesel exhaust fumes, solvents, animals, and UV radiation (EPA, 2017). The entire analysis can be likened to a "Devil's Advocate" position against claims of glyphosate associated with NHL. The EPA report concludes the section on NHL with the statement:

Based on the weight-of-evidence, the agency cannot exclude chance and/or bias as an explanation for observed associations in the database. Due to study limitation and contradictory result across studies of at least equal quality, a conclusion regarding the association between glyphosate exposure and risk of NHL cannot be determined based on the available data (EPA, 2017).

EXTERNAL INFLUENCES OF TOXICOLOGICAL SCIENCES

Whenever scientific groups exhibit substantial disagreement on the toxicological assessment of a chemical it is important to consider non-scientific factors that may have influence on the assessments. In the case of glyphosate, a chemical in commerce since the 1970s, which has been extremely lucrative to herbicide manufacturers, there has been a strong corporate lobbying effort to protect its regulatory approval in the United States and elsewhere throughout the world.

After IARC reported its finding that glyphosate was a probable human carcinogen, hundreds of lawsuits were filed in the United States against Monsanto on behalf of individuals who had contracted Non-Hodgkin's lymphoma, alleging glyphosate as the cause. Several hundred cases were consolidated by one judge in the U.S. District Court in San Francisco, California. Many other lawsuits are making their way through state courts. As part of the legal process, plaintiffs may request internal documents from Monsanto, called discovery documents. A substantial trove of these discovery documents has been placed on a publicly accessible database. Two French journalists, Stéphane Foucart and Stéphane Horel

Table 1. Comparison of EPA and IARC Assessment of Glyphosate

	EPA Report	IARC Monograph
Year Published	2017	2017
International Panel	No	Yes
Review of existing studies only	Yes	Yes
Number of specific articles referenced	114	269
Unpublished studies cited	Yes (30)	No (0)
Use of "weight of evidence"	Yes	Yes
Characterization of "weight of evidence"	Yes	No
Categorize quality of studies	Yes	No
Finding	Non-carcinogenic in humans	Probable human carcinogen

received the Varenne Award for their series published in *Le Monde* (Foucart and Horel, 2017). The Monsanto litigation documents were posted on an open access public website titled US Right to Know (US Right to Know, n.d.) One book has already been published citing the documents (Gillam, 2017).

The documents reveal an intense lobbying effort on the part of Monsanto that includes ghostwriting articles for scientific journals allegedly showing that glyphosate is safe for humans, undue influence on EPA regulators (Gillam, 2017a) and efforts to gain journal retractions on papers that are unfavorable to glyphosate health risks. The company hired contract researchers to write journal articles favorable to glyphosate that did not include Monsanto's funding source or its input. What we have found from these documents is that the regulatory process in the United States has been replete with corporate lobbying at the regulatory agencies, at journals, and at the Executive Branch of government to penalize the World Health Organization by withholding funds because of the IARC finding.

There have been studies published about ghostwriting in medical journals largely associated with pharmaceutical companies (McHenry, 2010; Sismondo, 2007). Also, much has been written about the efforts of the tobacco and lead industries to influence science. Lawsuits against pesticide manufacturers have generally not unshielded internal documents, which are placed under protective order, putatively to protect trade secrets. The glyphosate case is the exception. When the Roundup litigation documents were released to the public, we begin to see scholarly articles analyzing them for what they reveal about corporate influence on science. (McHenry, 2018; Krimsky and Gillam, 2018).

Among the things we learn from the internal documents from Monsanto is that the company ghost-wrote journal articles as a standard business practice. In addition, they cultivated relationships with journal editors by engaging them as consultants and expecting favors at the appropriate time. Monsanto also provided lecture notes for scientists who presented talks at scientific meetings. Their strategy was to seed the scientific and regulatory communities with a constructed consensus on the safety of glyphosate and in particular its product Roundup.

IMPEDIMENTS TO CONSENSUS OVER CHEMICAL RISK

As a field, toxicology's primary focus is to study the effects of chemicals on humans and other living things. There is no single test or methodology for obtaining such knowledge. Human population studies, when possible, provide the most direct evidence. Clinical trials, which are rarely acceptable for industrial chemicals, are used for pharmaceuticals that are designed for therapeutic purposes. The gold standard methodology for drug safety and efficacy is the randomized controlled trial with human subjects. In animal studies, randomization is not necessary because the animals are bred to be genetically similar. While animal studies offer great control for exposure and confounding variables, the results are often discounted by some stakeholders, courts and regulators because of the physiological differences between humans and animals.

EPA's "Revised Glyphosate Issue Paper" stated that there was insufficient evidence to establish glyphosate as a human carcinogen. In the EPA's glyphosate file, it refers to a general fact sheet that was produced by Oregon State University (Oregon State University, n.d.). The fact sheet stated: The U.S. EPA classified glyphosate as Group E, evidence of non-carcinogenicity in humans. The U.S. EPA does not consider glyphosate to be a human carcinogen based on studies of laboratory animals that did not produce compelling evidence of carcinogenicity. It then added: Researchers reviewed the scientific literature on glyphosate, its major metabolite AMPA, formulated Roundup products manufactured by Monsanto, and the surfactant POEA. They found that Roundup and its components did not cause mutations or tumor formation. The researchers concluded that glyphosate is not carcinogenic. The reference given for this claim is: Williams, Kroes and Munro. Safety evaluation and risk assessment of the herbicide Roundup and its active ingredient, glyphosate, for humans. This paper is now known from the Monsanto litigation internal documents as a ghostwritten paper. Yet, it was never retracted by the journal. After the publisher reviewed the allegations against so-called ghost-written or Monsanto-influenced papers, the journal published an "expression of concern" that proper disclosures were not made in the published articles.

Another edition of the fact sheet referred to in the EPA Internet site stated:

Is glyphosate likely to contribute to the development of cancer? When high doses were administered to laboratory animals, some studies suggest that glyphosate has carcinogenic potential. Studies on cancer rates in people have provided conflicting results on whether the use of glyphosate containing products is associated with cancer. Some studies have associated glyphosate use with non-Hodgkin lymphoma (http://npic.orst.edu/factsheets/glyphogen.html)

EPA's updated review of glyphosate is largely focused on showing every conceivable limitation of each study that has shown any positive association of glyphosate with NHL. The agency criticized the exposure data of the human studies, small sizes of animal studies, incommensurability of metadata, and the possible confounding effects from exposure to other pesticides. Animal experiments or human epidemiological studies involving low-dose exposures are vulnerable to all types of limitations, which are exploited by pesticide manufacturers who ask for consistent, replicable, dose-dependent and definitive results (Krimsky, 2014; Lanphear, 2017). There is no indication from the EPA analysis of what evidence it would accept to demonstrate that glyphosate exposure is associated with NHL. What we do know, is what evidence they would not accept.

The scientific assessment of the data on glyphosate, is not straight forward and requires lots of presuppositions such as "we assume glyphosate is safe unless proven unsafe" or "we assume glyphosate is unsafe unless proven safe." The assumption we begin with determines the relevant evidence.

Beyond the science, there are also the impediments from the politics. The appointment by President Donald Trump of Scott Pruitt to head the U.S. EPA has set a new goal for the agency. As reported by the *Guardian* in 2018, Pruitt promised polluters EPA will value their profits over American lives (Nuccitelli, 2018). Agency scientists would be given a signal that any chemical must be reviewed with the goal of demonstrating that the scientific evidence is not sufficient to declare the chemical unsafe. The agency can always appeal to the "weight of evidence." Most uses of "weight of evidence" (WOE) are subjective and do not reveal a methodology. One commentator notes:

...the frequent lack of definition of the term "weight of evidence," multiple uses of the term and a lack of consensus about its meaning, and the many different kinds of weights, both qualitative and quantitative, which can be used in RA [risk assessment]. A practical recommendation emerges: the WOE concept and its associated methods should be fully described when used. A research agenda should examine the advantages of quantitative versus qualitative weighting schemes, how best to improve existing methods, and how best to combine those methods (e.g., epidemiology's causal criteria with toxicology's quality criteria (Weed, 2005).

In an unusual consensus statement signed by fourteen scientists provides a list of uncertainties in the current state of knowledge on the toxicology of glyphosate (Myers et al., 2016). Concerns over use of glyphosate-based herbicides and risks associated with exposures: a consensus statement. These scientists were not emphasizing these uncertainties to dismiss the potential health effects. They understand that the uncertainties they raise are exploited by the commercial glyphosate interests, who argue against imposing any but the most minimal regulations on the herbicide. The consensus statement concludes that glyphosate should be given a high priority for full assessment.

Among the uncertainties cited in the consensus statement are:

- Because glyphosate is used in conjunction with other agricultural chemicals including insecticides, herbicides and fungicides, it is difficult to distinguish its effects from the effects of other substances in human studies. Since chemicals are not studies in mixtures, the synergistic effects of glyphosate with other chemicals is unknown.
- Adjuvants in glyphosate formulations are not tested independently. Either acting alone or in conjunction with other chemicals, the adjuvants might have unanticipated and untested effects.
- The vast majority of glyphosate toxicology studies used in regulatory assessments do not cover a sufficiently wide range of dose levels; some exclude low but environmentally relevant doses.
- Biomonitoring of glyphosate and its metabolites in the blood and urine of people have not been conducted. Without this information, you cannot estimate exposure risk.
- There is limited data on glyphosate pharmacokinetics in vertebrates, such as how it behaves in the organs, tissues and fluids and whether and where bioaccumulation occurs.

The EPA's classification of human carcinogens stated in its 2005 *Guidelines for Carcinogen Risk Assessment*, lists five categories: 1) carcinogenic to humans; 2) likely to be carcinogenic to humans; 3) suggestive evidence of carcinogenic potential; 4) inadequate information to assess carcinogenic potential; 5) not likely to be carcinogenic to humans. These categories closely match IARC's five categories, where its second category is a "probable human carcinogen."

The EPA report states that choosing one of the five categories is a matter of judgment and cannot be reduced to a formula, since each category is applicable to "a wide variety of potential data sets and weights of evidence." The report spends considerably more time on "weight of evidence" than is found in the IARC *Monograph.* The agency report concludes that, based on all the available data, the "weight of evidence" does not support the conclusion that glyphosate is either "carcinogenic to humans" or "likely to be carcinogenic to humans." Referring to its 2005 *Cancer Guidelines*, the criteria for a chemical to be "carcinogenic to humans" only when there is convincing epidemiological evidence of a causal association between human exposure to the chemical and cancer. And for the second category, "likely to be carcinogenic to humans," the weight of evidence must be adequate to reach carcinogenic potential to humans.

One can use this information in two ways. Because of the uncertainties, there is no definitive evidence of glyphosate cancer risk and therefore let the product remain in commerce as it has been. Or, as the consensus scientists state: a fresh and independent examination of GBH [glyphopsate-based herbicides] should be undertaken... accompanied by systematic efforts by relevant agencies to monitor GBH levels in people and in the food supply, none of which is occurring today (Myers et al., 2016).

As in the IARC study, the EPA analysis did not apply non-traditional models of carcinogenesis. They did select and emphasized different studies and it is likely, although not definitive, they used different criteria for human carcinogenicity than that of IARC, whose criteria was not as transparent as that of the EPA.

What we learn from this exercise is that glyphosate's commercial stakeholders accept the phrase "no evidence of risk" means allow the herbicide to remain on the market. In contrast, others may say "no evidence of risk" is not tantamount to "evidence of no risk." The standoff is between those individuals who believe a substance is safe unless you have conclusive evidence it is not safe and those who consider a substance unsafe until it can be proven safe. Unlike U.S. environmental law, the European Union has adopted the "Precautionary Principle" whereby a nation can (and perhaps should) take action if there is a chemical risk that remains inconclusive.

CONCLUSION

The current scientific controversy over glyphosate toxicology cannot be de-contextualized from the political circumstances in which it is embedded. Those groups and scientists that have a professional or financial interest in the continued use of glyphosate select the science that supports that conclusion and dismiss or discount the studies that do not. For example, a study that shows glyphosate is a chelating agent that can affect the micronutrients of plants and ultimately of humans has been ignored by regulators (Mertens et al., 2018). Another study found that glyphosate exposure in pregnancy shortened gestational length (Parvez et al., 2018). And when a non-peer reviewed report indicates that glyphosate was found to bioaccumulate in mother's breast milk, a peer-reviewed counter report by a pro-glyphosate consultant disputes the results (Bus, 2015). Of course, these studies do not demonstrate that glyphosate causes human cancer. IARC relied on animal studies that did find cancer and human studies that raised important suspicions that glyphosate could be the cause of non-Hodgkin's lymphoma. But the accumulation of studies, including one in rodents that shows glyphosate can impact the microbiome of vertebrates (Mao et al., 2018), or the teratogenic effects of glyphosate on frog embryos (Bonfanti et al., 2018) begin to build a case against the chemical.

This analysis shows that human toxicology, in the best of circumstances, has its own problematic features. When we add the uncertainties of low doses, difficulty of finding long-term effects, singling out one substance from cluster exposures to the financial interests that have become embedded in the practice of science, the results are understandably divergent across communities. Even the best and politically unencumbered toxicology will endure uncertainties. The question is whether the uncertainties should justify keeping a chemical in commerce, or prevent the chemical from entering commerce in the first place. After forty-four years in use, public health officials are asking for independent toxicological studies on the health effects of glyphosate-based herbicides. This fact alone underscores the failure of the "approve first, test later" principle of regulation. The toxicological debates are best resolved before a chemical has become part of the human diet, which is emblematic of the European Precautionary Principle.

REFERENCES

Baird, D. D., Upchurch, R. P., Homesley, W. B., & Franz, J. E. (1971). Introduction of a new broad-spectrum post emergence herbicide class with utility for herbaceous perennial weed control. *Proceedings of the North Central Weed Science Society, 26*, 64–68.

Benbrook, C.M. (2016). Impact of genetically engineered crops on pesticide use in U.S.—the first sixteen years. *Environmental Sciences Europe, 24*, 1-13.

Bonfanti, P., Saibene, M., Bacchetta, R., Mantecca, P., & Colombo, A. (2018). A glyphosate micro-emulsion formulation displays teratogenicity in *Xenopus leavis. Aquatic Toxicology (Amsterdam, Netherlands), 195*, 103–113. doi:10.1016/j.aquatox.2017.12.007 PMID:29306033

Bus, J. S. (2015). Analysis of Moms Across America report suggesting bioaccumulation of glyphosate in U.S. mother's breast milk: Implausibility based on inconsistency with available body of animal toxicokinetic human biomonitoring, and physico-chemical data. *Regulatory Toxicology and Pharmacology, 73*(3), 758–764. doi:10.1016/j.yrtph.2015.10.022 PMID:26520181

Dill, G. M., Sammons, R. D., Feng, P. C., Kohn, F., Kretzmer, K., Mehrsheikh, A., ... Haupfear, E. A. (2010). Glyphosate: discovery, development, applications, and properties. Glyphosate resistance in crops and weeds: history, development, and management, 1-33.

Environmental Protection Agency (EPA). (2017, December 12). *Office of Pesticide Programs, Revised Glyphosate Issue Paper: Evaluation of Carcinogenic Potential*. Author.

Foucart, S. & Horel, S. (2017). Monsanto papers: Les agencies sous l'influence de la firm. *La Monde*.

Gillam, C. (2017). *Whitewash*. Washington, DC: Island Press. doi:10.5822/978-1-61091-833-6

Gillam, C. (2017a, August 18). Collusion or coincidence? records show EPA efforts to slow herbicide review came in coordination with Monsanto. *Huffington Post*. Retrieved from https://www.huffingtonpost.com/entry/collusion-or-coincidence-records-show-epa-efforts_us_5994dad4e4b056a2b0ef02f1

US Right to Know. (n.d.). *The Monsanto Papers. (Glyphosate) Cancer Case Key Documents & Analysis*. Retrieved from https://usrtk.org/pesticides/mdl-monsanto-glyphosate-cancer-case-key-documents-analysis/

International Agency for Research on Cancer (IARC), IARC Working Group on the Evaluation of Carcinogenic Risks to Humans. (2017). *Some Organic Insecticides and Herbicides. IARC Monograph on the Evaluation of Carcinogenic Risks to Humans* (Vol. 112). Lyon, France: Monograph.

John, F. (1974). *U.S. Patent No. 3,799,758*. Washington, DC: U.S. Patent and Trademark Office.

Kishore, G. M., Padgette, S. R., & Fraley, R. T. (1992). History of herbicide-tolerant crops, methods of development and current state of the art—emphasis on glyphosate tolerance. Weed Technology, 6, 626-634.

Krimsky, S. (2014). Low-dose toxicology: Narratives from the science-transcience interface. In N. York (Ed.), *Powerless Science? Science and Politics in a Toxic World*. Berghahn.

Krimsky, S. (2017). The Unsteady State and Inertia of Chemical Regulation Under the US Toxic Substances Control Act. *PLoS Biology*, *15*(12), e2002404. doi:10.1371/journal.pbio.2002404 PMID:29252997

Krimsky, S., & Gillam, C. (2018). Roundup litigation discovery documents: Implications for public health and journal ethics. *Journal of Public Health Policy*, *39*(14). doi:10.105741271-018-0134-z PMID:29884897

Landrigan, P. J., & Belpoggi, F. (2018). The need for research on the health effects of glyphosate-based herbicides. *Environmental Health*, *17*(1), 51. doi:10.118612940-018-0392-z PMID:29843729

Lanphear, B. (2017). Low-level toxicity of chemicals: No acceptable levels? *PLOS Biology*, *15*(12).

Mao, Q., Manservisi, F., Panzacchi, S., Mandrioli, D., Menghetti, I., Vornoli, A., ... Hu, J. (2018). The Ramazzini Institute 13-week pilot study on glyphosate and roundup administered at human-equivalent dose to Sprague Dawley rats: Effects on the microbiome. *Environmental Health*, *17*(1), 50. doi:10.118612940-018-0394-x PMID:29843725

McHenry, L. (2010). Of sophists and spin-doctors: Industry sponsored ghostwriting and the crisis of academic medicine. *Mens Sana Monographs*, *8*(1), 129–145. doi:10.4103/0973-1229.58824 PMID:21327175

McHenry, L. (2018). The Monsanto papers: Poisoning the scientific well. *International Journal of Risk & Safety in Medicine*, *29*(3-4), 193–205. doi:10.3233/JRS-180028 PMID:29843257

Mertens, M., Höss, S., Neumann, G., Afzal, J., and Reichenbecher, W. (2018). Glyphosate, a chelating agent—relevant for ecological risk assessment. *Environmental Science and Pollution Research*. doi:10.100711356-017-1080-1

Myers, J. P., Antoniou, M. N., Blumberg, B., Carroll, L., Colborn, T., Everett, L. G., ... Benbrook, C. M. (2016). Concerns over use of glyphosate-based herbicides and risks associated with exposures: A consensus statement. *Environmental Health*, *15*(1), 19–31. doi:10.118612940-016-0117-0 PMID:26883814

Nuccitelli, D. (2018, April 23). Pruitt promised polluters EPA will value their profits over American lives; Pruitt is one of TIME's 100 most influential people for his efforts to maximize polluters' profits. *The Guardian*.

Oregon State University Fact Sheet on Glyphosate. (n.d.). Retrieved from http://npic.orst.edu/factsheets/archive/glyphotech.html

Parvez, S., Gerona, R. R., Proctor, C., Friesen, M., Ashby, J. L., Reiter, J. L., ... Winchester, P. D. (2018). Glyphosate exposure in pregnancy and shortened gestational length: A prospective Indiana birth cohort study. *Environmental Health, 17*(1), 23. doi:10.118612940-018-0367-0 PMID:29519238

Saracci, R., & Wild, C. P. (2015). *International Agency for Research on Cancer: The First 50 Years: 1965-2015*. Lyon, France: World Health Organization.

Sismondo, S. (2007). Ghost management. How much of the medical literature is shaped behind the scenes by the pharmaceutical industry? *PLoS Med* 4(9): e286.S.

Weed, D. L. (2005). Weight of Evidence: A review concept and methods. *Risk Analysis, 25*(6), 1545–1557. doi:10.1111/j.1539-6924.2005.00699.x PMID:16506981

Compilation of References

Abbott, N. J. (2000). Inflammatory mediators and modulation of blood-brain barrier permeability. *Cellular and Molecular Neurobiology*, *20*(2), 131–147. doi:10.1023/A:1007074420772 PMID:10696506

Abdul, K. S., Jayasinghe, S. S., Chandana, E. P., Jayasumana, C., & De Silva, P. M. (2015). Arsenic and human health effects: *A review. Environmental Toxicology and Pharmacology*, *40*(3), 828–846. doi:10.1016/j.etap.2015.09.016 PMID:26476885

Abernathy, C. O., Liu, Y. P., Longfellow, D., Aposhian, H. V., Beck, B., Fowler, B., ... Waalkes, M. (1999). Arsenic: Health effects, mechanisms of actions, and research issues. *Environmental Health Perspectives*, *107*(7), 593–597. doi:10.1289/ehp.99107593 PMID:10379007

Abernathy, C. O., Thomas, D. J., & Calderon, R. L. (2003). Health Effects and Risk Assessment of Arsenic. *The Journal of Nutrition*, *133*(5), 1536S–1538S. doi:10.1093/jn/133.5.1536S PMID:12730460

Abhinav, S., Navin, S., Verma, S. K., Kumar, R., Ali, M., Kumar, A., & Ghosh, A. K. (2016): Groundwater and blood samples assessment for arsenic toxicity in rural population of Darbhanga district of Bihar, India. In *Proceedings of the 6th International congress on arsenic in the environment*, Stockholm, Sweden, June 19-23 (pp. 418-420). London, UK: Taylor & Francis group.

Abrahams, B. S., & Geschwind, D. H. (2008). Advances in autism genetics: On the threshold of a new neurobiology. *Nature Reviews. Genetics*, *9*(5), 341–355. doi:10.1038/nrg2346 PMID:18414403

Acharyya, S. K., Chackraborty, P., Lahiri, S., Raymahashay, B. C., Guha, S., & Bhowmik, A. (1999). Arsenic poisoning in the Ganges delta. *Nature*, *401*(6753), 545. doi:10.1038/44052 PMID:10524619

Acharyya, S. K., Lahiri, S., Raymahashay, B. C., & Bhowmik, A. (2000). Arsenic toxicity of groundwater in parts of the Bengal basin in India and Bangladesh, the role of quaternary stratigraphy and Holocene sea-level fluctuation. *Environ. Geol.*, *39*(10), 1127–1137. doi:10.1007002540000107

Achenbach, T. M., & Rescorla, L. A. (2001). *Manual for the ASEBA school-age forms & profiles: an integrated system of mult-informant assessment*. Burlington: University of Vermont, Research Center for Children, Youth & Families.

Acid, S. A. (2004). Lehninger principles of biochemistry.

Action, P. (2007). *The Deadly Chemicals in Cotton. Environmental Justice Foundation in collaboration with Pesticide Action*. London, UK: Development House.

Adler, N. E., & Newman, K. (Ed.). (2002). Socioeconomic Disparities In Health: Pathways And Policies.

Adonis, M., Martínez, V., Marín, P., Berrios, D., & Gil, L. (2005). Smoking habit and genetic factors associated with lung cancer in a population highly exposed to arsenic. *Toxicology Letters*, *159*(1), 32–37. doi:10.1016/j.toxlet.2005.04.007 PMID:16099114

Adonis, M., Martínez, V., Marín, P., & Gil, L. (2005). CYP1A1 and GSTM1 genetic polymorphisms in lung cancer populations exposed to arsenic in drinking water. *Xenobiotica*, *35*(5), 519–530. doi:10.1080/00498250500057310 PMID:16012082

AfricaFocus Bulletin. (2009, January 22). Africa: Agricultural knowledge.

AfricaFocus Bulletin. (2012). Africa: The hidden issue of "gene grabbing."

AfricaFocus Bulletin. (2013). Africa: Monopolizing maize.

Agency for Cancer Research (IARC). (2004). Some drinking-water disinfectants and contaminants including arsenic. IARC.

Agency for Toxic Substances and Disease Registry (ATSDR). (2007). *Arsenic Toxicity*. Washington, DC, USA: U.S. Department of Health and Human Services.

Aguzzi, A., Barres, B. A., & Bennett, M. L. (2013). Microglia: Scapegoat, saboteur, or something else? *Science*, *339*(6116), 156–161. doi:10.1126cience.1227901 PMID:23307732

Ahamed, S., Kumar, S. M., Mukherjee, A., Amir, H. M., Das, B., Nayak, B., ... Chakraborti, D. (2006). Arsenic groundwater contamination and its health effects In the state of Uttar Pradesh (UP) in upper and middle Ganga plain, India: A severe danger. *The Science of the Total Environment*, *370*(2-3), 31022. doi:10.1016/j.scitotenv.2006.06.015 PMID:16899281

Ahmadi-Jouibari, T., & Fattahi, N. (2015). Speciation of inorganic arsenic species and total inorganic arsenic in rice using microwave-assisted dispersive liquid–liquid micro-extraction and electrothermal atomic absorption spectrometry. *Food Additives & Contaminants: Part A*, *32*(7), 1140–1147. doi:10.1080/19440049.2015.1049565 PMID:25959514

Ahmad, S. A., Sayed, M. H., Barua, S., Khan, M. H., Faruquee, M. H., Jalil, A., ... Talukder, H. K. (2001). Arsenic in drinking water and pregnancy outcomes. *Environmental Health Perspectives*, *109*(6), 629–631. doi:10.1289/ehp.01109629 PMID:11445518

Ahmed, F. E. (2002). Detection of Genetically Modified Organisms in Foods. *Trends in Biotechnology*, *20*(5), 215–223. doi:10.1016/S0167-7799(01)01920-5 PMID:11943377

Ahsan, H., Chen, Y., Parvez, F., Argos, M., Hussain, A. I., Momotaj, H., ... Graziano, J. (2006). Health effects of arsenic longitudinal study (heals): Description of a multidisciplinary epidemiologic investigation. *Journal of Exposure Science & Environmental Epidemiology*, *16*(2), 191–205. doi:10.1038j.jea.7500449 PMID:16160703

Ainsworth, E., & McGrath, J. (2010). Direct effects of rising atmospheric carbon dioxide and ozone on crop yields. In D. Lobell & M. Burke (Eds.), *Climate change and food security: Adapting agriculture to a warmer world* (pp. 109–130). New York, NY: Springer.

Alassane-Kpembi, I., Kolf-Clauw, M., Gauthier, T., Abrami, R., Abiola, F. A., Oswald, I. P., & Puel, O. (2013). New insights into mycotoxin mixtures: The toxicity of low doses of Type B trichothecenes on intestinal epithelial cells is synergistic. *Toxicology and Applied Pharmacology*, *272*(1), 191–198. doi:10.1016/j.taap.2013.05.023 PMID:23735874

Alavanja, M. C., Dosemeci, M., Samanic, C., Lubin, J., Lynch, C. F., Knott, C., ... Blair, A. (2004). Pesticides and lung cancer risk in the agricultural health study cohort. *American Journal of Epidemiology*, *160*(9), 876–885. doi:10.1093/aje/kwh290 PMID:15496540

Alavanja, M. C., Samanic, C., Dosemeci, M., Lubin, J., Tarone, R., Lynch, C. F., ... Blair, A. (2003). Use of agricultural pesticides and prostate cancer risk in the Agricultural Health Study cohort. *American Journal of Epidemiology*, *157*(9), 800–814. doi:10.1093/aje/kwg040 PMID:12727674

AlexandratosN.BruinsmaJ. (2012). World agriculture towards 2030/2050: the 2012 revision. Food and Agriculture Organization. Rome, Italy: Retrieved from http://www.fao.org/fileadmin/templates/esa/Global_persepctives/world_ag_2030_50_2012_rev.pdf

Ali, T., Ismail, M., Asad, F., Ashraf, A., Waheed, U., & Khan, Q. M. (2018). Pesticide genotoxicity in cotton picking women in Pakistan evaluated using comet assay. *Drug and Chemical Toxicology*, *41*(2), 213–220. doi:10.1080/01480545.2017.1343342 PMID:28721745

Alonso, A., Marsal, S., & Julia, A. (2015). Analytical methods in untargeted metabolomics: State of the art in 2015. *Frontiers in Bioengineering and Biotechnology*, *3*, 23. doi:10.3389/fbioe.2015.00023 PMID:25798438

Altieri, M. A., Rosset, P., & Thrupp, L. A. (1998). *The potential of agroecology to combat hunger in the developing world. A 2020 Vision for Food, Agriculture, and the Environment, 2020 Brief 55*. Washington, DC: International Food Policy Research Institute.

Alysandratos, K. D., Asadi, S., Angelidou, A., Zhang, B., Sismanopoulos, N., Yang, H., ... Theoharides, T. C. (2012). Neurotensin and CRH interactions augment human mast cell activation. *PLoS One*, *7*(11), e48934. doi:10.1371/journal.pone.0048934 PMID:23155429

Amaral, D. G., Bauman, M. D., & Schumann, C. M. (2003). The amygdala and autism: Implications from non-human primate studies. *Genes Brain & Behavior*, *2*(5), 295–302. doi:10.1034/j.1601-183X.2003.00043.x PMID:14606694

American Academy of Pediatrics. Committee on Environmental Health. (1998). Toxic effects of indoor molds. *Pediatrics, 101,* 712-714.

American Psychiatric Association. (2000). *Diagnostic and statistical manual of mental disorders*. Washington: American Psychiatric Association.

American Psychiatric Association. (2013). DSM-5 Autism Spectrum Disorder Fact Sheet. Retrieved from https://www.psychiatry.org/.../DSM/APA_DSM-5-Autism-Spectrum-Disorder.pdf

Ames, B. N., Durston, W. E., Yamasaki, E., & Lee, F. D. (1973). Carcinogens are mutagens: A simple test system combining liver homogenates for activation and bacteria for detection. *Proceedings of the National Academy of Sciences of the United States of America*, *70*(8), 2281–2285. doi:10.1073/pnas.70.8.2281 PMID:4151811

Ames, B. N., & Gold, L. S. (1998). The causes and prevention of cancer: The role of environment. *Biotherapy (Dordrecht, Netherlands)*, *11*(2-3), 205–220. doi:10.1023/A:1007971204469 PMID:9677052

Anderson, K., & Kuhn, K. (2017). *What the Health*. United States: A.U.M Films & Media.

Anderson, J. L., Bowden, E. F., & Pickup, P. G. (1996). Dynamic electrochemistry: Methodology and application. *Analytical Chemistry*, *68*(12), R379–R444. doi:10.1021/a1960015y PMID:11008788

Anderson, J. W., Johnstone, B. M., & Remley, D. T. (1999). Breast-feeding and cognitive development: A meta-analysis. *The American Journal of Clinical Nutrition*, *70*(4), 525–535. doi:10.1093/ajcn/70.4.525 PMID:10500022

Andersson, M. A., Nikulin, M., Koljalg, U., Andersson, M. C., Rainey, F., Reijula, K., & … . (1997). Bacteria, molds, and toxins in water-damaged building materials. *Applied and Environmental Microbiology*, *63*, 387–393. PMID:9023919

Andra, S. S., Charisiadis, P., Karakitsios, S., Sarigiannis, D. A., & Makris, K. C. (2015). Passive exposures of children to volatile trihalomethanes during domestic cleaning activities of their parents. *Environmental Research, 136*, 187–195. doi:10.1016/j.envres.2014.10.018 PMID:25460636

Andreji, J., Stránai, I., Massanyi, P. & Valent, M. (2005). Concentration of selected metals in muscle of various fish species. *Journal of environmental science and health, 40*, 899-912.

Andres, A., Cleves, M. A., Bellando, J. B., Pivik, R., Casey, P. H., & Badger, T. M. (2012). Developmental status of 1-year-old infants fed breast milk, cow's milk formula, or soy formula. *Pediatrics, 129*(6), 1134–1140. doi:10.1542/peds.2011-3121 PMID:22641754

Andrianou, X., & Makris, K. (2018). The framework pf urban exposome: Application of exposome concept in urban health studies. *The Science of the Total Environment, 636*, 963–967. doi:10.1016/j.scitotenv.2018.04.329 PMID:29729514

Angelova, R. A. (2018), Organic Cotton: Technological and Environmental Aspects. In *Proc. of XXIII Int. Scientific Conference FPEPM*, September 17 – 20 (pp. 351-356).

Ankley, G. T., Bennett, R. S., Erickson, R. J., Hoff, D. J., Hornung, M. W., Johnson, R. D., ... Villeneuve, D. L. (2010). Adverse outcome pathways: A conceptual framework to support ecotoxicology research and risk assessment. *Environmental Toxicology and Chemistry, 29*(3), 730–741. doi:10.1002/etc.34 PMID:20821501

Annett, M. (2002). *Handedness and brain asymmetry: the right shift theory. East Sussex BN3 2FA*. Psychology Press.

Antoshak, R. (2013). Sustainable Cotton, the e3 Program, and the Better Cotton Initiative. Retrieved from http://rantoshak.blogspot.com/2013/07/sustainable-cotton-e3-program-and.html

Anyanwu, E. C., Campbell, A. W., & Vojdani, A. (2003). Neurophysiological effects of chronic indoor environmental toxic mold exposure on children. *The Scientific World Journal, 3*, 281–290. doi:10.1100/tsw.2003.22 PMID:12806113

Aoyama, K., Watabe, M., & Nakaki, T. (2008). Regulation of neuronal glutathione synthesis. *Journal of Pharmacological Sciences, 108*(3), 227–238. doi:10.1254/jphs.08R01CR PMID:19008644

Arcus-Arth Broadwin, R. & Lam, R. (2001). Impacts of Socioeconomic Factors on Residential Indoor Air Quality and Human Health. *Environmental Toxicology and Human Health, 2*.

Argos, M., Ahsan, H., & Graziano, J. H. (2012). Arsenic and human health: Epidemiologic progress and public health implications. *Reviews on Environmental Health, 27*(4), 191–195. doi:10.1515/reveh-2012-0021 PMID:22962196

Argos, M., Kalra, T., Pierce, B. L., Chen, Y., Parvez, F., Islam, T., ... Ahsan, H. (2011). A prospective study of arsenic exposure from drinking water and incidence of skin lesions in Bangladesh. *American Journal of Epidemiology, 174*(2), 185–194. doi:10.1093/aje/kwr062 PMID:21576319

Argos, M., Kalra, T., Rathouz, P. J., Chen, Y., Pierce, B., Parvez, F., ... Ahsan, H. (2010). Arsenic exposure from drinking water, and all-cause and chronic-disease mortalities in Bangladesh (heals): A prospective cohort study. *Lancet, 376*(9737), 252–258. doi:10.1016/S0140-6736(10)60481-3 PMID:20646756

Armando, V. L., & Angel, A. O. (1979). Chronic arsenic poisoning. *Boletín Médico del Hospital Infantil de México, 36*(5), 849–861. PMID:157141

Armienta, M. A., & Segovia, N. (2008). Arsenic and fluoride in the groundwater of Mexico. *Environmental Geochemistry and Health, 30*(4), 345–353. doi:10.100710653-008-9167-8 PMID:18335171

Armstrong, B. K., White, E., & Saracci, R. (1992). Principles of exposure measurement in epidemiology. *Monographs in Epidemiology and Biostatistics, 1*(21).

Arora, S., Rana, R., Chhabra, A., Jaiswal, A., & Rani, V. (2013). miRNA-transcription factor 656 interactions: A combinatorial regulation of gene expression. *Molecular Genetics and Genomics*, *288*(3-4), 77–87. doi:10.100700438-013-0734-z PMID:23334784

Arrighi, M., & Herz-Picciotto, I. (1994). The evolving concept of the healthy worker survivor effect. *Epidemiology*, *5*(2), 189–195. doi:10.1097/00001648-199403000-00009 PMID:8172994

Arthur, G., & Yobo, K. (2014). Genetically Modified Crops in Africa. In M. Ahuja & K. Ramawat (Eds.), *Biotechnology and Biodiversity* (pp. 17–37). New York, NY: Springer.

Arya, D. (2015). *Genetically Modified Foods Benefits and Risks*. Massachusetts Medical Society. http://www.massmed.org/Patient-Care/Health-Topics/Nutrition-and-Physical-Activity/Genetically-Modified-Foods-(pdf)/

Asadi, S., Alysandratos, K. D., Angelidou, A., Miniati, A., Sismanopoulos, N., Vasiadi, M., ... Theoharides, T. C. (2012). Substance P (SP) induces expression of functional corticotropin-releasing hormone receptor-1 (CRHR-1) in human mast cells. *The Journal of Investigative Dermatology*, *132*(2), 324–329. doi:10.1038/jid.2011.334 PMID:22089831

Asadi, S., & Theoharides, T. C. (2012). Corticotropin-releasing hormone and extracellular mitochondria augment IgE-stimulated human mast-cell vascular endothelial growth factor release, which is inhibited by luteolin. *J Neuroinflam*, *9*(1), 85. doi:10.1186/1742-2094-9-85 PMID:22559745

Asadullah, M. N., & Chaudhury, N. (2011). Poisoning the mind: Arsenic contamination of drinking water wells and children's educational achievement in rural Bangladesh. *Economics of Education Review*, *30*(5), 873–888. doi:10.1016/j.econedurev.2011.05.001

Aschner, M., Yao, C. P., Allen, J. W., & Tan, K. H. (2000). Methylmercury alters glutamate transport in astrocytes. *Neurochemistry International*, *37*(2-3), 199–206. doi:10.1016/S0197-0186(00)00023-1 PMID:10812205

Asimina, S., Chapizanis, D., Karakitsios, S., Kontoroupis, P., Asimakopoulos, D. N., Maggos, T., & Sarigiannis, D. (2018). Assessing and enhancing the utility of low-cost activity and location sensors for exposure studies. *Environmental Monitoring and Assessment*, *190*(3), 155. doi:10.100710661-018-6537-2 PMID:29464404

Athreya, B. (2006). *Submission to US Department of Labor in response to Federal Register notice FR Doc. E6-20561 published November 29, 2006*. In Request for Information on Efforts by Certain Countries to Eliminate the Worst Forms of Child Labor.

Atmaca, M., Tezcan, E., & Ustundag, B. (2007). Plasma nitric oxide and leptin values in patients with olanzapine-induced weight gain. *Journal of Psychiatric Research*, *41*(1-2), 74–79. doi:10.1016/j.jpsychires.2005.12.003 PMID:16426639

Australian Water Association. (2018). *Antidepressant drugs in water affect fish behaviour.* Retrieved from http://www.awa.asn.au/AWA_MBRR/Publications/Latest_News/Antidepressant_drugs_in_water_affect_fish_behaviour.aspx

Avino, T. A., Barger, N., Vargas, M. V., Carlson, E. L., Amaral, D. G., Bauman, M. D., & Schumann, C. M. (2018). Neuron numbers increase in the human amygdala from birth to adulthood, but not in autism. *Proceedings of the National Academy of Sciences of the United States of America*, *115*(14), 3710–3715. doi:10.1073/pnas.1801912115 PMID:29559529

Ayala, A., & Meier, B. (2017). A human rights approach to the health implications of food and nutrition insecurity. *Public Health Reviews*, *38*(10), 1–22. doi:10.118640985-017-0056-5 PMID:29450082

Babenko, O., Kovalchuk, I., & Metz, G. A. (2015). Stress-induced perinatal and transgenerational epigenetic programming of brain development and mental health. *Neuroscience and Biobehavioral Reviews*, *48*, 70–91. doi:10.1016/j.neubiorev.2014.11.013 PMID:25464029

Bacher, J., Wenzig, K., & Vogler, M. (2004). SPSS twoStep cluster - a first evaluation. In *RC33 Sixth International Conference on Social Science Methodology: "Recent Developments and Applications in Social Research Methodology,"* Amsterdam, The Netherlands.

Badzakova-Trajkov, G., Häberling, I. S., & Corballis, M. C. (2010). Cerebral asymmetries in monozygotic twins: An fMRI study. *Neuropsychologia*, *48*(10), 3086–3093. doi:10.1016/j.neuropsychologia.2010.06.020 PMID:20600189

Bagasra, O., Golkar, Z., Garcia, M., Rice, L. N., & Pace, D. G. (2013). Role of perfumes in pathogenesis of Autism. *Medical Hypotheses*, *80*(6), 795–803. doi:10.1016/j.mehy.2013.03.014 PMID:23578362

Bagasra, O., & Heggen, C. (2018). *Autism and Environmental Factors*. Wiley Blackwell Press. doi:10.1002/9781119042280

Bagasra, O., & Pace, D. G. (2013). Smell of Autism: Synthetic Fragrances and Cause for Allergies, Asthma, Cancer and Autism. OA Publishing London Reviews. *OA Autism*, *1*(2), 15. doi:10.13172/2052-7810-1-2-611

Bagla, P., & Kaiser, J. (1996). India's spreading health crisis draws global arsenic experts. *Science*, *274*(5285), 174–175. doi:10.1126cience.274.5285.174 PMID:8927976

Baig, J. A., Kazi, T. G., Shah, A. Q., Kandhro, G. A., Kandhro, G. A., Afridi, H. I., ... Jalbani, N. (2010). Speciation and evaluation of Arsenic in surface water and groundwater samples: A multivariate case study. *Ecotoxicology and Environmental Safety*, *73*(5), 914–923. doi:10.1016/j.ecoenv.2010.01.002 PMID:20363500

Bailey, K. A., Hester, S. D., Knapp, G. W., Owen, R. D., & Thai, S. F. (2010). Gene expression of normal human epidermal keratinocytes modulated by trivalent arsenicals. *Molecular Carcinogenesis*, *49*(12), 981–998. doi:10.1002/mc.20677 PMID:20886546

Baird, D. D., Upchurch, R. P., Homesley, W. B., & Franz, J. E. (1971). Introduction of a new broad-spectrum post emergence herbicide class with utility for herbaceous perennial weed control. *Proceedings of the North Central Weed Science Society*, *26*, 64–68.

Baldo, J. V., Ahmad, L., & Ruff, R. (2002). Neuropsychological performance of patients following mold exposure. *Applied Neuropsychology*, *9*(4), 193–202. doi:10.1207/S15324826AN0904_1 PMID:12584073

Bali, A. (2017). Bioremediation of Pharmaceutical Wastes. In J. N. Bhakta (Ed.), *Handbook of Research on Inventive Bioremediation Techniques* (pp. 364–393). Hershey, PA: IGI Global. doi:10.4018/978-1-5225-2325-3.ch016

Banerjee, N., Paul, S., Sau, T. J., Das, J. K., Bandyopadhyay, A., Banerjee, S., & Giri, A. K. (2013). Epigenetic modifications of DAPK and p16 genes contribute to arsenic-induced skin lesions and nondermatological health effects. *Toxicological Sciences*, *135*(2), 300–308. doi:10.1093/toxsci/kft163 PMID:23872714

Bang du, Y., Lee, I.K. & Lee, B.M. (2011). Toxicological characterization of phthalic Acid. *Toxicological Research*, *4*, 191–203. doi:10.5487/TR.2011.27.4.191 PMID:24278572

Bardsley, D. K., & Wiseman, N. D. (2012). Climate change vulnerability and social development for remote indigenous communities of South Australia. *Global Environmental Change*, *22*(3), 713–723. doi:10.1016/j.gloenvcha.2012.04.003

Bardullas, U., Limo'n-Pacheco, J. H., Giordano, M., Carrizales, L., Mendoza-Trejo, M. S., & Rodrı'guez, V. M. (2009). Chronic low-level arsenic exposure causes gender-specific alterations in locomotor activity, dopaminergic systems, and thioredoxin expression in mice. *Toxicology and Applied Pharmacology*, *239*(2), 169–177. doi:10.1016/j.taap.2008.12.004 PMID:19121333

Bargossi, C., Fiorini, M. C., Montalti, M., Prodi, L., & Zaccheroni, N. (2000). Recent developments in transition metal ion detection by luminescent chemosensors. *Coordination Chemistry Reviews*, *208*(1), 17–32. doi:10.1016/S0010-8545(00)00252-6

Baron-Cohen, S., Auyeung, B., Nørgaard-Pedersen, B., Hougaard, D. M., Abdallah, M. W., Melgaard, L., ... Lombardo, M. V. (2015). Elevated fetal steroidogenic activity in autism. *Molecular Psychiatry*, *20*(3), 369–376. doi:10.1038/mp.2014.48 PMID:24888361

Baron, R. L. (1994). A carbamate insecticide: A case study of aldicarb. *Environmental Health Perspectives*, *102*(Suppl. 11), 23–27. doi:10.1289/ehp.94102s1123 PMID:7737038

Barraclough, S., & Utting, P. (1987). *Food security trends and prospects in Latin America, Working paper no. 99.* Helen Kellogg Institute for International Studies, University of Notre Dame, USA.

Barreau, F., Salvador-Cartier, C., Houdeau, E., Bueno, L., & Fioramonti, J. (2008). Long-term alterations of colonic nerve-mast cell interactions induced by neonatal maternal deprivation in rats. *Gut*, *57*(5), 582–590. doi:10.1136/gut.2007.126680 PMID:18194988

Barrett, B., Charles, J. W., & Temte, J. L. (2015, January). Climate change, human health, and epidemiological transition. *Preventive Medicine*, *70*, 69–75. doi:10.1016/j.ypmed.2014.11.013 PMID:25434735

Baskaran, R., Cullen, R., & Colombo, S. (2009). Estimating values of environmental impacts of dairy farming in New Zealand. *New Zealand Journal of Agricultural Research*, *52*(4), 377–389. Retrieved from https://www.tandfonline.com/doi/pdf/10.1080/00288230909510520?needAccess=true doi:10.1080/00288230909510520

Bates, M. N., Smith, A. H., & Hopenhayn-Rich, C. (1992). Arsenic Ingestion and Internal Cancers: A Review. *American Journal of Epidemiology*, *135*(5), 462–476. doi:10.1093/oxfordjournals.aje.a116313 PMID:1570813

Bauman, M. D., Lavenex, P., Mason, W. A., Capitanio, J. P., & Amaral, D. G. (2004). The development of mother-infant interactions after neonatal amygdala lesions in rhesus monkeys. *The Journal of Neuroscience*, *24*(3), 711–721. doi:10.1523/JNEUROSCI.3263-03.2004 PMID:14736857

Bauman, M. L. (2010). Medical comorbidities in autism: Challenges to diagnosis and treatment. *Neurotherapeutics; the Journal of the American Society for Experimental NeuroTherapeutics*, *7*(3), 320–327. doi:10.1016/j.nurt.2010.06.001 PMID:20643385

Bauman, M. L., & Kemper, T. L. (2003). The neuropathology of the autism spectrum disorders: What have we learned? *Novartis Foundation Symposium*, *251*, 112–122. PMID:14521190

Bawa, A. S., & Anilakumar, K. R. (2013). Genetically modified foods: Safety, risks and public concerns - a review. *Journal of Food Science and Technology*, *50*(6), 1035–1046. doi:10.100713197-012-0899-1 PMID:24426015

Bayley, N. (2006). *Bayley scales of infant and toddler development: administration manual.* Harcourt Assessment.

Beaudouin, R., Micallef, S., & Brochot, C. (2010). A stochastic whole-body physiologically based pharmacokinetic model to assess the impact of inter-individual variability on tissue dosimetry over the human lifespan. *Regulatory Toxicology and Pharmacology*, *57*(1), 103–116. doi:10.1016/j.yrtph.2010.01.005 PMID:20122977

Beischlag, T. V., Morales, J. L., Hollingshead, B. D., & Perdew, G. H. (2008). The Aryl Hydrocarbon Receptor Complex and the Control of Gene Expression. *Critical Reviews in Eukaryotic Gene Expression*, *18*(3), 207–250. doi:10.1615/CritRevEukarGeneExpr.v18.i3.20 PMID:18540824

Benbrook, C.M. (2016). Impact of genetically engineered crops on pesticide use in U.S.—the first sixteen years. *Environmental Sciences Europe, 24*, 1-13.

Benbrook, C. M. (2016). Trends in glyphosate herbicide use in the United States and globally. *Environmental Sciences Europe*, *28*(1), 3. doi:10.118612302-016-0070-0 PMID:27752438

Benjamini, Y., & Hochberg, Y. (1995). Controlling the false discovery rate: A practical and powerful approach to multiple testing. *Journal of the Royal Statistical Society. Series B. Methodological*, 289–300.

Bennett, J. W., & Klich, M. (2003). Mycotoxins. *Clinical Microbiology Reviews*, *16*(3), 497–516. doi:10.1128/CMR.16.3.497-516.2003 PMID:12857779

Bennett, R., Buthelezi, T. J., Ismael, Y., & Morse, S. (2003). Bt cotton, pesticides, labour and health: A case study of smallholder farmers in the Makhathini Flats, Republic of South Africa. *Outlook on Agriculture*, *32*(2), 123–128. doi:10.5367/000000003101294361

Bennike, N. H., Oturai, N. B., Müller, S., Kirkeby, C. S., Jørgensen, C., Christensen, A. B., ... Johansen, J. D. (2018). Fragrance contact allergens in 5588 cosmetic products identified through a novel smartphone application. *Journal of the European Academy of Dermatology and Venereology*, *1*(1), 79–85. doi:10.1111/jdv.14513 PMID:28796916

Beránek, M. (2005). POPs Pesticides in the Czech Republic. The International POPs Elimination Project Czech Republic.

Bercum, F. M., Rodgers, K. M., Benison, A. M., Smith, Z. Z., Taylor, J., Kornreich, E., ... Barth, D. S. (2015). Maternal Stress Combined with Terbutaline Leads to Comorbid Autistic-Like Behavior and Epilepsy in a Rat Model. *The Journal of Neuroscience*, *35*(48), 15894–15902. doi:10.1523/JNEUROSCI.2803-15.2015 PMID:26631470

Berkowicz, R., Ketzel, M., Jensen, S. S., Hvidberg, M., & Raaschou-Nielsen, O. (2008). Evaluation and application of OSPM for traffic pollution assessment for a large number of street locations. *Environmental Modelling & Software*, *23*(3), 296–303. doi:10.1016/j.envsoft.2007.04.007

Bernier, R., Golzio, C., Xiong, B., Stessman, H. A., Coe, B. P., Penn, O., ... Eichler, E. E. (2014). Article: Disruptive CHD8 Mutations Define a Subtype of Autism Early in Development. *Cell*, *158*(2), 263–276. doi:10.1016/j.cell.2014.06.017 PMID:24998929

Berry, H. L., Bowen, K., & Kjellstrom, T. (2010). Climate change and mental health: A causal pathways framework. *International Journal of Public Health*, *55*(2), 123–132. doi:10.100700038-009-0112-0 PMID:20033251

Berry, H. L., Waite, T. D., Dear, K. B., Capon, A. G., & Murray, V. (2018). The case for systems thinking about climate change and mental health. *Nature Climate Change*, *8*(4), 282–290. doi:10.103841558-018-0102-4

Better Cotton Principles and Criteria. (2018). Version 2.0, March 2018. Retrieved from https://bettercotton.org/about-better-cotton/better-cotton-standard-system/production-principles-and-criteria/

Beversdorf, D. Q., Manning, S. E., Hillier, A., Anderson, S. L., Nordgren, R. E., Walters, S. E., ... Bauman, M. L. (2005). Timing of prenatal stressors and autism. *Journal of Autism and Developmental Disorders*, *35*(4), 471–478. doi:10.100710803-005-5037-8 PMID:16134032

Bhattacharjee, S., Chakravarty, S., Maity, S., Dureja, V., & Gupta, K. K. (2005). Metal contents in the groundwater of Sahebgunj district, Jharkhand, India, with special reference to arsenic. *Chemosphere*, *58*(9), 1203–1217. doi:10.1016/j.chemosphere.2004.09.055 PMID:15667841

Bhattacharya, P., Jacks, G., Frisbie, S. H., Smith, E., Naidu, R., & Sarkar, B. (2002). Arsenic in the environment: a global perspective. In B. Sarkar (Eds.), Heavy Metals in the Environment (pp. 147-215). New York, NY: Marcel Dekker, Inc. doi:10.1201/9780203909300.ch6

Bhattacharya, P., Chatterjee, D., & Jacks, G. (1997). Occurrence of arsenic contaminated groundwater in alluvial aquifers from Delta plain, Eastern India: Options for a safe drinking water supply. *Water: Research and Development*, *13*, 79–92.

Bhattacharya, P., Samal, A. C., Majumdar, A., & Santra, S. C. (2010). Arsenic Contamination in Rice, Wheat, Pulses, and Vegetables: A Study in an Arsenic Affected Area of West Bengal, India. *Water, Air, and Soil Pollution*, *213*(1-4), 3–13. doi:10.100711270-010-0361-9

Bienkowski, B. (2018). Diabetes Drug Makes Male Minnows More Female. *Scientific American*. Retrieved from https://www.scientificamerican.com/article/diabetes-drug-makes-male-minnows-more-female/

Bilbo, S. D., Block, C. L., Bolton, J. L., Hanamsagar, R., & Tran, P. K. (2018). Beyond infection - Maternal immune activation by environmental factors, microglial development, and relevance for autism spectrum disorders. *Experimental Neurology*, *299*, 241–251. doi:10.1016/j.expneurol.2017.07.002 PMID:28698032

Billeci, L., Tonacci, A., Tartarisco, G., Ruta, L., Pioggia, G., & Gangemi, S. (2015). Association Between Atopic Dermatitis and Autism Spectrum Disorders: A Systematic Review. *American Journal of Clinical Dermatology*, *16*(5), 371–388. doi:10.100740257-015-0145-5 PMID:26254000

Biocyc.org. (2017). Pathway: inosine-5'-phosphate biosynthesis.

Birgersson, S., Karlsson, B. S., & Söderlund, L. (2009). *Soy milk – an attributional Life Cycle Assessment examining the potential environmental impact of soy milk*. Stockholm, Sweden: KTH Royal Institute of Technology.

Bissen, M., & Frimmel, H. F. (2003). Arsenic – a Review. Part I: Occurrence, Toxicity, Speciation, Mobility. *Clean- Soil, Air. Water (Basel)*, *31*, 9–18.

Bitanihirwe, B. K., & Cunningham, M. G. (2009). Zinc: The brain's dark horse. *Synapse (New York, N.Y.)*, *63*(11), 1029–1049. doi:10.1002yn.20683 PMID:19623531

Bjørklund, G., Skalny, A. V., Rahman, M. M., Dadar, M., Yassa, H. A., Aaseth, J., ... Tinkov, A. A. (2018). Toxic metal(loid)-based pollutants and their possible role in autism spectrum disorder. *Environmental Research*, *166*, 234–250. doi:10.1016/j.envres.2018.05.020 PMID:29902778

Black, M. D., Selk, D. E., Hitchcock, J., Wettstein, J. G., & Sorensen, S. M. (1999). On the effect of neonatal nitric oxide synthase inhibition in rats: A potential neurodevelopmental model of schizophrenia. *Neuropharmacology*, *38*(9), 1299–1306. doi:10.1016/S0028-3908(99)00041-6 PMID:10471083

Black, R., Victora, C., Walker, S., Bhutta, Z., Christian, P., de Onis, M., ... Uauay, R. (2013). Maternal and child undernutrition and overweight in low-income and middle-income countries. *Lancet*, *382*(9890), 427–451. doi:10.1016/S0140-6736(13)60937-X PMID:23746772

Blackwell, R. Q., Yang, T. H., & Ai, I. (1961). Preliminary report on arsenic level in water and food from the endemic Blackfoot area. *Journal of the Formosan Medical Association*, *60*, 1139–1140.

Blancke, S., Van Breusegem, F., De Jaeger, G., Braeckman, J., & Van Montagu, M. (2015). Fatal attraction: The intuitive appeal of GMO opposition. *Trends in Plant Science*, *20*(7), 414–418. doi:10.1016/j.tplants.2015.03.011 PMID:25868652

Blasi, D. A., & Drouillard, J. (2002). Composition and feeding value of cottonseed feed products for beef cattle. Kansas State University, Agricultural Experiment Station and Cooperative Extension Service.

Bliss-Moreau, E., Bauman, M. D., & Amaral, D. G. (2011a). Neonatal amygdala lesions result in globally blunted affect in adult rhesus macaques. *Behavioral Neuroscience*, *125*(6), 848–858. doi:10.1037/a0025757 PMID:21988521

Bliss-Moreau, E., Moadab, G., Santistevan, A., & Amaral, D. G. (2017). The effects of neonatal amygdala or hippocampus lesions on adult social behavior. *Behavioural Brain Research*, *322*, 123–137. doi:10.1016/j.bbr.2016.11.052 PMID:28017854

Bliss-Moreau, E., Toscano, J. E., Bauman, M. D., Mason, W. A., & Amaral, D. G. (2011b). Neonatal amygdala lesions alter responsiveness to objects in juvenile macaques. *Neuroscience*, *178*, 123–132. doi:10.1016/j.neuroscience.2010.12.038 PMID:21215794

Blue Diamond Launches "Almond Breeze" as Thailand's Brand Leader for the Dairy-Free Almond Milk Global Trend [Press release]. (2017, June 30). Retrieved from https://assets.ctfassets.net/99ef2wobcp71/6RHDBpFaSWMKMwsSSsm40G/7db7b31f9f185a3018715283541ddb84/Press_Release_Blue_Diamond_Almond_Milk_launch_En_Final_0617.pdf

Blue Diamond. (2018). Almond Breeze. Retrieved from https://www.bluediamond.com/brand/almond-breeze

Boehm, G., Cervantes, H., Georgi, G., Jelinek, J., Sawatzki, G., Wermuth, B., & Colombo, J.-P. (1998). Effect of increasing dietary threonine intakes on amino acid metabolism of the central nervous system and peripheral tissues in growing rats. *Pediatric Research*, *44*(6), 900–906. doi:10.1203/00006450-199812000-00013 PMID:9853925

Bojanowska-Czajka, A., Kciuk, G., Gumiela, M., Borowiecka, S., Nałęcz-Jawecki, G., Koc, A., ... Trojanowicz, M. (2015). Analytical, toxicological and kinetic investigation of decomposition of the drug diclofenac in waters and wastes using gamma radiation. *Environmental Science and Pollution Research International*, *22*(24), 20255–20270. doi:10.100711356-015-5236-6 PMID:26308920

Boleda, M. R., Galceran, M. T., & Ventura, F. J. (2007). Trace determination of cannabinoids and opiates in wastewater and surface waters by ultra-performance liquid chromatography-tandem mass spectrometry. *Journal of Chromatography. A*, *1175*(1), 38–48. doi:10.1016/j.chroma.2007.10.029 PMID:17980892

Bollati, V., & Baccarelli, A. (2010). Environmental epigenetics. *Heredity*, *105*(1), 105–112. doi:10.1038/hdy.2010.2 PMID:20179736

Bonchak, J. G., Prouty, M. E., & de la Feld, S. F. (2018). Prevalence of Contact Allergens in Personal Care Products for Babies and Children. *Dermatitis*, *29*(2), 81–84. doi:10.1097/DER.0000000000000348 PMID:29494392

Bondarenko, E., Hodgson, D. M., & Nalivaiko, E. (2014). Amygdala mediates respiratory responses to sudden arousing stimuli and to restraint stress in rats. *American Journal of Physiology. Regulatory, Integrative and Comparative Physiology*, *306*(12), R951–R959. doi:10.1152/ajpregu.00528.2013 PMID:24740655

Bondy, J. A., & Murty, U. S. R. (1976). *Graph theory with applications*. Citeseer. doi:10.1007/978-1-349-03521-2

Bonfanti, P., Saibene, M., Bacchetta, R., Mantecca, P., & Colombo, A. (2018). A glyphosate micro-emulsion formulation displays teratogenicity in *Xenopus leavis. Aquatic Toxicology (Amsterdam, Netherlands)*, *195*, 103–113. doi:10.1016/j.aquatox.2017.12.007 PMID:29306033

Bonham, M., O'Connor, J. M., Hannigan, B. M., & Strain, J. (2002). The immune system as a physiological indicator of marginal copper status? *British Journal of Nutrition*, *87*(05), 393–403. doi:10.1079/BJN2002558 PMID:12010579

Bonnefoi, M. S., Belanger, S. E., Devlin, D. J., Doerrer, N. G., Embry, M. R., Fukushima, S., ... van der Laan, J. W. (2010). Human and environmental health challenges for the next decade (2010–2020). *Critical Reviews in Toxicology*, *40*(10), 893–911. doi:10.3109/10408444.2010.506640 PMID:20854192

Bonting, S. L. (1992). Chemical sensors for space applications. Advances in Space Biology and Medicine. *Advances in Space Biology and Medicine*, *2*, 263–293. doi:10.1016/S1569-2574(08)60024-6 PMID:1342247

Bonvallot, N., Tremblay-Franco, M., Chevrier, C., Canlet, C., Warembourg, C., Cravedi, J.-P., & Cordier, S. (2013). Metabolomics tools for describing complex pesticide exposure in pregnant women in Brittany (France). *PLoS One*, *8*(5), e64433. doi:10.1371/journal.pone.0064433 PMID:23704985

Boonchai, W., Green, A., Ng, J., Dicker, A., & Chenevix-Trench, G. (2000). Basal cell carcinoma in chronic arsenicism occurring in Queensland, Australia, after ingestion of an asthma medication. *Journal of the American Academy of Dermatology*, *43*(4), 664–669. doi:10.1067/mjd.2000.107939 PMID:11004623

Borgoño, J. M., Vicent, P., Venturíno, H., & Infante, A. (1977). Arsenic in the drinking water of the city of Antofagasta: Epidemiological and clinical study before and after the installation of a treatment plant. [PubMed]. *Environmental Health Perspectives*, *19*, 103–105.

Bouchard, M. F., Chevrier, J., Harley, K. G., Kogut, K., Vedar, M., Calderon, N., ... Eskenazi, B. (2011). Prenatal exposure to organophosphate pesticides and IQ in 7-year-old children. *Environmental Health Perspectives*, *119*(8), 1189–1195. doi:10.1289/ehp.1003185 PMID:21507776

Bouldin, E. (2010). History and development of public health. In E. Andresen & E. Bouldin (Eds.), *Public health foundations: Concepts and practices* (pp. 3–24). San Francisco, CA: John Wiley & Sons, Inc.

Bou-Resli, M., Mathew, T., Dashti, H., & Al-Zaid, N. (2002). Brain selenium accumulation in rat pups of selenium supplemented mothers. *Anatomia, Histologia, Embryologia*, *31*(4), 228–231. doi:10.1046/j.1439-0264.2002.00400.x PMID:12196265

Braissant, O., Honegger, P., Loup, M., Iwase, K., Takiguchi, M., & Bachmann, C. (1999). Hyperammonemia: Regulation of argininosuccinate synthetase and argininosuccinate lyase genes in aggregating cell cultures of fetal rat brain. *Neuroscience Letters*, *266*(2), 89–92. doi:10.1016/S0304-3940(99)00274-8 PMID:10353334

Brammer, H. (2008). Threat of Arsenic to Agriculture in India, Bangladesh and Nepal. *Economic and Political Weekly*, 43.

Brasel, T. L., Campbell, A. W., Demers, R. E., Ferguson, B. S., Fink, J., Vojdani, A., & ... . (2004). Detection of trichothecene mycotoxins in sera from individuals exposed to Stachybotrys chartarum in indoor environments. *Archives of Environmental Health*, *59*, 317–323. PMID:16238166

Brasel, T. L., Douglas, D. R., Wilson, S. C., & Straus, D. C. (2005a). Detection of airborne Stachybotrys chartarum macrocyclic trichothecene mycotoxins on particulates smaller than conidia. *Applied and Environmental Microbiology*, *71*(1), 114–122. doi:10.1128/AEM.71.1.114-122.2005 PMID:15640178

Brasel, T. L., Martin, J. M., Carriker, C. G., Wilson, S. C., & Straus, D. C. (2005b). Detection of airborne Stachybotrys chartarum macrocyclic trichothecene mycotoxins in the indoor environment. *Applied and Environmental Microbiology*, *71*(11), 7376–7388. doi:10.1128/AEM.71.11.7376-7388.2005 PMID:16269780

Braun, J. M., Kalkbrenner, A. E., Just, A. C., Yolton, K., Calafat, A. M., Sjödin, A., ... Lanphear, B. P. (2014). Gestational exposure to endocrine-disrupting chemicals and reciprocal social, repetitive, and stereotypic behaviors in 4- and 5-year-old children: The HOME study. *Environmental Health Perspectives*, *122*(5), 513–520. doi:10.1289/ehp.1307261 PMID:24622245

Bray, F., Ferlay, J., Soerjomataram, I., Siegel, R. L., Torre, L. A., & Jemal, A. (2018, November). Global cancer statistics 2018: GLOBOCAN estimates of incidence and mortality worldwide for 36 cancers in 185 countries. *CA: a Cancer Journal for Clinicians*, *68*(6), 394–424. doi:10.3322/caac.21492 PMID:30207593

Breckpot, J., Thienpont, B., Vermeesch, J. R., Devriendt, K., Gewillig, M., & Allegaert, K. (2012). Differences in copy number variation between discordant monozygotic twins as a model for exploring chromosomal mosaicism in congenital heart defects. *Molecular Syndromology*, *2*(2), 81–87. doi:10.1159/000335284 PMID:22511896

Brook, R. D. (2008). Cardiovascular effects of air pollution. *Clinical Science*, *115*(6), 175–187. doi:10.1042/CS20070444 PMID:18691154

Brown, M. T., & Wicker, L. R. (2000). Discriminant analysis. In H.E.A. Tinsley & S.D. Brown (Eds.), handbook of applied multivariate statistics and mathematical modeling (Ch. 8, pp. 209-235). London, UK: Academic Press.

Brown, R. C., Lockwood, A. H., & Sonawane, B. R. (2005). Neurodegenerative diseases: An overview of environmental risk factors. *Environmental Health Perspectives*, *113*(9), 1250–1256. doi:10.1289/ehp.7567 PMID:16140637

Brundtland, G. H. (1987). *Our Common Future. World Commission on Environment and Development*. Oxford: Oxford University Press.

Buck Louis, G. M., Smarr, M. M., & Patel, C. J. (2017). The Exposome Research Paradigm: An Opportunity to Understand the Environmental Basis for Human Health and Disease. *Current Environmental Health Reports*, *4*(1), 89–98. doi:10.100740572-017-0126-3 PMID:28194614

Buckman, T. D., Sutphin, M. S., & Eckhert, C. D. (1993). A comparison of the effects of dietary selenium on selenoprotein expression in rat brain and liver. Biochimica et Biophysica Acta (BBA)-. *Protein Structure and Molecular Enzymology.*, *1163*(2), 176–184. doi:10.1016/0167-4838(93)90179-U PMID:8490049

Budavari, S. (1989). *An Encyclopedia of Chemicals, Drugs, and Biologicals. The Merck Index*. Rahway, NJ: Merck and Co. Inc.

Buehler, J. W., Berkelman, R. L., Hartley, D. M., & Peters, C. J. (2003). Syndromic surveillance and bioterrorism-related epidemics. *Emerging Infectious Diseases*, *9*(10), 1197–1204. doi:10.3201/eid0910.030231 PMID:14609452

Buie, T., Fuchs, G. J. III, Furuta, G. T., Kooros, K., Levy, J., Lewis, J. D., ... Winter, H. (2010). Recommendations for evaluation and treatment of common gastrointestinal problems in children with ASDs. *Pediatrics*, *125*(Suppl 1), S19–S29. doi:10.1542/peds.2009-1878D PMID:20048084

Burns, C. (2004). *A review of the literature describing the link between poverty, food insecurity and obesity with specific reference to Australia. Centre for Physical Activity and Nutrition Research School of Exercise and Nutrition Sciences, Deakin University Melbourne*. Australia: VicHealth.

Bushey, D. F., Bannon, G. A., Delaney, B. F., Graser, G., Hefford, M., Jiang, X., ... Harper, M. S. (2014). Characteristics and safety assessment of intractable proteins in genetically modified crops. *Regulatory Toxicology and Pharmacology*, *69*(2), 154–170. doi:10.1016/j.yrtph.2014.03.003 PMID:24662477

Bus, J. S. (2015). Analysis of Moms Across America report suggesting bioaccumulation of glyphosate in U.S. mother's breast milk: Implausibility based on inconsistency with available body of animal toxicokinetic human biomonitoring, and physico-chemical data. *Regulatory Toxicology and Pharmacology*, *73*(3), 758–764. doi:10.1016/j.yrtph.2015.10.022 PMID:26520181

Busnelli, M., & Chini, B. (2017). Molecular Basis of Oxytocin Receptor Signalling in the Brain: What we know and what we need to know. *Current Topics in Behavioral Neurosciences*. doi:10.1007/7854_2017_6

Butler, D., & Reichhardt, T. (1999). Long-term effect of GM crops serves up food for thought. *Nature*, *398*(6729), 651–653. doi:10.1038/19381 PMID:10227281

Byrne, P., Pendell, D., & Graff, G. (2014). *Labeling of Genetically Modified Foods. Food and Nutrition Series (Health). Colorado State University Extension.* Retrieved from https://extension.colostate.edu/docs/pubs/foodnut/09371.pdf

Byrne, S., Amarasiriwardena, D., Bandak, B., Bartkus, L., Kane, J., Jones, J., ... Cornejo, L. (2010). Were Chinchorros exposed to arsenic? Arsenic determination in Chinchorro Mummies' hair by laser ablation inductively coupled plasma-mass spectrometry (LA-ICP-MS). *Microchemical Journal*, *94*(1), 28–35. doi:10.1016/j.microc.2009.08.006

Calderon, J., Navarro, M. E., Jimenez-Capdeville, M. E., Santos-Diaz, M. A., Golden, A., Rodriguez-Leyva, I., ... Diaz-Barriga, F. (2001). Exposure to arsenic and lead and neuropsychological development in Mexican children. *Environmental Research*, *85*(2), 69–76. doi:10.1006/enrs.2000.4106 PMID:11161656

Cameron, P. J. (2007). Factors influencing the development of integrated pest management (IPM) in selected vegetable crops: A review. *New Zealand Journal of Crop and Horticultural Science*, *35*(3), 365–384. doi:10.1080/01140670709510203

Campbell, A. W., Thrasher, J. D., Gray, M. R., & Vojdani, A. (2004). Mold and mycotoxins: Effects on the neurological and immune systems in humans. *Advances in Applied Microbiology*, *55*, 375–406. doi:10.1016/S0065-2164(04)55015-3 PMID:15350803

Campbell, A. W., Thrasher, J. D., Madison, R. A., Vojdani, A., Gray, M. R., & Johnson, A. (2003). Neural autoantibodies and neurophysiologic abnormalities in patients exposed to molds in water-damaged buildings. *Archives of Environmental Health*, *58*(8), 464–474. doi:10.3200/AEOH.58.8.464-474 PMID:15259425

Campbell, T. C., & Campbell, T. M. (2004). *The China study: The most comprehensive study of nutrition ever conducted and the startling implications for diet, weight loss and long-term health.* Dallas, TX: BenBella Books.

Caplin, J. L., Hanlon, G. W., & Taylor, H. D. (2008). Presence of vancomycin and ampicillin-resistant *Enterococcus faecium* of epidemic clonal complex-17 in wastewaters from the south coast of England. *Environmental Microbiology*, *10*(4), 885–892. doi:10.1111/j.1462-2920.2007.01507.x PMID:18093157

Capuron, L., Ravaud, A., & Dantzer, R. (2001). Timing and specificity of the cognitive changes induced by interleukin-2 and interferon-alpha treatments in cancer patients. *Psychosomatic Medicine*, *63*(3), 376–386. doi:10.1097/00006842-200105000-00007 PMID:11382265

Carletto, C., & Banerjee, A. (2013). Towards better measurement of household food security: Harmonizing indicators and the role of household surveys. *Global Food Security*, *2*(1), 30–40. doi:10.1016/j.gfs.2012.11.006

Carlson, A. L., Xia, K., Azcarate-Peril, M. A., Goldman, B. D., Ahn, M., Styner, M. A., ... Knickmeyer, R. C. (2018). Infant Gut Microbiome Associated With Cognitive Development. *Biological Psychiatry*, *83*(2), 148–159. doi:10.1016/j.biopsych.2017.06.021 PMID:28793975

Carmin, J., & Agyeman, J. (Eds.). (2011). *Environmental Inequalities Beyond Borders: Local Perspectives on Global Injustices*. Boston, MA: MIT Press. doi:10.7551/mitpress/8759.001.0001

Carter, C.A., &. Gruere, G.P. (2003). Mandatory labeling of genetically modified foods: does it really provide consumer choice? *AgBioForum*, *6*(1 and 2), 68 – 70.

Casas, L., Torrent, M., Zock, J. P., Doekes, G., Forns, J., Guxens, M., ... Sunyer, J. (2013). Early life exposures to home dampness, pet ownership and farm animal contact and neuropsychological development in 4 year old children: A prospective birth cohort study. *International Journal of Hygiene and Environmental Health*, *216*(6), 690–697. doi:10.1016/j.ijheh.2012.12.013 PMID:23357052

Caspi, R., Altman, T., Billington, R., Dreher, K., Foerster, H., Fulcher, C. A., ... Karp, P. D. (2014). The MetaCyc database of metabolic pathways and enzymes and the BioCyc collection of Pathway/Genome Databases. *Nucleic Acids Research*, *42*(D1), D459–D471. doi:10.1093/nar/gkt1103 PMID:24225315

Castiglioni, S., Zuccato, E., Chiabrando, C., Fanelli, R., & Bagnati, R. (2008). Mass spectrometric analysis of illicit drugs in wastewater and surface water. *Mass Spectrometry Reviews*, *27*(4), 378–384. doi:10.1002/mas.20168 PMID:18421768

Castren, K., Ranki, A., Welsh, J. A., & Vähäkangas, K. H. (1998). Infrequent p53 mutations in arsenic-related skin lesions. *Oncology Research*, *10*(9), 475–482. PMID:10223623

Cataldo, I., Azhari, A., & Esposito, G. A. (2018, February 13). Review of Oxytocin and Arginine-Vasopressin Receptors and Their Modulation of Autism Spectrum Disorder. *Frontiers in Molecular Neuroscience*, *11*, 27. doi:10.3389/fnmol.2018.00027 PMID:29487501

Caussy, E., & World Health Organization. (2005). A field guide for detection, management and surveillance of arsenicosis cases. World Health Organization.

CDC. (2012): Principles of epidemiology in public health practice (3rd ed.). CDC USA.

Ceccarelli, S., Grando, S., Maatougui, M., Michael, M., Slash, M., Haghparast, R., ... Nachit, M. (2010). Plant breeding and climate changes. *The Journal of Agricultural Science*, *148*(06), 627–637. doi:10.1017/S0021859610000651

Centeno, J. A., Tchounwou, P. B., Patlolla, A. K., Mullick, F. G., Murakata, L., Meza, E., & Yedjou, C. G. (2006). Environmental pathology and health effects of arsenic poisoning. In *Managing Arsenic in the Environment: From Soil to Human Health* (pp. 311–327). Collingwood, Australia: Csiro Publishing.

Centers for Disease Control and Prevention. (2014). CDC estimates 1 in 68 children has been identified with autism spectrum disease. Retrieved from https://www.cdc.gov/media/releases/2014/p0327-autism-spectrum disorder.html

Centers for Disease Control and Prevention. (2018). Autism Spectrum Disorders. Retrieved from https://www.cdc.gov/ncbddd/autism/index.html

Centers for Disease Control and Prevention. (2018). CDC estimates 1 in 59 children has been identified with autism spectrum disorder. Retrieved from https://www.cdc.gov/features/new-autism-data/index.html

Cesarino, I., Moraes, F. C., Lanza, M. R. V., & Machado, S. A. S. (2012). Electrochemical detection of carbamate pesticides in fruit and vegetables with a biosensor based on acetylcholinesterase immobilised on a composite of polyaniline–carbon nanotubes. *Food Chemistry*, *135*(3), 873–879. doi:10.1016/j.foodchem.2012.04.147 PMID:22953799

Chadeau-Hyam, M., Campanella, G., Jombart, T., Bottolo, L., Portengen, L., Vineis, P., ... Vermeulen, R. C. H. (2013). Deciphering the complex: Methodological overview of statistical models to derive OMICS-based biomarkers. *Environmental and Molecular Mutagenesis*, *54*(7), 542–557. doi:10.1002/em.21797 PMID:23918146

Chae, M.-Y., & Czarnik, A. W. (1992). Fluorometric chemodosimetry. Mercury(II) and silver(I) indication in water via enhanced fluorescence signalling. *Journal of the American Chemical Society*, *114*(24), 9704–9705. doi:10.1021/ja00050a085

Chakraborti, D., Das, B., Rahman, M. M., Chowdhury, U. K., Biswas, B., Goswami, A. B., ... Das, D. (2009). Status of groundwater arsenic contamination in the state of West Bengal, India: A 20-year study report. *Molecular Nutrition & Food Research*, *53*(5), 542–551. doi:10.1002/mnfr.200700517 PMID:19382148

Chakraborti, D., Mukherjee, S. C., Pati, S., Sengupta, M. K., Rahman, M. M., Chowdhury, U. K., ... Basu, G. K. (2003). Arsenic groundwater contamination in Middle Ganga Plain, Bihar, India: A future danger? *Environmental Health Perspectives*, *111*(9), 1194–1201. doi:10.1289/ehp.5966 PMID:12842773

Chakraborti, D., Rahman, M. M., Ahamed, S., Dutta, R. N., Pati, S., & Mukherjee, S. C. (2016). Arsenic groundwater contamination and its health effects in Patna district (capital of Bihar) in the middle Ganga plain, India. *Chemosphere*, *152*, 520–529. doi:10.1016/j.chemosphere.2016.02.119 PMID:27011321

Chakraborti, D., Rahman, M. M., & Alauddin, M. (2015). Groundwater arsenic contamination in Bangladesh - 21 years of research. *Journal of Trace Elements in Medicine and Biology*, *31*, 237–248. doi:10.1016/j.jtemb.2015.01.003 PMID:25660323

Chakraborti, D., Rahman, M. M., Chowdhury, U. K., Paul, K., Chowdhury, U. K., Sengupta, M. K., ... Mukherjee, S. C. (2002). Arsenic calamity in the Indian subcontinent: What lessons have been learned? *Talanta*, *58*(1), 3–22. doi:10.1016/S0039-9140(02)00270-9 PMID:18968730

Chakraborti, D., Sengupta, M. K., Rahman, M. M., Ahamed, S., Chowdhury, U. K., & ... . (2004). Groundwater arsenic contamination and its health effects in the Ganga– Meghna–Brahmaputra Plain. *Journal of Environmental Monitoring*, *6*, 74N–83N. PMID:15241847

Chakraborti, D., Singh, S., Rahman, M., Dutta, R., Mukherjee, S., Pati, S., & Kar, P. (2018). Groundwater arsenic contamination in the Ganga River Basin: A future health danger. *International Journal of Environmental Research and Public Health*, *15*(2), 180.

Chandrasekharam, D., Karamakar, J., Berner, J., & Stuben, D. (2001). Arsenic contamination in groundwater, Murshidabad district, West Bengal. In R. Cidu (Ed.), *Proceeding 10th International Symposium on Water Rocks Interaction*, Villasimius, Italy (Vol. 2, pp. 1051-1054).

Charlet, L., & Polya, D. (2006). Arsenic in shallow reducing ground waters in southern Asia, an environmental health disaster. *Elements*, *2*(2), 91–96. doi:10.2113/gselements.2.2.91

Charpin-Kadouch, C., Maurel, G., Felipo, R., Queralt, J., Ramadour, M., Dumon, H., ... Charpin, D. (2006). Mycotoxin identification in moldy dwellings. *Journal of Applied Toxicology*, *26*(6), 475–479. doi:10.1002/jat.1164 PMID:17080403

Chaste, P., Roeder, K., & Devlin, B. (2017). The yin and yang of autism genetics: How rare de novo and common variations affect liability. *Annual Review of Genomics and Human Genetics*, *31*(18), 167–187. doi:10.1146/annurev-genom-083115-022647 PMID:28426285

Chattopadhyay, S., Bhaumik, S., Purkayastha, M., Basu, S., Nag Chaudhuri, A., & Das Gupta, S. (2002). Apoptosis and necrosis in developing brain cells due to arsenic toxicity and protection with antioxidants. *Toxicology Letters*, *136*(1), 65–76. doi:10.1016/S0378-4274(02)00282-5 PMID:12368058

Chemicals Program of the United Nations Environment Programme. (2004). *Childhood pesticide poisoning: information for advocacy and action*. Retrieved from http://www.who.int/ceh/publications/pestpoisoning.pdf

Chen, A. Y. Y., & Olsen, T. (2016). Chromated copper arsenate–treated wood: A potential source of arsenic exposure and toxicity in dermatology. *International Journal of Women's Dermatology*, *2*(1), 28–30. doi:10.1016/j.ijwd.2016.01.002 PMID:28491998

Chen, C. J., Chuang, Y. C., You, S. L., Lin, T. M., & Wu, H. Y. (1986). A retrospective study on malignant neoplasms of bladder, lung and liver in blackfoot disease endemic area in Taiwan. *British Journal of Cancer*, *53*(3), 399–405. doi:10.1038/bjc.1986.65 PMID:3964542

Chen, C. L., Chiou, H. Y., Hsu, L. I., Hsueh, Y. M., Wu, M. M., Wang, Y. H., & Chen, C.-J. (2010). Arsenic in drinking water and risk of urinary tract cancer: A follow-up study from north eastern Taiwan. *Cancer Epidemiology, Biomarkers & Prevention*, *19*(1), 101–110. doi:10.1158/1055-9965.EPI-09-0333 PMID:20056628

Chen, X. H., Wang, F. L., Zhang, R., Ji, L. L., Yang, Z. L., Lin, H., & Zhao, B. (2016). Evidences of inhibited arbuscular mycorrhizal fungal development and colonization in multiple lines of Bt cotton. *Agriculture, Ecosystems & Environment*, *230*, 169–176. doi:10.1016/j.agee.2016.05.008

Chen, Y., & Ahsan, H. (2004). Cancer burden from arsenic in drinking water in Bangladesh. *American Journal of Public Health*, *94*(5), 741–744. doi:10.2105/AJPH.94.5.741 PMID:15117692

Chen, Y., Graziano, J. H., Parvez, F., Hussain, I., Momotaj, H., van Geen, A., ... Ahsan, H. (2006). Modification of risk of arsenic-induced skin lesions by sunlight exposure, smoking, and occupational exposures in Bangladesh. *Epidemiology (Cambridge, Mass.)*, *17*(4), 459–467. doi:10.1097/01.ede.0000220554.50837.7f PMID:16755266

Chen, Y., Graziano, J. H., Parvez, F., Liu, M., Slavkovich, V., Kalra, T., ... Ahsan, H. (2011). Arsenic exposure from drinking water and mortality from cardiovascular disease in Bangladesh: Prospective cohort study. *BMJ (Clinical Research Ed.)*, 342. PMID:21546419

Chen, Y., & Karagas, M. R. (2013). Arsenic and Cardiovascular Disease: New Evidence From the United States. *Annals of Internal Medicine*, *159*, 713–714. PMID:24061555

Chen, Y., Shang, X., Li, C., Xue, Z., Chen, H., Wu, H., & Wang, T. (2018). The synthesis, crystal, hydrogen sulfide detection and cell assement of novel chemsensors based on coumarin derivatives. *Scientific Reports*, *8*(1), 16159. doi:10.103841598-018-34331-9 PMID:30385799

Chiorando, M. (2018). US Dairy Sales to Drop 11% by 2020. *Plant Based News*. Retrieved from https://www.plantbasednews.org/post/us-dairy-sales-drop-11-2020-other-positive-vegan-stats

Chiou, H. Y., Chiou, S. T., Hsu, Y. H., Chou, Y. L., Tseng, C. H., Wei, M. L., & Chen, C. J. (2001). Incidence of transitional cell carcinoma and arsenic in drinking water: A follow-up study of 8102 residents in a arseniasis endemic area in Northeastern Taiwan. *American Journal of Epidemiology*, *153*(5), 411–418. doi:10.1093/aje/153.5.411 PMID:11226969

Chiou, H. Y., Hsueh, Y. M., Liaw, K. F., Horng, S. F., Chiang, M. H., Pu, Y. S., ... & Chen, C. J. (1995). Incidence of internal cancers and ingested inorganic arsenic: A seven-year follow-up study in Taiwan. *Cancer Research*, *55*(6), 1296–1300. PMID:7882325

Choi, J. S., & Kim, J. J. (2010). Amygdala regulates risk of predation in rats foraging in a dynamic fear environment. *Proceedings of the National Academy of Sciences of the United States of America*, *107*(50), 21773–21777. doi:10.1073/pnas.1010079108 PMID:21115817

Chollet, M., Gille, D., Piccinali, P., Bütikofer, U., Schmid, A., Stoffers, H., ... Walther, B. (2014). Short communication: Dairy consumption among middle-aged and elderly adults in Switzerland. *Journal of Dairy Science*, *97*(9), 5387–5392. doi:10.3168/jds.2014-8193 PMID:24997665

Chown, N., & Hughes, L. (2016). History and first descriptions of autism: Asperger versus Kanner revisited. *Journal of Autism and Developmental Disorders*, *46*(6), 2270–2272. doi:10.100710803-016-2746-0 PMID:26883648

Christensen, D. L., Braun, K. V. N., Baio, J., Bilder, D., Charles, J., Constantino, J. N., ... Lee, L. C. (2018). Prevalence and characteristics of autism spectrum disorder among children aged 8 years—autism and developmental disabilities monitoring network, 11 sites, United States, 2012. *MMWR. Surveillance Summaries*, *65*(13). doi:10.15585/mmwr.ss6503a1

Christensen, F. M. (1998). Pharmaceuticals in the environment--a human risk? *Regulatory Toxicology and Pharmacology*, *28*(3), 212–222. doi:10.1006/rtph.1998.1253 PMID:10049792

Chrousos, G. P. (1995). The hypothalamic-pituitary-adrenal axis and immune-mediated inflammation. *The New England Journal of Medicine*, *332*(20), 1351–1362. doi:10.1056/NEJM199505183322008 PMID:7715646

Clara, A. M., Strenn, B., Gans, O., Martinez, E., Kreuzinger, N., & Kroiss, H. (2005). Removal of selected pharmaceuticals, fragrances and endocrine disrupting compounds in a membrane bioreactor and conventional wastewater treatment plants. *Water Research*, *39*(19), 4797–4807. doi:10.1016/j.watres.2005.09.015 PMID:16242170

Classen, H., Gröber, U., Löw, D., Schmidt, J., & Stracke, H. (2011). Zinc deficiency. Symptoms, causes, diagnosis and therapy. *Medizinische Monatsschrift fur Pharmazeuten*, *34*, 87–95. PMID:21736013

Clay, J. (2013). *World agriculture and the environment: a commodity-by-commodity guide to impacts and practices*. Washington, DC: Island Press.

Coates, J. (2013). Build it back better: Deconstructing food security for improved measurement and action. *Global Food Security*, *2*(3), 188–194. doi:10.1016/j.gfs.2013.05.002

Coggon, D., Barker, D. J., Cole, R. B., & Nelson, M. (1989). Stomach cancer and food storage. *Journal of the National Cancer Institute*, *81*(15), 1178–1182. doi:10.1093/jnci/81.15.1178 PMID:2746670

Cohen, R. (1998). *Milk the deadly poison*. New Jersey: Argus.

Cohn, B. A., Wolff, M. S., Cirillo, P. M., & Sholtz, R. I. (2007). DDT and breast cancer in young women: New data on the significance of age at exposure. *Environmental Health Perspectives*, *115*(10), 1406–1414. doi:10.1289/ehp.10260 PMID:17938728

Cole, P., Trichopoulos, D., Pastides, H., Starr, T., & Mandel, J. S. (2003). Dioxin and cancer: A critical review. *Regulatory Toxicology and Pharmacology*, *38*(3), 378–388. doi:10.1016/j.yrtph.2003.08.002 PMID:14623487

Collins, L. V., Hajizadeh, S., Holme, E., Jonsson, I. M., & Tarkowski, A. (2004). Endogenously oxidized mitochondrial DNA induces in vivo and in vitro inflammatory responses. *Journal of Leukocyte Biology*, *75*(6), 995–1000. doi:10.1189/jlb.0703328 PMID:14982943

Collotta, M., Bertazzi, P. A., & Bollati, V. (2013). Epigenetics and pesticides. *Toxicology*, *307*, 35–41. doi:10.1016/j.tox.2013.01.017 PMID:23380243

Colvert, E., Tick, B., McEwen, F., Stewart, C., Curran, S. R., Woodhouse, E., ... Bolton, P. (2015). Heritability of autism spectrum disorder in a UK population-based twin sample. *JAMA Psychiatry*, *72*(5), 415–423. doi:10.1001/jamapsychiatry.2014.3028 PMID:25738232

Combalbert, S., & Hernandez-Raquet, G. (2010). Occurrence, fate, and biodegradation of estrogens in sewage and manure. *Applied Microbiology and Technology*, *86*(6), 1671–1692. doi:10.100700253-010-2547-x PMID:20354692

Concha, G., Nermell, B., & Vahter, M. (1998). Metabolism of inorganic arsenic in children with chronic high arsenic exposure in northern Argentina. *Environmental Health Perspectives*, *106*(6), 355–359. doi:10.1289/ehp.98106355 PMID:9618352

Conner, A. J., & Jacobs, J. M. E. (1999). Genetic engineering of crops as potential source of genetic hazard in the human diet. *Mutation Research/Genetic Toxicology and Environmental Mutagenesis*, *443*(1-2), 223–234. doi:10.1016/S1383-5742(99)00020-4 PMID:10415441

Constantino, J. N., Przybeck, T., Friesen, D., & Todd, R. D. (2000). Reciprocal social behavior in children with and without pervasive developmental disorders. *Journal of Developmental and Behavioral Pediatrics*, *21*(1), 2–11. doi:10.1097/00004703-200002000-00002 PMID:10706343

Cordain, L. (2012). *The Paleo Answer: 7 days to lose weight, feel great, stay young*. Hoboken, NJ: JohnWiley & Sons.

Costa, B. E., Coelho, N. M., & Coelho, L. M. (2015). Determination of arsenic species in rice samples using CPE and ETAAS. *Food Chemistry*, *178*, 89–95. doi:10.1016/j.foodchem.2015.01.014 PMID:25704688

Costa, L. G., Aschner, M., Vitalone, A., Syversen, T., & Soldin, O. P. (2004). Developmental neuropathology of environmental agents. *Annual Review of Pharmacology and Toxicology*, *44*(1), 87–110. doi:10.1146/annurev.pharmtox.44.101802.121424 PMID:14744240

Costopoulou, D., Vassiliadou, I., Papadopoulos, A., Makropoulos, V., & Leondiadis, L. (2006). Levels of dioxins, furans and PCBs in human serum and milk of people living in Greece. *Chemosphere*, *65*(9), 1462–1469. doi:10.1016/j.chemosphere.2006.04.034 PMID:16765419

Cowan, C. S. M., Hoban, A. E., Ventura-Silva, A. P., Dinan, T. G., Clarke, G., & Cryan, J. F. (2018). Gutsy Moves: The Amygdala as a Critical Node in Microbiota to Brain Signaling. *BioEssays*, 40. PMID:29148060

Crafa, D., & Warfa, N. (2015). Maternal migration and autism risk: Systematic analysis. *International Review of Psychiatry (Abingdon, England)*, *27*(1), 64–71. doi:10.3109/09540261.2014.995601 PMID:25738316

Crago, B. R., Gray, M. R., Nelson, L. A., Davis, M., Arnold, L., & Thrasher, J. D. (2003). Psychological, neuropsychological, and electrocortical effects of mixed mold exposure. *Archives of Environmental Health*, *58*(8), 452–463. doi:10.3200/AEOH.58.8.452-463 PMID:15259424

Crespo-López, M. E., De Sa, A. L., Herculano, A. M., Burbano, R. R., & do Nascimento, J. L. M. (2007). Methylmercury genotoxicity: A novel effect in human cell lines of the central nervous system. *Environment International*, *33*(2), 141–146. doi:10.1016/j.envint.2006.08.005 PMID:17007929

Csardi, G., & Nepusz, T. (2006). The igraph software package for complex network research. InterJournal. *Complex Systems*, *1695*, 1–9.

Cui, Y., Balshaw, D. M., Kwok, R. K., Thompson, C. L., Collman, G. W., & Birnbaum, L. S. (2016). The Exposome: Embracing the Complexity for Discovery in Environmental Health. *Environmental Health Perspectives*, *124*(8), A137–A140. doi:10.1289/EHP412 PMID:27479988

Cullen, W. R., McBride, B. C., & Reglinski, J. (1984). The reaction of methylarsenicals with thiols: Some biological implications. *Journal of Inorganic Biochemistry*, *21*(3), 179–194. doi:10.1016/0162-0134(84)83002-0 PMID:6392480

Cutts, B. B., Darby, K. J., Boone, C. G., & Brewis, A. (2009). City structure, obesity, and environmental justice: An integrated analysis of physical and social barriers to walkable streets and park access. *Social Science & Medicine*, *69*(9), 1314–1322. doi:10.1016/j.socscimed.2009.08.020 PMID:19751959

Cuzick, J., Evans, S., Gillman, M., & Evans, D. A. P. (1982). Medicinal arsenic and internal malignancies. *British Journal of Cancer*, *45*(6), 904–911. doi:10.1038/bjc.1982.143 PMID:6212076

Cycoń, M., Borymski, S., Żołnierczyk, B., & Piotrowska-Seget, Z. (2016). Variable effects of non-steroidal anti-inflammatory drugs (NSAIDs) on selected biochemical processes mediated by soil microorganisms. *Frontiers in Microbiology*, *7*, 1969. doi:10.3389/fmicb.2016.01969 PMID:28018307

D'Haenens, J. P., McDonald, K. W., Langley, R. L., Higgins, S. A., Scott, R., Farquhar, P. N., & Meggs, W. J. (2013). Aldicarb: A case series of watermelon-borne carbamate toxicity. *Journal of Agromedicine*, *18*(2), 174–177. doi:10.1080/1059924X.2013.766141 PMID:23540307

da Rocha, M. E. B., da Chagas, O. F., Maia, F. E. F., Guedes, M. I. F., & Rondina, D. (2014). Mycotoxins and their effects on human and animal health. *Food Control*, *36*(1), 159-165.

Dahl, R. (2012). To Label or Not to Label, Environmental Health Perspectives. *Environmental Health Perspectives*, *120*(9), 359–361. Retrieved from http://ehp.niehs.nih.gov/wp-content/uploads/2012/09/ehp.120-a358.pdf PMID:23487845

Dairy and Dairy Alternative Beverage Trends in the U.S. (2017). 4th ed.). Retrieved from https://www.packagedfacts.com/Dairy-Alternative-Beverage-Trends-Edition-11000293/

Dairy foods and cancer. (2015). Cancer Council NSW. Retrieved from https://www.cancercouncil.com.au/1958/cancer-prevention/diet-exercise/nutrition-diet/fruit-vegetables/dairy-foods-and-cancer/

Dairy Sustainable Agriculture. (2018). World Wildlife Fund. Retrieved from https://www.worldwildlife.org/industries/dairy

Dairy, N. Z. (n.d.). Dairy NZ. Retrieved from https://www.dairynz.co.nz/

Damalas, C. A., & Hashemi, S. M. (2010). Pesticide risk perception and use of personal protective equipment among young and old cotton growers in northern Greece. *Agrociencia*, *44*(3).

DaMatta, F., Grandis, A., Arenque, B., & Buckeridge, M. (2010). Impacts of climate changes on crop physiology and food quality. *Food Research International*, *43*(7), 1814–1823. doi:10.1016/j.foodres.2009.11.001

Danaee, H., Nelson, H. H., Liber, H., Little, J. B., & Kelsey, K. T. (2004). Low dose exposure to sodium arsenite synergistically interacts with UV radiation to induce mutations and alter DNA repair in human cells. *Mutagenesis*, *19*(2), 143–148. doi:10.1093/mutage/geh010 PMID:14981161

Darbre, P. D. (2018). Overview of air pollution and endocrine disorders. *International Journal of General Medicine*, *11*, 191–207. doi:10.2147/IJGM.S102230 PMID:29872334

Dartey, E., Sarpong, k., Darko, G., & Acheampong-Marfo, M. (2013). Urinary arsenic and mercury levels in artisanal miners in some communities in the Obuasi Municipality of Ghana. *Journal of Environmental Chemistry and Ecotoxicology*, *55*, 113–118.

Das, D., Chatterjee, A., Mandal, B. K., Samanta, G., Chakraborti, D., & Chanda, B. (1995). Arsenic in groundwater in six districts of West Bengal, India: The biggest arsenic calamity in the world. Part 2. Arsenic concentration in drinking water, hair, nails, urine, skin-scale and liver tissue (biopsy) of the affected people. *Analyst (London)*, *120*(3), 917–924. doi:10.1039/an9952000917 PMID:7741255

Das, D., Samanta, G., Mandal, B. K., Chowdhury, T. R., Chanda, C. R., Chowdhury, P. P., & ... . (1996). Arsenic in groundwater in six districts of West Bengal, India. *Environmental Geochemistry and Health*, *18*(1), 5–15. doi:10.1007/BF01757214 PMID:24194364

Das, H., Mitra, A., Sengupta, P., Hossain, A., Islam, F., & Rabbani, G. (2004). Arsenic concentrations in rice, vegetables, and fish in Bangladesh: A preliminary study. *Environment International*, *30*(3), 383–387. doi:10.1016/j.envint.2003.09.005 PMID:14987870

Das, S., Thomas, K. G., Thomas, K. J., Kamat, P. V., & George, M. V. (1994). Photochemistry of squaraine dyes. Photophysical properties of crown ether squaraine fluorophore and their metal ion complexes. *Journal of Physical Chemistry*, *98*(37), 9291–9296. doi:10.1021/j100088a033

Datta, D. V., & Kaul, M. K. (1976). Arsenic content of drinking water in villages in northern India. A concept of arsenicosis. *The Journal of the Association of Physicians of India*, *24*, 599–604. PMID:1025145

Daughton, C. G. (2003). Cradle-to-cradle stewardship of drugs for minimizing their environmental disposition while promoting human health. I. Rationale for and avenues toward a green pharmacy. *Environmental Health Perspectives*, *111*(5), 757–774. doi:10.1289/ehp.5947 PMID:12727606

Davila-Esqueda, M. E., Jimenez-Capdeville, M. E., Delgado, J. M., De la Cruz, E., Aradillas Garcia, C., Jimenez-Suarez, V., ... Llerenas, J. R. (2012). Effects of arsenic exposure during the pre- and postnatal development on the puberty of female offspring. *Experimental and Toxicologic Pathology*, *64*(1-2), 25–30. doi:10.1016/j.etp.2010.06.001 PMID:20580540

Davis, C. D., & Milner, J. (2004). Frontiers in nutrigenomics, proteomics, metabolomics and cancer prevention. *Mutation Research*, *551*(1-2), 51–64. doi:10.1016/j.mrfmmm.2004.01.012 PMID:15225581

De Bleecker, J., Willems, J., Van Den Neucker, K., De Reuck, J., & Vogelaers, D. (1992). Prolonged toxicity with intermediate syndrome after combined parathion and methyl parathion poisoning. *Journal of Toxicology. Clinical Toxicology, 30*(3), 333–345. doi:10.3109/15563659209021548 PMID:1512808

De Chaudhuri, S., Kundu, M., Banerjee, M., Das, J., Majumdar, P., Basu, S., ... Giri, A. (2008). Arsenic-induced health effects and genetic damage in keratotic individuals: Involvement of p53 arginine variant and chromosomal aberrations in arsenic susceptibility. *Mutation Research, 659*(1-2), 118–125. doi:10.1016/j.mrrev.2007.11.008 PMID:18249029

De Santis, B., Brera, C., Mezzelani, A., Soricelli, S., Ciceri, F., Moretti, G., ... & Raggi, M. E. (2019). Role of mycotoxins in the pathobiology of autism: A first evidence. Nutritional neuroscience, 22(2), 132-144. PMID:28795659

de Vendômois, J. S., Roullier, F., Cellier, D., & Séralini, G. E. (2009). A Comparison of the Effects of Three GM Corn Varieties on Mammalian Health. *International Journal of Biological Sciences, 5*(7), 706–726. doi:10.7150/ijbs.5.706 PMID:20011136

de Winter-Sorkina, R., & Cassee, F. R. (2002). *From concentration to dose: factors influencing airborne particulate matter deposition in humans and rats.* Bilthoven: RIVM National Institute for Public Health and the Environment.

Defarge, N., Spirouxde Vendômois, J., & Séralini, G. E. (2018). Toxicity of formulants and heavy metals in glyphosate-based herbicides and other pesticides. *Toxicology Reports, 5*, 156–163. doi:10.1016/j.toxrep.2017.12.025 PMID:29321978

DEFRA. (2006). Food security and the UK: An evidence and analysis paper. Department for Environment, Food and Rural Affairs, Food Chain Analysis Group, London, UK.

Delaney, B. (2015). Safety assessment of foods from genetically modified crops in countries with developing economies. *Food and Chemical Toxicology, 86*, 132–143. doi:10.1016/j.fct.2015.10.001 PMID:26456807

Delicious, S. (n.d.). So Delicious. Retrieved from http://sodeliciousdairyfree.com/

Dennis, K. K., Marder, E., Balshaw, D. M., Cui, Y., Lynes, M. A., Patti, G. J., ... Barr, D. B. (2017). Biomonitoring in the Era of the Exposome. *Environmental Health Perspectives, 125*(4), 502–510. doi:10.1289/EHP474 PMID:27385067

Department for International Development (DFID). (2011, September). *Scaling up nutrition: The UK's position paper on undernutrition.* London, UK: DFID. Retrieved from https://assets.publishing.service.gov.uk/government/uploads/system/uploads/attachment_data/file/67466/scal-up-nutr-uk-pos-undernutr.pdf

Desbiolles, F., Malleret, L., Tiliacos, C., Wong-Wah-Chung, P., & Laffont-Schwob, I. (2018). Occurrence and eco-toxicological assessment of pharmaceuticals: Is there a risk for the Mediterranean aquatic environment? *The Science of theTotal Environment, 639*, 1334-1348.

Deth, R., Muratore, C., Benzecry, J., Power-Charnitsky, V. A., & Waly, M. (2008). How environmental and genetic factors combine to cause autism: A redox/methylation hypothesis. *Neurotoxicology, 29*(1), 190–201. doi:10.1016/j.neuro.2007.09.010 PMID:18031821

Dewan, A., Bhatnagar, V. K., Mathur, M. L., Chakma, T., Kashyap, R., Sadhu, H. G., ... Saiyed, H. N. (2004). Repeated episodes of endosulfan poisoning. *Journal of Toxicology. Clinical Toxicology, 42*(4), 363–369. doi:10.1081/CLT-120039542 PMID:15461244

Deziel, N. (2014). Pharmaceuticals in wastewater treatment plant effluent waters," *Scholarly Horizons: University of Minnesota, Morris Undergraduate Journal, 1*(2).

Dhar, R. K., Biswas, B. K., Samanta, G., Mandal, B. K., Chakraborti, D., Roy, S., ... & Khan, A. W. (1997). Groundwater arsenic calamity in Bangladesh. *Current Science, 73*, 48.

Díaz, J., Jordan, A., García, R., López, C., Alberdi, J., Hernández, E., & Otero, A. (2002). Heat waves in Madrid 1986–1997: Effects on the health of the elderly. *International Archives of Occupational and Environmental Health*, *75*(3), 163–170. doi:10.100700420-001-0290-4 PMID:11954983

Dich, J., & Wiklund, K. (1998). Prostate cancer in pesticide applicators in Swedish agriculture. *The Prostate*, *34*(2), 100–112. doi:10.1002/(SICI)1097-0045(19980201)34:2<100::AID-PROS4>3.0.CO;2-O PMID:9465941

Diels, J., Cunha, M., Manaia, C., Sabugosa-Madeira, B., & Silva, M. (2011). Association of financial or professional conflict of interest to research outcomes on health risks or nutritional assessment studies of genetically modified products. *Food Policy*, *36*(2), 197–203. doi:10.1016/j.foodpol.2010.11.016

Diet, nutrition and the prevention of chronic diseases. (2003). World Health Organization. Retrieved from http://www.who.int/dietphysicalactivity/publications/trs916/en/

Dill, G. M., Sammons, R. D., Feng, P. C., Kohn, F., Kretzmer, K., Mehrsheikh, A., ... Haupfear, E. A. (2010). Glyphosate: discovery, development, applications, and properties. Glyphosate resistance in crops and weeds: history, development, and management, 1-33.

Dixit, S., & Hering, J. G. (2003). Comparison of arsenic V and arsenic III sorption onto iron oxides minerals: implications for arsenic mobility: environmental science and technology. *Environmental Science & Technology*, *37*, 4182–4189. doi:10.1021/es030309t PMID:14524451

Doebler, J. A., Martin, L. J., Morse, J. D., Ballough, G. P., Strauss, J. A., & Anthony, A. (1992). Mesenteric mast cell degranulation in acute T-2 toxin poisoning. *Toxicology Letters*, *62*(1), 33–38. doi:10.1016/0378-4274(92)90075-U PMID:1509504

Doi, K., & Uetsuka, K. (2011). Mechanisms of mycotoxin-induced neurotoxicity through oxidative stress-associated pathways. *International Journal of Molecular Sciences*, *12*(8), 5213–5237. doi:10.3390/ijms12085213 PMID:21954354

Domingo, J. L. (2000). Health risks of GM foods: Many opinions but few data. *Science*, *288*(5472), 1748–1749. doi:10.1126cience.288.5472.1748 PMID:10877692

Domingo, J. L. (2007). Toxicity studies of genetically modified plants: A review of the published literature. *Critical Reviews in Food Science and Nutrition*, *47*(8), 721–733. doi:10.1080/10408390601177670 PMID:17987446

Domingo, J. L. (2011). Human health effects of genetically modified (GM) plants: Risk and perception. *Human and Ecological Risk Assessment*, *17*(3), 535–537. doi:10.1080/10807039.2011.571065

Domingo, J. L. (2016). Safety assessment of GM plants: An updated review of the scientific literature. *Food and Chemical Toxicology*, *95*, 12–18. doi:10.1016/j.fct.2016.06.013 PMID:27317828

Domingo, J. L., & Bordonaba, J. G. (2011). A literature review on the safety assessment of genetically modified plants. *Environment International*, *37*(4), 734–742. doi:10.1016/j.envint.2011.01.003 PMID:21296423

Domingo, J. L., & Gomez, M. (2000). Health risks of genetically modified foods: A literature review. *Revista Espanola de Salud Publica*, *74*, 255–261. PMID:10918812

Dominiak, A., Wilkaniec, A., Wroczynski, P., & Adamczyk, A. (2016). Selenium in the Therapy of Neurological Diseases. Where is it Going? *Current Neuropharmacology*, *14*, 282–299. doi:10.2174/1570159X14666151223100011 PMID:26549649

Donelan, J., Boucher, W., Papadopoulou, N., Lytinas, M., Papaliodis, D., & Theoharides, T. C. (2006). Corticotropin-releasing hormone induces skin vascular permeability through a neurotensin-dependent process. *Proceedings of the National Academy of Sciences of the United States of America*, *103*(20), 7759–7764. doi:10.1073/pnas.0602210103 PMID:16682628

Dong, Z., Yuan, G., & Hu, J. (2016). Uncertainty analysis in 2,3,7,8-tetrachlorodibenzo-p-dioxin (TCDD) cancer dose-response for three occupational cohorts. *Environment International*, *88*, 53–59. doi:10.1016/j.envint.2015.12.010 PMID:26708281

Donselaar, M. E., Bhatt, A. G., Bose, N., Bruining, J., & Ghosh, A. K. Entrapment of Arsenic Contaminated Groundwater in Point Bars: Case Study of Holocene Ganges River deposits, Bihar, India. In *Proceedings of 10th International Conference on Fluvial Sedimentology*, University of Leeds, UK.

Dotson, G. S., Maier, A., Siegel, P. D., Anderson, S. E., Green, B. J., Stefaniak, A. B., ... Kimber, I. (2015). Setting occupational exposure limits for chemical allergens—Understanding the challenges. *Journal of Occupational and Environmental Hygiene, 12*(sup1), S82-S98. doi:10.1093/acprof:oso/9780198509851.001.0001

Dotson, G. S., Maier, A., Siegel, P. D., Anderson, S. E., Green, B. J., Stefaniak, A. B., ... Kimber, I. (2015). Setting occupational exposure limits for chemical allergens—Understanding the challenges. *Journal of Occupational and Environmental Hygiene*, *12*(Suppl. 1), S82–S98.

Dowling, K. C., Costella, R. G., & Lemley, A. T. (2018). Modeling the Movement of a Rapidly Degrading Solute, Methomyl, in Dynamic Soil-Water Systems. *Mechanisms Of Pesticide Movement Into Ground Water, 101*.

Dream. (2018). Rice Dream. Retrieved from http://www.dreamplantbased.com/product/rice-dream-classic-original-organic-rice-drink/

Drinking Water –Specification (2nd Rev.). (2012). New Delhi. *Bureau of Indian Standards IS, 10500*, 2012.

Dujols, V., Ford, F., & Czarnik, A. W. (1997). A Long-Wavelength Fluorescent Chemodosimeter Selective for Cu(II) Ion in Water. *Journal of the American Chemical Society*, *119*(31), 7386–7387. doi:10.1021/ja971221g

Dumitrescu, E. I., & Hurlin, C. (2012). Testing for Granger non-causality in heterogeneous panels. *Economic Modelling*, *29*(4), 1450–1460. doi:10.1016/j.econmod.2012.02.014

DuPuis, E. M. (2002). Natures perfect food: How milk became Americas drink. New York: New York University Press.

Duval, B. D., Dijkstra, P., Natali, S. M., Megonigal, J. P., Ketterer, M. E., Drake, B. G., ... Hungate, B. A. (2011). Plant-soil distribution of potentially toxic elements in response to elevated atmospheric CO_2. *Environmental Science & Technology*, *45*(7), 2570–2574. doi:10.1021/es102250u PMID:21405117

E3 – Sustainable Grown Cotton. (2018). Retrieved from https://www.e3cotton.us/

EAA. (2015). Air Quality in Europe – *2015 Report*. Retrieved from https://www.eea.europa.eu/publications/air-quality-in-europe-2015

Edvinsson, L., Cervos-Navarro, J., Larsson, L. I., Owman, C., & Ronnberg, A. L. (1977). Regional distribution of mast cells containing histamine, dopamine or 5-hydroxytryptamine in the mammalian brain. *Neurology*, *27*(9), 878–884. doi:10.1212/WNL.27.9.878 PMID:408735

EFSA (European Food Safety Authority) Panel on Contaminants in the Food Chain. (2009). Scientific opinion on arsenic in food. *EFSA Journal*, *7*(10), 1351. doi:10.2903/j.efsa.2009.1351

Ehrlich, D. E., & Rainnie, D. G. (2015). Prenatal Stress Alters the Development of Socioemotional Behavior and Amygdala Neuron Excitability in Rats. *Neuropsychopharmacology*, *40*(9), 2135–2145. doi:10.1038/npp.2015.55 PMID:25716930

Eleršek, T., Milavec, S., Korošec, M., Brezovšek, P., Negreira, N., Zonja, B., ... Filipič, M. (2016). Toxicity of the mixture of selected antineoplastic drugs against aquatic primary producers and their behaviour under the applied exposure conditions. *Environmental Science and Pollution Research International*, *23*(15), 14780–14790. doi:10.100711356-015-6005-2 PMID:26755176

Ellis, J., Athersuch, T., Thomas, L., Teichert, F., Perez-Trujillo, M., Svendsen, C., ... Keun, H. C. (2012). Metabolic profiling detects early effects of environmental and lifestyle exposure to cadmium in a human population. *BMC Medicine*, *10*(1), 61. doi:10.1186/1741-7015-10-61 PMID:22713677

Emanuele, E. (2014). Can trehalose prevent neurodegeneration? Insights from experimental studies. *Current Drug Targets*, *15*(5), 551–557. doi:10.2174/1389450115666140225104705 PMID:24568549

Emirmahmutoglu, F., & Kose, N. (2011). Testing for granger causality in heterogeneous mixed panels. *Economic Modelling*, *28*(3), 870–876. doi:10.1016/j.econmod.2010.10.018

Emond, C., DeVito, M., Warner, M., Eskenazi, B., Mocarelli, P., & Birnbaum, L. S. (2016). An assessment of dioxin exposure across gestation and lactation using a PBPK model and new data from Seveso. *Environment International*, *92-93*, 23–32. doi:10.1016/j.envint.2016.03.015 PMID:27045706

Engel, R. R., Hopenhayn-Rich, C., Receveur, O., & Smith, A. H. (1994). Vascular effects of chronic arsenic exposure: A review. *Epidemiologic Reviews*, *16*(2), 184–209. doi:10.1093/oxfordjournals.epirev.a036150 PMID:7713176

Entine, J., & Wendel, J. (2013). 2000+ Reasons Why GMOs Are Safe to Eat and Environmentally Sustainable. *Forbes*. Retrieved from http://www.forbes.com/sites/jonentine/2013/10/14/2000-reasons-why-gmos-are-safe-to-eat-and-environmentally-sustainable

Environmental Protection Agency (EPA). (2017, December 12). *Office of Pesticide Programs, Revised Glyphosate Issue Paper: Evaluation of Carcinogenic Potential*. Author.

Environmental Protection Agency. Managing Pharmaceutical Waste: A 10-Step Blueprint for Healthcare Facilities in the United States, *U.S. Environmental Protection Agency*. Retrieved from http://www.hercenter.org/hazmat/tenstepblueprint.pdf

Epstein, P. R. (2001). Climate change and emerging infectious diseases. *Microbes and Infection*, *3*(9), 747–754. doi:10.1016/S1286-4579(01)01429-0 PMID:11489423

Erbs, M., Manderscheid, R., Jansen, G., Seddig, S., Pacholski, A., & Weigela, H. (2010). Effects of free-air CO_2 enrichment and nitrogen supply on grain quality parameters and elemental composition of wheat and barley grown in a crop rotation. *Agriculture, Ecosystems & Environment*, *136*(1-2), 59–68. doi:10.1016/j.agee.2009.11.009

Escher, B. I., Hackermüller, J., Polte, T., Scholz, S., Aigner, A., Altenburger, R., ... Wambaugh, J. F. (2017). From the exposome to mechanistic understanding of chemical-induced adverse effects. *Environment International*, *99*, 97–106. doi:10.1016/j.envint.2016.11.029 PMID:27939949

Esposito, P., Chandler, N., Kandere, K., Basu, S., Jacobson, S., Connolly, R., ... & Theoharides, T. C. (2002). Corticotropin-releasing hormone and brain mast cells regulate blood-brain-barrier permeability induced by acute stress. Journal of Pharmacology and Experimental Therapeutics, 303(3), 1061-1066. doi:10.1124/jpet.102.038497 PMID:12438528

Esquinas-Alcázar, J. (2005). Protecting crop genetic diversity for food security: Political, ethical and technical challenges. *Nature Reviews. Genetics*, *6*(12), 946–953. doi:10.1038/nrg1729 PMID:16341075

Etzel, R. A. (2002). Mycotoxins. *Journal of the American Medical Association*, *287*(4), 425–427. doi:10.1001/jama.287.4.425 PMID:11798344

European Chemicals Agency. (2012). *The status of industrial vegetable oils from genetically modified plants*. Retrieved from https://echa.europa.eu/documents/10162/22816103/the_status_of_industrial_vegetable_oils_from_genetically_modified_plants_expert_report_en.pdf/e6b0de1b-c9d5-4e07-8fc6-8f4dae318c55

European Environment Agency. (2013). *Environment and human health*. EEA Report No 5/2013. doi:10.2800/9092

European Food Safety Authority (EFSA). (2015). Conclusion on the peer review of the pesticide risk assessment of the active substance glyphosate. *EFSA Journal*, *13*(11), 4302.

European Union. (1997). EU 97/618/EC. Commission Recommendations 29 July 1997 concerning the scientific aspects and the presentation of information necessary to support applications for the placing on the market of novel foods and novel food ingredients and the preparation of initial assessment reports under Regulation EC 259/97 of the European Parliament and of the Council. *Official Journal of the European Communities*.

Everitt, B. S., Landau, S., Leese, M., & Stahl, D. (2011). *Cluster analysis* (5th ed.). United Kingdom: John Wiley & Sons, Ltd. doi:10.1002/9780470977811

Extension Toxicology Network. (2003). Exotoxnet—A Pesticide Information Project. U.S. Department of Agriculture, Extension Service, and the National Agricultural Pesticide Impact Assessment Program.

Eyer, F., Meischner, V., Kiderlen, D., Thiermann, H., Worek, F., Haberkorn, M., ... Eyer, P. (2003). Human parathion poisoning. *Toxicological Reviews*, *22*(3), 143–163. doi:10.2165/00139709-200322030-00003 PMID:15181664

Fanzo, J. (2014). Strengthening the engagement of food and health systems to improve nutrition security: Synthesis and overview of approaches to address nutrition. *Global Food Security*, *3*(3-4), 183–192. doi:10.1016/j.gfs.2014.09.001

Fanzo, J. (2015). Ethical issues for human nutrition in the context of global food security and sustainable development. *Global Food Security*, *7*, 15–23. doi:10.1016/j.gfs.2015.11.001

FAO/WHO. (1996). *Biotechnology and Food Safety. Report of a Joint.* FAO/WHO consultation, Rome, Italy, 1996. Retrieved from ftp://ftp.fao.org/es/esn/food/biotechnology.pdf

FAO/WHO. (2000). *Safety Aspects of Genetically Modified Foods of Plant Origin.* Report of a Joint FAO/WHO Expert Consultation on Foods Derived from Biotechnology, Geneva, Switzerland, 2000, Food and Agriculture Organisation of the United Nations, Rome. Retrieved from ftp://ftp.fao.org/es/esn/food/gmreport.pdf

FAO/WHO. (2001). *Allergenicity of Genetically Modified Foods. Report of a Joint FAO/WHO Expert Consultation on Foods Derived from Biotechnology.* Rome, 2001, Food and Agriculture Organisation of the United Nations, Rome. Retrieved from http://www.who.int/fsf/Documents/Biotech_Consult_Jan2001/report20.pdf

FAO/WHO. (2002). *Report of the Third Session of the Codex Ad Hoc Intergovernmental Task Force on Foods Derived from Biotechnology (ALINORM 01/34).* Codex Ad Hoc Intergovernmental Task Force on Foods Derived from Biotechnology, Food and Agriculture Organisation of the United Nations, Rome. Retrieved from ftp://ftp.fao.org/codex/alinorm03/Al03_34e.pdf

Farmer, T. D., Shaw, P. J., & Williams, I. D. (2015). Destined for indecision? A critical analysis of waste management practices in England from 1996 to 2013. *Waste Management (New York, N.Y.)*, *39*, 266–276. doi:10.1016/j.wasman.2015.02.023 PMID:25771762

Faro, L., do Nascimento, J., Campos, F., Vidal, L., Alfonso, M., & Durán, R. (2005). Protective effects of glutathione and cysteine on the methylmercury-induced striatal dopamine release in vivo. *Life Sciences*, *77*(4), 444–451. doi:10.1016/j.lfs.2004.11.033 PMID:15894013

Federal Environment Agency. (2013). *Pharmaceuticals in the Environment – A first Compilation of German Monitoring Data*. Retrieved from www.umweltbundesamt.de/sites/default/files/medien/377/dokumente/compilation-pharmaceuticalsintheenvironment_uba.pdf

Feinberg, A. P., & Tycko, B. (2004). The history of cancer epigenetics. *Nature Reviews. Cancer*, *4*(2), 143–153. doi:10.1038/nrc1279 PMID:14732866

Feinberg, J. I., Bakulski, K. M., Jaffe, A. E., Tryggvadottir, R., Brown, S. C., Goldman, L. R., ... Feinberg, A. P. (2015). Paternal sperm DNA methylation associated with early signs of autism risk in an autism-enriched cohort. *International Journal of Epidemiology*, *44*(4), 1199–1210. doi:10.1093/ije/dyv028 PMID:25878217

Felis, E., Marciocha, D., Surmacz-Gorska, J., & Miksch, K. (2007). Photochemical degradation of naproxen in the aquatic environment. *Water Science and Technology*, *55*(12), 281–286. doi:10.2166/wst.2007.417 PMID:17674860

Felis, E., & Miksch, K. (2007). Removal of analgesic drugs from the aquatic environment using photochemical methods. *Water Science and Technology*, *60*(9), 2253–2259. doi:10.2166/wst.2009.668 PMID:19901456

Ferguson, B. J., Marler, S., Altstein, L. L., Lee, E. B., Mazurek, M. O., McLaughlin, A., ... Beversdorf, D. Q. (2016). Associations between cytokines, endocrine stress response, and gastrointestinal symptoms in autism spectrum disorder. *Brain, Behavior, and Immunity*, *58*, 57–62. doi:10.1016/j.bbi.2016.05.009 PMID:27181180

Fernandez-Cornejo, J., & Caswell, M. (2006). The first Decade of Genetically Engineered Crops in the United States. *USDA ERS Economic Bulletin*. Retrieved from http://www.ers.usda.gov/publications/eib11/eib11.pdf

Fernando, Panozzo, J., Tausz, M., Norton, R., Fitzgerald, G., & Seneweera, S. (2012). Rising atmospheric CO_2 concentration affects mineral content and protein concentration of wheat grain. *Food Chemistry*, *133*(4), 1307–1311. doi:10.1016/j.foodchem.2012.01.105

Fernando, S., Jobst, K. J., Taguchi, V. Y., Helm, P. A., Reiner, E. J., & McCarry, B. E. (2014). Identification of the halogenated compounds resulting from the 1997 Plastimet Inc. fire in Hamilton, Ontario, using comprehensive two-dimensional gas chromatography and (ultra)high resolution mass spectrometry. *Environmental Science & Technology*, *48*(18), 10656–10663. doi:10.1021/es503428j PMID:25133985

Fillol, C., Dor, F., Labat, L., Boltz, P., Bouard, J. L., Mantey, K., ... Seta, N. (2010). Urinary arsenic concentrations and speciation in residents living in an area with naturally contaminated soils. *The Science of the Total Environment*, *408*(5), 1190–1194. doi:10.1016/j.scitotenv.2009.11.046 PMID:20004003

Fiorentino, M., Sapone, A., Senger, S., Camhi, S. S., Kadzielski, S. M., Buie, T. M., ... Fasano, A. (2016). Blood-brain barrier and intestinal epithelial barrier alterations in autism spectrum disorders. *Molecular Autism*, *7*(1), 49. doi:10.118613229-016-0110-z PMID:27957319

Fisher, A. T., López-Carrillo, L., Gamboa-Loira, B., & Cebrián, M. E. (2017). Standards for arsenic in drinking water: Implications for policy in Mexico. *Journal of Public Health Policy*, *38*(4), 395–406. doi:10.105741271-017-0087-7 PMID:28808298

Fisher, R. A. (1936). The use of multiple measurements in taxonomic problems. *Annals of Human Genetics*, *7*(2), 179–188.

Fitzpatrick, T. B. E. A., Wolff, K., & Freedberg, I. M. & Austen, K.F. (1993). Dermatology in General Medicine. New York: McGraw Hill.

Fog, N. K. (2003). Mycotoxin production by indoor molds. *Fungal Genetics and Biology*, *39*(2), 103–117. doi:10.1016/S1087-1845(03)00026-4 PMID:12781669

Fombonne, E. (2009). Epidemiology of pervasive developmental disorders. *Pediatric Research*, *65*(6), 591–598. doi:10.1203/PDR.0b013e31819e7203 PMID:19218885

Fontes, E. M. G., Pires, C. S. S., Sujii, E. R., & Panizzi, A. R. (2002). The environmental effects of genetically modified crops resistant to insects. *Neotropical Entomology*, *31*(4), 497–513. doi:10.1590/S1519-566X2002000400001

Food and Agricultural Organization (FAO). (1983). *World food security: A reappraisal of the concepts and approaches* [Director General's Report]. Rome, Italy: FAO.

Food and Agricultural Organization (FAO). (1996). *Rome declaration on world food security*. Rome, Italy: World Food Summit.

Forastiere, F., Stafoggia, M., Tasco, C., Picciotto, S., Agabiti, N., Cesaroni, G., & Perucci, C. A. (2007). Socioeconomic status, particulate air pollution, and daily mortality: Differential exposure or differential susceptibility. *American Journal of Industrial Medicine*, *50*(3), 208–216. doi:10.1002/ajim.20368 PMID:16847936

Forgacs, A. L., Kent, M. N., Makley, M. K., Mets, B., DelRaso, N., Jahns, G. L., ... Reo, N. V. (2012). Comparative metabolomic and genomic analyses of TCDD-elicited metabolic disruption in mouse and rat liver. *Toxicological Sciences*, *125*(1), 41–55. doi:10.1093/toxsci/kfr262 PMID:21964420

Foster, H. R., Burton, G. A., Basu, N., & Werner, E. E. (2010). Chronic exposure to fluoxetine (Prozac) causes developmental delays in Rana pipiens larvae. *Environmental Toxicology and Chemistry*, *29*(12), 2845–2850. doi:10.1002/etc.345 PMID:20836066

Foucart, S. & Horel, S. (2017). Monsanto papers: Les agencies sous l'influence de la firm. *La Monde*.

Frank, M. G., Weber, M. D., Watkins, L. R., & Maier, S. F. (2016). Stress-induced neuroinflammatory priming: A liability factor in the etiology of psychiatric disorders. *Neurobiology of Stress*, *4*, 62–70. doi:10.1016/j.ynstr.2015.12.004 PMID:27981190

Frewer, L. J., & Shepherd, R. (1995). Ethical concerns and risk perceptions associated with different applications of genetic engineering: Interrelationships with the perceived need for regulation of the technology. *Agriculture and Human Values*, *12*(1), 48–57. doi:10.1007/BF02218074

Fromme, H., Gareis, M., Volkel, W., & Gottschalk, C. (2016). Overall internal exposure to mycotoxins and their occurrence in occupational and residential settings--An overview. *International Journal of Hygiene and Environmental Health*, *219*(2), 143–165. doi:10.1016/j.ijheh.2015.11.004 PMID:26725999

Fuhrman, J. (2011). *Eat to live: The amazing nutrient-rich program for fast and sustained weight loss*. Little and Brown.

Fuhrman, J. (2015). *The end of dieting: How to live for life*. HarperOne.

Gabriel, H. E., Crott, J. W., Ghandour, H., Dallal, G. E., Choi, S. W., Keyes, M. K., ... Mason, J. B. (2006). Chronic cigarette smoking is associated with diminished folate status, altered folate form distribution, and increased genetic damage in the buccal mucosa of healthy adults. *The American Journal of Clinical Nutrition*, *83*(4), 835–841. doi:10.1093/ajcn/83.4.835 PMID:16600936

Gaffron, P. (2012). Urban transport, environmental justice and human daily activity patterns. *Transport Policy*, *20*, 114–127. doi:10.1016/j.tranpol.2012.01.011

Gailer, J. (2007). Arsenic–selenium and mercury–selenium bonds in biology. *Coordination Chemistry Reviews*, *251*(1-2), 234–254. doi:10.1016/j.ccr.2006.07.018

Gailer, J. (2009). Chronic toxicity of As III in mammals: The role of (GS) 2 AsSe−. *Biochimie*, *91*(10), 1268–1272. doi:10.1016/j.biochi.2009.06.004 PMID:19539009

Gajski, G., Gerić, M., Žegura, B., Novak, M., Nunić, J., Bajrektarević, D., ... & Filipič, M. (2016). Genotoxic potential of selected cytostatic drugs in zebrafish liver cell line, human hepatoma HepG2 cells and human lymphocytes. *Environmental Science and Pollution Research International*, *23*(15), 14739–14750. doi:10.100711356-015-4592-6 PMID:25943512

Gamble, M. V., Liu, X., Slavkovich, V., Pilsner, J. R., Ilievski, V., Factor-Litvak, P., ... Graziano, J. H. (2007). Folic acid supplementation lowers blood arsenic. *The American Journal of Clinical Nutrition*, *86*(4), 1202–1209. doi:10.1093/ajcn/86.4.1202 PMID:17921403

Gangwang, G., Liu, G., Liu, H., Zhang, N., & Wang, Y. (2012). Photodegradation of salicylic acid in aquatic environment: effect of different forms of nitrogen. *The Science of the Total Environment, 435-436*, 573-577.

Garai, R., Chakraborty, A. K., Dey, S. B., & Saha, K. C. (1984). Chronic arsenic poisoning from tube-well water. *Journal of the Indian Medical Association*, *82*, 34–35. PMID:6747321

Garry, V. F. (2004). Pesticides and children. *Toxicology and Applied Pharmacology*, *198*(2), 152–163. doi:10.1016/j.taap.2003.11.027 PMID:15236951

Garzanti, E., Vezzoli, G., Ando, S., France-Lanord, C., Singh, S. K., & Foster, G. (2004). Sand Petrology and focused erosion in collision orogens: The Brahmaputra case. *Earth and Planetary Science Letters*, *220*(1-2), 157–174. doi:10.1016/S0012-821X(04)00035-4

Garzillo, C., Pugliese, M., Loffredo, F., & Quarto, M. (2017). Indoor radon exposure and lung cancer risk: A meta-analysis of case-control studies. *Translational Cancer Research*, *6*(Supplement 5), S934–S943. doi:10.21037/tcr.2017.05.42

Gbaruko, B. C., Ogwo, E. I., Igwe, J. C., & Yu, H. (2009). Organophosphate induced chronic neurotoxicity: Health, environmental and risk exposure issues in developing nations of the world. *African Journal of Biotechnology*, *8*(20).

Georgin-Lavialle, S., Gaillard, R., Moura, D., & Hermine, O. (2016). Mastocytosis in adulthood and neuropsychiatric disorders. *Translational Research; the Journal of Laboratory and Clinical Medicine*, *174*, 77–85.

Georgin-Lavialle, S., Moura, D. S., Salvador, A., Chauvet-Gelinier, J. C., Launay, J. M., Damaj, G., ... Gaillard, R. (2016b). Mast cells' involvement in inflammation pathways linked to depression: Evidence in mastocytosis. *Molecular Psychiatry*, *21*(11), 1511–1516. doi:10.1038/mp.2015.216 PMID:26809839

Gerhardt, R. E. (1980). Moonshine-related arsenic poisoning. *Archives of Internal Medicine*, *140*(2), 211–213. doi:10.1001/archinte.1980.00330140069020 PMID:7352816

Geschwind, D. H., & State, M. W. (2015). Gene hunting in autism spectrum disorder: On the path to precision medicine. *Lancet Neurology*, *11*(11), 1109–1120. doi:10.1016/S1474-4422(15)00044-7 PMID:25891009

Ghai, D., & Vivian, J. M. (2014). *Grassroots environmental action: people's participation in sustainable development.* Routledge.

Ghosh, D., & Bhadury, P. (2018). Microbial Cycling of Arsenic in the Aquifers of Bengal Delta Plains (BDP). In T. K. Adhya, B. Lal, B. Mohapatra, D. Paul, & S. Das (Eds.), *Advances in Soil Microbiology: Recent Trends and Future Prospects* (pp. 91–108). Springer Singapore. doi:10.1007/978-981-10-6178-3_5

Ghosh, D., Bhadury, P., & Routh, J. (2014). Diversity of arsenite oxidizing bacterial communities in arsenic-rich deltaic aquifers in West Bengal, India. *Frontiers in Microbiology*, *5*, 602. doi:10.3389/fmicb.2014.00602 PMID:25484877

Ghosh, D., Bhadury, P., & Routh, J. (2018). Coping with arsenic stress: Adaptations of arsenite-oxidizing bacterial membrane lipids to increasing arsenic levels. *MicrobiologyOpen*, 594. PMID:29577673

Ghosh, D., Routh, J., & Bhadury, P. (2015a). Characterization and microbial utilization of dissolved lipid organic fraction in arsenic impacted aquifers (India). *Journal of Hydrology (Amsterdam)*, *527*, 221–233. doi:10.1016/j.jhydrol.2015.04.051

Ghosh, D., Routh, J., & Bhadury, P. (2017). Sub-surface biogeochemical characteristics and its effect on arsenic cycling in the Holocene grey sand aquifers of the Lower Bengal Basin. *Frontiers in Environmental Science*, *5*, 82. doi:10.3389/fenvs.2017.00082

Ghosh, D., Routh, J., Därio, M., & Bhadury, P. (2015b). Elemental and biomarker characteristics in a Pleistocene aquifer vulnerable to arsenic contamination in the Bengal Delta Plain, India. *Applied Geochemistry*, *61*, 87–98. doi:10.1016/j.apgeochem.2015.05.007

Ghosh, S. K., Bandyopadhyay, D., Bandyopadhyay, S. K., & Debbarma, K. (2013). Cutaneous malignant and premalignant conditions caused by chronic arsenicosis from contaminated ground water consumption: A profile of patients from eastern India. *Skinmed*, *11*(4), 211–216. PMID:24053006

Ghosh, S., & De, S. (1995). Sources of arseniferous sediments at Kauchua and Itina, Habra Block, North-24 Paragans, West Bengal, a case study. *Journal of Earth Science*, *22*, 183–189.

Gillam, C. (2017a, August 18). Collusion or coincidence? records show EPA efforts to slow herbicide review came in coordination with Monsanto. *Huffington Post*. Retrieved from https://www.huffingtonpost.com/entry/collusion-or-coincidence-records-show-epa-efforts_us_5994dad4e4b056a2b0ef02f1

Gillam, C. (2017). *Whitewash*. Washington, DC: Island Press. doi:10.5822/978-1-61091-833-6

Gillispie, E. C., Sowers, T. D., Duckworth, O. W., & Polizzotto, M. L. (2015). Soil Pollution Due to Irrigation with Arsenic-Contaminated Groundwater: Current State of Science. *Current Pollution Reports*, *1*(1), 1–12. doi:10.100740726-015-0001-5

Gilmore, T. D. (2006). Introduction to NF-κB: Players, pathways, perspectives. *Oncogene*, *51*(51), 6680–6684. doi:10.1038j.onc.1209954 PMID:17072321

Girolamo, F., Coppola, C., & Ribatti, D. (2017). Immunoregulatory effect of mast cells influenced by microbes in neurodegenerative diseases. *Brain, Behavior, and Immunity*, *65*, 68–89. doi:10.1016/j.bbi.2017.06.017 PMID:28676349

GlaxoSmithKline. (2016). *GSK Public policy positions: Pharmaceuticals in the environment*. US: GlaxoSmithKline Communications and Government Affairs.

Gleadow, R., Evans, J. R., McCaffery, S., & Cavagnaro, T. R. (2009). Growth and nutritive value of cassava are reduced when grown in elevated CO_2. *Plant Biology*, *11*(1), 76–82.

Glin, L. J., Kuiseau, J., Thiam, A., Vodouhé, D. S., Dinham, B., & Ferrigno, S. (2006). *Living with Poison: Problems of Endosulfan in West Africa cotton growing systems*. London: PAN UK.

Global Dairy Market Briefing 2018 - Milk and Butter, Cheese, Dry, Condensed, and Evaporated Dairy Product, Ice Cream and Frozen Dessert. (2018, January 22). *Business Wire*. Retrieved from https://www.businesswire.com/news/home/20180122006338/en/Global-Dairy-Market-Briefing-2018---Milk

GLOBOCAN. (2012). v1.0, cancer incidence and mortality worldwide: IARC CancerBase No. 11. International Agency for Research on Cancer Web site. Retrieved from http://globocan.iarc.fr

Godfray, H. C. J., Crute, I. R., Lawrence, D., Pretty, J. N., Thomas, S. M., Beddington, J. R., ... Toulmin, C. (2010). Food security: The challenge of feeding 9 billion people. *Science*, *327*(5967), 812–818. doi:10.1126cience.1185383 PMID:20110467

Godoy, A. A., Kummrow, F., & Pamplin, P. A. (2015a). Occurrence, ecotoxicological effects and risk assessment of antihypertensive pharmaceutical residues in the aquatic environment--A review. *Chemosphere*, *138*, 281–291. doi:10.1016/j.chemosphere.2015.06.024 PMID:26091869

Godoy, A. A., Kummrow, F., & Pamplin, P. A. (2015b). Ecotoxicological evaluation of propranolol hydrochloride and losartan potassium to Lemna minor L. (1753) individually and in binary mixtures. *Ecotoxicology (London, England)*, *24*(5), 1112–1123. doi:10.100710646-015-1455-3 PMID:25847105

Goff, H., & Griffiths, M. (2006). Major advances in fresh milk and milk products: Fluid milk products and frozen desserts. *Journal of Dairy Science*, *89*(4), 1163–1173. doi:10.3168/jds.S0022-0302(06)72185-3 PMID:16537949

Goldschmidt, R. C., Hough, L. B., Glick, S. D., & Padawer, J. (1984). Mast cells in rat thalamus: Nuclear localization, sex difference and left-right asymmetry. *Brain Research*, *323*(2), 209–217. doi:10.1016/0006-8993(84)90291-9 PMID:6084538

Gómez-Fernández, J., Tomás, C., Carrasco, J. A., Sánchez-Sánchez, R., González-Bulnes, A., Gómez-Izquierdo, E., & de Mercado, E. (2015). Use of "ChemSensor" as an early discrimination tool of Iberian pig semen according to their freezability. *ITEA*, *111*(1), 34–49.

Good Groceries Company. (n.d.) Suzie's Quinoa Milk. Retrieved from http://www.goodgroceries.com/quinoa-milk/

Gordon, W. A., Cantor, J. B., Johanning, E., Charatz, H. J., Ashman, T. A., Breeze, J. L., ... Abramowitz, S. (2004). Cognitive impairment associated with toxigenic fungal exposure: A replication and extension of previous findings. *Applied Neuropsychology*, *11*(2), 65–74. doi:10.120715324826an1102_1 PMID:15477176

Gore, A. C., Chappell, V. A., Fenton, S. E., Flaws, J. A., Nadal, A., Prins, G. S., ... Zoeller, R. T. (2015). Executive Summary to EDC-2: The Endocrine Society's Second Scientific Statement on Endocrine-Disrupting Chemicals. *Endocrine Reviews*, *36*(6), 593–602. doi:10.1210/er.2015-1093 PMID:26414233

Gorny, R. L., Reponen, T., Willeke, K., Schmechel, D., Robine, E., Boissier, M., & Grinshpun, S. A. (2002). Fungal fragments as indoor air biocontaminants. *Applied and Environmental Microbiology*, *68*(7), 3522–3531. doi:10.1128/AEM.68.7.3522-3531.2002 PMID:12089037

Gouveia, N. (2016). Addressing Environmental Health Inequalities. *International Journal of Environmental Research and Public Health*, *13*(9), 858. doi:10.3390/ijerph13090858 PMID:27618906

Grandjean, P., Berlin, A., Gilbert, M., & Penning, W. (1988). Preventing percutaneous absorption of industrial chemicals: The "skin" denotation. *American Journal of Industrial Medicine*, *14*(1), 97–107. doi:10.1002/ajim.4700140111 PMID:3044066

Granger, C. W. J., & Yoon, G. (2002). *Hidden cointegration*. University of California.

Granger, C. W. J. (1969). Investigating causal relations by econometric models and cross spectral methods. *Econometrica*, *37*(3), 424–438. doi:10.2307/1912791

Grant, J. (2017). List of foods containing GMOs. *Live Strong*. Retrieved from https://www.livestrong.com/article/314824-list-of-foods-containing-gmos/

Greber, J. F. (2003). Gallium and gallium compounds. In *Ullmann's Encyclopedia of Industrial Chemistry* (6th rev. Ed., Vol. 15, pp. 235–240). Weinheim: Wiley-VCH Verlag GmbH & Co.

Greger, M. S. (2015). *How not to die: Discover the foods scientifically proven to prevent and reverse disease*. PAN Books.

Grewal, S. I., & Jia, S. (2007). Heterochromatin revisited. *Nature Reviews. Genetics*, *8*(1), 35–46. doi:10.1038/nrg2008 PMID:17173056

Grinevich, V., Desarménien, M. G., Chini, B., Tauber, M., & Muscatelli, F. (2015). Ontogenesis of oxytocin pathways in the mammalian brain: Late maturation and psychosocial disorders. *Frontiers in Neuroanatomy*, *20*(8), 164. doi:10.3389/fnana.2014.00164 PMID:25767437

Groot, M. J., & Hooft, K. E. (2016). The hidden effects of dairy farming on public and environmental health in the Netherlands, India, Ethiopia, and Uganda, Considering the use of antibiotics and other agro-chemicals. *Frontiers in Public Health*, *4*. doi:10.3389/fpubh.2016.00012 PMID:26942171

Grossman, E. (2014, May 27). As Dairy Farms Grow Bigger, New Concerns About Pollution. Retrieved from https://e360.yale.edu/features/as_dairy_farms_grow_bigger_new_concerns_about_pollution

Gross-Sorokin, M. Y., Roast, S. D., & Brighty, G. C. (2006). Assessment of feminization of male fish in English rivers by the environment agency of England and Wales. *Environmental Health Perspectives*, *114*(Supplement 1), 147–151. doi:10.1289/ehp.8068 PMID:16818261

Group, E. (2016). GMO foods cause gut damage. *Global Healing Center*. Retrieved from https://www.globalhealingcenter.com/natural-health/gmo-foods-cause-gut-damage/

Gruere, A., & Plastina, A. (2010). Some Alternatives to Conventional Cotton: Organic Cotton, Fairtrade Cotton, Cotton Made In Africa and Better Cotton Initiative. *Cotton*, (May-June), 5-9.

Grzadzinski, R., Di Martino, A., Brady, E., Mairena, M. A., O'Neale, M., Petkova, E., ... Castellanos, F. X. (2011). Examining autistic traits in children with ADHD: Does the autism spectrum extend to ADHD? *Journal of Autism and Developmental Disorders*, *41*(9), 1178–1191. doi:10.100710803-010-1135-3 PMID:21108041

Grzesiuk, M., Mielecki, D., Pilżys, T., Garbicz, D., Marcinkowski, M., & Grzesiuk, E. (2018). How cyclophosphamide at environmentally relevant concentration influences Daphnia magna life history and its proteome. *PLoS One*, *13*(4), e0195366. doi:10.1371/journal.pone.0195366 PMID:29621334

Guidelines for Drinking-water Quality. (2011). Geneva: WHO Press.

Guo, H. R., Yu, H. S., Hu, H., & Monson, R. R. (2001). Arsenic in drinking water and skin cancers: Cell-type specificity (Taiwan, ROC). *Cancer Causes & Control*, *12*(10), 909–916. doi:10.1023/A:1013712203455 PMID:11808710

Guo, J. X., Hu, L., Yand, P. Z., Tanabe, K., Miyatalre, M., & Chen, Y. (2007). Chronic arsenic poisoning in drinking water in Inner Mongolia and its associated health effects. *Journal of Environmental Science and Health. Part A, Toxic/Hazardous Substances & Environmental Engineering*, *42*(12), 1853–1858. doi:10.1080/10934520701566918 PMID:17952786

Guo, J., Astrup, A., Lovegrove, J. A., Gijsbers, L., Givens, D. I., & Soedamah-Muthu, S. S. (2017). Milk and dairy consumption and risk of cardiovascular diseases and all-cause mortality: Dose–response meta-analysis of prospective cohort studies. [PubMed]. *European Journal of Epidemiology*, *32*(4), 269–287. doi:10.100710654-017-0243-1

Guo, X., Fujino, Y., Kaneko, S., Wu, K., Xia, Y., & Yoshimura, T. (2001). Arsenic contamination of groundwater and prevalence of arsenical dermatosis in the Hetao plain area, Inner Mongolia, China. *Molecular and Cellular Biochemistry*, *222*(1/2), 137–140. doi:10.1023/A:1017916826439 PMID:11678595

Guo, X., Zheng, C., & Xu, M. (2004). Characterization of Arsenic Emissions from a Coal-Fired Power Plant. *Energy & Fuels*, *18*(6), 1822–1826. doi:10.1021/ef049921b

Gupta, S., Ellis, S. E., Ashar, F. N., Moes, A., Bader, J. S., Zhan, J., ... Arking, D. E. (2014). Transcriptome analysis reveals dysregulation of innate immune response genes and neuronal activity-dependent genes in autism. *Nature Communications*, *5*(1), 5748. doi:10.1038/ncomms6748 PMID:25494366

Guriillot, S., & Charlet, L. (2007). Bengal arsenic, an archive of Himalaya orogeny and paleohydrology. *Journal of Environmental Science and Health*, *42*(12), 1785–1794. doi:10.1080/10934520701566702 PMID:17952779

Gutsell, S., & Russell, P. (2013). The role of chemistry in developing understanding of adverse outcome pathways and their application in risk assessment. *Toxicology Research*, *2*(5), 299–307. doi:10.1039/c3tx50024a

Guy, R. H. (2010). Predicting the rate and extent of fragrance chemical absorption into and through the skin. *Chemical Research in Toxicology*, *23*(5), 864–870. doi:10.1021/tx9004105 PMID:20392076

Haas, J., Storch-Hagenlocher, B., Biessmann, A., & Wildemann, B. (2002). Inducible nitric oxide synthase and argininosuccinate synthetase: Co-induction in brain tissue of patients with Alzheimer's dementia and following stimulation with β-amyloid 1–42 in vitro. *Neuroscience Letters*, *322*(2), 121–125. doi:10.1016/S0304-3940(02)00095-2 PMID:11958858

Häberling, I. S., Badzakova-Trajkov, G., & Corballis, M. C. (2013). Asymmetries of the arcuate fasciculus in monozygotic twins: Genetic and nongenetic influences. *PLoS One*, *8*(1).

Hacker, R. S., & Hatemi-J, A. (2006). Tests for causality between integrated variables using asymptotic and bootstrap distributions: Theory and application. *Applied Economics*, *38*(13), 1489–1500. doi:10.1080/00036840500405763

Hair, J. F., Black, W. C., Babin, B. J., & Anderson, R. E. (2010). *Multivariate data analysis: A global perspective*. New Jersey: Pearson.

Halder, G., & Johnson, R. L. (2011). Hippo signaling: Growth control and beyond. *Development.*, *138*(1), 9–22. doi:10.1242/dev.045500 PMID:21138973

Halling-Sørensen, B., Nors Nielsen, S., Lanzky, P. F., Ingerslev, F., Holten Lützhøft, H. C., & Jørgensen, S. E. (1998). Occurrence, fate and effects of pharmaceutical substances in the environment--a review. *Chemosphere*, *36*(2), 357–393. doi:10.1016/S0045-6535(97)00354-8 PMID:9569937

Hallmayer, J., Cleveland, S., Torres, A., Phillips, J., Cohen, B., Torigoe, T., ... Lotspeich, L. (2011). Genetic heritability and shared environmental factors among twin pairs with autism. *Archives of General Psychiatry*, *68*(11), 1095–1102. doi:10.1001/archgenpsychiatry.2011.76 PMID:21727249

Haluza, D., Kaiser, A., Moshammer, H., Flandorfer, C., Kundi, M., & Neuberger, M. (2012). Estimated health impact of a shift from light fuel to residential wood-burning in Upper Austria. *Journal of Exposure Science & Environmental Epidemiology*, *22*(4), 339–343. doi:10.1038/jes.2012.27 PMID:22569207

Hamadani, J. D., Tofail, F., Nermell, B., Gardner, R., Shiraji, S., Bottai, M., ... Vahter, M. (2011). Critical windows of exposure for arsenic-associated impairment of cognitive function in pre-school girls and boys: A population-based cohort study. *International Journal of Epidemiology*, *40*(6), 1593–1604. doi:10.1093/ije/dyr176 PMID:22158669

Haque, R., Mazumder, D. N., Samanta, S., Ghosh, N., Kalman, D., Smith, M. M., ... Smith, A. H. (2003). Arsenic in drinking water and skin lesions: Dose-response data from West Bengal, India. *Epidemiology (Cambridge, Mass.)*, *14*(2), 174–182. doi:10.1097/01.EDE.0000040361.55051.54 PMID:12606883

Harrell, F.E. Jr. & Dupont, M. C. (2006). The Hmisc Package. R package version. 3, 0-12.

Harrington, J. M., Middaugh, J. P., Morse, D. L., & Housworth, J. (1978). A survey of a population exposed to high concentrations of arsenic in well water in Fairbanks, Alaska. *American Journal of Epidemiology*, *108*(5), 377–385. doi:10.1093/oxfordjournals.aje.a112635 PMID:727207

Harvest, L. (n.d.). Living Harvest. Retrieved from https://livingharvest.com

Hassall, R. (2017). How should applied psychologists conceptualise an autism spectrum disorder diagnosis and its predictive validity? *Educational and Child Psychology*, *34*(4), 20–29.

Hatemi-J, A. (2012). Asymmetric causality tests with an application. *Empirical Economics*, *43*(1), 447–456. doi:10.100700181-011-0484-x

Hays, M. D., Geron, C. D., Linna, K. J., Smith, N. D., & Schauer, J. J. (2002). Speciation of gas-phase and fine particle emissions from burning of foliar fuels. *Environmental Science & Technology*, *36*(11), 2281–2295. doi:10.1021/es0111683 PMID:12075778

Health Concerns about Dairy Products. (2016, January 26). Physicians Committee for Responsible Medicine. Retrieved from http://www.pcrm.org/health/diets/vegdiets/health-concerns-about-dairy-products

Healthy Diet. (2015). World Health Organization. Retrieved from http://www.who.int/mediacentre/factsheets/fs394/en/

Healy, J. D. (2003). Excess winter mortality in Europe: A cross country analysis identifying key risk factors. *Journal of Epidemiology and Community Health*, *57*(10), 784–789. doi:10.1136/jech.57.10.784 PMID:14573581

Heaney, R. P. (2013). Dairy intake, dietary adequacy, and lactose intolerance. *Advances in Nutrition*, *4*(2), 151–156. doi:10.3945/an.112.003368 PMID:23493531

He, B. S., Wang, J., Liu, J., & Hu, X. M. (2017). Eco-pharmacovigilance of non-steroidal anti-inflammatory drugs: Necessity and opportunities. *Chemosphere*, *181*, 178–189. doi:10.1016/j.chemosphere.2017.04.084 PMID:28437743

Hecker, M., Sessa, W. C., Harris, H. J., Anggård, E., & Vane, J. R. (1990). The metabolism of L-arginine and its significance for the biosynthesis of endothelium-derived relaxing factor: Cultured endothelial cells recycle L-citrulline to L-arginine. *Proceedings of the National Academy of Sciences of the United States of America*, *87*(21), 8612–8616. doi:10.1073/pnas.87.21.8612 PMID:2236071

Heerboth, S., Lapinska, K., Snyder, N., Leary, M., Rollinson, S., & Sarkar, S. (2014). Use of Epigenetic Drugs in Disease: An Overview. *Genetics & Epigenetics*, *6*, 9–19. doi:10.4137/GEG.S12270 PMID:25512710

Hefferon, K.L. (2016*). Food Security of Genetically Modified Foods*. doi:10.1016/B978-0-08-100596-5.03532-0

Hendry, K. M., & Cole, E. C. (1993). A review of mycotoxins in indoor air. *Journal of Toxicology and Environmental Health*, *38*(2), 183–198. doi:10.1080/15287399309531711 PMID:8433402

Heneka, M. T., Wiesinger, H., Dumitrescu-Ozimek, L., Riederer, P., Feinstein, D. L., & Klockgether, T. (2001). Neuronal and glial coexpression of argininosuccinate synthetase and inducible nitric oxide synthase in Alzheimer disease. *Journal of Neuropathology and Experimental Neurology*, *60*(9), 906–916. doi:10.1093/jnen/60.9.906 PMID:11556547

Henessy, W., Gupta, A., & Kowalski, S. (2014). Practice driving policy: Agbiotech transfer as capacity building. In S. Smith, P. Philips, & D. Castle (Eds.), *Handbook on agriculture, biotechnology and development* (pp. 314–342). Cheltenham, UK: Edward Elgar Publishing Limited. doi:10.4337/9780857938350.00028

Henning, K. J. (2004). What is syndromic surveillance. *Morbidity and Mortality Weekly Report*, *53*(Supplement), 7–11.

Henry, C., Hugo, S., & Blackburn, J. (2006). Cumulative long-term effects of genetically modified (GM) crops on human/animal health and the environment: risk assessment methodologies. *European Union*. Retrieved from https://ec.europa.eu/food/sites/food/files/plant/docs/gmo_rep-stud_2006_report_lt-effects.pdf

Herbert, M. R. (2010). Contributions of the environment and environmentally vulnerable physiology to autism spectrum disorders. *Current Opinion in Neurology*, *23*(2), 103–110. doi:10.1097/WCO.0b013e328336a01f PMID:20087183

Herceg, Z. (2016). Epigenetic Mechanisms as an Interface Between the Environment and Genome. *Advances in Experimental Medicine and Biology*, *903*, 3–15. doi:10.1007/978-1-4899-7678-9_1 PMID:27343085

Heynen, M., Fick, J., Jonsson, M., Klaminder, J., & Brodin, T. (2016). Effect of bioconcentration and trophic transfer on realized exposure to oxazepam in 2 predators, the dragonfly larvae (*Aeshna grandis*) and the Eurasian perch (*Perca fluviatilis*). *Environmental Toxicology and Chemistry*, *35*(4), 930–937. doi:10.1002/etc.3368 PMID:26762222

High on Hemp Milk? Dr. Weil. (2016, December 01). Retrieved from https://www.drweil.com/diet-nutrition/nutrition/high-on-hemp-milk/

Hoddinot, J., Rosegrant, M., & Torero, M. (2012). *Investments to reduce hunger and undernutrition. Copenhagen Consensus 2012 Challenge Paper, Hunger and Malnutrition*. Washington, DC: International Food Policy Research Institute.

Hoddinott, J. (1999). *Operationalizing household food security in developing projects: An introduction Technical Guide no. 1*. Washington, DC: International Food Policy Research Institute.

Högy, P., Wieser, H., Köhler, P., Schwadorf, K., Breuer, J., Franzaring, J., ... Fangmeier, A. (2009). Effects of elevated CO_2 on grain yield and quality of wheat: Results from a 3-year free-air CO_2 enrichment experiment. *Plant Biology*, (Suppl. 1), 1160–1169. PMID:19778369

Hollocks, M. J., Howlin, P., Papadopoulos, A. S., Khondoker, M., & Simonoff, E. (2014). Differences in HPA-axis and heart rate responsiveness to psychosocial stress in children with autism spectrum disorders with and without co-morbid anxiety. *Psychoneuroendocrinology*, *46*, 32–45. doi:10.1016/j.psyneuen.2014.04.004 PMID:24882156

Holmes, N. M., Parkes, S. L., Killcross, A. S., & Westbrook, R. F. (2013). The basolateral amygdala is critical for learning about neutral stimuli in the presence of danger, and the perirhinal cortex is critical in the absence of danger. *The Journal of Neuroscience*, *33*(32), 13112–13125. doi:10.1523/JNEUROSCI.1998-13.2013 PMID:23926265

Holm, G., Snape, J. R., Murray-Smith, R., Talbot, J., Taylor, D., & Sörme, P. (2013). Implementing ecopharmacovigilance in practice: Challenges and potential opportunities. *Drug Safety*, *36*(7), 533–546. doi:10.100740264-013-0049-3 PMID:23620169

Hommer, R. E., & Swedo, S. E. (2015). Schizophrenia and autism-related disorders. *Schizophrenia Bulletin*, *41*(2), 313–314. doi:10.1093chbulbu188 PMID:25634913

Homola, J., Yee, S. S., & Gsuglitz, G. (1999). Surface Plasmon Resonance Sensors: Review. Sensors and Actuators B: Chemical. *Sensors and Actuators. B, Chemical*, *54*(1-2), 3–15. doi:10.1016/S0925-4005(98)00321-9

Hong, Y.-S., Song, K.-H., & Chung, J.-Y. (2014). Health Effects of Chronic Arsenic Exposure. *Journal of Preventive Medicine and Public Health*, *47*(5), 245–252. doi:10.3961/jpmph.14.035 PMID:25284195

Hooijdonk, T. V., & Hettinga, K. (2015). Dairy in a sustainable diet: A question of balance. *Nutrition Reviews*, *73*(Suppl 1), 48–54. doi:10.1093/nutrit/nuv040 PMID:26175490

Hope, J. (2013). A review of the mechanism of injury and treatment approaches for illness resulting from exposure to water-damaged buildings, mold, and mycotoxins. *The Scientific World Journal*, *2013*, 767482. doi:10.1155/2013/767482 PMID:23710148

Hope, J. H., & Hope, B. E. (2012). A review of the diagnosis and treatment of Ochratoxin A inhalational exposure associated with human illness and kidney disease including focal segmental glomerulosclerosis. *Journal of Environmental and Public Health*. doi:10.1155/2012/835059 PMID:22253638

Hopenhayn-Rich, C., Biggs, M. L., & Smith, A. H. (1998). Lung and kidney cancer mortality associated with arsenic drinking water in Ordoba, Argentina. *International Journal of Epidemiology*, *27*(4), 561–569. doi:10.1093/ije/27.4.561 PMID:9758107

Hopenhyan, C. (2006). Arsenic in Drinking Water: Impact on Human Health. *Elements*, *2*(2), 103–107. doi:10.2113/gselements.2.2.103

Hopton, J. L., & Hunt, S. M. (1996). Housing conditions and mental health in a disadvantaged area in Scotland. *Journal of Epidemiology and Community Health*, *50*(1), 56–61. doi:10.1136/jech.50.1.56 PMID:8762355

Horn, F., & Breeze, R. (n.d.). Agriculture and food security. Agricultural Research Service, United States Department of Agriculture, Washington, DC.

Horrigan, L., Lawrence, R. S., & Walker, P. (2002). How sustainable agriculture can address the environmental and human health harms of industrial agriculture. *Environmental Health Perspectives*, *110*(5), 445–456. doi:10.1289/ehp.02110445 PMID:12003747

Hou, J., Wan, W., Mao, D., Wang, C., Mu, Q., Qin, S., & Luo, Y. (2015). Occurrence and distribution of sulfonamides, tetracyclines, quinolones, macrolides, and nitrofurans in livestock manure and amended soils of Northern China. *Environmental Science and Pollution Research International*, *22*(6), 4545–4554. doi:10.100711356-014-3632-y PMID:25318415

Hsiao, E. Y., McBride, S. W., Hsien, S., Sharon, G., Hyde, E. R., McCue, T., ... Mazmanian, S. K. (2013). Microbiota modulate behavioral and physiological abnormalities associated with neurodevelopmental disorders. *Cell*, *155*(7), 1451–1463. doi:10.1016/j.cell.2013.11.024 PMID:24315484

Huang, Y., Yan, F., Fu, M., & Zhang, R. (2017). Silica-based optical chemosensors for detection and removal of metal ions. *Journal of the Indian Chemical Society*, *14*(1), 157–176.

Hughes, B. W., Sealey, L. A., & Bagasra, O. (2016). Mechanism of Male Gender Bias in Neuroblastoma Cell Lines Exposed to Fragrances: A Link to Autism Spectrum Disorder. *Expert Opinion on Environmental Biology*, *5*, 1–21.

Hughes, M. F., Beck, B. D., Chen, Y., Lewis, A. S., & Thomas, D. J. (2011). Arsenic Exposure and Toxicology: A Historical Perspective. *Toxicological Sciences*, *123*(2), 305–332. doi:10.1093/toxsci/kfr184 PMID:21750349

Huguet, G., Benabou, M., & Bourgeron, T. (2016). The genetics of autism spectrum disorders. In *A time for metabolism and hormones* (pp. 101–129). Springer International Publishing. doi:10.1007/978-3-319-27069-2_11

Hu, J., Fang, J., Dong, Y., Chen, S. J., & Chen, Z. (2005). Arsenic in cancer therapy. *Anti-Cancer Drugs*, *16*(2), 119–127. doi:10.1097/00001813-200502000-00002 PMID:15655408

Hundal, H. S., Singh, K., & Singh, D. (2009). Arsenic content in ground and canal waters of Punjab, North-West India. *Environmental Monitoring and Assessment*, *154*(1-4), 393–400. doi:10.100710661-008-0406-3 PMID:18568407

Hunt, K. M., Srivastava, R. K., Elmets, C. A., & Athar, M. (2014). The mechanistic basis of arsenicosis: Pathogenesis of skin cancer. *Cancer Letters*, *354*(2), 211–219. doi:10.1016/j.canlet.2014.08.016 PMID:25173797

Hyndman, S. J. (1990). Housing dampness and health amongst British Bengalis in east London. *Social Science & Medicine*, *30*(1), 131–141. doi:10.1016/0277-9536(90)90336-Q PMID:2305276

IDFA Calls on HHS to Challenge WHO Policies at World Health Assembly. (2018). Retrieved from https://www.idfa.org/news-views/headline-news/article/2018/05/16/idfa-calls-on-hhs-to-challenge-who-policies-at-world-health-assembly

Idso, S. B., & Idso, K. E. (2001). Effects of atmospheric CO_2 enrichment on plant constituents related to animal and human health. *Environmental and Experimental Botany*, *45*(2), 179–199. doi:10.1016/S0098-8472(00)00091-5 PMID:11275225

IMF. (2012). *World Economic outlook*. Washington, DC, U.S.A.: World Economic and Financial Surveys.

Infante-Rivard, C., & Weichenthal, S. (2007). Pesticides and childhood cancer: An update of Zahm and Ward's 1998 review. *Journal of Toxicology and Environmental Health. Part B*, *10*(1-2), 81–99.

International Agency for Research on Cancer (IARC), IARC Working Group on the Evaluation of Carcinogenic Risks to Humans. (2017). *Some Organic Insecticides and Herbicides. IARC Monograph on the Evaluation of Carcinogenic Risks to Humans* (Vol. 112). Lyon, France: Monograph.

International Agency for Research on Cancer (IARC). (2012). A Review of Human Carcinogens: Arsenic, Metals, Fibres, and Dusts.

International Agency for Research on Cancer. (2015). Some organophosphate insecticides and herbicides: Diazinon, Glyphosate, Malathion, parathion, and Tetrachlorvinphos. *IARC Monographs on the Evaluation of Carcinogenic Risks to Humans*, 112.

International Service for the Acquisition of Agri-Biotech Applications. (2010). *Global Status of Commercialized Biotech/GM crops: 2010. ISAAA Brief 42-2010: Executive Summary*. Retrieved from http://www.isaaa.org/resources/publications/briefs/42/executivesummary/default. asp

IOBE, Equating the Excise Duty Rates on Heating and Diesel Oil. Foundation for economic and industrial research, 2013.

Iossifov, I., O'Roak, B. J., Sanders, S. J., Ronemus, M., Krumm, N., Levy, D., ... Wigler, M. (2014). The contribution of de novo coding mutations to autism spectrum disorder. *Nature*, *515*(7526), 216–221. doi:10.1038/nature13908 PMID:25363768

ISAAA. (2009). Pocket K No. 3: Are the food derived from GM crops safe? Retrieved from http://www.isaaa.org/resources/publications/pocketk/3/default.asp

ISAAA. (2012). *Annual report Executive Summary*. International Service for the Acquisition of Agribiotech Applications.

Ishiguro, S. (1992). Industries using arsenic and arsenic compounds. *Applied Organometallic Chemistry*, *6*(4), 323–331. doi:10.1002/aoc.590060404

Ishizawa, Y. (2011). Special article: General anesthetic gases and the global environment. *Anesthesia and Analgesia*, *112*(1), 213–217. doi:10.1213/ANE.0b013e3181fe02c2 PMID:21048097

Isidori, M., Lavorgna, M., Nardelli, A., Parrella, A., Previtera, L., & Rubino, M. (2005). Ecotoxicity of naproxen and its phototransformation products. *The Science of the Total Environment*, *348*(1), 93–101. doi:10.1016/j.scitotenv.2004.12.068 PMID:16162316

Ismaiel, A. A., & Papenbrock, J. (2015). Mycotoxins [Agriculture.]. *Producing Fungi and Mechanisms of Phytotoxicity.*, *5*, 492–537.

Ismail, N. A. H., Wee, S. Y., & Aris, A. Z. (2017). Multi-class of endocrine disrupting compounds in aquaculture ecosystems and health impacts in exposed biota. *Chemosphere*, *188*, 375–388. doi:10.1016/j.chemosphere.2017.08.150 PMID:28892772

Iyyanki, V. M., & Manickam, V. (2017). Chapter Eight – Environmental Risk Assessment. In V. M. Iyyanki & V. Manickam (Eds.), *Environmental Management: Science and Engineering for Industry* (pp. 135–152). India: BS Publications. doi:10.1016/B978-0-12-811989-1.00008-7

Jabbar, A., Masud, S. Z., Parveen, Z., & Ali, M. (1993). Pesticide residues in cropland soils and shallow groundwater in Punjab Pakistan. *Bulletin of Environmental Contamination and Toxicology*, *51*(2), 268–273. doi:10.1007/BF00198891 PMID:8353391

Jackson, K. W., & Chen, G. (1996). Atomic Absorption, Atomic Emission, and Flame Emission Spectrometry. *Analytical Chemistry*, *68*(12), 231–256. doi:10.1021/a19600121 PMID:8092468

Jacobsen, B. K., Knutsen, S. F., & Fraser, G. E. (1998, December). Does high soy milk intake reduce prostate cancer incidence? The Adventist Health Study (United States). *NCBI*. Retrieved from https://www.ncbi.nlm.nih.gov/pubmed/10189040

Jager, T. (2016). Dynamic Modeling for Uptake and Effects of Chemicals. In J. Blasco, P. M. Chapman, O. Campana, & M. Hampel (Eds.), *Marine Ecotoxicology: Current Knowledge and Future Uses* (pp. 718–798). Academic Press. doi:10.1016/B978-0-12-803371-5.00003-5

James, K. A., Byers, T., Hokanson, J. E., Meliker, J. R., Zerbe, G. O., & Marshall, J. A. (2015). Association between lifetime exposure to inorganic arsenic in drinking water and coronary heart disease in Colorado residents. *Environmental Health Perspectives*, *123*(2), 128–134. doi:10.1289/ehp.1307839 PMID:25350952

Jang, Y.-C., Yashoda, S., & Hwidong, K. (2016). Source, Distribution, Toxicity and Remediation of Arsenic in the Environment – A review 2016. *International Journal of Applied Environmental Sciences*, *11*, 559–581.

Jeanneret, F., Boccard, J., Badoud, F., Sorg, O., Tonoli, D., Pelclova, D., ... Rudaz, S. (2014a). Human urinary biomarkers of dioxin exposure: Analysis by metabolomics and biologically driven data dimensionality reduction. *Toxicology Letters*, *230*(2), 234–243. doi:10.1016/j.toxlet.2013.10.031 PMID:24201000

Jedrychowski, W., Maugeri, U., Perera, F., Stigter, L., Jankowski, J., Butscher, M., ... Sowa, A.Ref Type. (2011). Cognitive function of 6-year old children exposed to mold-contaminated homes in early postnatal period. Prospective birth cohort study in Poland. *Physiology & Behavior*, *104*(5), 989–995. doi:10.1016/j.physbeh.2011.06.019 PMID:21763705

Jeste, S. S., & Geschwind, D. H. (2014). Disentangling the heterogeneity of autism spectrum disorder through genetic findings. *Nature Reviews. Neurology*, *10*(2), 74–81. doi:10.1038/nrneurol.2013.278 PMID:24468882

Jewison, T., Su, Y., Disfany, F. M., Liang, Y., Knox, C., Maciejewski, A., ... Wishart, D. S. (2014). SMPDB 2.0: Big improvements to the Small Molecule Pathway Database. *Nucleic Acids Research*, *42*(D1), D478–D484. doi:10.1093/nar/gkt1067 PMID:24203708

Ji, Y., Ferronato, C., Salvador, A., Yang, X, & Chovelon, J. M. (2014). Degradation of ciprofloxacin and sulfamethoxazole by ferrous-activated persulfate: implications for remediation of groundwater contaminated by antibiotics. *The Science of the Total Environment, 472,* 800-808.

Jiang, J. Q., Ashekuzzaman, S. M., Jiang, A., Sharifuzzaman, S. M., & Chowdhury, S. R. (2013). Arsenic contaminated groundwater and its treatment options in Bangladesh. *International Journal of Environmental Research and Public Health, 10*(1), 18–46. doi:10.3390/ijerph10010018 PMID:23343979

Jiao, X., Ashtari, N., Balaei, M. R., Chen, Q. M., Badbezanchi, I., Shojaei, S., ... Marzban, H. (2016). Mevalonate Cascade and Neurodevelopmental and Neurodegenerative Diseases: Future Targets for Therapeutic Application. *Current Molecular Pharmacology*. PMID:26758948

Ji, L., Fu, R., & Mitchell, E. W. (1992). Glutathione and antioxidant enzymes in skeletal muscle: Effects of fiber type and exercise intensity. *Journal of Applied Physiology, 73*(5), 1854–1859. doi:10.1152/jappl.1992.73.5.1854 PMID:1474061

Jin, S., Bluemling, B., & Mol, A. P. (2015). Information, trust and pesticide overuse: Interactions between retailers and cotton farmers in China. *NJAS Wageningen Journal of Life Sciences, 72*, 23–32. doi:10.1016/j.njas.2014.10.003

Ji, Y., Zeng, C., Ferronato, C., Chovelon, J. M., & Yang, X. (2012). Nitrate-induced photodegradation of atenolol in aqueous solution: Kinetics, toxicity and degradation pathways. *Chemosphere, 88*(5), 644–649. doi:10.1016/j.chemosphere.2012.03.050 PMID:22497785

Jobling, S., Burn, R. W., Thorpe, K., Williams, R., & Tyler, C. (2009). Statistical modeling suggests that antiandrogens in effluents from wastewater treatment works contribute to widespread sexual disruption in fish living in English rivers. *Environmental Health Perspectives, 117*(5), 797–802. doi:10.1289/ehp.0800197 PMID:19479024

John, F. (1974). *U.S. Patent No. 3,799,758*. Washington, DC: U.S. Patent and Trademark Office.

Johnson, C. H., Athersuch, T. J., Collman, G. W., Dhungana, S., Grant, D. F., Jones, D. P., ... Vasiliou, V. (2017). Yale school of public health symposium on lifetime exposures and human health: The exposome; summary and future reflections. *Human Genomics, 11*(1), 32. doi:10.118640246-017-0128-0 PMID:29221465

Johnston, F. H., Hanigan, I. C., Henderson, S. B., & Morgan, G. G. (2013). Evaluation of interventions to reduce air pollution from biomass smoke on mortality in Launceston, Australia: Retrospective analysis of daily mortality, 1994-2007. *BMJ (Clinical Research Ed.)*, 346. PMID:23299843

Joint Meeting on Pesticide Residues. (2004). *Report of the Joint Meeting of the FAO Panel of Experts on Pesticide Residues in Food and the Environment and the WHO Core Assessment Group on Pesticide Residues*. Retrieved from http://www.fao.org/home/en/

Kadono, T., Inaoka, T., Murayama, N., Ushijima, K., Nagano, M., Nakamura, S., ... Ohtsuka, R. (2002). Skin manifestations of arsenicosis in two villages in Bangladesh. *International Journal of Dermatology, 41*(12), 841–846. doi:10.1046/j.1365-4362.2002.01668.x PMID:12492966

Kalia, M. (2008). Brain development: Anatomy, connectivity, adaptive plasticity, and toxicity. *Metabolism: Clinical and Experimental, 57*, S2–S5. doi:10.1016/j.metabol.2008.07.009 PMID:18803960

Kalkbrenner, A. E., Schmidt, R. J., & Penlesky, A. C. (2014). Environmental chemical exposures and autism spectrum disorders: A review of the epidemiological evidence. *Current Problems in Pediatric and Adolescent Health Care, 44*(10), 277–318. doi:10.1016/j.cppeds.2014.06.001 PMID:25199954

Kalkstein, L. S., & Greene, J. S. (1997). An evaluation of climate/mortality relationships in large US cities and the possible impacts of a climate change. *Environmental Health Perspectives*, *105*(1), 84–93. doi:10.1289/ehp.9710584 PMID:9074886

Kalogeromitros, D., Syrigou, E. I., Makris, M., Kempuraj, D., Stavrianeas, N. G., Vasiadi, M., & Theoharides, T. C. (2007). Nasal provocation of patients with allergic rhinitis and the hypothalamic-pituitary-adrenal axis. *Annals of Allergy, Asthma & Immunology*, *98*(3), 269–273. doi:10.1016/S1081-1206(10)60717-X PMID:17378259

Kamatou, G. P., Vermaak, I., & Viljoen, A. M. (2012). Eugenol--from the remote Maluku Islands to the international market place: A review of a remarkable and versatile molecule. *Molecules (Basel, Switzerland)*, *17*(6), 6953–6981. doi:10.3390/molecules17066953 PMID:22728369

Kanehisa, M., Goto, S., Sato, Y., Furumichi, M., & Tanabe, M. (2012). KEGG for integration and interpretation of large-scale molecular data sets. *Nucleic Acids Research*, *40*(D1), D109–D114. doi:10.1093/nar/gkr988 PMID:22080510

Kanner, L. (1951). The conception of wholes and parts in early infantile autism. *The American Journal of Psychiatry*, *108*(1), 23–26. doi:10.1176/ajp.108.1.23 PMID:14838158

Kanungo, S., Soares, N., He, M., & Steiner, R. D. (2013). Sterol metabolism disorders and neurodevelopment-an update. *Developmental Disabilities Research Reviews*, *17*(3), 197–210. doi:10.1002/ddrr.1114 PMID:23798009

Kapaj, S., Peterson, H., Liber, K., & Bhattacharya, P. (2006). Human health effects from chronic As poisoning—A review. *Journal of Environmental Science and Health*, *41*(10), 2399–2428. doi:10.1080/10934520600873571 PMID:17018421

Karagas, M. R., Stukel, T. A., & Tosteson, T. D. (2002). Assessment of cancer risk and environmental levels of arsenic in New Hampshire. *International Journal of Hygiene and Environmental Health*, *205*(1-2), 85–94. doi:10.1078/1438-4639-00133 PMID:12018020

Karma, G. (2016). Good Karma. Retrieved from http://goodkarmafoods.com/products/?gclid=EAIaIQobChMIu4aLqarg2wIVyAOGCh1lqQYIEAAYASAAEgLF0_D_BwE

Karunasena, E., Larranaga, M. D., Simoni, J. S., Douglas, D. R., & Straus, D. C. (2010). Building-associated neurological damage modeled in human cells: A mechanism of neurotoxic effects by exposure to mycotoxins in the indoor environment. *Mycopathologia*, *170*(6), 377–390. doi:10.100711046-010-9330-5 PMID:20549560

Katajamaa, M., Miettinen, J., & Orešič, M. (2006). MZmine: Toolbox for processing and visualization of mass spectrometry based molecular profile data. *Bioinformatics (Oxford, England)*, *22*(5), 634–636. doi:10.1093/bioinformatics/btk039 PMID:16403790

Kattel, E., Kaur, B., Trapido, M., & Dulova, N. (2018). Persulfate-based photodegradation of a beta-lactam antibiotic amoxicillin in various water matrices. *Environmental Technology*, 1–28. doi:10.1080/09593330.2018.1493149 PMID:29932810

Kaviraj A., Unlu E., Gupta A., Nemr A. (2014). Biomarkers of environmental pollutants. *BioMed Research International*. doi:. doi:10.155/2014/806598

Keatinge, W. R., Donaldson, G. C., Cordioli, E., Martinelli, M., Kunst, A. E., Mackenbach, J. P., ... Vuori, I. (2000). Heat related mortality in warm and cold regions of Europe: Observational study. *BMJ (Clinical Research Ed.)*, *321*(7262), 670–673. doi:10.1136/bmj.321.7262.670 PMID:10987770

KEGG. (2017). *2-Oxobutanoate. Vol.* KEGG, Purine Metabolism.

KEGG. (n.d.). Citrate cycle (TCA cycle).

Kelbessa, W. (2005). *The utility of ethical dialogue for marginalized voices in Africa*. Retrieved from http://pubs.iied.org/pdfs/13508IIED.pdf?

Kelbessa, W. (2012). Environmental injustice in Africa. In H. McDonald (Ed.), *Pragmatism and Environmentalism 9* (Vol. 1, pp. 99–132). New York, NY: Rodopi.

Kelder, T., van Iersel, M. P., Hanspers, K., Kutmon, M., Conklin, B. R., Evelo, C. T., & Pico, A. R. (2012). WikiPathways: Building research communities on biological pathways. *Nucleic Acids Research*, *40*(D1), D1301–D1307. doi:10.1093/nar/gkr1074 PMID:22096230

Kerger, B. D., Leung, H.-W., Scott, P., Paustenbach, D. J., Needham, L. L., Patterson, D. G. Jr, ... Mocarelli, P. (2006). Age- and Concentration-Dependent Elimination Half-Life of 2,3,7,8-Tetrachlorodibenzo-p-dioxin in Seveso Children. *Environmental Health Perspectives*, *114*(10), 1596–1602. doi:10.1289/ehp.8884 PMID:17035149

Kessenides, D. (2016, October 20). Forget Organic, Retailers Increasingly Are Turning to Sustainable Cotton. *Bloomberg*. Retrieved from https://www.bloomberg.com/news/articles/2016-10-20/forget-organic-retailers-increasingly-are-turning-to-sustainable-cotton

Key, S., Ma, J. K. C., & Drake, P. M. W. (2008). Genetically modified plants and human health. *Journal of the Royal Society of Medicine*, *101*(6), 290–298. doi:10.1258/jrsm.2008.070372 PMID:18515776

Khanal, S. K., Xie, B., Thompson, M. L., Sung, S., Ong, S. K., & Van Leeuwent, J. (2006). Fate, transport, and biodegradation of natural estrogens in the environment and engineered systems. *Environmental Science & Technology*, *40*(21), 6537–6546. doi:10.1021/es0607739 PMID:17144275

Kilburn, K. H. (2003). Indoor mold exposure associated with neurobehavioral and pulmonary impairment: A preliminary report. *Archives of Environmental Health*, *58*(7), 390–398. doi:10.1080/00039896.2003.11879139 PMID:15143851

Kilburn, K. H., Thrasher, J. D., & Immers, N. B. (2009). Do terbutaline- and mold-associated impairments of the brain and lung relate to autism? *Toxicology and Industrial Health*, *25*(9-10), 703–710. doi:10.1177/0748233709348391 PMID:19793774

Kim, K. N. & Hong, Y. C. (2017). The exposome and the future of epidemiology: a vision and prospect.

Kim, H. J., Han, J. H., Kim, M. K., Lim, C. S., Kim, H. M., & Cho, B. R. (2010). Dual-Color Imaging of Sodium/Calcium Ion Activities with Two-Photon Fluorescent Probes. *Angewandte Chemie International Edition*, *49*(38), 6786–6789. doi:10.1002/anie.201002907 PMID:20715036

Kim, J. H., Kim, H. J., Kim, S. H., Lee, J. H., Do, J. H., Kim, H.-J., ... Kim, J. S. (2009). Fluorescent coumarinyl dithiane as a selective chemodosimeter for mercury (II) ion in aqueous solution. *Tetrahedron Letters*, *50*(43), 5958–5961. doi:10.1016/j.tetlet.2009.08.045

Kim, J. H., Lee, D., Lim, H., Kim, T., Suk, K., & Seo, J. (2018). Risk assessment to human health: Consumer exposure to ingredients in air fresheners. *Regulatory Toxicology and Pharmacology*, *98*, 31–40. doi:10.1016/j.yrtph.2018.05.015 PMID:29857116

Kim, Y. K., Amidfar, M., & Won, E. (2018). A review on inflammatory cytokine-induced alterations of the brain as potential neural biomarkers in post-traumatic stress disorder. *Progress in Neuro-Psychopharmacology & Biological Psychiatry*. doi:10.1016/j.pnpbp.2018.06.008 PMID:29932946

Kiossoglou, P., Borda, A., Gray, K., Martin-Sanchez, F., Verspoor, K., & Lopez-Campos, G. (2017). Characterising the Scope of Exposome Research: A Generalisable Approach. *Studies in Health Technology and Informatics*, *245*, 457–461. PMID:29295136

Kishore, G. M., Padgette, S. R., & Fraley, R. T. (1992). History of herbicide-tolerant crops, methods of development and current state of the art—emphasis on glyphosate tolerance. Weed Technology, 6, 626-634.

Kleter, G. A., Peijnenburg, A. A. C. M., & Aarts, H. J. M. (2005). Health Considerations Regarding Horizontal Transfer of Microbial Transgenes Present in Genetically Modified Crops. *Journal of Biomedicine & Biotechnology*, *2005*(4), 326–352. doi:10.1155/JBB.2005.326 PMID:16489267

Kocovska, E., Fernell, E., Billstedt, E., Minnis, H., & Gillberg, C. (2012). Vitamin D and autism: Clinical review. *Research in Developmental Disabilities*, *33*(5), 1541–1550. doi:10.1016/j.ridd.2012.02.015 PMID:22522213

Kok, E. J., & Kuiper, H. A. (2003). Comparative safety assessment for biotech crops. *Trends in Biotechnology*, *21*(10), 439–444. doi:10.1016/j.tibtech.2003.08.003 PMID:14512230

Kolpin, D. W., Furlong, E. T., Meyer, M. T., Thurman, E. M., Zaugg, S. D., Barber, L. B., & Buxton, H. T. (2002). Pharmaceuticals, Hormones, and Other Organic Wastewater Contaminants in U.S. Streams, 1999–2000: A National Reconnaissance. *Environmental Science & Technology*, *36*(6), 1202–1211. doi:10.1021/es011055j PMID:11944670

Komorowicz, I., & Barałkiewicz, D. (2016). Determination of total arsenic and arsenic species in drinking water, surface water, wastewater, and snow from Wielkopolska, Kujawy-Pomerania, and Lower Silesia provinces, Poland. *Environmental Monitoring and Assessment*, *188*(9), 504. doi:10.100710661-016-5477-y PMID:27488197

Koons, R. D., & Peters, C. A. (1994). Axial distribution of arsenic in individual human hairs by solid sampling graphite furnace AAS. *Journal of Analytical Toxicology*, *18*(1), 36–40. doi:10.1093/jat/18.1.36 PMID:8127082

Korte, E., & Fernando, Q. (1991). A review of arsenic (III) in groundwater. *Critical Reviews in Environmental Control*, *21*(1), 1–39. doi:10.1080/10643389109388408

Kotey, S., Ertel, K., & Whitcomb, B. (2014). Co-occurrence of autism and asthma in a nationally-representative sample of children in the United States. *Journal of Autism and Developmental Disorders*, *44*(12), 3083–3088. doi:10.100710803-014-2174-y PMID:24997632

Kovacs, R., Bakos, K., Urbnyi, B., Kovesi, J., Gazsi, G., Csepeli, A., ... Horvath, A. (2016). Acute and sub-chronic toxicity of four cytostatic drugs in zebrafish. *Environmental Science and Pollution Research International*, *23*(15), 14718–14729. doi:10.100711356-015-5036-z PMID:26201655

Kovacs, R., Csenki, Z., Bakos, K., Urbanyi, B., Horvath, A., Garaj-Vrhovac, V., ... Filipic, M. (2015). Assessment of toxicity and genotoxicity of low doses of 5-fluorouracil in zebrafish (*Danio rerio*) two-generation study. *Water Research*, *77*, 201–212. doi:10.1016/j.watres.2015.03.025 PMID:25889180

Koyama, R., & Ikegaya, Y. (2015). Microglia in the pathogenesis of autism spectrum disorders. *Neuroscience Research*, *100*, 1–5. doi:10.1016/j.neures.2015.06.005 PMID:26116891

Krackt, U. (1981). Food security for people in the 1980s. *Paper prepared for discussion at the North-South Food Roundtable Meeting*, Washington DC.

Krimsky, S. (2014). Low-dose toxicology: Narratives from the science-transcience interface. In N. York (Ed.), *Powerless Science? Science and Politics in a Toxic World.* Berghahn.

Krimsky, S. (2015). An illusory consensus behind GMO health assessment. *Science, Technology & Human Values*, *1*, 32. doi:10.1177/0162243915598381

Krimsky, S. (2017). The Unsteady State and Inertia of Chemical Regulation Under the US Toxic Substances Control Act. *PLoS Biology*, *15*(12), e2002404. doi:10.1371/journal.pbio.2002404 PMID:29252997

Krimsky, S., & Gillam, C. (2018). Roundup litigation discovery documents: Implications for public health and journal ethics. *Journal of Public Health Policy*, *39*(14). doi:10.105741271-018-0134-z PMID:29884897

Krista, H., Tamara, S., & Richard, F. (2009). Environmental justice and Roma communities in Central and Eastern Europe. *Environmental Policy and Governance*, *19*(4), 251–268. doi:10.1002/eet.511

Krupp, D. R., Barnard, R. A., Duffourd, Y., Evans, S. A., Mulqueen, R. M., Bernier, R., ... O'Roak, B. J. (2017). Article: Exonic Mosaic Mutations Contribute Risk for Autism Spectrum Disorder. *American Journal of Human Genetics*, *101*(3), 369–390. doi:10.1016/j.ajhg.2017.07.016 PMID:28867142

Kuhn, T. (1939). The Structure of Scientific Revolutions. In O. Neurath (Ed.), Foundations of the unity of science (Vol. 2). Chicago, IL: University of Chicago Press.

Kuiper, H. A., Kleter, G. A., Noteborn, H. P. J. M., & Kok, E. J. (2001). Assessment of the food safety issues related to genetically modified foods. *The Plant Journal*, *27*(6), 503–528. doi:10.1046/j.1365-313X.2001.01119.x PMID:11576435

Kulage, K., Smaldone, A., & Cohn, E. (2014). How will DSM-5 Affect Autism diagnosis? A Systematic literature review and meta-analysis. *Journal of Autism and Developmental Disorders*, *44*(8), 1918–1932. doi:10.100710803-014-2065-2 PMID:24531932

Kumagai, Y., & Sumi, D. (2007). Arsenic: Signal transduction, transcription factor, and biotransformation involved in cellular response and toxicity. *Annual Review of Pharmacology and Toxicology*, *47*(1), 243–262. doi:10.1146/annurev.pharmtox.47.120505.105144 PMID:17002598

Kumar, A., Ali, M., Rahman, S. M., Iqubal, A. M., Anand, G., Niraj, P. K., ... & Kumar, R. (2015). Ground Water Arsenic Poisoning in "Tilak Rai Ka Hatta" Village of Buxar District, Bihar, India Causing Severe Health Hazards and Hormonal Imbalance. *Journal of Environmental & Analytical Toxicology*, *5*, 290.

Kumar, A., Ghosh, A. K., & Singh, N. (2016c). Arsenic on drinking water: An emerging human right challenge in India. In N. Singh (Ed.), The Human Right to water – From concept to reality (Ch. 4). Springer International Publishing Switzerland.

Kumar, A., Kumar, R., Ali, M., Gahlot, V., & Ghosh, A. K. (2016b). Groundwater Arsenic poisoning in Buxar district of Bihar. In *Proceedings of the 6th International congress on arsenic in the environment*, Stockholm, Sweden, June 19-23 (pp. 378-379). London, UK: Taylor & Francis group.

Kumar, A., Xagoraraki, I. (2010). Pharmaceuticals, personal care products and endocrine-disrupting chemicals in U.S. surface and finished drinking waters: a proposed ranking system. *The Science of the Total Environment, 408*(28), 5972-5989.

Kumar, A., Rahman, M. S., Iqubal, M. A., Ali, M., Niraj, P. K., Anand, G., & Kumar, P. (2016a). Ground water arsenic contamination: A local survey in India. *International Journal of Preventive Medicine*, 7.

Kumar, R., Kranthi, S., Nitharwal, M., Jat, S. L., & Monga, D. (2012). Influence of pesticides and application methods on pest and predatory arthropods associated with cotton. *Phytoparasitica*, *40*(5), 417–424. doi:10.100712600-012-0241-5

Kummerer, K. (2009a). The presence of pharmaceuticals in the environment due to human use—Present knowledge and future challenges. *Journal of Environmental Management*, *90*(8), 2354–2366. doi:10.1016/j.jenvman.2009.01.023 PMID:19261375

Kummerer, K. (2009b). Antibiotics in the environment—a review—part II. *Chemosphere*, *75*(4), 435–441. doi:10.1016/j.chemosphere.2008.12.006 PMID:19178931

Kummerer, K. (2010). Pharmaceuticals in the environment. *Annual Review of Environment and Resources*, *35*(1), 57–75. doi:10.1146/annurev-environ-052809-161223

Kümmerer, K., Haiß, A., Schuster, A., Hein, A., & Ebert, I. (2016). Antineoplastic compounds in the environment—Substances of special concern. *Environmental Science and Pollution Research International*, *23*(15), 14791–14804. doi:10.100711356-014-3902-8 PMID:25475615

Kundi, M., Parrella, A., Lavorgna, M., Criscuolo, E., Russo, C., & Isidori, M. (2016). Prediction and assessment of ecogenotoxicity of antineoplastic drugs in binary mixtures. *Environmental Science and Pollution Research International*, *23*(15), 14771–14779. doi:10.100711356-015-4884-x PMID:26139396

Kurttio, P., Komulainen, H., Hakala, E., Kahelin, H., & Pekkanen, J. (1998). Urinary excretion of arsenic species after exposure to arsenic present in drinking water. *Archives of Environmental Contamination and Toxicology*, *34*(3), 297–305. doi:10.1007002449900321 PMID:9504979

Kushki, A., Drumm, E., Mobarak, M. P., Tanel, N., Dupuis, A., Chau, T., & Anagnostou, E. (2013). Investigating the autonomic nervous system response to anxiety in children with autism spectrum disorders. *PLoS One*, *8*(4), e59730. doi:10.1371/journal.pone.0059730 PMID:23577072

Laenge, R., Steger-Hartmann, T., & Schweinfurth, H. (2006). The environmental risk assessment of human pharmaceuticals in the overall EU regulatory affairs process. *Regulatory Toxicology and Pharmacology*, *45*(3), 223–228. doi:10.1016/j.yrtph.2006.04.001 PMID:16716476

Lai, M. C., Lombardo, M. V., & Baron-Cohen, S. (2014). Autism. *Lancet*, *383*(9920), 896–910. doi:10.1016/S0140-6736(13)61539-1 PMID:24074734

Lamichhane, S. A. (2014). Genetically Modified Foods-Solution for Food Security. *International Journal of Genetic Engineering and Biotechnology*, *5*(1), 43–48.

Lamm, S. H., & Kruse, M. B. (2004). Arsenic Ingestion and Bladder Cancer Mortality—What Do the Dose-Response Relationships Suggest About Mechanism? *Human and Ecological Risk Assessment*, *11*(2), 433–450. doi:10.1080/10807030590925678

Landesman, W. J., Allan, B. F., Langerhans, R. B., Knight, T. M., & Chase, J. M. (2007). Inter-annual associations between precipitation and human incidence of West Nile virus in the United States. *Vector Borne and Zoonotic Diseases (Larchmont, N.Y.)*, *7*(3), 337–343. doi:10.1089/vbz.2006.0590 PMID:17867908

Landi, M. T., Bertazzi, P. A., Baccarelli, A., Consonni, D., Masten, S., Lucier, G., ... Grassman, J. (2003). TCDD-mediated alterations in the AhR-dependent pathway in Seveso, Italy, 20 years after the accident. *Carcinogenesis*, *24*(4), 673–680. doi:10.1093/carcin/bgg002 PMID:12727795

Landrigan, P. J., & Belpoggi, F. (2018). The need for independent research on the health effects of glyphosate-based herbicides. *Environmental Health*, *17*(1), 51. doi:10.118612940-018-0392-z PMID:29843729

Langbein, T., Sonntag, H., Trapp, D., Hoffmann, A., Malms, W., Röth, E. P., ... Zellner, R. (1999). Volatile anaesthetics and the atmosphere: Atmospheric lifetimes and atmospheric effects of halothane, enflurane, isoflurane, desflurane and sevoflurane. *British Journal of Anaesthesia*, *82*(1), 66–73. doi:10.1093/bja/82.1.66 PMID:10325839

Lanphear, B. (2017). Low-level toxicity of chemicals: No acceptable levels? *PLOS Biology*, *15*(12).

Lari, S. Z., Khan, N. A., Gandhi, K. N., Meshram, T. S., & Thacker, N. P. (2014). Comparison of pesticide residues in surface water and ground water of agriculture intensive areas. *Journal of Environmental Health Science & Engineering*, *12*(1), 11. doi:10.1186/2052-336X-12-11 PMID:24398360

Larkin, A., & Hystad, P. (2017). Towards Personal Exposures: How Technology Is Changing Air Pollution and Health Research. *Current Environmental Health Reports*, *4*(4), 463–471. doi:10.100740572-017-0163-y PMID:28983874

Larsson, D. G. J. (2014). Antibiotics in the environment. *Upsala Journal of Medical Sciences*, *119*(2), 108–112. doi:10.3109/03009734.2014.896438 PMID:24646081

LaSalle, J. M. (2013). Epigenomic strategies at the interface of genetic and environmental risk factors for autism. *Journal of Human Genetics*, *58*(7), 396–401. doi:10.1038/jhg.2013.49 PMID:23677056

Layton, B. S., Lafontaine, S., & Renaud, L. P. (1981). Connections of medial preoptic neurons with the median eminence and amygdala. An electrophysiological study in the rat. *Neuroendocrinology*, *33*(4), 235–240. doi:10.1159/000123237 PMID:7290340

Leaderer, B. P., Naeher, L., Jankun, T., Balenger, K., Holford, T. R., Toth, C., ... Koutrakis, P. (1999). Indoor, outdoor, and regional summer and winter concentrations of PM10, PM2.5, SO42-, H+, NH4+, NO3-, NH3, and nitrous acid in homes with and without kerosene space heaters. *Environmental Health Perspectives*, *107*, 223–231. PMID:10064553

Lechtman, H., & Klein, S. (1999). The Production of Copper–Arsenic Alloys (Arsenic Bronze) by Copper smelting: Modern Experiment, Ancient Practice. *Journal of Archaeological Science*, *26*(5), 497–526. doi:10.1006/jasc.1998.0324

Lee, C. H., Yu, C. L., Liao, W. T., Kao, Y. H., Chai, C. Y., Chen, G. S., & Yu, H. S. (2004). Effects and interactions of low doses of arsenic and UVB on keratinocyte apoptosis. *Chemical Research in Toxicology*, *17*(9), 1199–1205.

Lee, K., Yanagisawa, Y., Spengler, J. D., & Billick, I. H. (1995). Classification of house characteristics based on indoor nitrogen dioxide concentrations. *Environment International*, *21*(3), 277–282. doi:10.1016/0160-4120(95)00025-G

Leeman, W. R., Van Den Berg, K. J., & Houben, G. F. (2007). Transfer of chemicals from feed to animal products: The use of transfer factors in risk assessment. *Food Additives and Contaminants*, *24*(1), 1–13. doi:10.1080/02652030600815512 PMID:17164211

Leenhouts, H. P., & Chadwick, K. H. (1989). The molecular basis of stochastic and nonstochastic effects. *Health Physics*, *57*(Suppl. 1), 343–348. doi:10.1097/00004032-198907001-00048 PMID:2606691

Lee, R., Margaritis, M. M., Channon, K., & Antoniades, C. (2012). Evaluating oxidative stress in human cardiovascular disease: Methodological aspects and considerations. *Current Medicinal Chemistry*, *19*, 2504–2520. doi:10.2174/092986712800493057 PMID:22489713

Lee, S. K., Ou, Y. C., Andersen, M. E., & Yang, R. S. H. (2007). A physiologically based pharmacokinetic model for lactational transfer of PCB 153 with or without PCB 126 in mice. *Archives of Toxicology*, *81*(2), 101–111. doi:10.100700204-006-0130-0 PMID:16858609

Lehmann, G. M., LaKind, J. S., Davis, M. H., Hines, E. P., Marchitti, S. A., Alcala, C., & Lorber, M. (2018). Environmental chemicals in breast milk and formula: Exposure and risk assessment implications. *Environmental Health Perspectives*, *126*(9), 096001. doi:10.1289/EHP1953 PMID:30187772

Lenard, L., Laszlo, K., Kertes, E., Ollmann, T., Peczely, L., Kovacs, A., ... Karádi, Z. (2018). Substance P and neurotensin in the limbic system: Their roles in reinforcement and memory consolidation. *Neuroscience and Biobehavioral Reviews*, *85*, 1–20. doi:10.1016/j.neubiorev.2017.09.003 PMID:28887225

Lengfelder, E., Hofmann, W., & Nowak, D. (2012). Impact of arsenic trioxide in the treatment of acute promyelocytic leukemia. *Leukemia*, *26*(3), 433–442. doi:10.1038/leu.2011.245 PMID:21904379

Lewis, D. R., Southwick, J. W., Ouellet-Hellstrom, R., Rench, J., & Calderon, R. L. (1999). Drinking water arsenic in Utah: A cohort mortality study. *Environmental Health Perspectives*, *107*(5), 359–365. doi:10.1289/ehp.99107359 PMID:10210691

Liao, T. C., Lien, Y. T., Wang, S., Huang, S. L., & Chen, C. Y. (2016). Comorbidity of Atopic Disorders with Autism Spectrum Disorder and Attention Deficit/Hyperactivity Disorder. *The Journal of Pediatrics*, *171*, 248–255. doi:10.1016/j.jpeds.2015.12.063 PMID:26846570

Liaw, J., Marshall, G., Yuan, Y., Ferreccio, C., Steinmaus, C., & Smith, A. H. (2008). Increased childhood liver cancer mortality and arsenic in drinking water in northern Chile. *Cancer Epidemiology, Biomarkers & Prevention*, *17*(8), 1982–1987. doi:10.1158/1055-9965.EPI-07-2816 PMID:18708388

Li, C., Srivastava, R. K., Elmets, C. A., Afaq, F., & Athar, M. (2013). Arsenic-induced cutaneous hyperplastic lesions are associated with the dysregulation of Yap, a Hippo signaling-related protein. *Biochemical and Biophysical Research Communications*, *438*(4), 607–612. doi:10.1016/j.bbrc.2013.08.008 PMID:23942117

Li, C., Xu, J., Li, F., Chaudhary, S. C., Weng, Z., Wen, J., ... Athar, M. (2011). Unfolded protein response signaling and MAP kinase pathways underlie pathogenesis of arsenic-induced cutaneous inflammation. *Cancer Prevention Research*, *4*(12), 2101–2109. doi:10.1158/1940-6207.CAPR-11-0343 PMID:21911445

Liebig, M., Moltmann, J. F., & Knacker, T. (2006). Evaluation of measured and predicted environmental concentrations of selected human pharmaceuticals and personal care products. *Environmental Science and Pollution Research International*, *13*(2), 110–119. doi:10.1065/espr2005.08.276 PMID:16612900

Liem, A. K. D., Fürst, P., & Rappe, C. (2000). Exposure of populations to dioxins and related compounds. *Food Additives and Contaminants*, *17*(4), 241–259. doi:10.1080/026520300283324 PMID:10912239

Lien, H. C., Tsai, T. F., Lee, Y. Y., & Hsiao, C. H. (1999). Merkel cell carcinoma and chronic arsenicism. *Journal of the American Academy of Dermatology*, *41*(4), 641–643. PMID:10495389

Lin, C.-H., & Pan, T.-M. (2016). Perspectives on genetically modified crops and food detection. *Journal of Food and Drug Analysis*, *24*(1), 1–8. doi:10.1016/j.jfda.2015.06.011 PMID:28911391

Lin, D., Liu, J., Hu, Z., Cottrell, J. E., & Kass, I. S. (2018). Neonatal anesthesia exposure impacts brain microRNAs and their associated neurodevelopmental processes. *Scientific Reports*, *8*(1), 10656. doi:10.103841598-018-28874-0 PMID:30006558

Lindberg, A.-L., Rahman, M., Persson, L.-A., & Vahter, M. (2008). The risk of arsenic induced skin lesions in Bangladeshi men and women is affected by arsenic metabolism and the age at first exposure. *Toxicology and Applied Pharmacology*, *230*(1), 9–16. doi:10.1016/j.taap.2008.02.001 PMID:18336856

Lioy, P. J., & Rappaport, S. M. (2011). Exposure science and the exposome: An opportunity for coherence in the environmental health sciences [Editorial]. *Environmental Health Perspectives*, *119*(11), A466–A467. doi:10.1289/ehp.1104387 PMID:22171373

Lisowska, K. (2011). Genetically modified crops and food: Pros and cons. *Chemik*, *65*, 1193–1203.

Liu, S., Wang, Y.-M., & Han, J. (2017). Fluorescent chemosensors for copper(II) ion: Structure, mechanism and application. *Journal of Photochemistry and Photobiology C, Photochemistry Reviews*, *32*, 78–103. doi:10.1016/j.jphotochemrev.2017.06.002

Li, W. C. (2014). Occurrence, sources, and fate of pharmaceuticals in aquatic environment and soil. *Environmental Pollution*, *187*, 193–201. doi:10.1016/j.envpol.2014.01.015 PMID:24521932

Li, Y., Missig, G., Finger, B. C., Landino, S. M., Alexander, A. J., Mokler, E. L., ... Bolshakov, V. Y. (2018). Maternal and Early Postnatal Immune Activation Produce Dissociable Effects on Neurotransmission in mPFC-Amygdala Circuits. *The Journal of Neuroscience*, *38*(13), 3358–3372. doi:10.1523/JNEUROSCI.3642-17.2018 PMID:29491010

Li, Y., & Zhang, J. (2007). Serum concentrations of antioxidant vitamins and carotenoids are low in individuals with a history of attempted suicide. *Nutritional Neuroscience*, *10*(1-2), 51–58. doi:10.1080/10284150701250747 PMID:17539483

Llorente-Mirandes, T., Rubio, R., & López-Sánchez, J. F. (2017). Inorganic Arsenic Determination in Food: A Review of Analytical Proposals and Quality Assessment Over the Last Six Years. *Applied Spectroscopy*, *71*(1), 25–69. doi:10.1177/0003702816652374 PMID:28033722

Löffler, D., Römbke, J., Meller, M., & Ternes, T. A. (2005). Environmental fate of pharmaceuticals in water/sediment systems. *Environmental Science & Technology*, *39*(14), 5209–5218. doi:10.1021/es0484146 PMID:16082949

Loh, M., Sarigiannis, D., Gotti, A., Karakitsios, S., Pronk, A., Kuijpers, E., ... Cherrie, J. (2017a). How Sensors Might Help Define the External Exposome. *International Journal of Environmental Research and Public Health*, *14*(4), 434. doi:10.3390/ijerph14040434 PMID:28420222

Longstreth, J. (1991). Anticipated public health consequences of global climate change. *Environmental Health Perspectives*, *96*, 139–144. doi:10.1289/ehp.9196139 PMID:1820256

Loomis, D., & Kromhout, H. (2004). Exposure variability: Concepts and applications in occupational epidemiology. American journal of industrial medicine, 45(1), 113-122. doi:10.1002/ajim.10324 PMID:14691975

Lorentzen, P., McMillan, J., & Wacziarg, R. (2008). Death and development. *Journal of Economic Growth*, *13*(2), 81–124. doi:10.100710887-008-9029-3

Louveau, A., Smirnov, I., Keyes, T. J., Eccles, J. D., Rouhani, S. J., Peske, J. D., ... Kipnis, J. (2015). Structural and functional features of central nervous system lymphatic vessels. *Nature*, *523*(7560), 337–341. doi:10.1038/nature14432 PMID:26030524

Lübbert, C., Baars, C., Dayakar, A., Lippmann, N., Rodloff, A. C., Kinzig, M., & Sörgel, F. (2017). Environmental pollution with antimicrobial agents from bulk drug manufacturing industries in Hyderabad, South India, is associated with dissemination of extended-spectrum beta-lactamase and carbapenemase-producing pathogens. *Infection*, *45*(4), 479–491. doi:10.100715010-017-1007-2 PMID:28444620

Lucier, G. W., Portier, C. J., & Gallo, M. A. (1993). Receptor mechanisms and dose-response models for the effects of dioxins. *Environmental Health Perspectives*, *101*(1), 36–44. doi:10.1289/ehp.9310136 PMID:8390353

Łuczaj, L., Pieroni, A., Tardío, J., Pardo-de-Santayana, M., Sõukand, R., Svanberg, I., & Kalle, R. (2012). Wild food plant use in 21st century Europe: The disappearance of old traditions and the search for new cuisines involving wild edibles. *Acta Societatis Botanicorum Poloniae*, *81*(4), 359–370. doi:10.5586/asbp.2012.031

Lyall, K., Van de Water, J., Ashwood, P., & Hertz-Picciotto, I. (2015). Asthma and Allergies in Children With Autism Spectrum Disorders: Results From the CHARGE Study. *Autism Research*, *8*(5), 567–574. doi:10.1002/aur.1471 PMID:25722050

Lytras, M. D., & Papadopoulou, P. (2018). *Applying Big Data Analytics in Bioinformatics and Medicine*. Hershey, PA: IGI Global. doi:10.4018/978-1-5225-2607-0

MacDonald, S. A., & Vollrath, T. L. (2005). *The forces shaping world cotton consumption after the multifiber arrangement*. Washington, DC: US Department of Agriculture.

Machuka, J. (2001). Agricultural biotechnology for Africa. African scientists and farmers must feed their own people. *Plant Physiology*, *126*(1), 16–19. doi:10.1104/pp.126.1.16 PMID:11351064

MacKinnon, N., Kingsbury, M., Mahedy, L., Evans, J., & Colman, I. (2018). The Association Between Prenatal Stress and Externalizing Symptoms in Childhood: Evidence From the Avon Longitudinal Study of Parents and Children. *Biological Psychiatry*, *83*(2), 100–108. doi:10.1016/j.biopsych.2017.07.010 PMID:28893381

Magaña-Gómez, J. A., & de la Barca, A. M. (2009). Risk assessment of genetically modified crops for nutrition and health. *Nutrition Reviews*, *67*(1), 1–16. doi:10.1111/j.1753-4887.2008.00130.x PMID:19146501

Ma, H., Sorokin, A., Mazein, A., Selkov, A., Selkov, E., Demin, O., & Goryanin, I. (2007). The Edinburgh human metabolic network reconstruction and its functional analysis. *Molecular Systems Biology*, *3*, 135–135. doi:10.1038/msb4100177 PMID:17882155

Ma, J., Sengupta, M. K., Yuan, D., & Dasgupta, P. K. (2014). Speciation and detection of arsenic in aqueous samples: A review of recent progress in non-atomic spectrometric methods. *Analytica Chimica Acta*, *831*, 1–23. doi:10.1016/j.aca.2014.04.029 PMID:24861967

Malisch, R., & Kotz, A. (2014). Dioxins and PCBs in feed and food - Review from European perspective. *The Science of the Total Environment*, *491-492*, 2–10. doi:10.1016/j.scitotenv.2014.03.022 PMID:24804623

Mancini, F., Van Bruggen, A. H., Jiggins, J. L., Ambatipudi, A. C., & Murphy, H. (2005). Acute pesticide poisoning among female and male cotton growers in India. *International Journal of Occupational and Environmental Health*, *11*(3), 221–232. doi:10.1179/oeh.2005.11.3.221 PMID:16130962

Mandal, B. K., & Suzuki, K. T. (2002). Arsenic round the world: A review. *Talanta*, *58*(1), 201–235. doi:10.1016/S0039-9140(02)00268-0 PMID:18968746

Manrai, A. K., Cui, Y., Bushel, P. R., Hall, M., Karakitsios, S., Mattingly, C. J., ... Patel, C. J. (2017). Informatics and Data Analytics to Support Exposome-Based Discovery for Public Health. *Annual Review of Public Health*, *38*(1), 279–294. doi:10.1146/annurev-publhealth-082516-012737 PMID:28068484

Mansfield, N. E., Grundy, J., Coles, M. P., Avent, A. G., & Hitchcock, P. B. (2006, October). A Conformational Study of Phospha(III)- and Phospha(V)-guanidine Compounds. *Journal of the American Chemical Society*, *128*(42), 13879–13893. doi:10.1021/ja064212t

Mao, Q., Manservisi, F., Panzacchi, S., Mandrioli, D., Menghetti, I., Vornoli, A., ... Hu, J. (2018). The Ramazzini Institute 13-week pilot study on glyphosate and roundup administered at human-equivalent dose to Sprague Dawley rats: Effects on the microbiome. *Environmental Health*, *17*(1), 50. doi:10.118612940-018-0394-x PMID:29843725

Marathias, K., Lambracht-Hall, M., Savala, J., & Theoharides, T. C. (1991). Endogenous regulation of rat brain mast cell serotonin release. *International Archives of Allergy and Applied Immunology*, *95*(4), 332–340. doi:10.1159/000235470 PMID:1720423

Marco, E. J., & Skuse, D. H. (2006). Autism-lessons from the X chromosome. *Social Cognitive and Affective Neuroscience*, *1*(3), 183–193. doi:10.1093can/nsl028 PMID:18985105

Marketon, J. I., & Sternberg, E. M. (2010). The glucocorticoid receptor: A revisited target for toxins. *Toxins*, *2*(6), 1357–1380. doi:10.3390/toxins2061357 PMID:22069642

Marques, P. E., Amaral, S. S., Pires, D. A., Nogueira, L. L., Soriani, F. M., Lima, B. H., ... Menezes, G. B. (2012). Chemokines and mitochondrial products activate neutrophils to amplify organ injury during mouse acute liver failure. *Hepatology (Baltimore, Md.)*, *56*(5), 1971–1982. doi:10.1002/hep.25801 PMID:22532075

Marshall, G., Ferreccio, C., Yuan, Y., Bates, M. N., Steinmaus, C., Selvin, S., ... Smith, A. H. (2007). Fifty-Year study of lung and bladder cancer mortality in Chile related to arsenic in drinking water. *Journal of the National Cancer Institute*, *99*(12), 920–928. doi:10.1093/jnci/djm004 PMID:17565158

Martens, W. J., Niessen, L. W., Rotmans, J., Jetten, T. H., & McMichael, A. J. (1995). Potential impact of global climate change on malaria risk. *Environmental Health Perspectives*, *103*(5), 458–464. doi:10.1289/ehp.95103458 PMID:7656875

Martin, C. J., Platt, S. D., & Hunt, S. M. (1987). Housing conditions and ill health. *British Medical Journal (Clinical Research Ed.)*, *294*(6580), 1125–1127. doi:10.1136/bmj.294.6580.1125 PMID:3107723

Martinez, V. D., Buys, T. P. H., Adonis, M., Benítez, H., Gallegos, I., Lam, S., ... Gil, L. (2010). Arsenic-related DNA copy-number alterations in lung squamous cell carcinomas. *British Journal of Cancer*, *103*(8), 1277–1283. doi:10.1038j.bjc.6605879 PMID:20842114

Martuzzi, M., Mitis, F., & Forastiere, F. (2010). Inequalities, inequities, environmental justice in waste management and health. *European Journal of Public Health*, *20*(1), 21–26. doi:10.1093/eurpub/ckp216 PMID:20061348

Masuda, J. R., Poland, B., & Baxter, J. (2010). Reaching for environmental health justice: Canadian experiences for a comprehensive research, policy and advocacy agenda in health promotion. *Health Promotion International*, *25*(4), 453–463. doi:10.1093/heapro/daq041 PMID:20615911

Maszkowska, J., Stolte, S., Kumirska, J., Łukaszewicz, P., Mioduszewska, K., Puckowski, A., ... Białk-Bielińska, A. (2014). Beta-blockers in the environment: Part II. Ecotoxicity study. *The Science of the Total Environment*, *15*(493), 1122–1126. doi:10.1016/j.scitotenv.2014.06.039 PMID:24975494

Matsubara, T., Tanaka, N., Krausz, K. W., Manna, S. K., Kang, D. W., Anderson, E. R., ... Gonzalez, F.J. (2012). Metabolomics identifies an inflammatory cascade involved in dioxin- and diet-induced steatohepatitis. *Cell Metabolism*, *16*(5), 634–644. doi:10.1016/j.cmet.2012.10.006 PMID:23140643

Matsumoto, I., Inoue, Y., Shimada, T., & Aikawa, T. (2001). Brain mast cells act as an immune gate to the hypothalamic-pituitary-adrenal axis in dogs. *The Journal of Experimental Medicine*, *194*(1), 71–78. doi:10.1084/jem.194.1.71 PMID:11435473

Matthiessen, P., & Weltje, L. (2015). A review of the effects of azole compounds in fish and their possible involvement in masculinization of wild fish populations. *Critical Reviews in Toxicology*, *45*(5), 453–467. doi:10.3109/10408444.2015.1018409 PMID:25899164

Maud, C., Ryan, J., McIntosh, J. E., & Olsson, C. A. (2018, May 29). The role of oxytocin receptor gene (OXTR) DNA methylation (DNAm) in human social and emotional functioning: A systematic narrative review. *BMC Psychiatry*, *18*(1), 154. doi:10.118612888-018-1740-9 PMID:29843655

Maxwell, S., & Smith, M. (1992). Part 1: Household food security: A conceptual review. In S. Maxwell & T.R. Frankenberger (Eds.), Household food security: Concepts, indicators, measurements: A technical review (pp. 4-72). United Nations Children's Fund, New York, NY.

Maxwell, S. (1996). Food security: A post-modern perspective. *Food Policy*, *21*(2), 155–170. doi:10.1016/0306-9192(95)00074-7

Mazumder, G. D. N. (2008). Chronic arsenic toxicity and human health. *The Indian Journal of Medical Research*, *128*, 436–447. PMID:19106439

McCall, R. B. (1977). Childhood IQ's as Predictors of Adult Educational and Occupational Status. *Science*, *197*(4302), 482–483. doi:10.1126cience.197.4302.482 PMID:17783247

McCarty, K. M., Hanh, H. T., & Kim, K. W. (2011). Arsenic geochemistry and human health in South East Asia. *Reviews on Environmental Health*, *26*(1), 71–78. doi:10.1515/reveh.2011.010 PMID:21714384

McCusker, R. H., & Kelley, K. W. (2013). Immune-neural connections: How the immune system's response to infectious agents influences behavior. *The Journal of Experimental Biology*, *216*(1), 84–98. doi:10.1242/jeb.073411 PMID:23225871

McDougall, J. A., & McDougall, M. A. (1983). *The McDougall plan*. Clinton, NJ: New Win Pub.

McHenry, L. (2010). Of sophists and spin-doctors: Industry sponsored ghostwriting and the crisis of academic medicine. *Mens Sana Monographs*, *8*(1), 129–145. doi:10.4103/0973-1229.58824 PMID:21327175

McHenry, L. (2018). The Monsanto papers: Poisoning the scientific well. *International Journal of Risk & Safety in Medicine*, *29*(3-4), 193–205. doi:10.3233/JRS-180028 PMID:29843257

McManus, I. C. (1980). Handedness in twins: A critical review. *Neuropsychologia*, *18*(3), 347–355. doi:10.1016/0028-3932(80)90130-X PMID:7191061

McMichael, A. J. (2013). Globalization, climate change, and human health. *The New England Journal of Medicine*, *368*(14), 1335–1343. doi:10.1056/NEJMra1109341 PMID:23550671

McMichael, A. J., & Haines, A. (1997). Global climate change: The potential effects on health. *BMJ: British Medical Journal*, *315*(7111), 805–809. doi:10.1136/bmj.315.7111.805 PMID:9345177

McMichael, A. J., Woodruff, R. E., & Hales, S. (2006). Climate change and human health: Present and future risks. *Lancet*, *367*(9513), 859–869. doi:10.1016/S0140-6736(06)68079-3 PMID:16530580

McMichael, P. (2004). Biotechnology and food security: Profiting on insecurity. In L. Beneria & S. Bisnath (Eds.), *Global tensions: Challenges and opportunities in the world economy* (pp. 137–154). New York, NY: Routledge.

McPartland, J. C., Reichow, B., & Volkmar, F. R. (2012). Sensitivity and specificity of proposed DSM-5 Diagnostic criteria for autism spectrum disorder. *Journal of the American Academy of Child and Adolescent Psychiatry*, *51*(4), 368–383. doi:10.1016/j.jaac.2012.01.007 PMID:22449643

McPartland, J., & Volkmar, F. R. (2012). Autism and related disorders. *Handbook of Clinical Neurology*, *106*, 407–418. doi:10.1016/B978-0-444-52002-9.00023-1 PMID:22608634

Meakin, C. J., Martin, E. M., & Fry, R. C. (2017). Epigenetic mechanisms underlying arsenic-induced toxicity. *Current Opinion in Toxicology*, *6*, 1–9. doi:10.1016/j.cotox.2017.06.003

Meharg, A. A., & Rahman, M. M. (2003). Arsenic Contamination of Bangladesh Paddy Field Soils: Implications for Rice Contribution to Arsenic Consumption. *Environmental Science & Technology*, *37*(2), 229–234. doi:10.1021/es0259842 PMID:12564892

Meliker, J. R., Goovaerts, P., Jacquez, G. M., & Nriagu, J. O. (2010). Incorporating individual-level distributions of exposure error in epidemiologic analyses: An example using arsenic in drinking water and bladder cancer. *Annals of Epidemiology*, *20*(10), 750–758. doi:10.1016/j.annepidem.2010.06.012 PMID:20816314

Melkonian, S., Argos, M., Chen, Y., Parvez, F., Pierce, B., Ahmed, A., ... Ahsan, H. (2012). Intakes of several nutrients are associated with incidence of arsenic-related keratotic skin lesions in Bangladesh. *The Journal of Nutrition*, *142*(12), 2128–2134. doi:10.3945/jn.112.165720 PMID:23077185

Melkonian, S., Argos, M., Pierce, B. L., Chen, Y., Islam, T., Ahmed, A., ... Ahsan, H. (2011). A prospective study of the synergistic effects of arsenic exposure and smoking, sun exposure, fertilizer use, and pesticide use on risk of premalignant skin lesions in Bangladeshi men. *American Journal of Epidemiology*, *173*(2), 183–191. doi:10.1093/aje/kwq357 PMID:21098630

Melloy, P., Hollaway, G., Norton, J. L., Norton, R., Aitken, E., & Chakraborty, S. (2010). Production and fitness of *Fusarium pseudogramearum inoculum* at elevated carbon dioxide in FACE. *Global Change Biology*, *16*(12), 3363–3373. doi:10.1111/j.1365-2486.2010.02178.x

Meng, Q., Wang, Y., Yang, M., Zhang, R., Wang, R., & Zhang, Z. (2015). A new fluorescent chemosensor for highly selective and sensitive detection of inorganic phosphate (Pi) in aqueous solution and living cells. *RSC Advances*, *5*(66), 53189–53197. doi:10.1039/C5RA08712K

Mennigen, J. A., Stroud, P., Zamora, J. M., Moon, T. W., & Trudeau, V. L. (2011). Pharmaceuticals as neuroendocrine disruptors: Lessons learned from fish on Prozac. *Journal of Toxicology and Environmental Health. Part B, Critical Reviews*, *14*(5-7), 387–412. doi:10.1080/10937404.2011.578559 PMID:21790318

Mertens, M., Höss, S., Neumann, G., Afzal, J., and Reichenbecher, W. (2018). Glyphosate, a chelating agent—relevant for ecological risk assessment. *Environmental Science and Pollution Research.* doi:10.100711356-017-1080-1

Merzhanova, G. K., Dolbakyan, E. E., & Khokhlova, V. N. (2000). Interactions between neurons in the amygdala and hypothalamus during conditioned reflex behavior involving choice of reinforcement quality in cats. *Neuroscience and Behavioral Physiology*, *30*(6), 695–702. doi:10.1023/A:1026654917886 PMID:11127797

Mesnage, R., Defarge, N., Spiroux de Vendomois, J., & Seralini, G.-E. (2015). Potential toxic effects of glyphosate and its commercial formulations below regulatory limits. *Food and Chemical Toxicology*, *84*, 133–153. doi:10.1016/j.fct.2015.08.012 PMID:26282372

Michaëlsson, K., Wolk, A., Langenskiöld, S., Basu, S., Lemming, E. W., Melhus, H., & Byberg, L. (2014). Milk intake and risk of mortality and fractures in women and men: Cohort studies. *BMJ (Clinical Research Ed.)*, *349*. Retrieved from https://www.bmj.com/Content/349/bmj.g6015 PMID:25352269

Michalek, J. E., & Tripathi, R. C. (1999). Pharmacokinetics of TCDD in veterans of Operation Ranch Hand: 15-year follow-up. *Journal of Toxicology and Environmental Health. Part A.*, *57*(6), 369–378. doi:10.1080/009841099157584 PMID:10478820

Michalke, B., & Berthele, A. (2011). Contribution to selenium speciation in cerebrospinal fluid samples. *Journal of Analytical Atomic Spectrometry*, *26*(1), 165–170. doi:10.1039/C0JA00106F

Michopoulos, V., Powers, A., Gillespie, C. F., Ressler, K. J., & Jovanovic, T. (2017). Inflammation in Fear- and Anxiety-Based Disorders: PTSD, GAD, and Beyond. *Neuropsychopharmacology*, *42*(1), 254–270. doi:10.1038/npp.2016.146 PMID:27510423

Milbrath, M. O., Wenger, Y., Chang, C. W., Emond, C., Garabrant, D., Gillespie, B. W., & Jolliet, O. (2009). Apparent half-lives of dioxins, furans, and polychlorinated biphenyls as a function of age, body fat, smoking status, and breast-feeding. *Environmental Health Perspectives*, *117*(3), 417–425. doi:10.1289/ehp.11781 PMID:19337517

Milk Life? How About Milk Destruction: The Shocking Truth About the Dairy Industry and the Environment. (2018, April 13). *OnegreenPlanet.* Retrieved from http://www.onegreenplanet.org/animalsandnature/the-dairy-industry-and-the-environment

Milk, A. (2018). Alberta Milk. Retrieved from https://albertamilk.com/

Milkadamia. (n.d.) Milkadamia. Retrieved from http://www.milkadamia.com/#products

Miller, G. W. (2014). The Exposome: Purpose, Definition, and Scope. In G. W. Miller (Ed.), *The Exposome* (pp. 1–12). San Diego, CA: Academic Press. doi:10.1016/B978-0-12-417217-3.00001-X

Miller, G. W., & Jones, D. P. (2014). The nature of nurture: Refining the definition of the exposome. *Toxicological Sciences*, *137*(1), 1–2. doi:10.1093/toxsci/kft251 PMID:24213143

Millett, C., Lee, J. T., Laverty, A. A., Glantz, S. A., & Majeed, A. (2013). Hospital admissions for childhood asthma after smoke-free legislation in England. *Pediatrics*, *131*(2), 495–501. doi:10.1542/peds.2012-2592 PMID:23339216

Milliman, J. D., & Sivitsli, J. P. M. (1992). Geomorphyc/tectonic control of sediment discharge to the ocean: The importance of small mountainous rivers. *The Journal of Geology*, *100*(5), 525–544. doi:10.1086/629606

Millum, J. (2010). How should the benefits of bioprospecting be shared? *The Hastings Center Report*, *40*(1), 24–33. doi:10.1353/hcr.0.0227 PMID:20169653

Milton, A. H., Hore, S. K., Hossain, M. Z., & Rahman, M. (2012). Bangladesh arsenic mitigation programs: Lessons from the past. *Emerging Health Threats Journal*, 5. PMID:22558005

Milton, A. H., Smith, W., Rahman, B., Hasan, Z., Kulsum, U., Dear, K., ... Ali, A. (2005). Chronic arsenic exposure and adverse pregnancy outcomes in Bangladesh. *Epidemiology (Cambridge, Mass.)*, *16*(1), 82–86. doi:10.1097/01.ede.0000147105.94041.e6 PMID:15613949

Milton, M. D., Singh, J. D., & Butcher, R. J. (2004). Synthesis of b-ketoenamine donors having O, N, Se/Te donor functionalities and their reaction chemistry with Pd(II) and Pt(II) metal ions. *Tetrahedron Letters*, *45*(36), 6745–6747. doi:10.1016/j.tetlet.2004.07.057

Ministry of Water Resources, Government of India. (2010). Groundwater quality in shallow aquifers of India, Central Groundwater Board, Faridabad, India.

Modabbernia, A., Velthorst, E., & Reichenberg, A. (2017). Environmental risk factors for autism: An evidence-based review of systematic reviews and meta-analyses. *Molecular Autism*, *8*(1), 13. doi:10.118613229-017-0121-4 PMID:28331572

Moe, B., Peng, H., Lu, X., Chen, B., Chen, L. W., Gabos, S., ... Le, X. C. (2016). Comparative cytotoxicity of fourteen trivalent and pentavalent arsenic species determined using real-time cell sensing. *Journal of Environmental Sciences (China)*, *49*, 113–124. doi:10.1016/j.jes.2016.10.004 PMID:28007166

Moffitt, T. E., Gabrielli, W. F., Mednick, S. A., & Schulsinger, F. (1981). Socioeconomic status, IQ, and delinquency. *Journal of Abnormal Psychology*, *90*(2), 152–156. doi:10.1037/0021-843X.90.2.152 PMID:7288005

Mohai, P., Lantz, P. M., Morenoff, J., House, J. S., & Mero, R. P. (2009). Racial and Socioeconomic Disparities in Residential Proximity to Polluting Industrial Facilities: Evidence From the Americans' Changing Lives Study. *American Journal of Public Health*, *99*(S3), S649–S656. doi:10.2105/AJPH.2007.131383 PMID:19890171

Mohapatra, D. P., Brar, S. K., Daghrir, R., Tyagi, R. D., Picard, P., Surampalli, R. Y., & Drogui, P. (2014). Photocatalytic degradation of carbamazepine in wastewater by using a new class of whey-stabilized nanocrystalline TiO_2 and ZnO. *The Science of the Total Environment*, *485-486*, 263–269. doi:10.1016/j.scitotenv.2014.03.089 PMID:24727044

Mohapatra, D. P., Brar, S. K., Tyagi, R. D., Picard, P., & Surampalli, R. Y. (2014). Analysis and advanced oxidation treatment of a persistent pharmaceutical compound in wastewater and wastewater sludge-carbamazepine. *The Science of the Total Environment*, *470-471*, 58–75. doi:10.1016/j.scitotenv.2013.09.034 PMID:24140682

Moneim, A. E. A. (2015). Mercury-induced neurotoxicity and neuroprotective effects of berberine. *Perspective*, *10*, 881–882. PMID:26199596

Monteiro, H. P., Bechara, E. J., & Abdalla, D. S. (1991). Free radicals involvement in neurological porphyrias and lead poisoning. *Molecular and Cellular Biochemistry*, *103*(1), 73–83. doi:10.1007/BF00229595 PMID:1857346

Moreno Ávila, C. L., Limón-Pacheco, J. H., Giordano, M., & Rodríguez, V. M. (2016). Chronic exposure to arsenic in drinking water causes alterations in locomotor activity and decreases striatal mRNA for the D2 dopamine receptor in CD1 male mice. *Journal of Toxicology*.

Morley, W.A. & Seneff, S. (2014). Diminished brain resilience syndrome: A modern day neurological pathology of increased susceptibility to mild brain trauma, concussion, and downstream neurodegeneration. *Surgical Neurology International*, *5*, 97.

Mortensen, J. D. (1983). A Study of Age Specific Human Respiratory Morphometry: Final Report. University of Utah Research Institute.

Mortensen, J. D. (1988). *Age related morphometric analysis of human lung casts. Extrapolation of Dosimetric Relationships for Inhaled Particles and Gases*. San Diego, CA: Academic Press.

Mortensen, J. D., Young, J. D., Stout, L., Stout, A., Bagley, B., & Schaap, R. N. (1983). A numerical identification system for airways in the lung. *The Anatomical Record*, *206*(1), 103–114. doi:10.1002/ar.1092060112 PMID:6881547

Moscarello, J. M., & LeDoux, J. E. (2013). Active avoidance learning requires prefrontal suppression of amygdala-mediated defensive reactions. *The Journal of Neuroscience*, *33*(9), 3815–3823. doi:10.1523/JNEUROSCI.2596-12.2013 PMID:23447593

Mostafa, M. G., McDonald, J. C., & Cherry, N. M. (2008). Lung cancer and exposure to arsenic in rural Bangladesh. *Occupational and Environmental Medicine*, *65*(11), 765–768. doi:10.1136/oem.2007.037895 PMID:18417558

Moura, D. S., Sultan, S., Georgin-Lavialle, S., Barete, S., Lortholary, O., Gaillard, R., & Hermine, O. (2012). Evidence for cognitive impairment in mastocytosis: Prevalence, features and correlations to depression. *PLoS One*, *7*(6), e39468. doi:10.1371/journal.pone.0039468 PMID:22745762

Moyano, A., Garcia-Sanchez, A., Mayorga, P., Anawar, H. M., & Alvarez-Ayuso, E. (2009). Impact of irrigation with arsenic-rich groundwater on soils and crops. *Journal of Environmental Monitoring*, *11*(3), 498–502. doi:10.1039/B817634E PMID:19280028

Muehlhoff, E., Bennett, A., & McMahon, D. (2013). *Milk and dairy products in human nutrition*. Rome: Food and Agriculture Organization of the United Nations.

Mukai, K., Tsai, M., Saito, H., & Galli, S. J. (2018). Mast cells as sources of cytokines, chemokines, and growth factors. *Immunological Reviews*, *282*(1), 121–150. doi:10.1111/imr.12634 PMID:29431212

Mukherjee, S. C., Rahman, M. M., Chowdhury, U. K., Sengupta, M. K., Lodh, D., Chanda, C. R., ... Chakraborti, D. (2003). Neuropathy in arsenic toxicity from groundwater arsenic contamination in West Bengal, India. *Journal of Environmental Science and Health. Part A*, *38*, 165–183. PMID:12635825

Mundey, M. K., Roy, M., Roy, S., Awasthi, M. K., & Sharma, R. (2013). Antioxidant potential of Ocimum sanctum in arsenic induced nervous tissue damage. *Brazilian Journal of Veterinary Pathology*, *6*, 95–101.

Murcott, S. (2012). *Arsenic Contamination in the World: an International Sourcebook 2012*. IWA Publishing.

Murnaghan, I. (2018). *The long-term effects of GM foods*. Retrieved from www.geneticallymodifiedfoods.co.uk/longterm-effects-gm-foods.html

Murunga, E., & Zawada, E. (2007). Environmental and Occupational Causes of Toxic Injury to the Kidneys and Urinary Tract. In *Environmental and occupational medicine* (pp. 800–812). Lippincott Williams & Wilkins.

Musa, S., Gichuki, J. W., Raburu, P. O., & Mul, C. (2011). Organochlorine and organophosphorus pesticide residues in water and sediment from Yala/Nzoia River within Lake Victoria basin, Kenya. *Journal of Ecology and the Natural Environment*, *3*(12), 392–399.

Myasoedova, T. N., Mikhailova, T. S., Yalovega, G. E., & Plugotarenko, N. K. (2018). Resistive Low-Temperature Sensor Based on the SiO_2ZrO_2 Film for Detection of High Concentrations of NO_2 Gas. *Chemosensors*, *6*(4), 67. doi:10.3390/chemosensors6040067

Myers, J. P., Antoniou, M. N., Blumberg, B., Carroll, L., Colborn, T., Everett, L. G., ... Benbrook, C. M. (2016). Concerns over use of glyphosate-based herbicides and risks associated with exposures: A consensus statement. *Environmental Health*, *15*(1), 19–31. doi:10.118612940-016-0117-0 PMID:26883814

Myers, N., & Kent, J. (1995). *Environmental exodus: an emergent crisis in the global arena*. New York: Climate Institute.

Myszka, D. G. (1999). Improving Biosensor analysis. *Journal of Molecular Recognition*, *12*, 390–408. doi:10.1002/(SICI)1099-1352(199911/12)12:6<390::AID-JMR482>3.0.CO;2-8 PMID:10556875

Naeher, L. P., Brauer, M., Lipsett, M., Zelikoff, J. T., Simpson, C. D., Koenig, J. Q., & Smith, K. R. (2007). Woodsmoke health effects: A review. *Inhalation Toxicology*, *19*(1), 67–106. doi:10.1080/08958370600985875 PMID:17127644

Nałecz-Jawecki, G. (2007). Evaluation of the in vitro biotransformation of fluoxetine with HPLC, mass spectrometry and eco-toxicological tests. *Chemosphere*, *70*(1), 29–35. doi:10.1016/j.chemosphere.2007.07.035 PMID:17764718

Nanda, S., Kumar, M., Kumar, A., Behal, S., & Nanda, S. (2016). Malwa region, The focal point of cancer cases in Punjab: A Review study. *International Journal of Current Research in Multidisciplinary*, *1*(3), 41–45.

Narang, A. P. S., Chawla, L. S., & Khurana, S. B. (1987). Levels of arsenic in Indian opium eaters. *Drug and Alcohol Dependence*, *20*(2), 149–153. doi:10.1016/0376-8716(87)90064-0 PMID:2824159

NASA. (2014). What is climate change? Retrieved from https://www.nasa.gov/audience/forstudents/k-4/stories/nasa-knows/what-is-climate-change-k4.html

Naujokas, M. F., Anderson, B., Ahsan, H., Aposhian, H. V., Graziano, J. H., Thompson, C., & Suk, W. A. (2013). The broad scope of health effects from chronic arsenic exposure: Update on a worldwide public health problem. *Environmental Health Perspectives*, *121*(3), 295–302. doi:10.1289/ehp.1205875 PMID:23458756

Nehru, B., & Dua, R. (1997). The effect of dietary selenium on lead neurotoxicity. *Journal of Environmental Pathology, Toxicology and Oncology*, *16*(1), 47–50.

Neidell, M. J. (2004). Air pollution, health, and socio-economic status: The effect of outdoor air quality on childhood asthma. *Journal of Health Economics*, *23*(6), 1209–1236. doi:10.1016/j.jhealeco.2004.05.002 PMID:15556243

Nematollahi, N., Doronila, A., Mornane, P. J., Duan, A., Kolev, S. D., & Steinemann, A. (2018). Volatile chemical emissions from fragranced baby products. *Air Quality, Atmosphere & Health*, *11*(7), 785–790. doi:10.100711869-018-0593-1 PMID:30147808

Neveu, V., Moussy, A., Rouaix, H., Wedekind, R., Pon, A., Knox, C., ... Scalbert, A. (2017). Exposome-Explorer: A manually-curated database on biomarkers of exposure to dietary and environmental factors. *Nucleic Acids Research, 45*(D1), 979–984. doi:10.1093/nar/gkw980 PMID:27924041

Nickson, R., McArthur, J., Ravenscroft, P., Burgess, W., & Ahmed, I. K. M. (2000). Mechanism of arsenic poisoning of groundwater in Bangladesh and West Bengal. *Applied Geochemistry, 15*(4), 403–413. doi:10.1016/S0883-2927(99)00086-4

Nicolli, H. B., O'Connor, T. E., & Suriano, J. M. (1985). Geoquimica del arsenico y de otros oligoelementos en aguas subterraneas de la llanura Sudoriental de la provinda de Cordoba. *Miscelanea, 71*, 1–112.

Niedzwiecki, M. M., & Miller, G. W. (2017). The Exposome Paradigm in Human Health: Lessons from the Emory Exposome Summer Course. *Environmental Health Perspectives, 125*(6), 064502. doi:10.1289/EHP1712 PMID:28669935

Niehoff, N. M., Nichols, H. B., White, A. J., Parks, C. G., D'aloisio, A. A., & Sandler, D. P. (2016). Childhood and adolescent pesticide exposure and breast cancer risk. *Epidemiology (Cambridge, Mass.), 27*(3), 326–333. doi:10.1097/EDE.0000000000000451 PMID:26808595

Nielson Report. (2015). We are what we eat: Healthy eating trends around the world. Retrieved from https://www.nielsen.com/content/dam/nielsenglobal/eu/nielseninsights/pdfs/Nielsen%20Global%20Health%20and%20Wellness%20Report%20-%20January%202015.pdf

Nieuwenhuijsen, I. M. (2015). *Exposure Assessment in Environmental Epidemiology* (2nd ed.). Oxford University Press. doi:10.1093/med/9780199378784.001.0001

Noonan, C. W., & Balmes, J. R. (2010). Biomass smoke exposures: Health outcomes measures and study design. *Inhalation Toxicology, 22*(2), 108–112. doi:10.3109/08958370903008888 PMID:20044883

Nordstrom, D. K. (2002). Public health. Worldwide occurrences of arsenic in ground water. *Science, 296*(5576), 2143–2145. doi:10.1126cience.1072375 PMID:12077387

Novarino, G., El-Fishawy, P., Kayserili, H., Meguid, N., Scott, E., Schroth, J., ... Gleeson, J. (2012). Mutations in BCKD-kinase Lead to a Potentially Treatable Form of Autism with Epilepsy. *Science, 338*(6105), 394–397. doi:10.1126cience.1224631 PMID:22956686

NRC. (2001). Arsenic in drinking water: 2001 update. Washington, DC: The National academies press.

Ntow, W. J. (2005). Pesticide residues in Volta Lake, Ghana. *Lakes and Reservoirs: Research and Management, 10*(4), 243–248. doi:10.1111/j.1440-1770.2005.00278.x

Nuccitelli, D. (2018, April 23). Pruitt promised polluters EPA will value their profits over American lives; Pruitt is one of TIME's 100 most influential people for his efforts to maximize polluters' profits. *The Guardian.*

Nuckols, J. R., Ward, M. H., & Jarup, L. (2004). Using Geographic Information Systems for Exposure Assessment in Environmental Epidemiology Studies. *Environmental Health Perspectives, 112*(9), 1007–1015. doi:10.1289/ehp.6738 PMID:15198921

Nussbaumer, T., Czasch, C., Klippel, N., Johansson, L., & Tullin, T. (2008). Particulate Emissions from Biomass Combustion in IEA Countries. International Energy Agency (IEA) Bioenergy, Zürich, Switzerland.

Nynas, P., Pukkala, E., Vainio, H., & Oksa, P. (2017). Cancer incidence in asbestos- exposed workers: An ubdate on four Finnish cohorts. *Safety and Health at Work, 8*(20), 169–174. doi:10.1016/j.shaw.2016.11.003 PMID:28593073

O'Bryant, S. E., Edwards, M., Menon, C. V., Gong, G., & Barber, R. (2011). Long-term low-level arsenic exposure is associated with poorer neuropsychological functioning: A Project FRONTIER study. *International Journal of Environmental Research and Public Health*, *8*(3), 861–874. doi:10.3390/ijerph8030861 PMID:21556183

O'Roak, B. J., Vives, L., Fu, W., Egertson, J. D., Stanaway, I. B., Phelps, I. G., ... Munson, J. (2012). Multiplex targeted sequencing identifies recurrently mutated genes in autism spectrum disorders. *Science*, *338*(6114), 1619–1622.

O'Roak, B. J., Vives, L., Girirajan, S., Karakoc, E., Krumm, N., Coe, B. P., ... Eichler, E. E. (2012). Sporadic autism exomes reveal a highly interconnected protein network of de novo mutations. *Nature*, *485*(7397), 246–250. doi:10.1038/nature10989 PMID:22495309

Oaks, J. L., Gilbert, M., Virani, M. Z., Watson, R. T., Meteyer, C. U., Rideout, B. A., ... Khan, A. A. (2004). Diclofenac residues as the cause of vulture population decline in Pakistan. *Nature*, *427*(6975), 630–633. doi:10.1038/nature02317 PMID:14745453

OECD. (1993). *Safety Evaluation of Foods Derived by Modern Biotechnology: Concepts and Principles*. Organisation for Economic Co-operation and Development. Retrieved from http://www.oecd.org/pdf/M00034000/M00034525.pdf

OECD. (1996). *Food Safety Evaluation*. Paris: Organization for Economic Cooperation and Development.

Ogada, D. L., Keesing, F., & Virani, M. Z. (2012). Dropping dead: Causes and consequences of vulture population declines worldwide. *Annals of the New York Academy of Sciences*, *1249*(1), 57–71. doi:10.1111/j.1749-6632.2011.06293.x PMID:22175274

Oguamanam, C. (2013). Intellectual Property, Ag-biotech and the Right to Adequate Food: A Critical African Perspective.

Ogwu, M. C., Osawaru, M. E., & Ahana, C. M. (2014). Challenges in conserving and utilizing plant genetic resources (PGR). *International Journal of Genetics and Molecular Biology*, *6*(2), 16–22. doi:10.5897/IJGMB2013.0083

Olexova, L., Stefanik, P., & Krskova, L. (2016). Increased anxiety-like behaviour and altered GABAergic system in the amygdala and cerebellum of VPA rats - An animal model of autism. *Neuroscience Letters*, *629*, 9–14. doi:10.1016/j.neulet.2016.06.035 PMID:27353514

Olguin, A., Jauge, P., Cebrián, M., & Albores, A. (1983). Arsenic levels in blood, urine, hair, and nails from a chronically exposed human population. *Proceedings of the Western Pharmacology Society*, *26*, 175–177. PMID:6889337

Oliver, M. (2014). Why we need GMO crops in agriculture. *Missouri Medicine*, *111*, 492–507. PMID:25665234

Oracle. (2011). Oracle Crystal Ball Fusion Edition, version 11.0.

Oregon State University Fact Sheet on Glyphosate. (n.d.). Retrieved from http://npic.orst.edu/factsheets/archive/glyphotech.html

Organic Facts. (2018, April 265 Proven Benefits of Hemp Milk. Retrieved from https://www.organicfacts.net/hemp-milk.html

Osawaru, M. E., & Ogwu, M. C. (2014). Conservation and Utilization of Plant Genetic Resources. In: K. Omokhafe, & J. Odewale (Eds), *Proceedings of 38th Annual Conference of the Genetics Society of Nigeria*. (pp 105 -119). Nigeria: Empress Prints Nigeria Ltd.

Oski, F. A. (1996). *Don't drink your milk!: The frightening new medical facts about the worlds most overrated nutrient*. Ringgold, GA: TEACH Services.

Osredkar, J., & Sustar, N. (2011). Copper and zinc, biological role and significance of copper/zinc imbalance. *J. Clinic. Toxicological Sciences*, *3*, 2161–0495.

Ozonoff, S. (2012). Editorial Perspective: Autism Spectrum Disorders in DSM-5 – an historical perspective and the need for change. *Journal of Child Psychology and Psychiatry, and Allied Disciplines*, *53*(10), 1092–1094. doi:10.1111/j.1469-7610.2012.02614.x PMID:22970941

Pacific Foods. (2018). Pacific Foods. Retrieved from https://www.pacificfoods.com/

Packer, C. N., Stewart-Brown, S., & Fowle, S. E. (1994). Damp housing and adult health: Results from a lifestyle study in Worcester, England. *Journal of Epidemiology and Community Health*, *48*(6), 555–559. doi:10.1136/jech.48.6.555 PMID:7830009

Painter, M. M., Buerkley, M. A., Julius, M. L., Vajda, A. M., Norris, D. O., Barber, L. B., ... Schoenfuss, H. L. (2009). Antidepressants at environmentally relevant concentrations affect predator avoidance behavior of larval fathead minnows (*Pimephales promelas*). *Environmental Toxicology and Chemistry*, *28*(12), 2677–2684. doi:10.1897/08-556.1 PMID:19405782

Pandey, J. S., Kumar, R., & Devotta, S. (2005). Health risks of NO2, SPM and SO_2 in Delhi (India). *Atmospheric Environment*, *39*(36), 6868–6874. doi:10.1016/j.atmosenv.2005.08.004

Pang, X., Letourneau, R., Rozniecki, J. J., Wang, L., & Theoharides, T. C. (1996). Definitive characterization of rat hypothalamic mast cells. *Neuroscience*, *73*(3), 889–902. doi:10.1016/0306-4522(95)00606-0 PMID:8809807

Panigrahy, D., Kaipainen, A., Greene, E. R., & Huang, S. (2010). Cytochrome P450-derived eicosanoids: The neglected pathway in cancer. *Cancer and Metastasis Reviews*, *29*(4), 723–735. doi:10.100710555-010-9264-x PMID:20941528

Pan, W., Stone, K. P., Hsuchou, H., Manda, V. K., Zhang, Y., & Kastin, A. J. (2011). Cytokine signaling modulates blood-brain barrier function. *Current Pharmaceutical Design*, *17*, 3729–3740. doi:10.2174/138161211798220918 PMID:21834767

Papadopoulou, P., Lytras, M., & Marouli, C. (2018). Bioinformatics as Applied to Medicine: Challenges Faced Moving from Big Data to Smart Data to Wise Data. In M. Lytras & P. Papadopoulou (Eds.), *Applying Big Data Analytics in Bioinformatics and Medicine* (pp. 1–25). Hershey, PA: IGI Global. doi:10.4018/978-1-5225-2607-0.ch001

Parratt, J. R., & Sturgess, R. M. (1977). The possible roles of histamine, 5-hydroxytryptamine and prostaglandin F_{2alpha} as mediators of the acute pulmonary effects of endotoxin. *British Journal of Pharmacology*, *60*, 209–219. doi:10.1111/j.1476-5381.1977.tb07743.x PMID:328105

Parvez, F., Chen, Y., Brandt-Rauf, P. W., Slavkovich, V., Islam, T., Ahmed, A., ... Haque, S. E. (2010). A prospective study of respiratory symptoms associated with chronic arsenic exposure in Bangladesh: Findings from the Health Effects of Arsenic Longitudinal Study (HEALS). *Thorax*, *65*(6), 528–533. doi:10.1136/thx.2009.119347 PMID:20522851

Parvez, S., Gerona, R. R., Proctor, C., Friesen, M., Ashby, J. L., Reiter, J. L., ... Winchester, P. D. (2018). Glyphosate exposure in pregnancy and shortened gestational length: A prospective Indiana birth cohort study. *Environmental Health*, *17*(1), 23. doi:10.118612940-018-0367-0 PMID:29519238

Pastor Ciscato, C. H., Gebara, A. B., & de Souza Spinosa, H. (2002). Pesticide residues in cow milk consumed in Sao Paulo City (Brazil). *Journal of Environmental Science and Health. Part. B, Pesticides, Food Contaminants, and Agricultural Wastes*, *37*(4), 323–330. doi:10.1081/PFC-120004473 PMID:12081024

Patel, A. B., Tsilioni, I., Leeman, S. E., & Theoharides, T. C. (2016). Neurotensin stimulates sortilin and mTOR in human microglia inhibitable by methoxyluteolin, a potential therapeutic target for autism. *Proceedings of the National Academy of Sciences of the United States of America, 113*(45), E7049–E7058. doi:10.1073/pnas.1604992113 PMID:27663735

Patel, S. (2017). Fragrance compounds: The wolves in sheep's clothings. *Medical Hypotheses, 102*, 106–111. doi:10.1016/j.mehy.2017.03.025 PMID:28478814

Patz, J. A. (2002). A human disease indicator for the effects of recent global climate change. *Proceedings of the National Academy of Sciences of the United States of America, 99*(20), 12506–12508. doi:10.1073/pnas.212467899 PMID:12271143

Patz, J. A., Campbell-Lendrum, D., Holloway, T., & Foley, J. A. (2005). Impact of regional climate change on human health. *Nature, 438*(7066), 310–317. doi:10.1038/nature04188 PMID:16292302

Paulsen, F., Mai, S., Zellmer, U., & Alsen-Hinrichs, C. (1996). Blood and hair arsenic, lead and cadmium analysis of adults and correlation analysis with special reference to eating habits and other behavioral influences. *Gesundheitswesen (Bundesverband der Arzte des Offentlichen Gesundheitsdienstes (Germany)), 58*, 459–464. (in German) PubMed PMID:9011262

Pay, E. (2009). *The market for organic and fair-trade cotton fibre and cotton fibre products*. Rome, Italy: Food and Agriculture Organization of the United Nations.

Pazou, E. Y. A., Lalèyè, P., Boko, M., Van Gestel, M. A., Ahissou, H., Akpona, S., ... Van Straalen, N. M. (2006). Contamination of fish by organochlorine pesticide residues in the Ouémé River catchment in the Republic of Bénin. *Environment International, 32*(5), 594–599. doi:10.1016/j.envint.2006.01.007 PMID:16494946

Pearce, N. (2016). *Analysis of matched case-control studies*. Academic Press.

Pearce, D. C., Dowling, K., & Sim, M. R. (2012). Cancer incidence and soil arsenic exposure in a historical gold mining area in Victoria, Australia: A geospatial analysis. *Journal of Exposure Science & Environmental Epidemiology, 22*(3), 248–257. doi:10.1038/jes.2012.15 PMID:22434113

Pedersen, J. M., Mortensen, E. L., Christensen, D. S., Rozing, M., Brunsgaard, H., Meincke, R. H., ... Lund, R. (2018). Prenatal and early postnatal stress and later life inflammation. *Psychoneuroendocrinology, 88*, 158–166. doi:10.1016/j.psyneuen.2017.12.014 PMID:29291495

Pediatrics, A. A. o. (2000). Guide to Your Child's Allegies and Asthma. New York: V. Books.

Peltola, J., Andersson, M. A., Haahtela, T., Mussalo-Rauhamaa, H., Rainey, F. A., Kroppenstedt, R. M., ... Salkinoja-Salonen, M. S. (2001). Toxic-metabolite-producing bacteria and fungus in an indoor environment. *Applied and Environmental Microbiology, 67*(7), 3269–3274. doi:10.1128/AEM.67.7.3269-3274.2001 PMID:11425751

Pereira, B. V. R., Matus, G. N., Costa, M. J., Santos, A. C. A. D., Silva-Zacarin, E. C. M., do Carmo, J. B., & Nunes, B. (2018). Assessment of biochemical alterations in the neotropical fish species *Phalloceros harpagos* after acute and chronic exposure to the drugs paracetamol and propranolol. *Environmental Science and Pollution Research International, 25*(15), 14899–14910. doi:10.100711356-018-1699-6 PMID:29546518

Pesaran, M. H. (2004). General Diagnostic Tests for Cross Section Dependence in Panels. *CESifo*. Retrieved from https://ssrn.com/abstract=572504

Pesaran, H. M. (2007). A Simple Panel Unit Root Test in the Presence of Cross Section Dependence. *Journal of Applied Econometrics, 22*(2), 265–312. doi:10.1002/jae.951

Pesatori, A. C., Sontag, J. M., Lubin, J. H., Consonni, D., & Blair, A. (1994). Cohort mortality and nested case-control study of lung cancer among structural pest control workers in Florida (United States). *Cancer Causes & Control*, *5*(4), 310–318. doi:10.1007/BF01804981 PMID:8080942

Pesticide Action Network UK. (2000). *Methyl parathion*. Pesticide News No 36. Retrieved from http://www.pan-uk.org/pestnews/actives/methylpa.htm

Petherick, A. (2016). Milk consumption around the world. *Splash! Milk science update. International Milk Genomics Consortium*. Retrieved from http://milkgenomics.org/wp-content/uploads/2016/01/January-2016-SPLASH.pdf

Petra, A. I., Panagiotidou, S., Hatziagelaki, E., Stewart, J. M., Conti, P., & Theoharides, T. C. (2015). Gut-Microbiota-Brain Axis and Its Effect on Neuropsychiatric Disorders With Suspected Immune Dysregulation. *Clinical Therapeutics*, *37*(5), 984–995. doi:10.1016/j.clinthera.2015.04.002 PMID:26046241

Petrat, F., Boengler, K., Schulz, R., & de Groot, H. (2012). Glycine, a simple physiological compound protecting by yet puzzling mechanism (s) against ischaemia–reperfusion injury: Current knowledge. *British Journal of Pharmacology*, *165*(7), 2059–2072. doi:10.1111/j.1476-5381.2011.01711.x PMID:22044190

Pfizer. (2018). *Pharmaceuticals in the environment (PIE)*. US: Pfizer Inc.

Philip, R. C., Whalley, H. C., Stanfield, A. C., Sprengelmeyer, R., Santos, I. M., Young, A. W., ... Hall, J. (2010). Deficits in facial, body movement and vocal emotional processing in autism spectrum disorders. *Psychological Medicine*, *40*(11), 1919–1929. doi:10.1017/S0033291709992364 PMID:20102666

Phillips, T. (2008). Genetically modified organisms (GMOs): Transgenic crops and recombinant DNA technology. *Nature Education*, *1*(1), 213.

Pighin, J. (2003). Transgenic crops: how genetics is providing new ways to envision agriculture. *The Science Creative Quarterly*. Retrieved from http://www.scq.ubc.ca/transgenic-crops-how-genetics-is-providing-new-ways-to- envision-agriculture/

Pikki, K., Vorne, V., Ojanpera, K., & Pleijel, H. (2017). Impact of elevated O_3 and CO_2 exposure on potato tuber micronutrients. *Agriculture, Ecosystems & Environment*, *118*(1-4), 55–64. doi:10.1016/j.agee.2006.04.012

Pimparkar, B. D., & Bhave, A. (2010). Arsenicosis: Review of recent advances. *The Journal of the Association of Physicians of India*, *58*, 617–624. PMID:21510113

Pinstrup-Anderson, P. (2009). Food security: Definition and measurement. *Food Security*, *1*(1), 5–7. doi:10.100712571-008-0002-y

Plum, L. M., Rink, L., & Haase, H. (2010). The essential toxin: Impact of zinc on human health. *International Journal of Environmental Research and Public Health*, *7*(4), 1342–1365. doi:10.3390/ijerph7041342 PMID:20617034

Poduri, A., & Christopher, A. (2013). Somatic Mutation, Genomic Variation, and Neurological Disease. *Science*, *341*(6141), 1237758. doi:10.1126cience.1237758 PMID:23828942

Poiger, T., Buser, H., & Müller, M. D. (2001). Photodegradation of the pharmaceutical drug diclofenac in a lake: Pathway, field measurements, and mathematical modelling. *Environmental Toxicology and Chemistry*, *20*(2), 256–263. doi:10.1002/etc.5620200205 PMID:11351424

Polańska, K., Hanke, W., Gromadzińska, J., Ligocka, D., Gulczyńska, E., Sobala, W., & Wąsowicz, W. (2009). Polish mother and child cohort study - Defining the problem, the aim of the study and methodological assumptions. *International Journal of Occupational Medicine and Environmental Health*, *22*(4), 383–391. doi:10.2478/v10001-009-0037-0 PMID:20053622

Polańska, K., Hanke, W., Jurewicz, J., Sobala, W., Madsen, C., Nafstad, P., & Magnus, P. (2011). Polish mother and child cohort study (REPRO-PL) -Methodology of follow-up of the children. *International Journal of Occupational Medicine and Environmental Health*, *24*(4), 391–398. doi:10.247813382-011-0026-y PMID:22086452

Polanska, K., Hanke, W., Krol, A., Gromadzinska, J., Kuras, R., Janasik, B., ... Calamandrei, G. (2017). Micronutrients during pregnancy and child psychomotor development: Opposite effects of Zinc and Selenium. *Environmental Research*, *158*, 583–589. doi:10.1016/j.envres.2017.06.037 PMID:28715787

Polanska, K., Hanke, W., Sobala, W., Trzcinka-Ochocka, M., Ligocka, D., Brzeznicki, S., ... Magnus, P. (2013). Developmental effects of exposures to environmental factors: The polish mother and child cohort study. *BioMed Research International*. PMID:24191247

Polańska, K., Hanke, W., Sobala, W., Trzcinka-Ochocka, M., Ligocka, D., Strugała-Stawik, H., & Magnus, P. (2014). Predictors of environmental lead exposure among pregnant women - A prospective cohort study in Poland. *Annals of Agricultural and Environmental Medicine*, *21*, 49–54. PMID:24738496

Polanska, K., Ligocka, D., Sobala, W., & Hanke, W. (2014). Phthalate exposure and child development: The Polish Mother and Child Cohort Study. *Early Human Development*, *90*(9), 477–485. doi:10.1016/j.earlhumdev.2014.06.006 PMID:25038557

Polanska, K., Ligocka, D., Sobala, W., & Hanke, W. (2016). Effect of environmental phthalate exposure on pregnancy duration and birth outcomes. *International Journal of Occupational Medicine and Environmental Health*, *29*(4), 683–697. doi:10.13075/ijomeh.1896.00691 PMID:27443763

Polydoro, M., Schröder, N., Lima, M. N. M., Caldana, F., Laranja, D. C., Bromberg, E., ... Dal-Pizzol, F. (2004). Haloperidol-and clozapine-induced oxidative stress in the rat brain. *Pharmacology, Biochemistry, and Behavior*, *78*(4), 751–756. doi:10.1016/j.pbb.2004.05.018 PMID:15301931

Pompella, A., Visvikis, A., Paolicchi, A., De Tata, V., & Casini, A. F. (2003). The changing faces of glutathione, a cellular protagonist. *Biochemical Pharmacology*, *66*(8), 1499–1503. doi:10.1016/S0006-2952(03)00504-5 PMID:14555227

Pope, C. A. III, Ezzati, M., & Dockery, D. W. (2009). Fine-particulate air pollution and life expectancy in the United States. *The New England Journal of Medicine*, *360*(4), 376–386. doi:10.1056/NEJMsa0805646 PMID:19164188

Porter, J. R., Liyong, X., Challinor, A. J., Cochrane, K., Howden, S. M., Iqbal, M. M., … Ziska, L. (2014). Food security and food production systems. In C. Field et al. (Eds.), Climate change 2014: Impacts, adaptation, and vulnerability, Part A: Global and Sectoral Aspects (pp. 485-533). New York, NY: Cambridge University Press.

Portier, C. J., Tart, K. T., Carter, S. R., Dilworth, C. H., Grambsch, A. E., Gohlke, J., ... Maslak, T. (2013). A human health perspective on climate change: A report outlining the research needs on the human health effects of climate change. *Journal of Current Issues in Globalization*, *6*(4), 621–710.

Pournara, A., Kippler, M., Holmlund, T., Ceder, R., Grafstrom, R., Vahter, M., ... Wallberg, A. E. (2016). Arsenic alters global histone modifications in lymphocytes in 616 vitro and in vivo. *Cell Biology and Toxicology*, *32*(4), 275–284. doi:10.100710565-016-9334-0 PMID:27165195

Powell, C. (2015). How to make a GMO. Retrieved from http://sitn.hms.harvard.edu/flash/2015/how-to-make-a-gmo/

Powell, S. R. (2000). The antioxidant properties of zinc. *The Journal of Nutrition*, *130*(5), 1447S–1454S. doi:10.1093/jn/130.5.1447S PMID:10801958

Pritchett, L., & Summers, L. H. (1993). *Wealthier is healthier* (Vol. 1150). World Bank Publications.

Prüss-Üstün, A., Wolf, J., Corvalán, C. F., Bos, R., & Neira, M. P. (2016). *Preventing disease through healthy environments: a global assessment of the burden of disease from environmental risks*. World Health Organization. Retrieved from http://www.who.int/iris/handle/10665/204585

Public Health Information Systems. (2017). *Registries - Routine and Public*. Retrieved from www.coursera.org/learn/epidemiology-public-health/lecture/pYnBq/public-health-information-systems-July-24

Qaim, M., & Kouser, S. (2013). Genetically Modified Crops and Food Security. *PLoS One*, *8*(6), e64879. doi:10.1371/journal.pone.0064879 PMID:23755155

Qian, R. C., & Long, Y. T. (2017). Wearable Chemosensors: A Review of Recent Progress. *ChemistryOpen*. doi:10.1002/o00pen.2017159 PMID:29435397

Quadrelli, R., & Peterson, S. (2007). The energy–climate challenge: Recent trends in CO_2 emissions from fuel combustion. *Energy Policy*, *35*(11), 5938–5952. doi:10.1016/j.enpol.2007.07.001

Quinn, B., Schmidt, W., O'Rourke, K., & Hernan, R. (2011). Effects of the pharmaceuticals gemfibrozil and diclofenac on biomarker expression in the zebra mussel (*Dreissena polymorpha*) and their comparison with standardised toxicity tests. *Chemosphere*, *84*(5), 657–663. doi:10.1016/j.chemosphere.2011.03.033 PMID:21489596

Radjenović, J., Petrović, M., & Barceló, D. (2009). Fate and distribution of pharmaceuticals in wastewater and sewage sludge of the conventional activated sludge (CAS) and advanced membrane bioreactor (MBR) treatment. *Water Research*, *43*(3), 831–841. doi:10.1016/j.watres.2008.11.043 PMID:19091371

Raessler, M. (2018). The Arsenic Contamination of Drinking and Groundwaters in Bangladesh: Featuring Biogeochemical Aspects and Implications on Public Health. *Archives of Environmental Contamination and Toxicology*, *75*(1), 1–7. doi:10.100700244-018-0511-4 PMID:29520432

Raghavan, U. N., Albert, R., & Kumara, S. (2007). Near linear time algorithm to detect community structures in large-scale networks. *Physical Review. E*, *76*(3), 036106. doi:10.1103/PhysRevE.76.036106 PMID:17930305

Rahman, M. M., Ng, J. C., & Naidu, R. (2009). Chronic exposure of arsenic via drinking water and its adverse health impacts on humans. *Environmental Geochemistry and Health*, *31*(S1), 189–200. doi:10.100710653-008-9235-0 PMID:19190988

Raie, R. M. (1996). Regional variation in As, Cu, Hg, and Se and interaction between them. *Ecotoxicology and Environmental Safety*, *35*(3), 248–252. doi:10.1006/eesa.1996.0107 PMID:9007001

Rampersaud, G. C., Pereira, M. A., Girard, B. L., Adams, J., & Metzl, J. D. (2005). Breakfast habits, nutritional status, body weight, and academic performance in children and adolescents. *Journal of the American Dietetic Association*, *105*(5), 743–760. doi:10.1016/j.jada.2005.02.007 PMID:15883552

Ransohoff, R. M., & Brown, M. A. (2012). Innate immunity in the central nervous system. *The Journal of Clinical Investigation*, *122*(4), 1164–1171. doi:10.1172/JCI58644 PMID:22466658

Rappaport, S. M. (2011). Implications of the exposome for exposure science. *Journal of Exposure Science & Environmental Epidemiology*, *21*(1), 5–9. doi:10.1038/jes.2010.50 PMID:21081972

Rappaport, S. M. (2018). Redefining environmental exposure for disease etiology. *NPJ Syst Biol Appl.*, *4*(1), 30. doi:10.103841540-018-0065-0 PMID:30181901

Rappaport, S. M., Barupal, D. K., Wishart, D., Vineis, P., & Scalbert, A. (2014). The Blood Exposome and Its Role in Discovering Causes of Disease. *Environmental Health Perspectives*, *122*(8), 769–774. doi:10.1289/ehp.1308015 PMID:24659601

Rappaport, S. M., & Smith, M. T. (2010). Environment and disease risks. *Science*, *330*(6003), 460–461. doi:10.1126cience.1192603 PMID:20966241

Ratnaike, R.H. (2003). Acute and chronic arsenic toxicity. *Post Graduate Medical Journal*, *79*, 391-396.

Ratnaseelan, A. M., Tsilioni, I., & Theoharides, T. C. (2018). Effects of Mycotoxins on Neuropsychiatric Symptoms and Immune Processes. *Clinical Therapeutics*, *40*(6), 903–917. doi:10.1016/j.clinthera.2018.05.004 PMID:29880330

Ravenscroft, P., Brammer, H., & Richards, K. (2011). Health Effects of Arsenic in Drinking Water and Food. In *Arsenic pollution: A global synthesis*. Chichester: Wiley-Blackwell.

Rea, W. J., Didriksen, N., Simon, T. R., Pan, Y., Fenyves, E. J., & Griffiths, B. (2003). Effects of toxic exposure to molds and mycotoxins in building-related illnesses. *Archives of Environmental Health*, *58*(7), 399–405. doi:10.1080/00039896.2003.11879140 PMID:15143852

Recombinant Bovine Growth Hormone. (2018). American Cancer Society. Retrieved from https://www.cancer.org/cancer/cancer-causes/recombinant-bovine-growth-hormone.html

Reece, J. B., Urry, L. A., Cain, M. L., Wasserman, S. A., Minorsky, P. V., & Jackson, R. B. (2011). *Campbell biology*. Pearson Boston.

Regal, P. J. (1986). Models of genetically engineered organisms and their ecological impact. In H. A. Mooney & J. K. Drake (Eds.), *Ecology of Biological Invasions of North America and Hawaii* (pp. 111–129). New York: Springer. doi:10.1007/978-1-4612-4988-7_7

Regnault, T., Friedman, J., Wilkening, R., Anthony, R., & Hay, W. Jr. (2005). Fetoplacental transport and utilization of amino acids in IUGR—A review. *Placenta*, *26*, S52–S62. doi:10.1016/j.placenta.2005.01.003 PMID:15837069

Reichard, J. F., & Puga, A. (2010). Effects of arsenic exposure on DNA methylation and epigenetic gene regulation. *Epigenomics*, *2*(1), 87–104. doi:10.2217/epi.09.45 PMID:20514360

Remans, R., Wood, S., Saha, N., Anderman, T., & DeFries, R. (2014). Measuring nutritional diversity of national food supplies. *Global Food Security*, *3*(3-4), 174–182. doi:10.1016/j.gfs.2014.07.001

Renub Research. (2018). Global Dairy Alternatives Market to cross US $34 Billion by the year 2024. Retrieved from https://www.renub.com/global-dairy-alternatives-market-nd.php

Renzaho, A., & Mellor, D. (2010). Food security measurement in cultural pluralism: Missing the point or conceptual misunderstanding? *Nutrition (Burbank, Los Angeles County, Calif.)*, *26*(1), 1–9. doi:10.1016/j.nut.2009.05.001 PMID:19804955

Reports of the Joint Meeting of the FAO Panel of Experts on Pesticide Residues in Food and the WHO Core Assessment Group. (2003). Retrieved from http://www.fao.org/ag/AGP/AGPP/Pesticid

Responsible Environment Enhanced Livelihoods. (2016). REEL COTTON Code of Conduct, Version 1.0. Retrieved from http://cottonconnect.org/wp-content/uploads/reel-code-1.0.pdf

Ressler, K. J. (2010). Amygdala activity, fear, and anxiety: Modulation by stress. *Biological Psychiatry*, *67*(12), 1117–1119. doi:10.1016/j.biopsych.2010.04.027 PMID:20525501

Reutlinger, S., & Knapp, K. (1980). *Food security in deficit countries*. World Bank.

Riaz, L., Mahmood, T., Khalid, A., Rashid, A., Ahmed Siddique, M. B., Kamal, A., & Coyne, M. S. (2018). Fluoroquinolones (FQs) in the environment: A review on their abundance, sorption and toxicity in soil. *Chemosphere*, *191*, 704–720. doi:10.1016/j.chemosphere.2017.10.092 PMID:29078193

Ribeiro, L. D. O. P., Vargas-Pinilla, P., Kappel, D. B., Longo, D., Ranzan, J., Becker, M. M., ... & Schuch, J. B. (2018, June 1). Evidence for Association Between OXTR Gene and ASD Clinical Phenotypes. *Journal of Molecular Neuroscience*. doi:10.100712031-018-1088-0

Rice, S. A. (2003). Health effects of acute and prolonged CO2 exposure in normal and sensitive populations. In *Second Annual Conference on Carbon Sequestration* (pp. 5-8).

Richard, J., & Thomas, R. J. (2013). Particle size and pathogenicity in the respiratory tract. *Virulence*, *4*(8), 847–858. doi:10.4161/viru.27172 PMID:24225380

Richards, C., Jones, C., Groves, L., Moss, J., & Oliver, C. (2015). Prevalence of autism spectrum disorder phenomenology in genetic disorders: A systematic review and meta-analysis. *The Lancet. Psychiatry*, *2*(10), 909–916. doi:10.1016/S2215-0366(15)00376-4 PMID:26341300

Ripple Foods. (2017). Ripple Foods. Retrieved from https://www.ripplefoods.com/

Rivas, M., Garay, R. P., Escanero, J. F., Cia, J. R., Cia, P., & Alda, J. O. (2002, July). Soy milk lowers blood pressure in men and women with mild to moderate essential hypertension. NCBI. Retrieved from https://www.ncbi.nlm.nih.gov/pubmed/12097666

Robbins, T. W., & Sahakian, B. J. (2002). *Computer Methods of Assessment of Cognitive Function. In Principles and Practice of Geriatric Psychiatry* (pp. 147–151). John Wiley & Sons, Ltd. doi:10.1002/0470846410.ch28

Robertson, K., Stafford, T., Benedicto, J., & Hocking, N. (2013). Autism assessment: The Melton health model. *Journal of Paediatrics and Child Health*, *49*(12), 1057–1062. doi:10.1111/jpc.12303 PMID:23782166

Robinson, O., & Vrijheid, M. (2015). The Pregnancy Exposome. *Current Environmental Health Reports*, *2*(2), 204–213. doi:10.100740572-015-0043-2 PMID:26231368

Rodgers, A. B., Morgan, C. P., Bronson, S. L., Revello, S., & Bale, T. L. (2013). Paternal stress exposure alters sperm microRNA content and reprograms offspring HPA stress axis regulation. *The Journal of Neuroscience*, *33*(21), 9003–9012. doi:10.1523/JNEUROSCI.0914-13.2013 PMID:23699511

Rodgers, J., Glod, M., Connolly, B., & McConachie, H. (2012). The relationship between anxiety and repetitive behaviours in autism spectrum disorder. *Journal of Autism and Developmental Disorders*, *42*(11), 2404–2409. doi:10.100710803-012-1531-y PMID:22527704

Rodier, P. M. (1994). Vulnerable periods and processes during central nervous system development. *Environmental Health Perspectives*, *102*(Suppl. 2), 121–124. PMID:7925182

Rodriguez-Barranco, M., Gil, F., Hernández, A. F., Alguacil, J., Lorca, A., Mendoza, R., ... Lacasaña, M. (2016). Postnatal arsenic exposure and attention impairment in school children. *Cortex*, *74*, 370–382. doi:10.1016/j.cortex.2014.12.018 PMID:25682472

Rodriguez, J. I., & Kern, J. K. (2011). Evidence of microglial activation in autism and its possible role in brain underconnectivity. *Neuron Glia Biology*, *7*(2-4), 205–213. doi:10.1017/S1740925X12000142 PMID:22874006

Roede, J. R., Uppal, K., Park, Y., Tran, V., & Jones, D. P. (2014). Transcriptome–metabolome wide association study (TMWAS) of maneb and paraquat neurotoxicity reveals network level interactions in toxicologic mechanism. *Toxicology Reports*, *1*, 435–444. doi:10.1016/j.toxrep.2014.07.006 PMID:27722094

Rogan, W. J., & Gladen, B. C. (1993). Breast-feeding and cognitive development. *Early Human Development*, *31*(3), 181–193. doi:10.1016/0378-3782(93)90194-Y PMID:8444137

Rogers, C. E., Tomita, A. V., Trowbridge, P. R., Gone, J. K., Chen, J., Zeeb, P., ... Durant, J. L. (1997). Hair analysis does not support hypothesized arsenic and chromium exposure from drinking water in Woburn, Massachusetts. *Environmental Health Perspectives, 105*(10), 1090–1097. doi:10.1289/ehp.971051090 PMID:9349834

Role of Dairy in the Diet. (2018). Think USA dairy by the U.S. Dairy Export Council. Retrieved from http://www.thinkusadairy.org/health-and-wellness/role-of-dairy-in-the-diet

Ronald, A., Pennell, C. E., & Whitehouse, A. J. (2010). Prenatal maternal stress associated with ADHD and autistic traits in early childhood. *Frontiers in Psychology, 1*, 223. PMID:21833278

Ronzoni, S., Marconi, A. M., Cetin, I., Paolini, C. L., Teng, C., Pardi, G., & Battaglia, F. C. (1999). Umbilical amino acid uptake at increasing maternal amino acid concentrations: Effect of a maternal amino acid infusate. *American Journal of Obstetrics and Gynecology, 181*(2), 477–483. doi:10.1016/S0002-9378(99)70581-8 PMID:10454703

Ronzoni, S., Marconi, A. M., Paolini, C. L., Teng, C., Pardi, G., & Battaglia, F. C. (2002). The effect of a maternal infusion of amino acids on umbilical uptake in pregnancies complicated by intrauterine growth restriction. *American Journal of Obstetrics and Gynecology, 187*(3), 741–746. doi:10.1067/mob.2002.124291 PMID:12237657

Rooney, C., McMichael, A. J., Kovats, R. S., & Coleman, M. P. (1998). Excess mortality in England and Wales, and in Greater London, during the 1995 heatwave. *Journal of Epidemiology and Community Health, 52*(8), 482–486. doi:10.1136/jech.52.8.482 PMID:9876358

Rosanò, L., & Bagnato, A. (2016). β-arrestin1 at the cross-road of endothelin-1 signaling in cancer. *Journal of Experimental & Clinical Cancer Research: CR., 35*(1), 121. doi:10.118613046-016-0401-4 PMID:27473335

Rossignol, D. A., & Frye, R. E. (2012). A review of research trends in physiological abnormalities in autism spectrum disorders: Immune dysregulation, inflammation, oxidative stress, mitochondrial dysfunction and environmental toxicant exposures. *Molecular Psychiatry, 17*(4), 389–401. doi:10.1038/mp.2011.165 PMID:22143005

Rossman, T. G. (2003). Mechanism of arsenic carcinogenesis: An integrated approach. *Mutation Research, 533*(1-2), 37–65. doi:10.1016/j.mrfmmm.2003.07.009 PMID:14643412

Rossman, T. G., Uddin, A. N., & Burns, F. J. (2004). Evidence that arsenite acts as a cocarcinogen in skin cancer. *Toxicology and Applied Pharmacology, 198*(3), 394–404. doi:10.1016/j.taap.2003.10.016 PMID:15276419

Rother, H. A. (2000). Influences of pesticide risk perception on the health of rural South African women and children. *African Newsletter on Occupational Health and Safety, 10*(2), 11.

Rothman, K. J. (1993). Methodologic frontiers in environmental epidemiology. *Environmental Health Perspectives, 101*(suppl. 4), 19–21.

Rozniecki, J. J., Sahagian, G., Jacobson, S., Kempuraj, D., & Theoharides, T. C. (in press). Acute restraint stress induces brain metastases of luciferase-tagged breast cancer cells in mice. *Brain, Behavior, and Immunity.*

Rubasinghege, G., Gurung, R., Rijal, H., Maldonado-Torres, S., Chan, A., Acharya, S., ... Piyasena, M. (2017). Abiotic degradation and environmental toxicity of ibuprofen: Roles of mineral particles and solar radiation. *Water Research, 131*, 22–32. doi:10.1016/j.watres.2017.12.016 PMID:29258002

Rubin, C., Esteban, E., Kieszak, S., Hill, R. H. Jr, Dunlop, B., Yacovac, R., ... Pearce, K. (2002). Assessment of human exposure and human health effects after indoor application of methyl parathion in Lorain County, Ohio, 1995-1996. *Environmental Health Perspectives, 110*(Supplement 6), 1047–1051. doi:10.1289/ehp.02110s61047 PMID:12634138

Rüchardt, A. F. (2017). *Cotton Made in Africa, Annual Report*. Hamburg, Germany: Aid by Trade Foundation.

Ruel, M., Garrett, J., Yosef, S., & Olivier, M. (2017). Urbanization, food security and nutrition. In Se. de Pee et al. (Eds.), *Nutrition and Health*. New York, NY: Springer. doi:10.1007/978-3-319-43739-2

Ruggeri, B., Sarkans, U., Schumann, G., & Persico, A. M. (2014). Biomarkers in autism spectrum disorder: The old and the new 1. *Psychopharmacology, 231*(6), 1201–1216. doi:10.100700213-013-3290-7 PMID:24096533

Ruhoy, I. S. & Daughtonm C. G. (2007). Types and quantities of leftover drugs entering the environment *via* disposal to sewage—revealed by coroner records. *The Science of the Total Environment, 388*, 137–148.

Ruiz-Hernandez, A., Kuo, C. C., Rentero-Garrido, P., Tang, W. Y., Redon, J., Ordovas, J. M., ... Tellez-Plaza, M. (2015). Environmental chemicals and DNA methylation in adults: A systematic review of the epidemiologic evidence. *Clinical Epigenetics, 7*(1), 55. doi:10.118613148-015-0055-7 PMID:25984247

Rundle-Thiele, S., Kubacki, K., Tkaczynski, A., & Parkinson, J. (2015). Using two-step cluster analysis to identify homogeneous physical activity groups. *Marketing Intelligence & Planning, 33*(4), 522–537. doi:10.1108/MIP-03-2014-0050

Rush, E. (2013). Ethics of food security. In Q. Farmar-Bowers, V. Higgins, & J. Millar (Eds.), *Food security in Australia* (pp. 35–48). Boston, MA: Springer. doi:10.1007/978-1-4614-4484-8_3

Ryan, S. M., & Nielsen, C. J. (2010). Global warming potential of inhaled anesthetics: Application to clinical use. *Anesthesia and Analgesia, 111*(1), 92–98. doi:10.1213/ANE.0b013e3181e058d7 PMID:20519425

Ryland, L. K., Fox, T. E., Liu, X., Loughran, T. P., & Kester, M. (2011). Dysregulation of sphingolipid metabolism in cancer. *Cancer Biology & Therapy, 11*(2), 138–149. doi:10.4161/cbt.11.2.14624 PMID:21209555

Rzhetsky, A., Bagley, S. C., Wang, K., Lyttle, C. S., Cook, E. H. Jr, Altman, R. B., & Gibbons, R. D. (2014). Environmental and state-level regulatory factors affect the incidence of autism and intellectual disability. *PLoS Computational Biology, 10*(3), e1003518. doi:10.1371/journal.pcbi.1003518 PMID:24625521

Saari, G. N., Scott, W. C., & Brooks, B. W. (2017). Global scanning assessment of calcium channel blockers in the environment: Review and analysis of occurrence, ecotoxicology and hazards in aquatic systems. *Chemosphere, 189*, 466–478. doi:10.1016/j.chemosphere.2017.09.058 PMID:28957764

Saha, D. (2009). Arsenic groundwater contamination in parts of middle Ganga plain, Bihar. *Current Science, 97*(6), 753–755.

Saha, J. C., Dikshit, A. K., Bandyopadhyay, M., & Saha, K. C. (1999). A Review of Arsenic Poisoning and its Effects on Human Health. *Critical Reviews in Environmental Science and Technology, 29*(3), 281–313. doi:10.1080/10643389991259227

Saha, K. C. (2003). Diagnosis of arsenicosis. *Journal of Environmental Science and Health Part A, 38*(1), 255–272. doi:10.1081/ESE-120016893 PMID:12635831

Sahn, D. (1989). A conceptual framework for examining the seasonal aspects of household food security. In D. Sahn (Ed.), *Seasonal variability in third world agriculture: The consequences for food security* (pp. 67–77). Baltimore, MD: John Hopkins University Press.

Saluja, R., Metz, M., & Maurer, M. (2012). Role and relevance of mast cells in fungal infections. *Frontiers in Immunology, 3*, 146. doi:10.3389/fimmu.2012.00146 PMID:22707950

Sampson, T. R., & Mazmanian, S. K. (2015). Control of brain development, function, and behavior by the microbiome. *Cell Host & Microbe, 17*(5), 565–576. doi:10.1016/j.chom.2015.04.011 PMID:25974299

Samsonov, Y. N., & Pokrovskii, L. M. (2001). Sensitized photodecomposition of high disperse pesticide chemicals exposed to sunlight and irradiation from halogen or mercury lamp. *Atmospheric Environment, 35*(12), 2133–2141. doi:10.1016/S1352-2310(00)00494-5

Sancha, A. M., & O'Ryan, R. (2008). Managing Hazardous Pollutants in Chile: Arsenic. *Reviews of Environmental Contamination and Toxicology Reviews of Environmental Contamination and Toxicology, 196*, 123–146. PMID:19025095

Sánchez, M. A., & León, G. (2016). Status of market, regulation and research of genetically modified crops in Chile. *New Biotechnology, 33*(6), 815–823. doi:10.1016/j.nbt.2016.07.017 PMID:27474111

Sanchez-Pena, L. C., Petrosyan, P., Morales, M., Gonzalez, N. B., Gutierrez-Ospina, G., Del Razo, L. M., & Gonsebatt, M. E. (2010). Arsenic species, AS3MT amount, and AS3MT gene expression in different brain regions of mouse exposed to arsenite. *Environmental Research, 110*(5), 428–434. doi:10.1016/j.envres.2010.01.007 PMID:20138265

Sanders, J. (2009). Qualitative or quantitative differences between Asperger's disorder and Autism? Historical Considerations. *Journal of Autism and Developmental Disorders, 39*(11), 1560–1567. doi:10.100710803-009-0798-0 PMID:19548078

Sandin, S., Lichtenstein, P., Kuja-Halkola, R., Larsson, H., Hultman, C. M., & Reichenberg, A. (2014). The familial risk of autism. *Journal of the American Medical Association, 311*(17), 1770–1777. doi:10.1001/jama.2014.4144 PMID:24794370

Santhakumar, M., & Balaji, M. (2000). Acute toxicity of an organophosphorus insecticide monocrotophos and its effects on behaviour of an air-breathing fish, Anabas testudineus (Bloch). *Journal of Environmental Biology, 21*(2), 121–123.

Saracci, R., & Wild, C. P. (2015). *International Agency for Research on Cancer: The First 50 Years: 1965-2015*. Lyon, France: World Health Organization.

Sarantis, H., Naidenko, O. V., Gray, S., Houlihan, J., & Malkan, S. (2010). Not so sexy: The health risks of secret chemicals in fragrance. Breast Cancer Fund, Commonwealth and Environmental Working Group. Retrieved from https://www.ewg.org/sites/default/files/report/SafeCosmetics_FragranceRpt.pdf

Sarigiannis, D. A., Hansen, U. (2012). Considering the cumulative risk of mixtures of chemicals - A challenge for policy makers. *Environmental Health: A Global Access Science Source*.

Sarigiannis, D., Karakitsios, S., Gotti, A., Loizou, G., Cherrie, J., Smolders, R., . . . Sleeuwenhoek, A. (2014). Integra: From global scale contamination to tissue dose. In *Proceedings - 7th International Congress on Environmental Modelling and Software: Bold Visions for Environmental Modeling, iEMSs 2014* (Vol. 2, pp. 1001-1008). Academic Press.

Sarigiannis, D. (2015a). Exposome science for public health protection and innovation. *Toxicology Letters, 238*(2), S12–S13. doi:10.1016/j.toxlet.2015.08.154

Sarigiannis, D. (2015b). Unravelling the Exposome through integrated exposure biology. *Toxicology Letters, 238*(2), S229–S230. doi:10.1016/j.toxlet.2015.08.680

Sarigiannis, D. A. (2017). Assessing the impact of hazardous waste on children's health: The exposome paradigm. *Environmental Research, 158*, 531–541. doi:10.1016/j.envres.2017.06.031 PMID:28711809

Sarigiannis, D. A., Gotti, A., Handakas, E., & Karakitsios, S. P. (2018). Informatics and Data Analytics to Support Exposome-Based Discovery: Part 2 - Computational Exposure Biology. In M. Lytras & P. Papadopoulou (Eds.), *Applying Big Data Analytics in Bioinformatics and Medicine* (pp. 145–187). Hershey, PA: IGI Global. doi:10.4018/978-1-5225-2607-0.ch007

Sarigiannis, D. A., Gotti, A., & Karakitsios, S. P. (2019a). Indoor Air and Public Health. In B. Roig & ... (Eds.), *Management of Emerging Public Health Issues and Risks* (pp. 3–29). Academic Press. doi:10.1016/B978-0-12-813290-6.00001-9

Sarigiannis, D. A., & Karakitsios, S. P. (2018a). Addressing complexity of health impact assessment in industrially contaminated sites via the exposome paradigm. *Epidemiologia e Prevenzione*, *42*, 37–48. PMID:30322234

Sarigiannis, D. A., & Karakitsios, S. P. (2018b). Modeling Complex Exposures. In C. V. Rider & J. E. Simmons (Eds.), *Chemical Mixtures and Combined Chemical and Nonchemical Stressors: Exposure, Toxicity, Analysis, and Risk* (pp. 81–125). Cham: Springer International Publishing. doi:10.1007/978-3-319-56234-6_4

Sarigiannis, D. A., Karakitsios, S. P., Gotti, A., Papaloukas, C. L., Kassomenos, P. A., & Pilidis, G. A. (2009). Bayesian algorithm implementation in a real time exposure assessment model on benzene with calculation of associated cancer risks. *Sensors (Basel)*, *9*(2), 731–755. doi:10.339090200731 PMID:22399936

Sarigiannis, D. A., Karakitsios, S. P., Handakas, E., Papadaki, K., Chapizanis, D., & Gotti, A. (2018). Informatics and Data Analytics to Support Exposome-Based Discovery: Part 1 - Assessment of External and Internal Exposure. In M. Lytras & P. Papadopoulou (Eds.), *Applying Big Data Analytics in Bioinformatics and Medicine* (pp. 115–144). Hershey, PA: IGI Global. doi:10.4018/978-1-5225-2607-0.ch006

Sarigiannis, D. A., Karakitsios, S. P., Handakas, E., Simou, K., Solomou, E., & Gotti, A. (2016). Integrated exposure and risk characterization of bisphenol-A in Europe. *Food and Chemical Toxicology*, *98*, 134–147. doi:10.1016/j.fct.2016.10.017 PMID:27769850

Sarigiannis, D. A., Karakitsios, S. P., Kermenidou, M., Nikolaki, S., Zikopoulos, D., Semelidis, S., ... Tzimou, R. (2014). Total exposure to airborne particulate matter in cities: The effect of biomass combustion. *The Science of the Total Environment*, *493*, 795–805. doi:10.1016/j.scitotenv.2014.06.055 PMID:25000575

Sarigiannis, D. A., Karakitsios, S. P., Zikopoulos, D., Nikolaki, S., & Kermenidou, M. (2015b). Lung cancer risk from PAHs emitted from biomass combustion. *Environmental Research*, *137*, 147–156. doi:10.1016/j.envres.2014.12.009 PMID:25543545

Sarigiannis, D. A., & Salifoglou, A. (2016). Research directives toward deciphering adverse outcome pathways induced by environmental metallotoxins. *Current Opinion in Chemical Engineering*, *13*, 161–169. doi:10.1016/j.coche.2016.09.010

Sarigiannis, D. A., Soulakellis, N. A., & Sifakis, N. I. (2004). Information Fusion for Computational Assessment of Air Quality and Health Effects. *Photogrammetric Engineering and Remote Sensing*, *70*(2), 235–245. doi:10.14358/PERS.70.2.235

Sarigiannis, D. A., Soulakellis, N., Schäfer, K., Tombrou, M., Sifakis, N. I., Assimakopoulos, D., ... Saisana, M. (2002). ICAROS: An integrated computational environment for the assimilation of environmental data and models for urban and regional air quality. *Water Air and Soil Pollution Focus*, *2*(5/6), 641–654. doi:10.1023/A:1021357417913

Sarigiannis, D. A., Tratnik, J. S., Mazej, D., Kosjek, T., Heath, E., Horvat, M., ... Karakitsios, S. P. (2019b). Risk characterization of bisphenol-A in the Slovenian population starting from human biomonitoring data. *Environmental Research*, *170*, 293–300. doi:10.1016/j.envres.2018.12.056 PMID:30605834

Sarigiannis, D., Gotti, A., Karakitsios, S., Kontoroupis, P., & Nikolaki, S. (2012). Intera Platform: A Tool for Mechanistic Risk Assessment of Indoor Air Pollutants. *Epidemiology (Cambridge, Mass.)*, 23.

Sarigiannis, D., Karakitsios, S., Gotti, A., Handakas, E., & Papadaki, K. (2015a). INTEGRA: Advancing risk assessment using internal dosimetry metrics. *Toxicology Letters*, *238*(2), S110–S111. doi:10.1016/j.toxlet.2015.08.359

Sarigiannis, D., Marafante, E., Gotti, A., & Reale, G. C. (2009). Reflections on new directions for risk assessment of environmental chemical mixtures. *International Journal of Risk Assessment and Management*, *13*(3/4), 216–241. doi:10.1504/IJRAM.2009.030697

Sarigiannis, D., Papadaki, K., Kontoroupis, P., & Karakitsios, S. (2015b). Advanced QSAR models for use in toxicokinetic modelling. *Toxicology Letters*, *238*(2), S166–S167. doi:10.1016/j.toxlet.2015.08.568

Sattar, A., Xie, S., Hafeez, M. A., Wang, X., Hussain, H. I., Iqbal, Z., ... Yuan, Z. (2016). Metabolism and toxicity of arsenicals in mammals. *Environmental Toxicology and Pharmacology*, *48*, 214–224. doi:10.1016/j.etap.2016.10.020 PMID:27829199

Saugstad, O. D. (2005). Oxidative stress in the newborn–a 30-year perspective. *Neonatology*, *88*(3), 228–236. doi:10.1159/000087586 PMID:16210845

Sava, V., Reunova, O., Velasquez, A., Harbison, R., & Sanchez-Ramos, J. (2006a). Acute neurotoxic effects of the fungal metabolite ochratoxin-A. *Neurotoxicology*, *27*(1), 82–92. doi:10.1016/j.neuro.2005.07.004 PMID:16140385

Sava, V., Reunova, O., Velasquez, A., & Sanchez-Ramos, J. (2006b). Can low level exposure to ochratoxin-A cause parkinsonism? *Journal of the Neurological Sciences*, *249*(1), 68–75. doi:10.1016/j.jns.2006.06.006 PMID:16844142

Scafuri, B., Varriale, A., Facchiano, A., D'Auria, S., Raggi, M. E., & Marabotti, A. (2017). Binding of mycotoxins to proteins involved in neuronal plasticity: A combined in silico/wet investigation. *Scientific Reports*, *7*(1), 15156. doi:10.103841598-017-15148-4 PMID:29123130

Schindler, B. K., Esteban, M., Koch, H. M., Castano, A., Koslitz, S., Canas, A., ... Angerer, J. (2014). The European COPHES/DEMOCOPHES project: Towards transnational comparability and reliability of human biomonitoring results. *International Journal of Hygiene and Environmental Health*, *217*(6), 653–661. doi:10.1016/j.ijheh.2013.12.002 PMID:24405937

Schlett, A. & Beke, J. (2015). Food security and GMOS. *Studia Mundi – Economica, 2*(1), 94-102. doi:. doi:10.18531/Studia.Mundi.2015.02.01

Schmid, R. F., & Fallon, S. (2003). *The untold story of milk: Green pastures, contented cows and raw dairy foods.* Washington, DC: New Trends Pub.

Schmidt, W., O'Rourke, K., Hernan, R., & Quinn, B. (2011). Effects of the pharmaceuticals gemfibrozil and diclofenac on the marine mussel (*Mytilus* spp.) and their comparison with standardized toxicity tests. *Marine Pollution Bulletin*, *62*(7), 1389–1395. doi:10.1016/j.marpolbul.2011.04.043 PMID:21652050

Schmutz, J., Wheeler, J., Grimwood, J., Dickson, M., Yang, J., Caoile, C., ... Myers, R. M. (2004). Quality assessment of the human genome sequence. *Nature*, *429*(6990), 365–368. doi:10.1038/nature02390 PMID:15164052

Schneider, K. R., Schneider, R. G., & Richardson, S. (2017). *Genetically Modified Food. FSHN02-2 series Food Science and Human Nutrition Department*. UF/IFAS Extension.

Schopler, E., Mesibov, G. B., & Kunce, L. (1998). *Asperger Syndrome or High-Functioning Autism? Current Issues in Autism*. Berlin, Germany: Plenum Press. doi:10.1007/978-1-4615-5369-4

Schulman, H. (1997). Nitric oxide: A spatial second messenger. *Molecular Psychiatry*, *2*(4), 296–299. doi:10.1038j.mp.4000197 PMID:9246669

Schultz, M. M., Furlong, E. T., Kolpin, D. W., Werner, S. L., Schoenfuss, H. L., Barber, L. B., ... Vajda, A. M. (2010). Antidepressant pharmaceuticals in two U.S. effluent-impacted streams--Occurrence and fate in water and sediment, and selective uptake in fish neural tissue. *Environmental Science & Technology*, *44*(6), 1918–1925. doi:10.1021/es9022706 PMID:20121081

Scire, J., Robe, F. R., Fernau, M. E., & Yamartino, R. J. (2000b). *A user's Guide for the CALMET Meteorological Model (Version 5)*. Concord: Earth Tech Inc.

Scire, J., Strimaitis, D. G., & Yamartino, R. J. (2000a). *A user's Guide for the CALPUFF Dispersion Model (Version 5)*. Concord: Earth Tech Inc.

Sealey, L. A., Hughes, B. W., Sriskanda, A. N., Guest, J. R., Gibson, A. D., Johnson-Williams, L., ... Bagasra, O. (2016). Environmental factors in the development of autism spectrum disorders. *Environment International*, *88*, 288–298. doi:10.1016/j.envint.2015.12.021 PMID:26826339

Sealey, L. A., Hughes, B. W., Steinemann, A., Pestaner, J. P., Pace, D. G., & Bagasra, O. (2015). Role of Environmental Factors in Autism Development and Male Bias: Neuromodifying Effects of Fragrance. *Environmental Research*, *142*, 731–738. doi:10.1016/j.envres.2015.08.025 PMID:26408793

Semple, B.D., Blomgren, K., Gimlin, K. & Ferriero, D.M. (2013). Brain development in rodents and humans: Identifying benchmarks of maturation and vulnerability to injury across species. *Progress in Neurobiology, 106*, 1-16.

Seralini, G. E., Mesnage, R., Defarge, N., & Spiroux de Vendômois, J. (2014). Conclusiveness of Toxicity Data and Double Standards. *Food and Chemical Toxicology*, *69*(7), 357–359. doi:10.1016/j.fct.2014.04.018 PMID:24747919

Séralini, G.-E., Clair, E., Mesnage, R., Gress, S., Defarge, N., Malatesta, M., ... Spiroux de Vendômois, J. (2014). Republished study: Long-term toxicity of a Roundup herbicide and a Roundup-tolerant genetically modified maize. *Environmental Sciences Europe*, *26*(1), 14. doi:10.118612302-014-0014-5 PMID:27752412

Sethi, S., Tyagi, S. K., & Anurag, R. K. (2016). Plant-based milk alternatives an emerging segment of functional beverages: A review. [PubMed]. *Journal of Food Science and Technology*, *53*(9), 3408–3423. doi:10.100713197-016-2328-3

Seyma, T., Fueki, K., Shiokawa, J., & Suzuki, S. (Eds.). (1983). *Proceedings of the International Meeting on Chemical Sensors*, Fukuoka, Japan, September 19-22. Tokyo, Japan: Elsevier-Kodanscha.

Shankar, S., Shanker, U., & Shikha. (2014). Arsenic Contamination of Groundwater: A Review of Sources, Prevalence, Health Risks, and Strategies for Mitigation. *The Scientific World Journal*. doi:10.1155/2014/304524 PMID:25374935

Shapira, J. R. (1973). In D.L. Klayman & W.H. Gunther (Eds.), Organic selenium compounds: Their Chemistry and Biology. John Wiley & Sons Inc.

Sharma, M., Sharma, S., Arora, M., & Kaul, D. (2013). Regulation of cellular Cyclin D1 gene by arsenic is mediated through miR-2909. *Gene*, *522*(1), 60–64. doi:10.1016/j.gene.2013.03.058 PMID:23562784

Sharma, S. (1996). *Applied multivariate techniques*. USA: John Wiley & Sons.

Sheldon, R. A. (2007). The E factor: Fifteen years on. *Green Chemistry*, *9*(12), 1273–1283. doi:10.1039/b713736m

Shen, H., Xu, W., Zhang, J., Chen, M., Martin, F. L., Xia, Y., ... Zhu, Y. G. (2013). Urinary metabolic biomarkers link oxidative stress indicators associated with general arsenic exposure to male infertility in a Han Chinese population. *Environmental Science & Technology*, *47*, 8843–8851. PMID:23841501

Shepherd, D., Dirks, K., Welch, D., Dride, D., & Landon, J. (2016). The covariance between air pollution annoyance and noise annoyance, and its relationship with health-related quality of life. *International Journal of Environmental Research and Public Health*, *13*(8), 792. doi:10.3390/ijerph13080792 PMID:27509512

Sherwin, R. P. (1983). What is an adverse health effect? *Environmental Health Perspectives*, *52*, 177–182. PMID:6653520

Shivanand, P., & Noopur, S. (2010). Recombinant DNA technology: Applications in the field of biotechnology and crime sciences. *International Journal of Pharmaceutical Sciences Review and Research*, *1*(1), 43–49.

Shope, R. (1991). Global climate change and infectious diseases. *Environmental Health Perspectives*, *96*, 171–174. doi:10.1289/ehp.9196171 PMID:1820262

Shrestha, R. R., Shrestha, M. P., Upadhyay, N. P., Pradhan, R., Khadka, R., Maskey, A., ... Shrestha, K. (2003). Groundwater arsenic contamination, its health impact and mitigation program in Nepal. *Journal of Environmental Science and Health. Part A*, *38*(1), 185–200.

Shrestha, R., Flacke, J., Martinez, J., & van Maarseveen, M. (2016). Environmental Health Related Socio-Spatial Inequalities: Identifying "Hotspots" of Environmental Burdens and Social Vulnerability. *International Journal of Environmental Research and Public Health*, 13. PMID:27409625

Siamwalla, A., & Valdes, A. (1980). Food security in developing countries. *Food Policy*, *5*(4), 258–272. doi:10.1016/0306-9192(80)90055-X

Siddiqui, M. F., Kim, S., Jeon, H., Kim, T., Joo, C., & Park, S. (2018). Miniaturized Sample Preparation and Rapid Detection of Arsenite in Contaminated Soil Using a Smartphone. *Sensors (Basel)*, *18*(3), 777. doi:10.339018030777 PMID:29510538

Sidman, R. L., Taksir, T., Fidler, J., Zhao, M., Dodge, J. C., Passini, M. A., ... Shihabuddin, L. S. (2008). Temporal neuropathologic and behavioral phenotype of 6neo/6neo Pompe disease mice. *Journal of Neuropathology and Experimental Neurology*, *67*(8), 803–818. doi:10.1097/NEN.0b013e3181815994 PMID:18648322

Signes-Pastor, A. J., Carey, M., & Meharg, A. A. (2016). Inorganic arsenic in rice-based products for infants and young children. *Food Chemistry*, *191*, 128–134. doi:10.1016/j.foodchem.2014.11.078 PMID:26258711

Siirila, E. R., Navarre-Sitchler, A. K., Maxwell, R. M., & McCray, J. E. (2012). A quantitative methodology to assess the risks to human health from CO_2 leakage into groundwater. *Advances in Water Resources*, *36*, 146–164. doi:10.1016/j.advwatres.2010.11.005

Silberman, S. (2016). *NeuroTribes*. New York: Avery.

Silk. (2018). Silk. Retrieved from https://www.silk.com/

Silva, C. P., Otero, M., & Esteves, V. (2012). Processes for the elimination of estrogenic steroid hormones from water: A review. *Environmental Pollution*, *165*, 38–58. doi:10.1016/j.envpol.2012.02.002 PMID:22402263

Simcock, G., Kildea, S., Elgbeili, G., Laplante, D. P., Cobham, V., & King, S. (2017). Prenatal maternal stress shapes children's theory of mind: The QF2011 Queensland Flood Study. *Journal of Developmental Origins of Health and Disease*, *8*(04), 483–492. doi:10.1017/S2040174417000186 PMID:28337952

Simmonds, H., Webster, D., Lingam, S., & Wilson, J. (1985). An inborn error of purine metabolism, deafness and neurodevelopmental abnormality. *Neuropediatrics*, *16*(02), 106–108. doi:10.1055-2008-1052552 PMID:2989725

Singh, D. K., & Agarwal, R. A. (1983). Inhibition kinetics of certain organophosphorus and carbamate pesticides on acetylcholinesterase from the snail Lymnaeaacuminate. *Toxicology Letters*, *19*(3), 313–319. doi:10.1016/0378-4274(83)90136-4 PMID:6658844

Singh, S. K. (2017). An analysis of the cost-effectiveness of arsenic mitigation technologies: Implications for public policy. *International Journal of Sustainable Built Environment*, *6*(2), 522–535. doi:10.1016/j.ijsbe.2017.10.004

Singh, S. K. (2017). Groundwater arsenic contamination in Bihar: Causes, issues, and challenges. *International Journal of Current Research*, *9*(08), 56787–56790.

Singh, S. K., Ghosh, A. K., Kumar, A., Kislay, K., Kumar, C., Tiwari, R. R., ... Imam, M. D. (2014). Groundwater Arsenic contamination and associated health risks in Bihar, India. *International Journal of Environmental of Research*, *8*(1), 49–60.

Sismondo, S. (2007). Ghost management. How much of the medical literature is shaped behind the scenes by the pharmaceutical industry? *PLoS Med* 4(9): e286.S.

Skaper, S. D., Facci, L., & Giusti, P. (2014). Neuroinflammation, microglia and mast cells in the pathophysiology of neurocognitive disorders: A review. *CNS & Neurological Disorders - Drug Targets*, *13*(10), 1654–1666. doi:10.2174/1871527313666141130224206 PMID:25470401

Slominski, A.T., Zmijewski, M.A., Skobowiat, C., Zbytek, B., Slominski, R.M., Steketee, J.D. (2012). Sensing the environment: regulation of local and global homeostasis by the skin's neuroendocrine system. *Adv Anat Embryol Cell Biol., 212*, 1-115.

Slominski, A. T., Hardeland, R., Zmijewski, M. A., Slominski, R. M., Reiter, R. J., & Paus, R. (2018). Melatonin: A cutaneous perspective on its production, metabolism and functions. *The Journal of Investigative Dermatology*, *138*(3), 490–499. doi:10.1016/j.jid.2017.10.025 PMID:29428440

Slominski, A. T., Manna, P. R., & Tuckey, R. C. (2015). On the role of skin in the regulation of local and systemic steroidogenic activities. *Steroids*, *103*, 72–78. doi:10.1016/j.steroids.2015.04.006 PMID:25988614

Slominski, A. T., Zmijewski, A. M., Plonka, P., Szaflarski, J., & Paus, R. (2018). How ultraviolet light touches the brain and endocrine system through skin, and why. *Endocrinology*, *159*(5), 1992–2007. doi:10.1210/en.2017-03230 PMID:29546369

Slominski, A., Majewska, M. A., Skobowiat, C., Zbytek, B., Slominski, R. M., & Steketee, J. D. (2012). Sensing the environment: Regulation of local and global homeostasis by the skin neuroendocrine system. *Advances in Anatomy, Embryology, and Cell Biology*, *212*, 1–115. doi:10.1007/978-3-642-19683-6_1 PMID:22894052

Slominski, A., & Wortsman, J. (2000). Neuroendocrinology of the skin. *Endocrine Reviews*, *21*, 457–487. PMID:11041445

Slominski, A., Zmijewski, M., Zbytek, B., Tobin, D., Tobin, D. J., Theoharides, T. C., & Rivier, J. (2013). Key Role of CRF in the Skin Stress Response System. *Endocrine Reviews*, *34*(6), 827–884. doi:10.1210/er.2012-1092 PMID:23939821

Smedley, P. L., Kinniburgh, D. G., Macdonald, D. M. J., Nicolli, H. B., Barros, A. J., Tullio, J. O., ... Alonso, M. S. (2005). Arsenic associations in sediments from the loess aquifer of La Pampa, Argentina. *Applied Geochemistry*, *20*(5), 989–1016. doi:10.1016/j.apgeochem.2004.10.005

Smedman, A., Lindmark-Månsson, H., Drewnowski, A., & Edman, A. M. (2010). Nutrient density of beverages in relation to climate impact. *Food & Nutrition Research*, *54*(1), 5170. doi:10.3402/fnr.v54i0.5170

Smith, A. (2002). Public health. Arsenic epidemiology and drinking water standards. *Science*, *296*(5576), 2145–2146. doi:10.1126cience.1072896 PMID:12077388

Smith, A. H., Lingas, E. O., & Rahman, M. (2000). Contamination of drinking-water by arsenic in Bangladesh: A public health emergency. *Bulletin of the World Health Organization*, *78*(9), 1093–1103. PMID:11019458

Smith, A. H., Marshall, G., Yuan, Y., Ferreccio, C., Liaw, J., von Ehrenstein, O., ... Selvin, S. (2006). Increased mortality from lung cancer and bronchiectasis in young adults after exposure to arsenic in utero and in early childhood. *Environmental Health Perspectives*, *114*(8), 1293–1296. doi:10.1289/ehp.8832 PMID:16882542

Smith, E., Naidu, R., & Alston, A. M. (1998). Arsenic in the soil environment: A review. *Advances in Agronomy*, 64.

Smith, M., Pointing, J., & Maxwell, S. (1993). *Household food security, concepts and definitions: An annotated bibliography. Development Bibliography No. 8*. Brighton, UK: Institute of Development Studies, University of Sussex.

Snoj Tratnik, J., Falnoga, I., Trdin, A., Mazej, D., Fajon, V., Miklavčič, A., ... Horvat, M. (2017). Prenatal mercury exposure, neurodevelopment and apolipoprotein E genetic polymorphism. *Environmental Research*, *152*, 375–385. doi:10.1016/j.envres.2016.08.035 PMID:27616663

Snyder, S. A., & Benotti, M. J. (2010). Endocrine disruptors and pharmaceuticals: Implications for water sustainability. *Water Science and Technology*, *61*(1), 145–154. doi:10.2166/wst.2010.791 PMID:20057100

Snyder, S. A., Villeneuve, D. L., Snyder, E. M., & Giesy, J. P. (2001). Identification and quantification of estrogen receptor agonists in wastewater effluents. *Environmental Science & Technology*, *35*(18), 3620–3625. doi:10.1021/es001254n PMID:11783637

So Good Beverage. (2018). So Good. Retrieved from https://sogoodbeverage.com/

Sollome, J., Martin, E., Sethupathy, P., & Fry, R. C. (2016). Environmental contaminants and microRNA regulation: Transcription factors as regulators of toxicant-altered microRNA expression. *Toxicology and Applied Pharmacology*, *312*, 61–66. doi:10.1016/j.taap.2016.06.009 PMID:27292125

Solomon, D. J., Henry, R. C., Hogan, J. G., Van Amburg, G. H., & Taylor, J. (1991). Evaluation and implementation of public health registries. *Public Health Reports (Washington, D.C.)*, *106*(2), 142–150. PMID:1902306

SoNice. (2014). So Nice. Retrieved from https://sonice.ca/

SOT (Society of Toxicology). (2003). The safety of genetically modified foods produced through biotechnology. *Toxicological Sciences*, *71*(1), 2–8. doi:10.1093/toxsci/71.1.2 PMID:12520069

Soubbotina, T. P. (2004). *Beyond Economic Growth: An Introduction to Sustainable Development* (2nd ed.). Washington, DC: World Bank. doi:10.1596/0-8213-5933-9

Sousa, L. R., & Larson, J. M. (1977). Crown ether model systems for the study of photoexcited state response to geometrically oriented perturbers. The effect of alkali metal ions on emission from naphthalene derivatives. *Journal of the American Chemical Society*, *99*(1), 307–310. doi:10.1021/ja00443a084

Southgate, E. M., Davey, M. R., Power, J. B., & Merchant, R. (1995). Factors affecting the genetic engineering of plants by microprojectile bombardment. *Biotechnology Advances*, *13*(4), 631–657. doi:10.1016/0734-9750(95)02008-X PMID:14536367

Sowndhararajan, K., & Kim, S. (2016). Influence of Fragrances on Human Psychophysiological Activity: With Special Reference to Human Electroencephalographic Response. *Scientia Pharmaceutica*, *84*(4), 724–751. doi:10.3390cipharm84040724 PMID:27916830

Soy facts & data. (2017). Worldwide Fund for Nature. Retrieved from http://wwf.panda.org/our_work/food/agriculture/soy/facts/

Sparks, D. L. (2003). *Environmental soil chemistry*. Boston: Academic. doi:10.1016/B978-012656446-4/50001-3

Spengler, J., Neas, L., Nakai, S., Dockery, D., Speizer, F., Ware, J., & Raizenne, M. (1994). Respiratory symptoms and housing characteristics. *Indoor Air*, *4*(2), 72–82.

Spratt, E. G., Nicholas, J. S., Brady, K. T., Carpenter, L. A., Hatcher, C. R., Meekins, K. A., ... Charles, J. M. (2012). Enhanced cortisol response to stress in children in autism. *Journal of Autism and Developmental Disorders*, *42*(1), 75–81. doi:10.100710803-011-1214-0 PMID:21424864

Spruit, M., & Lammertink, M. (2018). Effective and Efficient Business Intelligence Dashboard Design: Gestalt Theory in Dutch Long-Term and Chronic Healthcare. In M. Lytras & P. Papadopoulou (Eds.), *Applying Big Data Analytics in Bioinformatics and Medicine* (pp. 243–271). Hershey, PA: IGI Global. doi:10.4018/978-1-5225-2607-0.ch010

Statista. (2018a). Global Cotton Production 1990-217. Retrieved from https://www.statista.com/statistics/259392/cotton-production-worldwide-since-1990/

Statista. (2018b). Global Cotton Price Since 1990. Retrieved from https://www.statista.com/statistics/259431/global-cotton-price-since-1990/

Statista. (2018c). Global Cotton Production 2017/2018, by country. Retrieved from https://www.statista.com/statistics/263055/cotton-production-worldwide-by-top-countries/

Statista. (2018d). Top Cotton Exporting Countries 2017/2018. Retrieved from https://www.statista.com/statistics/191895/leading-cotton-exporting-countries/

Statista. (2018e). Top Cotton Importing Countries 2017/2018. Retrieved from https://www.statista.com/statistics/191896/leading-cotton-importing-countries/

Statista. (2018f). Vegetable Oils: Global Consumption by oil type 2013/14 to 2017/2018. Retrieved from https://www.statista.com/statistics/263937/vegetable-oils-global-consumption

Stayner, L., Collins, J., Guo, Y., Heederik, D., Kogevinas, M., Steenland, K., ... Demers, P. (2017). Challenges and Opportunities for Occupational Epidemiology in the Twenty-first Century. *Current Environmental Health Reports*, *3*(3), 319–324. doi:10.100740572-017-0154-z PMID:28803393

Steiling, W., Bascompta, M., Carthew, P., Catalano, G., Corea, N., D'Haese, A., ... Singal, M. (2014). Principle considerations for the risk assessment of sprayed consumer products. *Toxicology Letters*, *227*(1), 41–49. doi:10.1016/j.toxlet.2014.03.005

Steinemann, A. (2018). National Prevalence and Effects of Multiple Chemical Sensitivities. *Journal of Occupational and Environmental Medicine*, *60*(3), e152–e156. doi:10.1097/JOM.0000000000001272 PMID:29329146

Stingone, J. A., Buck Louis, G. M., Nakayama, S. F., Vermeulen, R. C., Kwok, R. K., Cui, Y., ... Teitelbaum, S. L. (2017). Toward Greater Implementation of the Exposome Research Paradigm within Environmental Epidemiology. *Annual Review of Public Health*, *20*(38), 315–327. Epub2017Jan6. doi:10.1146/annurev-publhealth-082516-012750 PMID:28125387

Story, E. N., Kopec, R. E., Schwartz, S. J., & Harris, G. K. (2010). An update on the health effects of tomato lycopene. *Annual Review of Food Science and Technology*, *1*(1), 189–210. doi:10.1146/annurev.food.102308.124120 PMID:22129335

Straif, K., Benbrahim-Tallaa, L., Baan, R., Grosse, Y., Secretan, B., El Ghissassi, F., ... Cogliano, V. (2009). A review of human carcinogens–part C: Metals, arsenic, dusts, and fibres. *The Lancet Oncology*, *10*(5), 453–454. doi:10.1016/S1470-2045(09)70134-2 PMID:19418618

Street, M., Angelini, S., Bernasconi, S., Burgio, E., Cassio, A., Catellani, C., ... Gargano, G. (2018). Current knowledge on endocrine disrupting chemicals (EDCs) from animal biology to humans, from pregnancy to adulthood: Highlights from a national Italian meeting. *International Journal of Molecular Sciences*, *19*(6), 1647. doi:10.3390/ijms19061647

Striepe, B. (2011). Cotton: The dirty truth about "The Fabric of our Lives." *Crafting a Green World.* Retrieved from http://craftingagreenworld.com/2011/10/11/the-dirty-side-of-cotton/

Stuben, D., Berner, Z., Chandrasekharam, D., & Karamakar, J. (2003). Arsenic enrichment in groundwater of west Bengal, India: Geochemical evidence for mobilization of As under reducing conditions. *Applied Geochemistry*, *18*(9), 1417–1434. doi:10.1016/S0883-2927(03)00060-X

Sukul, P., & Spiteller, M. (2007). Fluoroquinolone antibiotics in the environment. *Reviews of Environmental Contamination and Toxicology*, *191*, 131–162. doi:10.1007/978-0-387-69163-3_5 PMID:17708074

Sun, S., Sursal, T., Adibnia, Y., Zhao, C., Zheng, Y., Li, H., ... Itagaki, K. (2013). Mitochondrial DAMPs increase endothelial permeability through neutrophil dependent and independent pathways. *PLoS One*, *8*(3), e59989. doi:10.1371/journal.pone.0059989 PMID:23527291

Sustainable Cotton Project. (2018). Media Kit. Retrieved from https://www.keepandshare.com/doc/6827338/media-kit-pdf-7-1-meg?da=y

Su, Z., Chen, K., Guo, Y., Qi, H., Yang, X. F., & Zhao, M. (2010). A coumarin-based fluorescent chemosensor for Zn 2+ in aqueous ethanol media. *Journal of Fluorescence*, *20*(4), 851–856.

Suzuki, T., Yamashita, S., Ushijima, T., Takumi, S., Sano, T., Michikawa, T., & Nohara, K. (2013). Genome-wide analysis of DNA methylation changes induced by gestational arsenic exposure in liver tumors. *Cancer Science*, *104*(12), 1575–1585. doi:10.1111/cas.12298 PMID:24118411

Swanson, N. L. (2013). *Genetically modified organisms and the deterioration of health in the United States.* Retrieved from https://people.csail.mit.edu/seneff/glyphosate/NancySwanson.pdf

Swart, R., Robinson, J., & Cohen, S. (2003). Climate change and sustainable development: Expanding the options. *Climate Policy*, *3*, S19–S40. doi:10.1016/j.clipol.2003.10.010

Szklo, M., & Nieto, F. J. (2007). *Epidemiology beyond the Basics* (2nd ed.). Boston, MA: Jones and Bartlett Publishers.

Tabachnick, B. G., & Fidell, L. S. (2013). *Using multivariate statistics* (6th ed.). USA: Pearson Education.

Taiwo, O. B., Kovacs, K. J., Sun, Y., & Larson, A. A. (2005). Unilateral spinal nerve ligation leads to an asymmetrical distribution of mast cells in the thalamus of female but not male mice. *Pain*, *114*(1), 131–140. doi:10.1016/j.pain.2004.12.002 PMID:15733638

Takagi, Y., Matsuda, S., Imai, S., Ohmori, Y., Masuda, T., Vinson, J. A., ... Kaniewski, A. (1988). Survey of trace elements in human nails: An international comparison. *Bulletin of Environmental Contamination and Toxicology*, *41*(4-6), 690–695. doi:10.1007/BF02021020 PMID:3233368

Takano, T. (2015). Role of Microglia in Autism: Recent Advances. *Developmental Neuroscience*, *37*(3), 195–202. doi:10.1159/000398791 PMID:25998072

Tamil Selvan, G., Varadaraju, C., Tamil Selvan, R., Enoch, I. V., & Mosae Selvakumar, P. (2018). On/off fluorescent chemosensor for selective detection of divalent iron and copper ions: Molecular logic operation and protein binding. *ACS Omega*, *3*(7), 7985–7992.

TanD. (2017). Cotton. Retrieved from https://greenstitched.com/tag/cotton/

Tang, B., Ding, B., Xu, K., & Tong, L. (2009). Use of selenium to detect mercury in water and cells: An enhancement of the sensitivity and specificity of a seleno fluorescent probe. *Chemistry*, *15*(13), 3147–3151. doi:10.1002/chem.200802165 PMID:19204963

Tariq, M. I., Afzal, S., & Hussain, I. (2004). Pesticides in shallow groundwater of bahawalnagar, Muzafargarh, DG Khan and Rajan Pur districts of Punjab, Pakistan. *Environment International*, *30*(4), 471–479. doi:10.1016/j.envint.2003.09.008 PMID:15031006

Tariq, M. I., Afzal, S., & Hussain, I. (2006). Degradation and persistence of cotton pesticides in sandy loam soils from Punjab, Pakistan. *Environmental Research*, *100*(2), 184–196. doi:10.1016/j.envres.2005.05.002 PMID:16009361

Taub, D., Miller, B., & Allen, H. (2008). Effect of elevated CO_2 on the protein concentration of food crops: A meta-analysis. *Global Change Biology*, *14*(3), 565–575. doi:10.1111/j.1365-2486.2007.01511.x

Taurines, R., Schwenck, R. B., Lyttwin, B., Schecklmann, M., Jans, T., Reefschlager, L., ... Romanos, M. (2016). Oxytocin plasma concentrations in children and adolescents with autism spectrum disorder: Correlation with autistic symptomatology. *Attention Deficit and Hyperactivity Disorders*, *6*(3), 231–239. doi:10.100712402-014-0145-y PMID:24989441

Taylor, K. M., Weisskopf, M., & Shine, J. (2014). Human exposure to nitro musks and the evaluation of their potential toxicity: An overview. *Environmental Health*, *13*(1), 14. doi:10.1186/1476-069X-13-14 PMID:24618224

Tchounwou, P. B., Patlolla, A. K., & Centeno, J. A. (2003). Carcinogenic and systemic health effects associated with arsenic exposure--a critical review. *Toxicologic Pathology*, *31*, 575–588. PMID:14585726

Teschke, K., Olshan, A., Daniels, J., De Roos, A., Parks, C., Schulz, M., & Vaughan, T. (2002). Occupational exposure in case-control studies: Opportunities for improvement. *Occupational and Environmental Medicine*, *59*(9), 575–594. doi:10.1136/oem.59.9.575 PMID:12205230

Teutsch, S., & Churchil, E. (2000). *Principles and practice of public health surveillance* (2nd ed.). Oxford University Press.

Textile Exchange. (2017). *Preferred Fiber & Materials Market Report*. Retrieved from https://textileexchange.org/downloads/2017-preferred-fiber-materials-market-report/

The Royal Society. (2002). Genetically modified plants for food use and human health— an update. Policy document 4/02. Retrieved from https://royalsociety.org/~/media/royal_society_content/policy/publications/2002/9 960.pdf

The World Bank. (1986). Poverty and hunger: Issues and options for food security in developing countries. World Bank Policy Study.

Theoharides, T. C. (2009). Autism spectrum disorders and mastocytosis 1. *International Journal of Immunopathology and Pharmacology*, *22*(4), 859–865. doi:10.1177/039463200902200401 PMID:20074449

Theoharides, T. C. (2016). Danger Signals and Inflammation. *Clinical Therapeutics*, *38*(5), 996–999. doi:10.1016/j.clinthera.2016.03.036 PMID:27101818

Theoharides, T. C. (2017). Neuroendocrinology of mast cells: Challenges and controversies. *Experimental Dermatology*, *26*(9), 751–759. doi:10.1111/exd.13288 PMID:28094875

Theoharides, T. C. (2018). Mold and Immunity. *Clinical Therapeutics*, *40*(6), 882–884. doi:10.1016/j.clinthera.2018.05.005 PMID:29859636

Theoharides, T. C., Alysandratos, K. D., Angelidou, A., Delivanis, D. A., Sismanopoulos, N., Zhang, B., ... Kalogeromitros, D. (2012). Mast cells and inflammation. *Biochimica et Biophysica Acta*, *1822*(1), 21–33. doi:10.1016/j.bbadis.2010.12.014 PMID:21185371

Theoharides, T. C., Asadi, S., Panagiotidou, S., & Weng, Z. (2013). The "missing link" in autoimmunity and autism: Extracellular mitochondrial components secreted from activated live mast cells. *Autoimmunity Reviews*, *12*(12), 1136–1142. doi:10.1016/j.autrev.2013.06.018 PMID:23831684

Theoharides, T. C., Donelan, J., Kempuraj, D., & Matsui, M. (in press). Skin mast cells as key sensors of environmental and psychological stress. *Current Opinion in Immunology*.

Theoharides, T. C., & Doyle, R. (2008). Autism, gut-blood-brain barrier and mast cells. *Journal of Clinical Psychopharmacology*, *28*(5), 479–483. doi:10.1097/JCP.0b013e3181845f48 PMID:18794641

Theoharides, T. C., Doyle, R., Francis, K., Conti, P., & Kalogeromitros, D. (2008). Novel therapeutic targets for autism. *Trends in Pharmacological Sciences*, *29*(8), 375–382. doi:10.1016/j.tips.2008.06.002 PMID:18606459

Theoharides, T. C., Stewart, J. M., Hatziagelaki, E., & Kolaitis, G. (2015a). Brain "fog," inflammation and obesity: Key aspects of 2 neuropsychiatric disorders improved by luteolin. *Frontiers in Neuroscience*, *9*, 225. doi:10.3389/fnins.2015.00225 PMID:26190965

Theoharides, T. C., Stewart, J. M., Panagiotidou, S., & Melamed, I. (2015b). Mast cells, brain inflammation and autism. *European Journal of Pharmacology*, *778*, 96–102. doi:10.1016/j.ejphar.2015.03.086 PMID:25941080

Theoharides, T. C., Tsilioni, I., Patel, A. B., & Doyle, R. (2016). Atopic diseases and inflammation of the brain in the pathogenesis of autism spectrum disorders. *Translational Psychiatry*, *6*(6), e844. doi:10.1038/tp.2016.77 PMID:27351598

Theoharides, T. C., Valent, P., & Akin, C. (2015c). Mast Cells, Mastocytosis, and Related Disorders. *The New England Journal of Medicine*, *373*(2), 163–172. doi:10.1056/NEJMra1409760 PMID:26154789

Thompson, S. (2017). How GM crops can help us feed a fast-growing world. *The Conversation*. Retrieved from http://theconversation.com/how-gm-crops-can-help-us-to-feed-a-fast-growing-world-71112

Thompson, P., & Hannah, W. (2008). Food and agricultural biotechnology: A summary and analysis of ethical concerns. In U. Stahl, U. Donalies, & E. Nevoigt (Eds.), *Advances in biochemical engineering/biotechnology* (pp. 229–264). Berlin, Germany: Springer.

Thomson, J. (2008). The role of biotechnology for agricultural sustainability in Africa. *Philosophical Transactions of the Royal Society*, *363*(1492), 905–913. doi:10.1098/rstb.2007.2191 PMID:17761472

Thrasher, J. D., & Crawley, S. (2009). The biocontaminants and complexity of damp indoor spaces: More than what meets the eyes. *Toxicology and Industrial Health*, *25*(9-10), 583–615. doi:10.1177/0748233709348386 PMID:19793773

Thurman, E. M., Zimmerman, L. R., Scribner, E. A., & Coupe, R. H. (1998). Occurrence of cotton pesticides in surface water of the Mississippi embayment. *U.S. Geological Survey Fact Sheet*, *4*, 22–98.

Tick, B., Bolton, P., Happé, F., Rutter, M., & Rijsdijk, F. (2016). Heritability of autism spectrum disorders: A meta-analysis of twin studies. *Journal of Child Psychology and Psychiatry, and Allied Disciplines*, *57*(5), 585–595. doi:10.1111/jcpp.12499 PMID:26709141

Tirone, T. A., & Brunicardi, F. C. (2001). Overview of glucose regulation. *World Journal of Surgery*, *25*(4), 461–467. doi:10.1007002680020338 PMID:11344399

Toda, H. Y., & Yamamoto, T. (1995). Statistical inference in vector autoregressions with possibly integrated processes. *Journal of Econometrics*, *66*(12), 225–250. doi:10.1016/0304-4076(94)01616-8

Toghill, K. E., & Richard, G. (2010). Compton Electrochemical Non-enzymatic Glucose Sensors: A Perspective and an Evaluation. *International Journal of Electrochemical Science*, *5*, 1246–1301.

Tomova, A., Husarova, V., Lakatosova, S., Bakos, J., Vlkova, B., Babinska, K., & Ostatnikova, D. (2015). Gastrointestinal microbiota in children with autism in Slovakia. *Physiology & Behavior*, *138*, 179–187. doi:10.1016/j.physbeh.2014.10.033 PMID:25446201

Top Trends in Prepared Foods 2017: Exploring trends in meat, fish and seafood; pasta, noodles and rice; prepared meals; savory deli food; soup; and meat substitutes. (2017). Retrieved from https://www.reportbuyer.com/product/4959853/top-trends-in-prepared-foods-2017-exploring-trends-in-meat-fish-and-seafood-pasta-noodles-and-rice-prepared-meals-savory-deli-food-soup-and-meat-substitutes.html

Tordjman, S., Somogyi, E., Coulon, N., Kermarrec, S., Cohen, D., Bronsard, G., ... Xavier, J. (2014). Gene x Environment interactions in autism spectrum disorders: Role of epigenetic mechanisms. *Frontiers in Psychiatry*, *5*, 53. doi:10.3389/fpsyt.2014.00053 PMID:25136320

Tottenham, N., & Sheridan, M. A. (2009). A review of adversity, the amygdala and the hippocampus: A consideration of developmental timing. *Frontiers in Human Neuroscience*, *3*, 68. PMID:20161700

Townsend, T. (1997, May). World Cotton Outlook. International Cotton Advisory Committee (ICAC). In *Proceedings of the 73 rd Annual Convention of the American Crop Shippers Association* (pp. 22-24).

Townsend, M., Peck, C., Meng, W., Heaton, M., Robison, R., & O'Neill, K. (2017). Evaluation of various glyphosate concentrations on DNA damage in human Raji cells and its impact on cytotoxicity. *Regulatory Toxicology and Pharmacology*, *85*, 79–85. doi:10.1016/j.yrtph.2017.02.002 PMID:28185844

Tran, N. V., & Miyake, K. (2017). Neurodevelopmental Disorders and Environmental Toxicants: Epigenetics as an Underlying Mechanism. *International Journal of Genomics*, *7526592*. doi:10.1155/2017/7526592 PMID:28567415

Tripathi, R., Raghunath, R., Mahapatra, S., & Sadasivan, S. (2001). Blood lead and its effect on Cd, Cu, Zn, Fe and hemoglobin levels of children. *The Science of the Total Environment*, *277*(1-3), 161–168. doi:10.1016/S0048-9697(00)00871-8 PMID:11589396

Trouba, K. J., Wauson, E. M., & Vorce, R. L. (2000). Sodium arsenite-induced dysregulation of proteins involved in proliferative signaling. *Toxicology and Applied Pharmacology*, *164*(2), 161–170. doi:10.1006/taap.1999.8873 PMID:10764629

Truitt, W. A., Sajdyk, T. J., Dietrich, A. D., Oberlin, B., McDougle, C. J., & Shekhar, A. (2007). From anxiety to autism: Spectrum of abnormal social behaviors modeled by progressive disruption of inhibitory neuronal function in the basolateral amygdala in Wistar rats. *Psychopharmacology*, *191*(1), 107–118. doi:10.100700213-006-0674-y PMID:17277936

Tsai, S. Y., Chou, H. Y., The, H.-W., Chen, C.-M., & Chen, C.-J. (2003). The HW, Chen CM, Chen CJ.The effects of chronic arsenic exposure from drinking water on the neuro behavioral development in adolescence. *Neurotoxicology*, *24*(4–5), 747–753. doi:10.1016/S0161-813X(03)00029-9 PMID:12900089

Tsatsakis, A. M., Nawaz, M. A., Kouretas, D., Balias, G., Savolainen, K., Tutelyan, V. A., ... Chung, G. (2017). Environmental impacts of genetically modified plants: A review. *Environmental Research*, *156*, 818–833. doi:10.1016/j.envres.2017.03.011 PMID:28347490

Tseng, C. H., Huang, Y. K., Huang, Y. L., Chung, C. J., Yang, M. H., Chen, C. J., & Hsueh, Y. M. (2005). Arsenic exposure, urinary arsenic speciation, and peripheral vascular disease in black foot disease-hyperendemic villages in Taiwan. *Toxicology and Applied Pharmacology*, *206*(3), 299–308. doi:10.1016/j.taap.2004.11.022 PMID:16039941

Tseng, W. P. (1977). Effects and dose response relationships of skin cancer and blackfoot disease with arsenic. *Environmental Health Perspectives*, *19*, 109–119. doi:10.1289/ehp.7719109 PMID:908285

Tsien, R. Y. (1980). New calcium indicators and buffers with high selectivity against magnesium and protons: Design, synthesis, and properties of prototype structures. *Biochemistry*, *19*(11), 2396–2404. doi:10.1021/bi00552a018 PMID:6770893

Tsoi, M. F., Cheung, C. L., Cheung, T. T., & Cheung, B. M. Y. (2016). Continual decrease in blood lead level in Americans: United States National Health Nutrition and Examination Survey 1999-2014. *The American Journal of Medicine*, *129*(11), 1213–1218. doi:10.1016/j.amjmed.2016.05.042 PMID:27341956

Tsuda, T., Babazono, A., Yamamoto, E., Kurumatani, N., Mino, Y., Ogawa, T., ... Aoyama, H. (1995). Ingested arsenic and internal cancer: A historical cohort study followed for 33 years. *American Journal of Epidemiology*, *141*(3), 198–209. doi:10.1093/oxfordjournals.aje.a117421 PMID:7840093

Turner, M. C., Nieuwenhuijsen, M., Anderson, K., Balshaw, D., Cui, Y., Dunton, G., ... Turner, M. C. (2017). Assessing the Exposome with External Measures: Commentary on the State of the Science and Research Recommendations. *Annual Review of Public Health*, *20*(38), 215–239. doi:10.1146/annurev-publhealth-082516-012802 PMID:28384083

Tutelyan, V. A. (2013). *Safety Assessment and Control* (1st ed.). Academic Press. doi:10.1016/C2011-0-08818-X

Twardowski, T., & Małyska, A. (2015). Uninformed and disinformed society and the GMO market. *Trends in Biotechnology*, *33*(1), 1–3. doi:10.1016/j.tibtech.2014.11.006 PMID:25528967

Tyler, L. N., Ai, L., Zuo, C., Fan, C. Y., & Smoller, B. R. (2003). Analysis of promoter hypermethylation of death associated protein kinase and p16 tumor suppressor genes in actinic keratoses and squamous cell carcinomas of the skin. *Modern Pathology*, *16*(7), 660–664. doi:10.1097/01.MP.0000077516.90063.7D PMID:12861061

Union of Concerned Scientists (UCS). *Why does CO_2 get most of the attention when there are so many other heat-trapping gases?* UCS.

United Nations. (1948). *Universal declaration of human rights.* Adopted by the General Assembly of the United Nations on December 10, 1948. Retrieved from http://www.un.org/en/universal-declaration-human-rights/index.html

United Nations. (1966). *The international covenant on economic, social and cultural rights.* Adopted by the General Assembly of the United Nations on December 16, 1966.

United Nations. (1974). *Report of the World Food Conference.* New York, NY: United Nations.

United Nations. (1975). *Report of the World Food Conference*. Rome: UN.

United Nations. (1992). *Sales No. E.73.II.A.14 and corrigendum.* Rio de Janeiro, Brazil: United Nations.

United Nations. (2015). *World population projected to reach 9.7 billion by 2050.* Department of Economic and Social Affairs, UN.

United Nations. (2017). *World Mortality 2017: Data Booklet.* Retrieved from http://www.un.org/en/development/desa/population/publications/pdf/mortality/World-Mortality-2017-Data-Booklet.pdf

United States Department of Agriculture (USDA). (2014). *Genetically Engineered Crops in the United States, February 2014.*

United States Environmental Protection Agency. (1999). Analytical methods support document for arsenic in drinking water.

United States Environmental Protection Agency. (2004). Monitoring arsenic in the environment: a review of science and technologies for field measurements and sensors.

US Department of Agriculture, National Agricultural Statistics Service. (2004). *Agricultural Chemical Usage, 2003 Field Crops Summary 2004.* Collingdale, PA: Diane Publishing Co.

US Right to Know. (n.d.). *The Monsanto Papers. (Glyphosate) Cancer Case Key Documents & Analysis.* Retrieved from https://usrtk.org/pesticides/mdl-monsanto-glyphosate-cancer-case-key-documents-analysis/

USDA ChooseMyPlate.gov. (n.d.). Choose My Plate. Retrieved from https://www.choosemyplate.gov/food-groups/dairy-amount.html

USDA. (2013). *Biotechnology Frequently Asked Questions*. Retrieved from http://www.usda.gov/wps/portal/usda/usdahome?navid=AGRICULTURE&contentid=BiotechnologyFAQs.xml

USEPA, U.S. Environmental Protection Agency. (1985). Health Assessment Document for Polychlorinated Dibenzo-p-Dioxin. Environmental Criteria and Assessment Office, Office of Health and Environmental Assessment, Office of Research and Development, Cincinnati, OH.

Usher, S., Han, L., Haslam, R. P., Michaelson, L. V., Sturtevant, D., Aziz, M., ... Napier, J. A. (2017). Tailoring seed oil composition in the real world: Optimising omega-3 long chain polyunsaturated fatty acid accumulation in transgenic *Camelina sativa. Scientific Reports*, *7*(1), 6570. doi:10.103841598-017-06838-0 PMID:28747792

Vahidnia, A., van der Voet, G. B., & de Wolff, F. A. (2007). Arsenic neurotoxicity--a review. *Human and Experimental Toxicology*, *26*(10), 823–832. doi:10.1177/0960327107084539 PMID:18025055

Valko, M., Rhodes, C. J., Moncol, J., Izakovic, M., & Mazur, M. (2006). Free radicals, metals and antioxidants in oxidative stress induced cancer. *Chemico-Biological Interactions*, *160*(1), 1–40. doi:10.1016/j.cbi.2005.12.009 PMID:16430879

Van Arman, S. A., & Czarnik, A. W. (1990). A general fluorescence assay for enzyme catalyzed polyanion hydrolysis based on template directed excimer formation. Application to heparin and polyglutamate. *Journal of the American Chemical Society*, *112*(13), 5376–5377. doi:10.1021/ja00169a070

Van den Berg, M., Birnbaum, L., Bosveld, A. T., Brunstrom, B., Cook, P., Feeley, M., ... Zacharewski, T. (1998). Toxic equivalency factors (TEFs) for PCBs, PCDDs, PCDFs for humans and wildlife. *Environmental Health Perspectives*, *106*(12), 775–792. doi:10.1289/ehp.98106775 PMID:9831538

van Duijn, H., & Maas, M. (2017). Organic Cotton's Threshold Moment. *Organic Cotton Accelerator*. Retrieved from http://www.organiccottonaccelerator.org/wp-content/uploads/dlm_uploads/2017/03/OCA-Organic-Cottons-Threshold-Moment-2017.pdf

van Steensel, F. J., Bogels, S. M., & Perrin, S. (2011). Anxiety disorders in children and adolescents with autistic spectrum disorders: A meta-analysis. *Clinical Child and Family Psychology Review*, *14*(3), 302–317. doi:10.100710567-011-0097-0 PMID:21735077

Velasco-Santamaría, Y. M., Korsgaard, B., Madsen, S. S., & Bjerregaard, P. (2011). Bezafibrate, a lipid-lowering pharmaceutical, as a potential endocrine disruptor in male zebrafish (Danio rerio). *Aquatic Toxicology (Amsterdam, Netherlands)*, *105*(1-2), 107–118. doi:10.1016/j.aquatox.2011.05.018 PMID:21703979

Verner, M. A., Charbonneau, M., Lopez-Carrillo, L., & Haddad, S. (2008). Physiologically based pharmacokinetic modeling of persistent organic pollutants for lifetime exposure assessment: A new tool in breast cancer epidemiologic studies. *Environmental Health Perspectives*, *116*(7), 886–892. doi:10.1289/ehp.10917 PMID:18629310

Vienna, A., Capucci, E., Wolfsperger, M., & Hauser, G. (1995). Heavy metals in hair of students in Rome. *Anthropologischer Anzeiger*, *53*, 27–32. PMID:7755371

Vieno, N., & Sillanpää, M. (2014). Fate of diclofenac in municipal wastewater treatment plant - a review. *Environment International*, *69*, 28–39. doi:10.1016/j.envint.2014.03.021 PMID:24791707

Vinceti, M., Wei, E. T., Malagoli, C., Bergomi, M., & Vivoli, G. (2001). Adverse health effects of selenium in humans. *Reviews on Environmental Health*, *16*(4), 233–252. doi:10.1515/REVEH.2001.16.4.233 PMID:12041880

Vineis, P., van Veldhoven, K., Chadeau-Hyam, M., & Athersuch, T. J. (2013). Advancing the application of omics-based biomarkers in environmental epidemiology. *Environmental and Molecular Mutagenesis*, *54*(7), 461–467. doi:10.1002/em.21764 PMID:23519765

Vineis, P., & Wild, C. P. (2014). Global cancer patterns: Causes and prevention. *Lancet*, *383*(9916), 549–557. doi:10.1016/S0140-6736(13)62224-2 PMID:24351322

Vitousek, P. M., Mooney, H. A., Lubchenco, J., & Melillo, J. M. (1997). Human domination of Earth's ecosystems. *Science*, *277*(5325), 494–499. doi:10.1126cience.277.5325.494

Volk, H. E., Kerin, T., Lurmann, F., Hertz-Picciotto, I., McConnell, R., & Campbell, D. B. (2014). Autism spectrum disorder: Interaction of air pollution with the MET receptor tyrosine kinase gene. *Epidemiology (Cambridge, MA)*, *25*(1), 44–47. doi:10.1097/EDE.0000000000000030 PMID:24240654

von Tobel, J. S., Antinori, P., Zurich, M. G., Rosset, R., Aschner, M., Gluck, F., ... Monnet-Tschudi, F. (2014). Repeated exposure to Ochratoxin A generates a neuroinflammatory response, characterized by neurodegenerative M1 microglial phenotype. *Neurotoxicology*, *44*, 61–70. doi:10.1016/j.neuro.2014.04.005 PMID:24792326

Vrijheid, M. (2014). The exposome: A new paradigm to study the impact of environment on health. *Thorax*, *69*(9), 876–878. doi:10.1136/thoraxjnl-2013-204949 PMID:24906490

Vrijheid, M., Slama, R., Robinson, O., Chatzi, L., Coen, M., van den Hazel, P., ... Nieuwenhuijsen, M. J. (2014). The Human Early-Life Exposome (HELIX): Project Rationale and Design. *Environmental Health Perspectives*, *122*(6), 535–544. doi:10.1289/ehp.1307204 PMID:24610234

Vulava, V. M., Cory, W. C., Murphey, V. L., & Ulmer, C. Z. (2016). Sorption, photodegradation, and chemical transformation of naproxen and ibuprofen in soils and water. *The Science of the Total Environment*, *565*, 1063–1070. doi:10.1016/j.scitotenv.2016.05.132 PMID:27262983

Walia, A. (2014, October 30). Most Human Beings Are Lactose Intolerant: Here's Why. Collective-evolution. Retrieved from http://www.collective-evolution.com/2013/04/03/over-75-of-earths-population-is-lactose-intolerant-for-a-reason-dairy-is-harmful/

Waliszewski, S. M., Pardio, V. T., Waliszewski, K. N., Chantiri, J. N., Aguirre, A. A., Infanzon, R. M., & Rivera, J. (1997). Organochlorine pesticide residues in cow's milk and butter in Mexico. *The Science of the Total Environment*, *208*(1-2), 127–132. doi:10.1016/S0048-9697(97)00270-2 PMID:9496657

Walker, G. (2012). *Environmental Justice: Concepts, Evidence and Politics*. Routledge. doi:10.4324/9780203610671

Wang, J., He, B., Yan, D., Hu, X. (2017). Implementing ecopharmacovigilance (EPV) from a pharmacy perspective: A focus on non-steroidal anti-inflammatory drugs. *The Science of the Total Environment, 15,* 603-604, 772-784.

Wang, C. T., Chang, W. T., Huang, C. W., Chou, S. S., Lin, C. T., Liau, S. J., & Wang, R. T. (1994). Studies on the concentrations of arsenic, selenium, copper, zinc, and iron in the hair of blackfoot disease patients in different clinical stages. *European Journal of Clinical Chemistry and Clinical Biochemistry*, *32*(3), 107–111. PMID:8031959

Wang, J. (1990). *New Approaches to metal speciation in natural waters Based on Modified and Microvoltametric Electrodes*. La Cruces, NM: Department of Chemistry, New Mexico State University.

Wang, J., Zhao, S. Q., Zhang, M. Y., & He, B. S. (2018). Targeted eco-pharmacovigilance for ketoprofen in the environment: Need, strategy and challenge. *Chemosphere*, *194*, 450–462. doi:10.1016/j.chemosphere.2017.12.020 PMID:29227893

Warnick, E. M., Bracken, M. B., & Kasl, S. (2008). Screening Efficiency of the Child Behavior Checklist and Strengths and Difficulties Questionnaire: A Systematic Review. *Child and Adolescent Mental Health*, *13*(3), 140–147. doi:10.1111/j.1475-3588.2007.00461.x

Wartenberg, D. (1994). *When is a Cluster Really a Cluster? The competing agendas of science, society and social programs. Environmental Epidemiology: Science for society or science in society?* Hamilton, Canada: McMaster University.

Wasserman, G. A., Liu, X., Loiacono, N. J., Kline, J., Factor-Litvak, P., van Geen, A., ... Graziano, J. H. (2014). A cross-sectional study of well water arsenic and child IQ in Maine school children. *Environmental Health*, *13*(1), 23. doi:10.1186/1476-069X-13-23 PMID:24684736

Wasserman, G. A., Liu, X., Parvez, F., Ahsan, H., Factor-Litvak, P., van Geen, A., ... Hussain, I. (2004). Water arsenic exposure and children's intellectual function in Araihazar, Bangladesh. *Environmental Health Perspectives*, *112*(13), 1329–1333. doi:10.1289/ehp.6964 PMID:15345348

Waterhouse, L., London, R., & Gillberg, C. (2016). ASD Validity *Rev. Journal of Autism and Developmental Disorders*, *3*(4), 302–329. doi:10.100740489-016-0085-x

Watkinson, A. J., Murby, E. J., & Costanzo, S. D. (2007). Removal of antibiotics in conventional and advanced wastewater treatment: Implications for environmental discharge and wastewater recycling. *Water Research*, *41*(18), 4164–4176. doi:10.1016/j.watres.2007.04.005 PMID:17524445

We Are What We Eat. (2015). Nielsen Report. Retrieved from http://www.nielsen.com/us/en/insights/reports/2015/we-are-what-we-eat.html

Webster, L. R., McKenzie, G. H., & Moriarty, H. T. (2002). Organophosphate-based pesticides and genetic damage implicated in bladder cancer. *Cancer Genetics and Cytogenetics*, *133*(2), 112–117. doi:10.1016/S0165-4608(01)00576-3 PMID:11943336

Wechsler, D. (2003). *Wechsler Intelligence Scale for Children*. San Antonio, TX: Psychological Corporation.

Weed, D. L. (2005). Weight of Evidence: A review concept and methods. *Risk Analysis*, *25*(6), 1545–1557. doi:10.1111/j.1539-6924.2005.00699.x PMID:16506981

Weedon, D. (2010). *Weedon's skin pathology*. Churchill Livingstone Elsevier.

Welsh, J. A., Lundeen, E. A., & Stein, A. D. (2013). The sugar-sweetened beverage wars. *Current*Opinion in Endocrinology & Diabetes and Obesity, 20(5), 401-406. PMID:23974767

Weston, A., Caminada, D., Galicia, H., & Fent, K. (2009). Effects of lipid-lowering pharmaceuticals bezafibrate and clofibric acid on lipid metabolism in fathead minnow (*Pimephales promelas*). *Environmental Toxicology and Chemistry*, *28*(12), 2648–2655. doi:10.1897/09-087.1 PMID:19522550

What is Agricultural Biotechnology? (2004). U.S. Agency for International Development, Agricultural Biotechnology Support Project II, and the Program for Biosafety Systems.

White, N. J. (1996). The treatment of malaria. *The New England Journal of Medicine*, *335*(11), 800–806. doi:10.1056/NEJM199609123351107 PMID:8703186

WHO. (2007). Health relevance of particulate matter from various sources.

WHO. (2008). Guidelines for drinking-water quality (3rd ed., Vol. 1). Geneva, World Health Organization.

WHO-UNICEF-USAID. (2015). *Improving nutrition outcomes with better water, sanitation and hygiene: practical solutions for policies and programs.* Retrieved from https://www.unicef.org/media/files/IntegratingWASHandNut_WHO_UNICEF_USAID_Nov2015.pdf

Wickre, J. B., Folt, C. L., Sturup, S., & Karagas, M. R. (2004). Environmental Exposure and Fingernail Analysis of Arsenic and Mercury in Children and Adults in a Nicaraguan Gold Mining Community. *Archives of Environmental Health: An International Journal, 59*(8), 400–409. doi:10.3200/AEOH.59.8.400-409 PMID:16268116

Wieczorek, A. (2013). History of Agricultural Biotechnology: How Crop Development has Evolved. *Nature*. Retrieved from http://www.nature.com/scitable/knowledge/library/history-of-agricultural-biotechnology-how-crop-development-25885295

Wild, C. P. (2005). Complementing the genome with an "exposome": The outstanding challenge of environmental exposure measurement in molecular epidemiology. *Cancer Epidemiology, Biomarkers & Prevention, 14*(8), 1847–1850. doi:10.1158/1055-9965.EPI-05-0456 PMID:16103423

Wild, C. P., Scalbert, A., & Herceg, Z. (2013). Measuring the exposome: A powerful basis for evaluating environmental exposures and cancer risk. *Environmental and Molecular Mutagenesis, 54*(7), 480–499. doi:10.1002/em.21777 PMID:23681765

Willsey, A. J., & State, M. W. (2015). Autism spectrum disorders: From genes to neurobiology. *Current Opinion in Neurobiology, 30*, 92–99. doi:10.1016/j.conb.2014.10.015 PMID:25464374

Wilson, J. G. (1973). *Environment and Birth Defects*. New York: Academic Press.

Winkel, L., Berg, M., Amini, M., Hug, S. J., & Annette Johnson, C. (2008). Predicting groundwater arsenic contamination in Southeast Asia from surface parameters. *Nature Geoscience, 1*(8), 536–542. doi:10.1038/ngeo254

Wishart, D., Mandal, R., Stanislaus, A., & Ramirez-Gaona, M. (2016). Cancer Metabolomics and the Human Metabolome Database. *Metabolites, 6*(1), 10. doi:10.3390/metabo6010010 PMID:26950159

Wolch, J., Byrne, J., & Newell, J. P. (2014). Urban green space, public health, and environmental justice: The challenge of making cities 'just green enough.' *Landscape and Urban Planning, 125*, 234–244. doi:10.1016/j.landurbplan.2014.01.017

Wolff, S. (2004). The history of autism. *European Child & Adolescent Psychiatry, 13*(4), 201–207. doi:10.100700787-004-0363-5 PMID:15365889

Wolfsperger, M., Hauser, G., Gössler, W., & Schlagenhaufen, C. (1994). Heavy metals in human hair samples from Austria and Italy: Influence of sex and smoking habits. *The Science of the Total Environment, 156*(3), 235–242. doi:10.1016/0048-9697(94)90190-2 PMID:7801110

Wolkoff, P., & Nielsen, G. D. (2017). Effects by inhalation of abundant fragrances in indoor air - An overview. *Environment International, 101*, 96–107. doi:10.1016/j.envint.2017.01.013 PMID:28126407

Wong S. S., Tan K. C., and Goh C. L. (1998). Cutaneous manifestations of chronic arsenicism: review of seventeen cases. *Journal of the American Academy of Dermatology, 38*(2), 179-185.

Wong, C. T., Wais, J., & Crawford, D. A. (2015). Prenatal exposure to common environmental factors affects brain lipids and increases risk of developing autism spectrum disorders. *The European Journal of Neuroscience, 42*(10), 2742–2760. doi:10.1111/ejn.13028 PMID:26215319

Wong, D. (2003). *Genetically Modified Food Labelling*. Hong Kong: Research and Library Services Division Legislative Council Secretariat. Retrieved from http://www.legco.gov.hk/yr02-03/english/sec/library/0203rp05e.pdf

Wong, H. H., & Wang, J. (2010). Merkel cell carcinoma. *Archives of Pathology & Laboratory Medicine, 134*(11), 1711–1716. PMID:21043828

World Health Organization (WHO). (2008). *Climate change and health.* Retrieved from http://www.who.int/iris/handle/10665/126809

World Health Organization (WHO). (2012). *Atlas of health and climate.* Retrieved from http://www.who.int/globalchange/publications/atlas/en/

World Health Organization (WHO). (2014). *Gender, climate change and health.* Retrieved from http://www.who.int/globalchange/publications/reports/gender_climate_change/en/

World Health Organization. (2001). Arsenic and arsenic compounds (2nd ed.). Geneva, International Programme on Chemical Safety.

World-Bank. (2013). *World Development Indicators database* (Vol. 2014). World Bank.

Wu, J. S., Ku, Y. H., Li, L. S., Lu, Y. C., Ding, X., & Wang, Y. G. (1999). Corticotropin releasing factor and substance P mediate the nucleus amygdaloideus centralis-nucleus ventromedialis-nucleus dorsomedialis pressor system. *Brain Research, 842*(2), 392–398. doi:10.1016/S0006-8993(99)01862-4 PMID:10526135

Wu, S., Zhang, L., & Chen, J. (2012). Paracetamol in the environment and its degradation by microorganisms. *Applied Microbiology and Technology, 96*(4), 875–884. doi:10.100700253-012-4414-4 PMID:23053075

Xi, S., Guo, L., Qi, R., Sun, W., Jin, Y., & Sun, G. (2010). Prenatal and early life arsenic exposure induced oxidative damage and altered activities and mRNA expressions of neurotransmitter metabolic enzymes in offspring rat brain. *Journal of Biochemical and Molecular Toxicology, 24*(6), 368–378. doi:10.1002/jbt.20349 PMID:20376865

Yadav, I. C., Devi, N. L., Syed, J. H., Cheng, Z., Li, J., Zhang, G., & Jones, K. C. (2015). Current status of persistent organic pesticides residues in air, water, and soil, and their possible effect on neighboring countries: A comprehensive review of India. *The Science of the Total Environment, 511*, 123–137. doi:10.1016/j.scitotenv.2014.12.041 PMID:25540847

Yamazoe, N., & Miura, N. (1992). New Approaches in the Design of Gas Sensors. In G. Sberveglieri (Ed.), *Gas Sensors.* Dordrecht: Springer. doi:10.1007/978-94-011-2737-0_1

Yao, L., Shen, B., Cao, C., Feng, W., & Li, F. (2014). Chemodosimeter functionalized magnetic silica yolk–shell nanocomposite for sensing and removal of Hg^{2+}. *RSC Advances, 4*(39), 20252–20255. doi:10.1039/c4ra02410a

Yarom, R., Bergmann, F., & Yagen, B. (1987). Cutaneous injury by topical T-2 toxin: Involvement of microvessels and mast cells. *Toxicon, 25*(2), 167–174. doi:10.1016/0041-0101(87)90238-8 PMID:3576633

Yarsan, E., Tanyuksel, M., Celik, S., & Aydin, A. (1999). Effects of aldicarb and malathion on lipid peroxidation. *Bulletin of Environmental Contamination and Toxicology, 63*(5), 575–581. doi:10.1007001289901019 PMID:10541675

Yoshida, T., Yamauchi, H., & Sun, G. F. (2004). Chronic health effects in people exposed to arsenic via the drinking water: Dose-response relationships in review. *Toxicology and Applied Pharmacology, 198*(3), 243–252. doi:10.1016/j.taap.2003.10.022 PMID:15276403

Yuan, Y., Marshall, G., Ferreccio, C., Steinmaus, C., Liaw, J., Bates, M., & Smith, A. H. (2010). Kidney cancer mortality: Fifty-year latency patterns related to arsenic exposure. *Epidemiology (Cambridge, Mass.), 21*(1), 103–108. doi:10.1097/EDE.0b013e3181c21e46 PMID:20010213

Yu, C. P., Deeb, R. A., & Chu, K. H. (2013). Microbial degradation of steroidal estrogens. *Chemosphere, 91*(9), 1225–1235. doi:10.1016/j.chemosphere.2013.01.112 PMID:23517889

Yu, H. S., Lee, C. H., Jee, S. H., Ho, C. K., & Guo, Y. L. (2001). Environmental and occupational skin diseases in Taiwan. *The Journal of Dermatology*, *28*(11), 628–631. doi:10.1111/j.1346-8138.2001.tb00049.x PMID:11770720

Yu, H. S., Liao, W. T., & Chai, C. Y. (2006). Arsenic carcinogenesis in the skin. *Journal of Biomedical Science*, *13*(5), 657–666. doi:10.100711373-006-9092-8 PMID:16807664

Yunus, F. M., Khan, S., Chowdhury, P., Milton, A. H., Hussain, S., & Rahman, M. (2016). A Review of Groundwater Arsenic Contamination in Bangladesh: The Millennium Development Goal Era and Beyond. International Journal of Environmental Research and Public Health, 13(2).

Yu, X., Deng, T., Guo, Y., & Wang, Q. (2014). Arsenic Species Analysis in Freshwater Using Liquid Chromatography Combined to Hydride Generation Atomic Fluorescence Spectrometry. *Journal of Analytical Chemistry*, *69*(1), 88–93. doi:10.1134/S1061934814010146

Zablotsky, B., Black, L. I., Maenner, M. J., Schieve, L. A., & Blumberg, S. J. (2015). Estimated prevalence of autism and other developmental disabilities following questionnaire changes in the 2014 National Health Interview Survey. *National Health Statistics Reports*. Retrieved from https://stacks.cdc.gov/view/cdc/38790

Zachos, J. C., Dickens, G. R., & Zeebe, R. E. (2008). An early cenozoic perspective on greenhouse warming and carbon-cycle dynamics. *Nature*, *451*(7176), 279–283. doi:10.1038/nature06588 PMID:18202643

Zahm, S. H., & Ward, M. H. (1998). Pesticides and childhood cancer. *Environmental Health Perspectives*, *106*(Supplement 3), 893. PMID:9646054

Zaidan, H., Leshem, M., & Gaisler-Salomon, I. (2013). Prereproductive stress to female rats alters corticotropin releasing factor type 1 expression in ova and behavior and brain corticotropin releasing factor type 1 expression in offspring. *Biological Psychiatry*, *74*(9), 680–687. doi:10.1016/j.biopsych.2013.04.014 PMID:23726318

Zaldivar, R., Prunes, L., & Ghai, G. L. (1981). Arsenic dose in patients with cutaneous carcinomata and hepatic haemangio-endothelioma after environmental and occupational exposure. *Archives of Toxicology*, *47*(2), 145–154. doi:10.1007/BF00332356 PMID:7271443

Zapata, A. M., Santamaría, M. R., Alvarez, M. I., Salazar, S. V., & Müller, U. (1996). Organochlorine pesticide residues in cow's milk, Nicaragua. *Boletin de la Oficina Sanitaria Panamericana. Pan American Sanitary Bureau*, *120*(6), 483–490.

Zerbe, N. (2004). Feeding the famine? American food aid and the GMO debate in Southern Africa. *Food Policy*, *29*(6), 593–608. doi:10.1016/j.foodpol.2004.09.002

Zhang, B., Angelidou, A., Alysandratos, K. D., Vasiadi, M., Francis, K., Asadi, S., ... Theoharides, T. C. (2010). Mitochondrial DNA and anti-mitochondrial antibodies in serum of autistic children. *Journal of Neuroinflammation*, *7*(1), 80. doi:10.1186/1742-2094-7-80 PMID:21083929

Zhang, B., Asadi, S., Weng, Z., Sismanopoulos, N., & Theoharides, T. C. (2012). Stimulated human mast cells secrete mitochondrial components that have autocrine and paracrine inflammatory actions. *PLoS One*, *7*(12), e49767. doi:10.1371/journal.pone.0049767 PMID:23284625

Zhang, J., & Kesteloot, H. (2005). Milk consumption in relation to incidence of prostate, breast, colon, and rectal cancers: Is there an independent effect? *Nutrition and Cancer*, *53*(1), 65–72. doi:10.120715327914nc5301_8 PMID:16351508

Zhang, N., Liu, G., Liu, H., Wang, Y., He, Z., & Wang, G. (2011). Diclofenac photodegradation under simulated sunlight: Effect of different forms of nitrogen and kinetics. *Journal of Hazardous Materials*, *192*(1), 411–418. PMID:21664047

Zhang, P. (2017). On arsenic trioxide in the clinical treatment of acute promyelocytic leukemia. *Leukemia Research Reports*, *7*, 29–32. doi:10.1016/j.lrr.2017.03.001 PMID:28462082

Zhang, X., Wang, Y., Dong, H., Xu, Y., & Zhang, S. (2016). Induction of Microglial Activation by Mediators Released from Mast Cells. *Cellular Physiology and Biochemistry*, *38*(4), 1520–1531. doi:10.1159/000443093 PMID:27050634

Zhang, Z., Kim, D. S., Lin, C. Y., Zhang, H., Lammer, A. D., Lynch, V. M., ... Sessler, J. L. (2015). Expanded porphyrin-anion supramolecular assemblies: Environmentally responsive sensors for organic solvents and anions. *Journal of the American Chemical Society*, *137*(24), 7769–7774. doi:10.1021/jacs.5b03131

Zhan, K., Chen, X., Lin, Z., & Bennian, I. (2006). Implementation of optical chemsensors based on HF etched fibre bragg grating structures. *Measurement Science & Technology*, *5*, 17.

Zhao, B., Ye, X., Yu, J., Li, L., Li, W., Li, S., ... Guan, K. L. (2008). TEAD mediates YAP- dependent gene induction and growth control. *Genes & Development*, *22*(14), 1962–1971. doi:10.1101/gad.1664408 PMID:18579750

Zhao, S., & Yu, G. (2017). A new image registration algorithm using SDTR. *Neurocomputing*, *234*, 174–184. doi:10.1016/j.neucom.2016.12.055

Zhou, B., Wang, J., & Ressom, H. W. (2012). MetaboSearch: Tool for Mass-Based Metabolite Identification Using Multiple Databases. *PLoS One*, *7*(6), e40096. doi:10.1371/journal.pone.0040096 PMID:22768229

Zhou, J., & Parada, L. F. (2012). PTEN signaling in autism spectrum disorders. *Current Opinion in Neurobiology*, *22*(5), 873–879. doi:10.1016/j.conb.2012.05.004 PMID:22664040

Zhu, X., Van Wesenbeeck, L., & Van Ierland, E. C. (2006). Impacts of Novel Protein Foods on Sustainable Food Production and Consumption: Lifestyle Change and Environmental Policy. *Environmental and Resource Economics*, *35*(1), 59–87. doi:10.100710640-006-9006-2

Zia, M. S., Khan, M. J., Qasim, M., & Rehman, A. (2009). Pesticide residue in the food chain and human body inside Pakistan. *Journal of the Chemical Society of Pakistan*, *31*, 284–291.

Ziats, M. N., Grosvenor, L. P., & Rennert, O. M. (2015). Functional genomics of human brain development and implications for autism spectrum disorders 1. *Translational Psychiatry*, *5*(10), e665. doi:10.1038/tp.2015.153 PMID:26506051

Zwolak, I., & Zaporowska, H. (2012). Selenium interactions and toxicity: A review. *Cell Biology and Toxicology*, *28*(1), 31–46. doi:10.100710565-011-9203-9 PMID:21913064

About the Contributors

Paraskevi Papadopoulou is Professor of Biology at Deree -The American College of Greece. She holds Biology degrees from the University of California, Los Angeles and from the University of Athens and a PhD in Biophysics and Cell Biology from the University of Athens. She has served as Head of the department of Science, Technology and Mathematics at Deree -The American University of Greece for 6 years. Her research interests are focused in the fields of Structural Biology/Molecular Biophysics and Bioinformatics, on structural and self-assembly studies of fibrous proteins. She has also contributed to the development of genetic testing protocols for genetic diseases such as Tuberous Sclerosis and of Neurofibromatosis type 1. Her current research engagement is on environmental health issues, sexually transmitted diseases, Mediterranean biodiversity and green roofs, and innovative ways of teaching and learning in STEM disciplines plus on big data analytics in bioinformatics and medicine. In addition, she teaches introductory and advanced courses in biology such as molecular biology, human genetics and cell and molecular neurobiology and environmental studies courses such as natural sciences research methods for the environmental studies program.

Christina Marouli studied biochemistry, urban and environmental policy (M.A.) and sociology (M.A and PhD) in the USA – with a specialisation on the environment, health and social inequalities. Her present research interests include education for sustainability, sustainable, healthy, smart cities, environmental behaviors and social change. She is teaching the Environmental Studies Program of Deree – American College of Greece (ACG) and she is the founder and ex-Director of the Center of Excellence for Sustainability at ACG. She is also a recipient of a Fulbright award in the context of which she did research on multicultural environmental education programmes in the USA in collaboration with a Turkish professor. She has extensive consulting experience on environmental and occupational health issues. She has also worked in NGOs on women's and children's issues as Director or expert and she was a co-founder of the Emergency Research Center.

Anastasia Misseyanni is Associate Professor of Environmental Studies at Deree – The American College of Greece (ACG). She holds a Chemistry degree from the University of Athens and graduate degrees in Biochemistry from the University of Paris 7 (DEA) and the University of Marburg (PhD). She has a long career in teaching during which she has developed and taught a significant number of undergraduate natural science and environmental studies courses with emphasis on chemistry, biological chemistry, environmental science, ecology, water resources and methodology for environmental studies. She has conducted research in the fields of protein-DNA interactions and hormone-regulated gene expression. She has also been active in the scholarship of teaching. Her present research interests include Mediterranean biodiversity and green roofs, environmental health issues, sustainability initiatives in higher education, innovative teaching and learning strategies in STEM disciplines, active and experiential learning. She coordinated the development of the Deree Environmental Studies program and has served as its program coordinator since 2010. Since fall 2014, she has served as the Head of the Department of Science and Mathematics at Deree-ACG. She has contributed to efforts and initiatives to promote sustainability at ACG.

* * *

Radostina A. Angelova (M.Sc., Ph.D., D.Sc.) is an associate professor at the Department of Textiles, Technical University of Sofia (Bulgaria). She also works at the Centre for Research and Design in Human Comfort, Energy, and Environment (CERDECEN).

Anisah Bagasra, PhD teaches a wide-range of psychology courses and mentors students on undergraduate research projects. Dr. Bagasra works in the area of mental health disparities, focusing on perception of mental illness and barriers to help-seeking. Her research interests include mental health issues affecting religious and ethnic minorities in the United States, acculturation issues, and cross-cultural and interfaith dialogue. Much of her research has been conducted in the Muslim American and African American faith communities in the South. She established Claflin's Psychology Major in 2013 and developed and taught the first fully-online courses at the University. As Interim Director of Online Education, she worked to launch four fully online undergraduate and two fully online master's degree programs.

Omar Bagasra is a Pakistani-American Molecular Biologist, Biotechnologist and author, known for his innovations in the Polymerase Chain Reaction method and popular public and scientific talks in biotechnology. He is also known for his role as an independent investigator in the HIV trial in Libya, an important event of international significance in immunology, medical criminology and human rights. He is a researcher and Professor of Biology at Claflin University.

Alka Bali, Dr., is working as an Associate Professor of Pharmaceutical Chemistry at the University Institute of Pharmaceutical Sciences (UIPS), Panjab University, Chandigarh. She did her B. Pharm., M. Pharm. (Pharmaceutical Chemistry) and Ph. D. from the same institute. She has a rich academic and research experience spanning more than 21 years of undergraduate and postgraduate teaching. She has expertise in the fields of pharmaceutical analysis and medicinal chemistry. Her research areas of interest include pharmaceutical analysis with focus on method development and validation, spectroscopic characterization of impurities in drugs and drug products, synthetic medicinal chemistry encompassing computer-aided drug designing (CADD), QSAR, synthesis and pharmacological evaluation of new chemical entities in the area of antipsychotics, anti-inflammatory agents and angiotensin II antagonists. She has two books, three book chapters, over 40 research and review articles in reputed international and national journals and 60 conference papers to her credit. She is an avid participant in many national and international conferences and is on reviewer panel of several reputed international journals.

Reyhan Cafri is an Assistant Professor in Economics at Iskenderun Technical University. Her research interests include development economics, spatial econometrics, and panel data econometrics. Her publications have appeared in such journals as *Social Indicators Research, Tourism Economics, Journal of Applied Sciences, Inte'rnational Journal of Management Economics and Business.*

Arpitha Chikkanna works on the study of microbial roles in bio-mineralization and bio-weathering of rocks. Research area includes microbiological cultures and their applications in bio-geochemistry.

Ashok Kumar Ghosh, Dr., is working as Professor and HoD, Research at Mahavir Cancer Institute and Research Centre since 1st July 2016. He is the Professor-in-Charge of Department of Environment and Water Management, A.N. College, Patna, India on 30th June after 44 years of active service. He is an adviser of East Zone Water partnership, an affiliate of Global Water Partnership (GWP). Currently he is working on a DST supported research project on bioremediation of arsenic sludge, and also a multinational (Indo-Dutch) research project DELTAP for arsenic mobilization in Gangetic floodplains of Bihar supported by NWO-Wotro – The funding agency of The Netherlands Government. Dr. Ghosh is also working on DST-UKIERI supported project Nutri-SAM jointly with University of Salford, UK and another Indo-German project INNOWATER supported by DST, Government of India. In October 2017, Dr. Ghosh was awarded another international project from Newton-Bhabha Fund in collaboration with the University of Manchester, UK. Dr. Ghosh has published more than 50 research papers and presented his research findings in international seminars/conferences in India and abroad (USA, UK, Australia, Ireland, Bangladesh, Spain, Germany, Turkey, The Netherlands and Sweden). He has also authored five book chapters published by international publishers. Dr. Ghosh is one of the coordinators of European Commission sponsored project "Erasmus Mundus Eurindia and India4EU II Program" - a worldwide cooperation and mobility that aims to enhance quality in higher education and promote intercultural understanding. Dr. Ghosh has been awarded Erasmus Mundus Fellowship in 2010,2 014 and 2015 for collaborative research with University of Applied Sciences, Karlsruhe, Germany and Royal Institute of Technology, Sweden. Dr. Ghosh has been nominated as Chairman of SEAC, Bihar (State Environmental Impact Assessment Authority) by Government of India in 2014.He is also Chairman of Bihar State Pollution Control Board since January 2018 and member of Regional Empowered Committee of MoEF&CC, Government of India since 2015.He was awarded for Excellence in Water Showcase Final at 7th World Water Forum in 2015 held at Daegu, South Korea for his research related to arsenic mitigation in rural Bihar.

Devanita Ghosh is a biogeochemistry enthusiast, fascinated by the microbial diversity and their interaction, participation in various biogeochemical cycles, evolution of life and biodiversity on Earth. Her research is based on studying the role of arsenite oxidizing bacterial assemblages in arsenic contaminated aquifers and to understand how the sedimentary organic matter that leaches into the aquifers during recharge, and what shapes those indigenous microbial populations.

Maria-Eleni Giota was born in Athens, Greece, in 1996. From a very young age, she had an interest in life and earth sciences, and the universe. In 2015, she started studying Chemistry at the National and Kapodistrian University of Athens. In the meantime, she completed a Minor in Biology at Deree-The American College of Greece.

Alberto Gotti, Dr., is a physicist of the University of Milan with over 25 years of experience in environment and health impact assessment, data assimilation and exposure modelling. In the last fifteen years, he has worked for the European Commission's Joint Research Centre (EC-DG-JRC), for the Centre for Research and Technology Hellas (CERTH). From 2013 he is a scientific associate of the Laboratory of Environmental Engineering of Aristotle University of Thessaloniki, focusing mainly on exposure to environmental hazards and their impact on health, and since 2015, he works as a researcher at the Eucentre Foundation - European Center for Training and Research in Mechanical Earthquakes (Centro Europeo di Formazione e Ricerca in Ingegneria Sismica) in Pavia, Italy. Dr. Gotti has extensive experience on environments and health impact assessment, exposure modelling including biologically-based toxicokinetics/dynamic models (PBTK/PD), development of dose-response relationships based on both mechanistic Biology-Based Dose Response (BBDR) modelling, uncertainty in human health risk assessment, data fusion comprising the assimilation and integration of data from different information sources and air quality assessment using satellite data. He is co-author of 35 papers and has participated in the implementation of 15 European projects related to environmental quality and human health.

Ike Iyioke has an extensive work experience both at MSU and abroad that spans almost two decades. His multidisciplinary backgrounds include a BPhil. in Philosophy from Pontifical University, Rome; a teaching certificate from University of Nigeria, Nsukka (UNN); a Master of Science in International Relations from UNN; a Master of Art in Environmental Science Writing from Michigan State University (MSU); and a PhD in Health Ethics from MSU. He likes to explore questions pertaining to moral philosophy, particularly bioethics. His research interests include issues about research subject/participant selection; biomedical research partnerships between Africa & the West; environmental science and public policy; environmental justice/racism; eugenics; science of life extension; and morality in primitive cultures. Iyioke has authored several publications including a book titled, Clinical Trials and the African Person: A Quest to Re-Conceptualize Responsibility.

Spyros Karakitsios, Dr., is specialized in environmental pollution, environmental risk, data synthesis and validation and health impact assessment. Dr. Karakitsios is involved in the analysis of environmental pollution data in order to more accurately map the exposure (and the relative internal dose) of the population to a large number of pollutants that end up in humans with multiple exposure mechanisms. Since 2011 he has been a scientific collaborator at the Laboratory of Environmental Engineering, Department of Chemical Engineering, Engineering School of Aristotle University of Thessaloniki, with the main object of chemicals risk assessment. From 2008 to 2011, he worked as a post-doctoral researcher at the Joint Research Center of the European Commission in Ispra, Italy, on issues related to chemical risk assessment, and from 2002 to 2008 Postgraduate and Ministry Doctoral researcher at the University of Ioannina on issues related to human exposure. He is the co-author of 66 papers and he has participated in the implementation of 11 European projects related to environment and health, including NEUROSOME, HBM4EU, HEALS, CROME, CheRRIE, BlueHealth, TRANSPHORM, URGENCHE, INTEGRA, INTERA and TAGS. In 2017 he won the Innovation Award for Chemical Risk Analysis by the European Chemical Industry Council.

Pınar Kaya Samut, Ph.D., is an Associate Professor in Quantitative Methods at Atılım University, Ankara, Turkey. Her research interests include fuzzy logic, uncertainty, Multi-Criteria Decision Making Techniques, mathematical programming, project management, total factor productivity. Her publications have appeared in such journals as Social Indicators Research, Journal of Business Economics and Management, Journal of Intellectual Disability Research, International Journal of Applied Decision Sciences.

Sheldon Krimsky is a Lenore Stern Professor of Humanities and Social Sciences in the Department of Urban & Environmental Policy and Planning and Adjunct Professor in Public Health and Community Medicine in the School of Medicine at Tufts University. He received his bachelors and master's degrees in physics from Brooklyn College, CUNY and Purdue University respectively, and a masters and doctorate in philosophy at Boston University. Professor Krimsky's research has focused on the linkages between science/technology, ethics/values and public policy. He is the author of 16 books including: Genetic Alchemy: The Social History of the Recombinant DNA Controversy (MIT Press) and Biotechnics and Society: The Rise of Industrial Genetics (Praeger). He is co-author of Environmental Hazards: Communicating Risks as a Social Process (Auburn House), and Agricultural Biotechnology and the Environment: Science, Policy and Social Values (Univ. Illinois), and co-editor of a collection of papers titled Social Theories of Risk (Praeger). Professor Krimsky has published over 100 essays and reviews that have appeared in many books and journals. His current book is about endocrine disrupters and is titled Hormonal Chaos: The Scientific and Social Origins of the Environmental Endocrine Hypothesis (Johns Hopkins Univ. Press, 1999). Professor Krimsky served on the National Institutes of Health's Recombinant DNA Advisory Committee from 1978-1981. He was a consultant to the Presidential Commission for the Study of Ethical Problems in Medicine and Biomedical and Behavioral Research and to the Congressional Office of Technology Assessment. He participated on a special study panel for the American Civil Liberties Union that formulated a policy on civil liberties and scientific research. Professor Krimsky was chairperson of the Committee on Scientific Freedom and Responsibility for the American Association for the Advancement of Science for 1988-1992. Currently he serves on the Board of Directors for the Council for Responsible Genetics and as a Fellow of the Hastings Center on Bioethics. Professor Krimsky has been elected Fellow of the American Association for the Advancement of Science for "seminal scholarship exploring the normative dimensions and moral implications of science in its social context."

Arun Kumar, Dr., has received his PhD in August 2008 from Patna University, Patna, Bihar, India. Currently, he is working as Scientist - I in Mahavir Cancer Institute & Research Centre, Patna, Bihar, India since August 2007. His research has been in the field of Environment Toxicology, Animal Toxicology, Medicinal Chemistry and Cancer biology. Based on this research and fellowship training he has received several awards and honors, such as: Prof. G.P. Talwar Gold Medal, New Delhi, Shradha Suman Award -2013, Patna, etc. He has authored and co-authored 98 peer-reviewed research articles and 3 books and one book chapter. He is serving as an editorial member & expert reviewer of several reputed journals. He has co-supervised 5 PhD students and supervised 92 M.Sc. dissertations. He is a member of the Indian Science Congress & Association, India. He has been principal investigator of a major project granted from Department of Science & Technology, New Delhi, Government of India and co-PI in the International bilateral DST- UKIERI Project.

Danielle McKain is a High School Mathematics Teacher at Beaver Area High School. She has taught a variety of courses including Algebra I, Algebra II, Integrated Math, Probability and Statistics, Trigonometry, and Computer Assisted Algebra. Additionally, she has years of experience preparing students for the SAT. Dr. McKain earned her PhD in Instructional Management and Leadership from Robert Morris University. She holds a Master of Science degree in Instructional Leadership with a concentration in Mathematics Education and a Bachelor of Science degree in Applied Mathematics. Her research interests include real world math, test preparation, math anxiety, remedial math, and preparing future teachers.

Luv Mehan has a B.Tech in Biochemical Engineering, an M.Tech in Earth Sciences. She works on microbial cultivation and applications. Her research area includes carbon sequestration, wastewater treatment, and biofuels.

Matthew Chidozie Ogwu is a doctoral researcher in the School of Biological Sciences, Seoul National University, Korea Republic. Matthew holds a master's degree in Plant Diversity and Conservation with distinction as well as a bachelor's degree in Plant Biology and Biotechnology (First Class Honours). He is a Lecturer at the University of Benin, Nigeria. His research focusses on sustainable development issues arising from various scales of biogeographical interactions. Matthew has published over 50 peer-reviewed scientific works and have presented his results at different international conferences. He has received many awards and scholarships.

Sarath P. K. is currently a master's student at Biological Science, Indian Institute of Science. She works on paleo-ecology and microbial metabolism and environmental proxies.

Jaanvi Sant is an undergraduate at Tufts University majoring in Biopsychology. She has an interest in the pathogenesis of neurodevelopmental disorders, especially autism. She wants to be a part of the movement toward finding a cure, so that people of all abilities can lead more joyful and empowered lives.

Dimosthenis Sarigiannis is a Professor of Environmental Engineering at the Aristotle University of Thessaloniki in Greece, Associate Professor of Environmental Health Engineering at the Institute for Advanced Study (IUSS) in Pavia, Italy, and Director of the PhD program on Environmental Chemical Risk at the Institute of Advanced Studies (IUSS) of Pavia in Italy and visiting Professor at the University of Paris Descartes. He is President of the Mediterranean Scientific Association for Environmental Protection, Vice-President of the Hellenic Society of Toxicology, member of the Expert Committee on Air Pollution of the Greek Ministry of Health and advisor to the WHO European Centre for Environment and Health. In 2015 he received the Bo Holmstedt award from EUROTOX and the Bo Holmstedt Foundation for his contributions to the safety of drugs and chemicals. His research focuses on the unraveling of the human exposome to improve the health risk assessment of industrial and environmental toxicants and on internalizing health aspects into cyclical economy strategies. He is the author or co-author of more than 110 scientific papers published in the peer-reviewed literature and has led or contributed to 40 international research projects in the above areas.

Richa Saxena, Dr. is working as an Asst. Prof., Chemistry, ITM University, Gwalior for eight years. She is actively involved in academics and research activities for almost 10 years. Her field of research is organometallic and coordination chemistry and has published research papers in journals of national and international repute. She is an avid participants in many national, international conferences and workshops and is a reviewer of few reputed journals.

Theoharis Theoharides, Dr., is Professor of Pharmacology and Internal Medicine, as well as Director of Molecular Immunopharmacology and Drug Discovery, in the Department of Immunology at Tufts University School of Medicine, Boston, MA. He was born in Thessaloniki, Greece, and graduated with Honors from Anatolia College. He received all his degrees with Honors from Yale University, and was awarded the Dean's Research Award and the Winternitz Price in Pathology. He trained in internal medicine at New England Medical Center, which awarded him the Oliver Smith Award "recognizing excellence, compassion and service." He also received a Certificate in Global Leadership from the Tufts Fletcher School of Law and Diplomacy and a Fellowship at the Harvard Kennedy School of Government. He has been serving as the Clinical Pharmacologist of the Massachusetts Drug Formulary Commission continuously since 1986. In Greece, he served on the Supreme Advisory Health Councils of the Ministries of Health and of Social Welfare, as well as on the Board of Directors of the Institute of Pharmaceutical Research and Technology. He Chaired an International Committee appointed by the Hellenic Ministries of Education and Health for the establishment of an independent medical school in Greece, and he is a member of the International Advisory Committee for the University of Cyprus School of Medicine. He is a member of 15 academies and scientific societies. He was inducted into the Alpha Omega Alpha National Medical Honor Society and the Rare Diseases Hall of Fame. He has received the Tufts Excellence in Teaching ten times, the Tufts Distinguished Faculty Recognition Award twice, the Tufts Alumni Award for Faculty Excellence, Boston Mayor's Community Award, and the Dr. George Papanicolau Award, as well as Honorary Doctor of Medicine from Athens University, Honorary Doctor of Sciences from Hellenic-American University., and the 2018 Albert Nelson Marquis Lifetime Achievement Award (Marquis Who is Who) and the 2018 Albert Nelson Marquis Distinguished Humanitarian Award. He is "Archon" of the Ecumenical Patriarchate of Constantinople. He first showed that mast cells, known for causing allergic reactions, are critical for inflammation, especially in the brain, and are involved in a number of inflammatory conditions that worsen by stress such as allergies, asthma, eczema, psoriasis, migraines, multiple sclerosis and most recently autism spectrum disorder. He has also shown that corticotropin-releasing hormone (CRH), neurotensin and substance P, peptides secreted under stress, act together, and with the cytokine IL-33, to trigger mast cells and microglia to secrete inflammatory molecules. These processes are inhibited by the novel flavonoids, luteolin and tetramethoxyluteolin that he has helped formulate in unique dietary supplements and a skin lotion. He has published over 410 scientific papers (JBC, JACI, JPET, NEJM, Nature, PNAS, Science) and 3 textbooks with 30,274 citations (h-factor 86) and he is in the top 5% of authors most cited in pharmacological and immunological journals. He has received 37 patents and trademarks, including three patents covering the use of luteolin in brain inflammation and autism: US 8,268,365 (09/18/12); US 9,050,275 (06/09/15); US 9,176,146 (11/03/15). He is also the President of Theta Biomedical Consulting and Development Co., Inc., of BiomedAdvice, LLC, of Algonot, LLC and of the nonprofit Brain-Gain.org.

Emmanouil Velonakis, M.D., Occupational physician, Professor of prevention and environmental Hygiene Department of Nurse. Faculty of Health Sciences. National and Kapodistrian University of Athens.

Index

F

G

H

I

L

M

N

O

P

Q

R

S

T

U

V

W

www.ingramcontent.com/pod-product-compliance
Lightning Source LLC
LaVergne TN
LVHW081415021026
849161LV00011BA/2730
* 9 7 8 1 5 2 2 5 7 6 3 5 8 *